Cytopathology of the Head and Neck
Ultrasound Guided FNAC

Cytopathology of the Head and Neck

Ultrasound Guided FNAC

Second Edition

Author: Gabrijela Kocjan, MBBS, Spec Clin Cyt, FRCPath

Senior Lecturer/Honorary Consultant,
Department of Cellular Pathology
University College London/University College Hospitals London

Contributor: Simon Morley, MA, BM, BCh, MRCP, FRCR

Consultant Radiologist
Department of Imaging
University College Hospitals London

WILEY Blackwell

This edition first published 2017 © 2017 by John Wiley & Sons Ltd
First edition published in 2001 by Greenwich Medical Medai Limited (London)

Registered Office
John Wiley & Sons Ltd, The Atrium, Southern Gate, Chichester, West Sussex, PO19 8SQ, UK

Editorial Offices
9600 Garsington Road, Oxford, OX4 2DQ, UK
The Atrium, Southern Gate, Chichester, West Sussex, PO19 8SQ, UK
111 River Street, Hoboken, NJ 07030-5774, USA

For details of our global editorial offices, for customer services and for information about how to apply for permission to reuse the copyright material in this book please see our website at www.wiley.com/wiley-blackwell

The right of Gabrijela Kocjan to be identified as the author of this work has been asserted in accordance with the UK Copyright, Designs and Patents Act 1988.

Library of Congress Cataloging-in-Publication Data

Names: Kocjan, Gabrijela, author.
Title: Cytopathology of the head and neck : ultrasound guided FNAC / Gabrijela Kocjan.
Other titles: Clinical cytopathology of the head and neck.
Description: Second edition. | Chichester, West Sussex ; Hoboken, NJ : John Wiley & Sons Inc., 2016. | Preceded by Clinical cytopathology of the head and neck : a text and atlas / Gabrijela Kocjan. 2001. | Includes bibliographical references and index.
Identifiers: LCCN 2016049896 | ISBN 9781118076026 (cloth) | ISBN 9781118560846 (Adobe PDF) | ISBN 9781118560792 (epub)
Subjects: | MESH: Head and Neck Neoplasms–diagnosis | Head and Neck Neoplasms–pathology | Biopsy, Fine-Needle–methods | Cyst Fluid–cytology | Cysts–pathology | Atlases
Classification: LCC RC280.H4 | NLM WE 17 | DDC 616.99/491–dc23
LC record available at https://lccn.loc.gov/2016049896

A catalogue record for this book is available from the British Library.

Wiley also publishes its books in a variety of electronic formats. Some content that appears in print may not be available in electronic books.

Cover image: courtesy of the author
Cover design: Wiley

Set in 9/11pt Minion by SPi Global, Pondicherry, India
Printed and bound in Singapore by Markono Print Media Pte Ltd

1   2017

MAXIMUM EFFECT WITH MINIMUM INTERVENTION

To all those striving to optimize diagnostic process and realize efficiency in the health service

Contents

Preface to the first edition, ix

Preface to the second edition, x

About the companion website, xi

1 Introduction, 1
1.1 Introduction, 1
1.2 Fine needle aspiration cytology of the head and neck, 1
1.3 Ultrasound guided FNAC, 1
1.4 A Combined US/FNAC approach, 2
1.5 Sampling technique, 2
References, 8

2 Salivary gland, 9
2.1 Introduction, 9
    2.1.1 Ultrasound guided FNAC, 10
    2.1.2 Diagnostic accuracy, 10
    2.1.3 Diagnostic pitfalls, 11
    2.1.4 Ultrasound versus other imaging modalities, 12
    2.1.5 FNAC versus frozen section and core biopsy, 12
    2.1.6 Cost effectiveness, 12
2.2 Diagnostic imaging of salivary glands, 13
    2.2.1 Normal Ultrasound appearance of salivary gland, 13
    2.2.2 Imaging Pitfalls and scanning issues, 13
2.3 Cytology of the salivary gland, 14
    2.3.1 Normal salivary gland cytology, 14
    2.3.2 Sialadenosis, 14
    2.3.3 Salivary gland cysts, 17
    2.3.4 Sialadenitis, 21
    2.3.5 Lymphoid proliferations of the salivary gland, 23
2.4 Salivary gland tumours, 29
    2.4.1 Pleomorphic adenoma, 29
    2.4.2 Adenolymphoma (Warthin's tumour), 35
    2.4.3 Basal cell adenoma, 37
    2.4.4 Oncocytoma, 39
    2.4.5 Rare benign tumours, 40
2.5 Malignant tumours of the salivary gland, 42
    2.5.1 Acinic cell carcinoma, 42
    2.5.2 Mucoepidermoid carcinoma, 44
    2.5.3 Adenoid cystic carcinoma, 48
    2.5.4 Polymorphous low grade adenocarcinoma, 51
    2.5.5 Epithelial myoepithelial carcinoma, 52
    2.5.6 Basal cell adenocarcinoma, 53
    2.5.7 Papillary cystadenocarcinoma, 54
    2.5.8 Mucinous adenocarcinoma, 54
    2.5.9 Oncocytic carcinoma, 54
    2.5.10 Salivary duct carcinoma, 55
    2.5.11 Adenocarcinoma (not otherwise specified), 57
    2.5.12 Carcinoma ex PLA, 57

    2.5.13 Primary squamous cell carcinoma of the salivary gland, 58
    2.5.14 Small cell carcinoma, 58
    2.5.15 Undifferentiated carcinoma of the salivary gland, 59
2.6 Miscellaneous tumours, 59
    2.6.1 Lymphoepithelial carcinoma, 59
    2.6.2 Mammary analogue secretory carcinoma, 59
    2.6.3 Cribriform adenocarcinoma of minor salivary gland, 60
    2.6.4 Soft tissue lesions, 61
    2.6.5 Granulocytic sarcoma, 61
    2.6.6 Paediatric lesions, 61
    2.6.7 Lymphomas, 61
    2.6.8 Primitive neuroectodermal tumour, 62
    2.6.9 Metastatic tumours in salivary gland, 63
2.7 Clinical management of salivary gland lesions, 64
References, 65

3 Thyroid, 71
3.1 Introduction, 71
    3.1.1 Ultrasound and FNAC procedure, 72
    3.1.2 FNAC reporting categories, 74
    3.1.3 Diagnostic accuracy, 74
    3.1.4 Diagnostic pitfalls, 76
    3.1.5 The role of FNAC thyroid in clinical management, 76
    3.1.6 FNAC versus frozen section and core biopsy histology, 77
    3.1.7 Ancillary techniques, 78
    3.1.8 Complications of FNAC, 78
3.2 Non-neoplastic and inflammatory conditions, 79
    3.2.1 Colloid goitre (non-toxic goitre, adenomatous hyperplasia, multinodular goitre), 79
    3.2.2 Cysts, 81
    3.2.3 Hyperactive goitre (toxic goitre, thyrotoxicosis, primary hyperthyroidism, Graves' disease), 83
    3.2.4 Thyroiditis, 85
3.3 Indeterminate cytological findings: follicular lesions, 87
    3.3.1 Atypia of uncertain significance (AUS)/Follicular lesion of uncertain significance (FLUS) (TBSRTC III, UK Thy 3a), 87
    3.3.2 'Follicular lesions' (TBSTRC IV: Follicular neoplasm or suspicious for a follicular neoplasm) (UK: Thy 3f), 90
3.4 Malignant tumours, 94
    3.4.1 Papillary carcinoma, 94
    3.4.2 Follicular carcinoma, 101
    3.4.3 Medullary carcinoma, 101
    3.4.4 Anaplastic carcinoma, 103

3.4.5   Thyroid lymphoma, 103
3.4.6   Metastatic tumours, 105
References, 106

4 Lymph nodes, 112
4.1   Introduction, 112
   4.1.1   Distribution of lymph node pathology, 112
   4.1.2   Diagnostic accuracy, 113
   4.1.3   Diagnostic pitfalls, 113
   4.1.4   Ancillary techniques, 113
   4.1.5   Core biopsy or FNAC?, 117
   4.1.6   Elastography or FNAC?, 117
4.2   Non-neoplastic lymphoproliferative conditions, 118
   4.2.1   Follicular hyperplasia, 118
   4.2.2   Sinus histiocytosis with massive
        lymphadenopathy (Rosai Dorfman), 119
   4.2.3   Granulomatous lymphadenitis, 122
   4.2.4   Chronic lymphadenitis, 128
   4.2.5   Drug reactions, 131
   4.2.6   Miscellaneous lymphadenopathies, 131
4.3   Hodgkin's lymphoma, 137
   4.3.1   Nodular Lymphocyte Predominant
        Hodgkin's lymphoma, 139
4.4   Non-Hodgkin's lymphoma, 139
   4.4.1   Introduction, 139
   4.4.2   Obtaining appropriate material, 142
   4.4.3   Classification of Non-Hodgkin's lymphoma, 142
   4.4.4   Precursor lesions, 142
   4.4.5   B-cell lymphomas, 143
   4.4.6   Mantle zone lymphoma, 144
   4.4.7   Follicular lymphoma, 147
   4.4.8   Marginal zone lymphoma (MALT type), 148
   4.4.9   Diffuse large B-cell lymphoma, 150
   4.4.10 Primary effusion lymphoma, 151
   4.4.11 Burkitt's lymphoma, 152
   4.4.12 T/NK-cell lymphomas, 154
   4.4.13 Anaplastic large cell lymphoma, 154
4.5   Metastatic carcinoma in lymph nodes, 160
References, 170

5 Miscellaneous lesions of the head and neck, 176
5.1   Introduction, 176
5.2   Benign soft tissue lesions, 176
   5.2.1   Lipoma, 176
   5.2.2   Fibromatosis colli, 176
   5.2.3   Nodular fasciitis, 178
   5.2.4   Proliferative fasciitis and proliferative myositis, 178
   5.2.5   Benign nerve sheath tumour (neurilemmoma,
        schwannoma), 180
5.3   Cysts of the head and neck, 181
   5.3.1   Thyroglossal cysts, 181
   5.3.2   Branchial cyst, 181
   5.3.3   Mucous retention cyst, 182
   5.3.4   Intraosseous cysts and other lesions, 183
   5.3.5   Rare cysts and differential diagnosis of cystic
        lesions of the head and neck, 183
5.4   Small round cell tumours, 184
   5.4.1   Rhabdomyosarcoma, 185
   5.4.2   Ewing's sarcoma/peripheral neuroectodermal
        tumour/Askin tumour, 186
   5.4.3   Olfactory neuroblastoma, 187
   5.4.4   Lymphoma, 187
5.5   Locally arising miscellaneous tumours, 189
   5.5.1   Carotid body tumours, 189
   5.5.2   Epithelioid sarcoma-like
        hemangioendothelioma, 190
   5.5.3   Meningioma, 190
   5.5.4   Ethmoid sinus intestinal type adenocarcinoma, 191
   5.5.5   Granular cell tumour, 192
References, 195

Index, 198

Preface to the first edition

The past century has seen Cytopathology as a discipline, and Fine Needle Aspiration Cytology as a method of obtaining material, become established. From the pioneering work of Martin and Ellis, through the enthusiasm of Zajicek and his colleagues, to the perseverance of numerous cytopathologists throughout the world, this simple technique has become part of the routine diagnostic investigations. To this end, this book summarises recent experiences with the role Cytopathology is playing in current clinical practice, particularly in relation to Head and Neck. This work is based on the experience drawn from a large referral practice from ear, nose and throat, maxillofacial and general surgeons, endocrinologists, oncologists and others. From sceptical beginnings the FNAC service has grown and developed, to the extent that it is now accepted as a routine investigation and cytopathologists are considered as the best people to deliver the service. Mutual understanding and trust between clinical colleagues and cytopathologists has led to the further development of skills and a desire for further improvement in respective disciplines. Clinically oriented work is a valuable source for the education and training of laboratory and junior pathology staff. To a cytopathologist, who meets new patients daily, this work is enormously satisfying. In the new millennium, our efforts should not be spent any more at proving the validity of FNAC. Instead, with the advances in new technologies, our aim should be the refinement of morphological diagnoses in order to match the existing or improve future treatment options.

My sincere thanks for producing this book go, firstly, to the patients who posed for the, sometimes, unflattering photographs; to the medical and technical colleagues in the Cytopathology Laboratory, University College Hospital London, to eminent clinical colleagues for their advice and support and to Mr Paratian for processing the photographs. Lastly, I would like to thank Tony and Arabella for putting up with my absences during the long gestation of this book.

Gabrijela Kocjan
London, May 2000

Preface to the second edition

The idea for the second edition of this book arose through realization that the working practices of Head and Neck (HN) diagnostic and clinical teams have changed dramatically in the last 15 years, not only in terms of organization of health service with its aims for provision of HN cancer care but also in their diagnostic input. The publication of high profile professional guidance documents highlighted the importance of specialist Multidisciplinary Teams (MDT) with the intention that these should bring together all the services and organizations to provide high quality care. Written protocols, that specify investigations for each type of presentation of possible HN cancer as well as specific guidelines for investigation and diagnosis of each form of HN cancer, have emerged. The aim of reducing cancer waiting times meant that Rapid Access (One stop) diagnostic clinics have become a requirement not only in the base hospital of the specialist multidisciplinary teams (MDT) but also in many District General Hospitals and that these clinics are required to provide same day diagnosis by Ultrasound and Fine Needle Aspiration Cytology (FNAC), tissue/cell sampling thus becoming an essential function of these clinics. Pathologists within the HN networks now have to ensure that conditions under which FNAC and rapid diagnosis clinics services are provided follow the professional guidelines and are also part of the local network guidelines.

The initial experience with One stop Clinics found widespread diagnostic difficulties including a high non-diagnostic rate highlighting the need for a particularly high level of expertise required to achieve a precise and reliable diagnosis in HN through the involvement of specialist radiologists and cytopathologists. To achieve high levels of diagnostic accuracy, special training and commitment to cytopathology are required in addition to histopathology. There is a need for recognition of the new skills expected of practicing pathologists and a comprehensive approach to cytopathology training, to include performing FNAC, with or without ultrasound guidance and interpreting them on site, as is the case with frozen section specimen training in histopathology. Ancillary techniques that have become available in the past 10 years are now a mainstream requirement for diagnosis and sometimes prognosis of various conditions and can be applied to FNAC material. Trainee pathologists specializing in cytopathology require a secondment to centres where on site evaluation and rapid access clinics are in place and where molecular techniques are available. This may require pathologists to be absent from routine work at their institution in order to learn new skills and adopt different ways of working.

Ultrasound (US) guidance has emerged as an essential adjunct to either FNAC or needle core biopsy, and its use is expected to increase. US combined with US guided FNAC can be recommended as a method for evaluating regional metastases in HN patients, for both those with and those without palpable lumps. US and, if necessary, FNAC should continue to be the investigation method of first choice for HN lesions. US-guided FNAC sessions benefit from attendance of cytopathology medical and non-medical staff to perform the procedure, assess adequacy of the samples and make decisions about collecting appropriate material for ancillary tests.

In our own practice, the emergence of MDT Meetings (MDM) where radiologists, oncologists, radiotherapists, surgeons, speech and language therapists, pathologists and other support staff meet regularly once a week and discuss individual cases in a formal meeting, meant a significant improvement in HN service. MDMs contributed to the understanding of the role each discipline plays in the clinical management and helped improve patient outcomes. This collaboration in a quest for successful outcomes has also helped drive the progress in using ancillary techniques in diagnosis thus enabling the so called personalised medicine. One stop HN clinics and MDMs are a model of service delivery that hopefully can be used as an example in successful health management.

My thanks for the publication of this book go primarily to all patients whose conditions served as an inspiration for education, training and research. I am extremely appreciative of all members of the MDT for their input, patience and support; our sessions were as much fun as they were informative. Thanks to my colleagues Simon Morley, a contributor to this book, and Timothy Beale, both radiologists, I managed to obtain a desk and a chair in the One Stop Clinic. Collaboration with surgeons, in particular Paul O'Flynn and Francis Vaz, went beyond the HN to tennis and golf tournaments. My gratitude goes to all my colleagues and staff in the Department of Cellular Pathology, who skeptically tolerated my indulgence in cytology, provided there was a Summer Party at the end. It is through cells that I met so many wonderful people, travelled around the world and made lasting friendships. It is a testament to Wiley editorial and production teams, headed by Claire Bonnet and Eswari Maruthu that this book is presented in such a clear and constructive manner which I am proud of and thankful for. Finally, my lasting devotion goes to my family who were a source of pride and encouragement throughout. I hope that this textbook justifies the sacrifice they made.

As I am approaching the end of my working life, this book represents forty years of experience working as a diagnostic cytopathologist in a prestigious institution, a tertiary referral and a Cancer Centre. As such, it is a summary of the most interesting clinical examples where FNAC made a real difference to the management. It is my life long ambition that this legacy continues and that, by using cells alone, maximum diagnostic effect is achieved with minimum of intervention. I believe that this is achievable in not too distant future.

Gabrijela Kocjan
Cavtat, January 2017

About the companion website

This book is accompanied by a companion website:

www.wiley.com/go/kocjan/clinical_cytopathology_head_neck2e

The website includes:

- Over 20 exclusive to website studies of head and neck ultrasound case histories, with description of essential diagnostic features and differential diagnosis, compiled by Dr Simon Morley.
- Powerpoints of all figures from the book

The password for the site is the last word in the caption for Figure 4.1.

CHAPTER 1

Introduction

Chapter contents

1.1 Introduction, 1
1.2 Fine needle aspiration cytology of the head and neck, 1
1.3 Ultrasound guided FNAC, 1

1.4 A combined US/FNAC approach, 2
1.5 Sampling technique, 2
References, 8

1.1 Introduction

The Head and Neck (HN) area is one of the most complex regions of the body because of its anatomical and functional diversity. Diseases of the HN, both primary and systemic, rarely go unnoticed; patients either notice changes themselves, or are alerted to them by the diagnostic investigations, often done for unrelated conditions.

HN cancer is the ninth most common cancer in the USA, accounting for 3.3 % of all cancers. The incidence of HN cancer has plateaued recently; however, morbidity and mortality continue to remain high. Despite the decline in overall mortality rates since 2001 a ratial disparity between the whites and the African Americans, both in incidence and mortality, still exists [1].

Tobacco and alcohol use are the most important risk factors for most HN cancers. In addition, infection with certain types of human papillomavirus (HPV) is thought to be the cause of an escalating incidence of HPV-related oropharyngeal squamous cell carcinoma predominantly among middle-aged adults [2].

1.2 Fine needle aspiration cytology of the head and neck

Fine needle aspiration cytology (FNAC) has been recognised as one of the core activities for the management of HN disease [3–23]. Sites in the HN that are amenable to FNAC include the thyroid, cervical masses and nodules, salivary glands, intraoral lesions and lesions in the paraspinal area and base of skull [24].

FNAC has a high overall diagnostic accuracy: 85–95% for all HN masses, 95% for benign lesions, and 87% for malignant ones [25, 26]. Diagnostic accuracy is dependent on the site of aspiration as well as the skill of the individual performing and interpreting the FNAC [24]. Each site undergoing FNAC within the HN is associated with its own set of differential diagnoses and diagnostic challenges. There are virtually no contraindications, and complications are minimal [27].

FNAC allows an immediate diagnosis to be available to the clinician so that appropriate treatment can be discussed with the patient. It is recommended as a first line of investigation in palpable HN masses. FNAC is the preferred first-line pathological

investigation of salivary gland and thyroid lumps because of the risk of recurrence and complications, respectively, associated with tissue biopsies [28].

The majority of aspirates from the HN will be to confirm an otherwise suspected diagnosis, for example a reactive lymphadenopathy or to confirm clinical staging for a metastatic carcinoma. However, there are a number of occasions where an unsuspected condition may be revealed, such as lymphoma or a salivary gland tumour. Whilst the diagnosis of lymphoma may need further tissue work up, the diagnosis of salivary gland lesions is often definitive in that it guides the surgical or non-surgical management. FNAC can diagnose majority of thyroid enlargements and help reduce the rate of surgery for benign thyroid disease. Ancillary techniques, namely immunocytochemistry, flow cytometry and molecular techniques, can greatly broaden the diagnostic range and specificity of FNAC. They are particularly useful in the diagnosis of lymphoproliferative processes and in determining the precise nature of lesions as variable as rhabdomyosarcoma, olfactory neuroblastoma and granular cell tumour. The prudent use of these techniques can be cost-effective and avoid the need for more invasive diagnostic procedures [29].

1.3 Ultrasound guided FNAC

Ultrasound imaging is a dynamic and readily available technique that is particularly useful in the examination of superficial structures. Modern machines combined with high frequency linear probes (7.5–12 MHz) produce high definition images in multiple planes. The spatial resolution that is achieved surpasses that of both multislice computed tomography (CT) and magnetic resonance imaging (MRI). Images are rapidly acquired, artefacts are few, and the technique is highly acceptable to most patients. As an adjunct to structural imaging, colour (directional) and power Doppler (non-directional but more sensitive) are often used to assess blood flow and the vascularity of tissue. These techniques add value in detecting abnormal peripheral or chaotic flow patterns in malignant lymph nodes, in assessing the patency of normal vessels, and in the investigation of vascular and lymphatic malformations.

Cytopathology of the Head and Neck: Ultrasound Guided FNAC, Second Edition. Gabrijela Kocjan.
© 2017 John Wiley & Sons Ltd. Published 2017 by John Wiley & Sons Ltd.
Companion website: www.wiley.com/go/kocjan/clinical_cytopathology_head_neck2e

Ultrasound (US) guidance is a useful adjunct to either FNAC or needle core biopsy (CB), and its use is expected to increase. US combined with US guided FNAC, rather than a tissue biopsy, can be recommended as a method for evaluating possible regional metastases in HN cancer patients, for both those with and those without a known primary tumour [30, 31].

US and, if necessary, FNAC, should continue to be the investigation method of first choice for HN lesions. The main indication for CB is after repeated failures of FNAC to provide a diagnosis. It can also be performed in patients who are not surgical candidates or in those who refuse surgery. Kraft et al. found CB was superior to FNAC in providing a specific diagnosis (90 vs 66%), and achieved a higher accuracy in identifying true neoplasms (100 vs 93%) and detecting malignancy (99 vs 90%). However, the sensitivity and specificity did not differ significantly between the two methods [32]. Khalid et al. found that the use of US-guided FNAC as the initial modality for tissue sampling of a thyroid nodule is more effective than traditional FNAC at an additional cost of $289 per additional correct diagnosis [33].

In our own experience, the adequacy rate of US guided FNAC is critical for the success of the service. In our institution the adequacy of US guided FNAC in the HN clinic is 97% [34]. Computed tomography and magnetic resonance imaging do not appear to add any advantage to FNAC in terms of specificity, sensitivity or accuracy of a malignant diagnosis [34]. As with rapid-diagnosis clinics, US-guided FNAC sessions benefit from attendance of cytopathology medical and non-medical staff to assess adequacy of the samples and make decisions about collecting appropriate material for ancillary tests.

1.4 A Combined US/FNAC approach

Recently, some cytopathologists have learned to use ultrasound machines to assist them in performing FNAC procedures. The sensitivity, specificity, positive predictive value (PPV), negative predictive value (NPV), and accuracy were 96, 50, 98, 33 and 94% in palpation guided (PGFNAC) versus 100, 86, 97, 100 and 97% in the US guided (USGFNAC) group, respectively. USGFNACs performed by a cytopathologist could significantly improve the specificity and NPV (P = 0.04) while preserving virtually the same excellent sensitivity and PPV as those of PGFNACs. With US guidance, a cytopathologist is able to perform FNACs in smaller, non-palpable lesions and target complex lesions with confidence and accuracy, thus achieving a better outcome [36].

In our experience, even better results are obtained when an experienced radiologist takes the FNAC and has a cytopathologist close by to process the material and interpret the slides (Fig. 1.1).

According to the British Society for Clinical Cytology (BSCC) Code of Practice, the combination of physical examination/clinical history, radiological assessment, careful needle sampling, appropriate cell preparation, subsequent interpretation and multidisciplinary clinical discussion are essential for a successful outcome [37]. The lack of skill, clinical information and communication can be detrimental to the result.

1.5 Sampling technique

Sample collection is a major factor influencing both the adequacy and the accuracy of FNAC [38,39]. It is our experience and experience of others that a good sampling technique is essential for

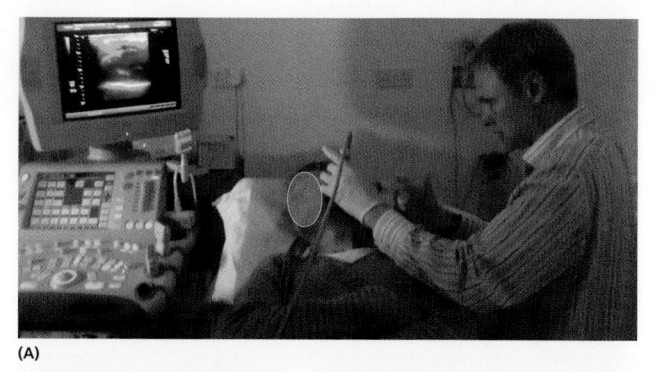

(A)

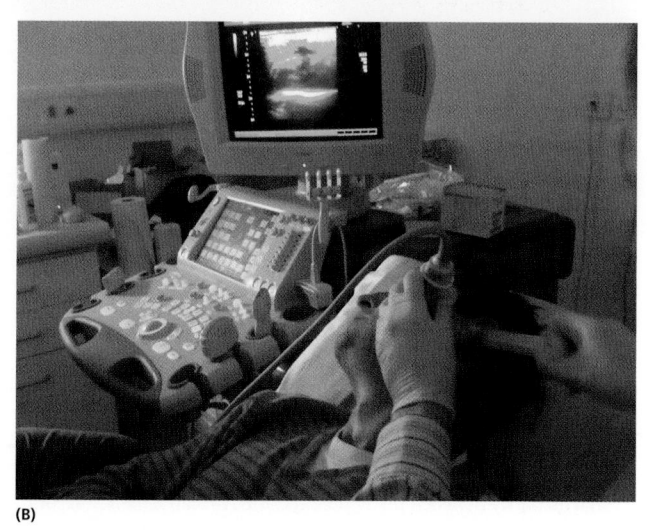

(B)

Figure 1.1 Ultrasound guided FNAC. (A) The radiologist, Dr Morley, uses the ultrasound probe in the left hand and injects the anesthetic into the lesion with the right hand. (B) Observing the monitor and using the ultrasound probe for guidance, the aspirator uses negative pressure to extract cystic fluid from the parotid gland lesion.

successful interpretation of FNAC. Comparing the material obtained by the cytopathologist with the material sent from various aspirators, Wu et al. found that the sensitivity of HN FNAC procedures is significantly better in the cytopathologist-performed group than in the non-cytopathologist-performed group (96 versus 67%) [40, 41]. Greater experience of the operator appears to improve the accuracy rate [42–44]. In experienced hands, palpation-guided FNAC is an excellent diagnostic tool. However, there is a movement towards using imaging guidance to target all masses [45].

The best results are obtained with a cytopathologist-led FNAC service, where the pathologist reviews the specimen immediately, in relation to the clinical context, thereby deciding on adequacy and the need for further sampling (Fig. 1.2) [46, 47].

With the FNAC procedure having been explained (Fig. 1.3), the patient is put in a supine position. The choice of whether to apply anaesthetic or not largely depends on the patient, the site involved and the extent of FNAC sampling planned. Since the average FNAC does not involve more than one pass with a 22+ G needle, most patients do not require local anaesthetic. However, if the patient is needle-phobic or a child, or if the site is particularly tender, for example, lip, nose, areola, or if it is expected that several passes will be necessary, a local anaesthetic is applied in the form of subcutaneous injection of 0.5 ml of 2% lignocaine. More recently we have

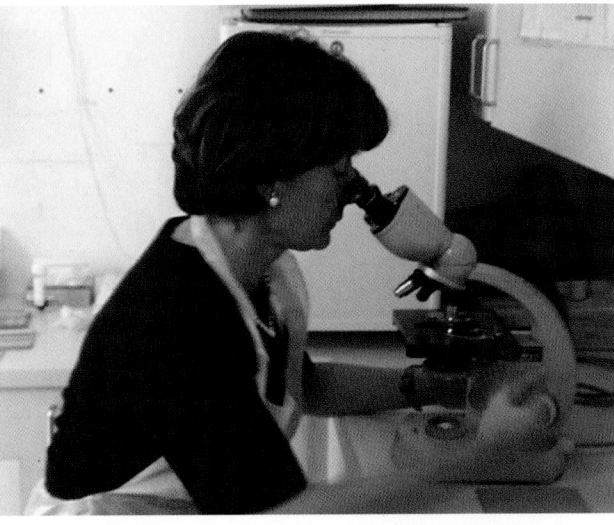

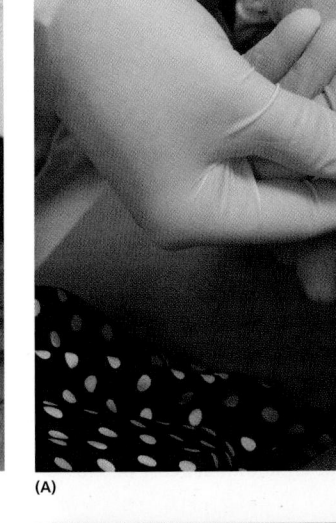

(A)

Figure 1.2 Examination of the glass slides in the clinic. This gives an orientation of adequacy and indicates whether further samples need to be taken for special techniques and/or for microbiology cultures. Results are usually not discussed with the patient at this preliminary stage of the investigations.

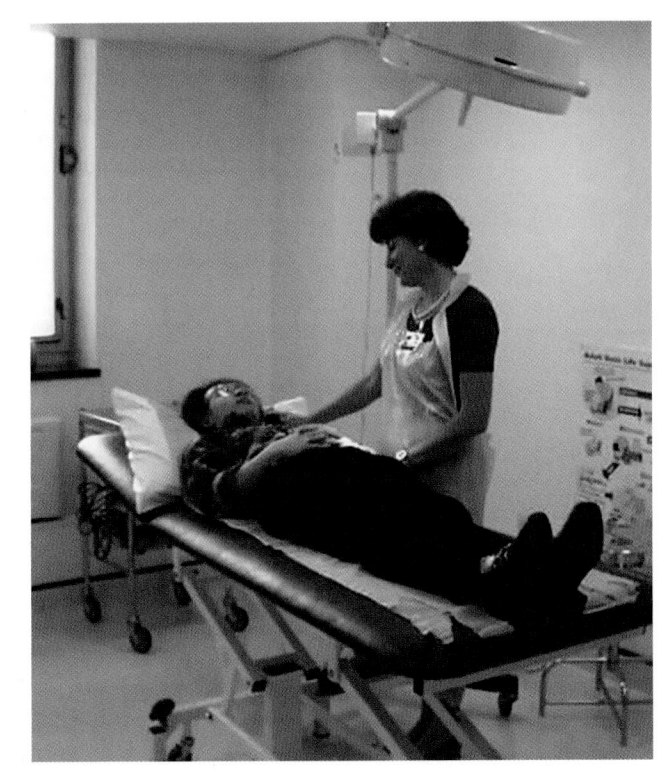

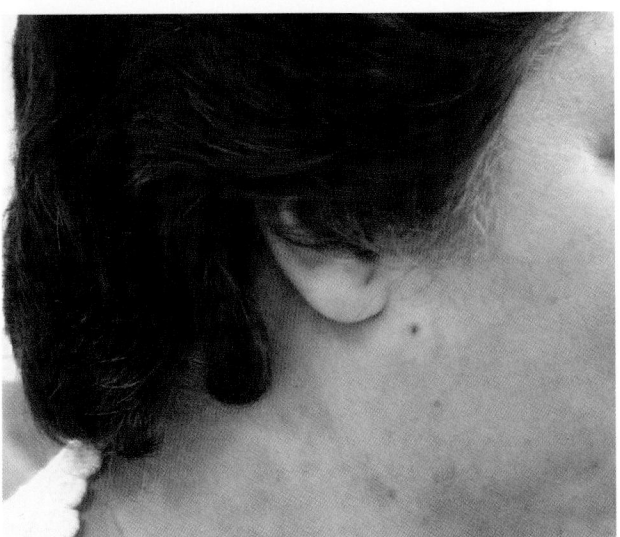

(B)

Figure 1.3 Clinical history and examination. The pathologist at the bedside examines the area referred to by the specialist and also asks the patient further relevant questions about the duration of the swelling, level of pain and any other associated systemic symptoms.

Figure 1.4 (A) Needle free anaesthetic system. Designed for patients who need daily injections, e.g. insulin, but also applicable to the local anaesthesia. This is particularly useful in children, in needle-phobic patients, in sensitive sites and where multiple needle passes are anticipated. (B) Needle-free anaesthetic system. A pale ring indicates the area of subdermal infiltration. A test needle should be passed through this area.

been using a needle free syringe where the pressurised air expels the anaesthetic, penetrating the skin, without the needle (Fig. 1.4A) [48]. Anaesthetic forms a small white ring through which the subsequent test needle is applied, once or more (Fig. 1.4B). Patients do not experience any pain on application of the anaesthetic and experience no or minimal pain at FNAC.

The palpable area in question is cleaned with an antiseptic agent and fixed between the two fingers of the non-dominant hand. 22 G, 23 G or smaller needle is then passed into the lump using a non-aspiration technique (capillary sampling) with the aid of a needle only (without the syringe attachment) (Fig. 1.5). In a meta analysis comprising over 2000 thyroid FNAC samples, there was no difference between the aspiration and non aspiration technique in assessing thyroid nodules [29]. In cases where a fluid aspirate is expected, a syringe and a syringe holder are attached to the needle to help aspiration (Fig. 1.6) [29, 49–54]. The needle is passed round in a fan-shaped manner several times in the cases of non-thyroid lumps. In the case of thyroid, several vertical movements in the same direction are usually sufficient to gain representative material. When exiting the lump, if using syringe attachment, it is important

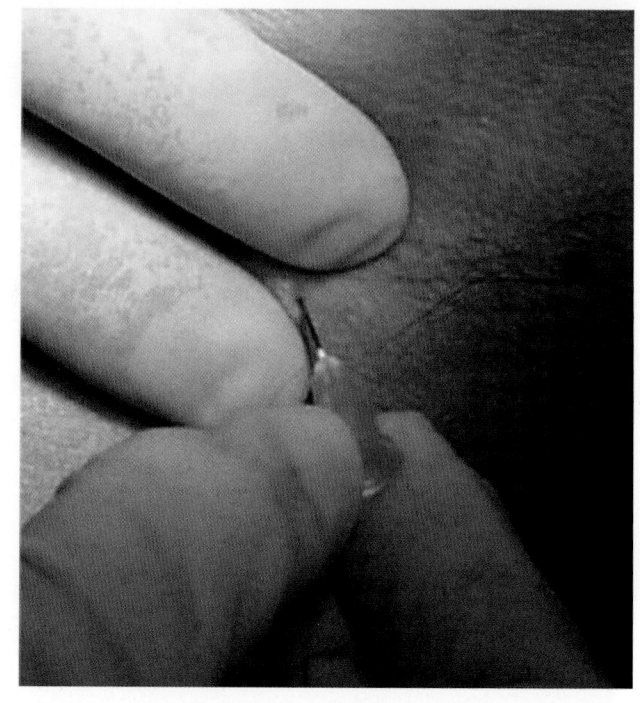

Figure 1.5 Free needle FNAC procedure. This, so called 'capillary technique', is particularly useful in very small, mobile lesions, e.g. lymph nodes. An aspirator has a much better feel of the tip of the needle and better control of the area sampled. It is not the method of choice for cystic or very sclerosed lesions.

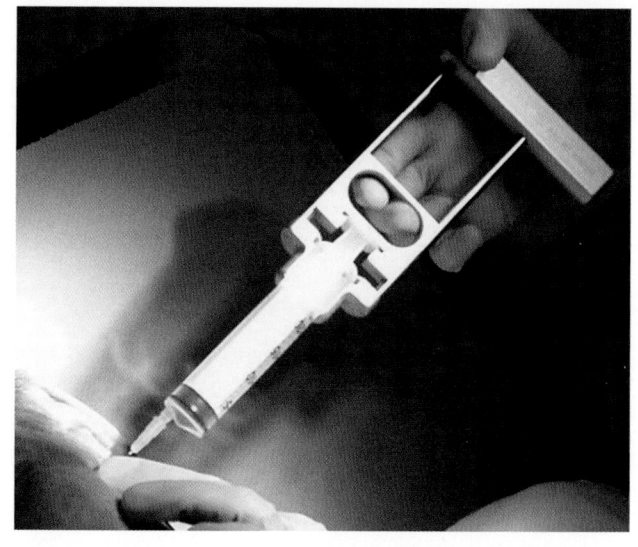

Figure 1.6 FNAC of fluids. A 20 ml syringe attached to a CAMECO (BELPRO MEDICAL, Canada), syringe holder A 23 G needle is used.

to release the negative pressure before exiting, otherwise the material is aspirated into the syringe and can only be retrieved by the aid of a needle wash.

Whilst adhering to the traditional technique of smearing the material ejected from the needle onto a slide and then either air drying or fixing it in alcohol, if necessary we also suspend the material from a separate needle pass in a liquid medium that can then be used for ancillary techniques including cell block

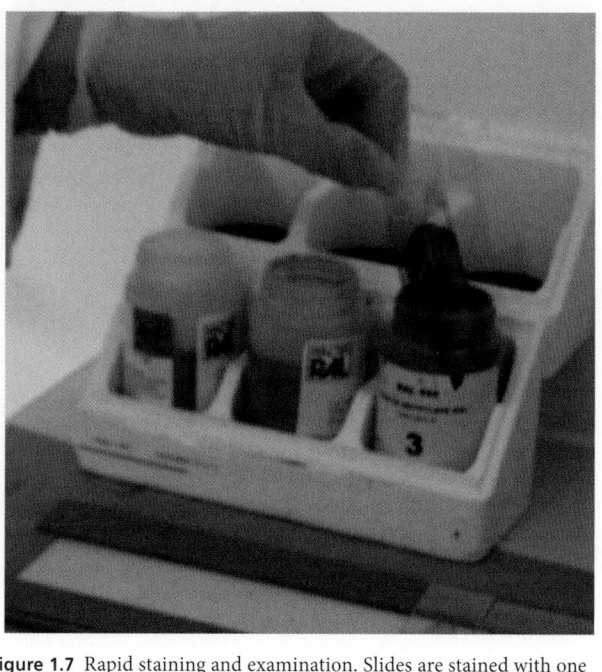

Figure 1.7 Rapid staining and examination. Slides are stained with one of the rapid stains and examined under the microscope for cellularity. This gives a good orientation if more material is needed or if different cell preparation technique should be applied.

(CBL). Air dried smears can be stained by a rapid staining technique to assess material adequacy in the One Stop clinic (Fig. 1.7). CBL provide a method for immunocytochemistry (ICC) that has revolutionised cytopathology by making it possible to apply panels of antibodies to multiple sequential sections of aspirated or exfoliated cellular material [55]. CBL can be prepared from virtually all varieties of cytological samples. CBL sections offer advantages over conventional cytological smears with respect to cellular architecture and archival storage. They also provide several sections, which can be utilised to perform special stains, immunophenotypic analysis, ultrastructural studies and molecular tests, including cytogenetic and polymerase chain reaction (PCR)-based techniques [56–59]. In today's era of personalised medicine, the ability to perform these tests augment the utility of cytological samples in analysing the molecular alterations as effectively as surgical biopsies or resection specimens. With the availability of molecular targeted therapy for many cancers, a large number of recent studies have used cytological material or CBL for molecular characterisation. Jain et al. described various methods of preparations of CBL and their application in cytology. The advantages and disadvantages of various methods of cell preparation are outlined in Table 1.1 [50].

One of the easiest way to prepare a CBL is the so-called 'Poor Man's cell block'. This method should be available to any laboratory and is able to produce very good results (Fig. 1.8) [61].

The final cytopathology report should be clear, written with the knowledge of the ultrasound and clinical findings, morphology and ancillary techniques (Fig. 1.9). Difficult cases should be discussed at the intradepartmental and multidisciplinary meetings and are also an important source of education and training [62] (Fig. 1.10).

Table 1.1 Comparison of different cytological preparation methods.

Direct smear[13]		Cytospin[25]		Cell block[2-4]		Liquid-based cytology[26]	
For	Against	For	Against	For	Against	For	Against
Diagnosis							
Fast		Optimal for cysts, urine and effusions	Cellular crowding	Additional to other slides	Needs time and histology skill	Easy to transport, collect and process	Low cellularity
Inexpensive	Needle handling	Multiple slides	Limited cellularity	Increased diagnostic yield		Reduced screening area	Cell shrinkage (methanol)
Routine process	Multiple slides	Air dried and/or alcohol fixed		More architecture		No air-drying artefacts	Less architecture
Permits rapid evaluation	Obscuring background			Archival storage		Clean background	Reduced or altered background material
Excellent cellular detail	Air-drying artefacts					Monolayer of cells	
ICC possible on fresh or destained slides	Adverse effect of stripped nuclei and cytoplasmic background	Routine laboratory method	Risk of FNs due to focal antigen expression	Easy to perform and compare with histology	Variable staining due to different fixatives	Equal or stronger than direct smears	Alcohol-based: may differ from formalin-fixed slides
Suitable for nuclear antibodies	Potential increased FNs			Routine histology controls Dual ICC possible		Equal distribution of staining Clean background	All antibodies not yet evaluated
Cytogenetic and molecular testing							
Potentially effective for preparation and storage	May be diluted by normal cells	Suitable for FISH	Cell crowding may hamper nuclear signals	Optimal results with current methods	Depends on cellular yield and fixation methods	Suitable for FISH and molecular analysis	Limited studies so far available
Routinely available and cost-effective	Cells of interest may be enriched by microdissection	DNA extraction possible	May be diluted by normal cells	Cells of interest may be enriched by microdissection	Partial cells in sections	Avoids cross-linkage of formalin fixation	May be affected by alcohol fixation (e.g. PR)
Whole cells	Whole cells	Whole cells	Whole cells	Sections	Whole cells	Whole cells	Whole cells

FISH, fluorescence in situ hybridization; FN, false negative; ICC, immunocytochemistry; PR, progesterone receptors.

Source: Jain D, Mathur SR, Iyer VK. Cell blocks in cytopathology: a review of preparative methods, utility in diagnosis and role in ancillary studies. *Cytopathology*. 2014 Dec; 25(6): 356–71.

Cytology Report

Department of Histopathology
University College London Medical School
Rockefeller Building, University St, London WC1E 6JJ

Lab No.: NG00-0404   Hospital No.: 0000000
Name : XXXXX,YYYYYY   Age/Sex : 18Y M
Cons/GP : Doctor X   Ward : Maxillofacial Unit,

....

SPECIMEN : Neck Fine needle aspirate

EXAMINED BY: DR T HATTER

SPECIMEN OBTAINED BY: DR G KOCJAN

CLINICAL DATA:
Swelling left neck and post auricular region.
Fluctuant below angle mandible.

MATERIAL RECEIVED:
Nineteen slides from FNA 2 different sites in the
left neck (see illustration).

MICROSCOPIC DESCRIPTION:
Smears show numerous single and small
aggregates of cells. The cells have large oval
nuclei with fine chromatin pattern, indistinct
nucleoli, and scanty basophilic cytoplasm with
prominent vacuolation.

Immunocytochemistry: LCA and CD20 positive. Tdt, desmin, SMA, myoglobin, MYC2 negative.

CYTOLOGICAL DIAGNOSIS:
FNA left neck. High grade B cell non Hodgkin's lymphoma (? Burkitt's). Biopsy is advised.

SNOMED :   TY0600;M095903

Signed :   Pathologist : DR G KOCJAN

Date : 14/02/2000

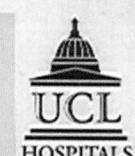

PATHOLOGY DIRECTORATE

Figure 1.8 Cytopathology report should contain patient's details, clinical history, number and position of the site(s) sampled (preferably illustrated by a photograph or a diagram), indicate the name of the aspirator, date of sample, number of slides made and/or other material obtained, microscopic description, special techniques used, cytological diagnosis, diagnostic code, pathologist's signature and date. This report is just an example for illustration. Today we would use flow cytometry and cell block immunocytochemistry to confirm and specify the diagnosis of lymphoma on FNAC.

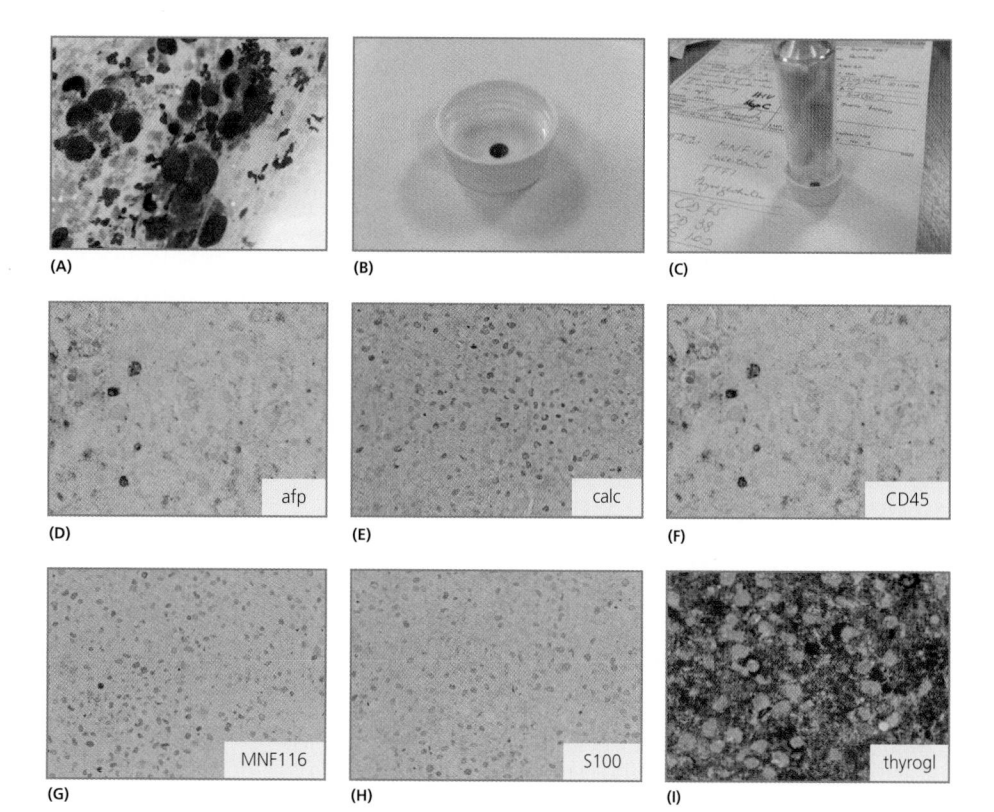

Figure 1.9 Images demonstrating the main steps in the preparation of a vapour fixed cell block. (A) The FNAC material from the thyroid is stained with May Grunwald Giemsa (MGG) and shows undifferentiated tumour cells. (B) The material is expelled from the needle into the well of the lid in a universal container. (C) It is left inverted for at least 6 h to allow the formalin vapours to fix it until solid after which it is handled as a histological sample. (D) afp negative, (E) calcitonin negative, (F) CD45 negative, (G) MNF 116 negative, (H) S100 negative and (I) Thyroglobulin positive. The conclusion was that this is anaplastic carcinoma arising from the thyroid.

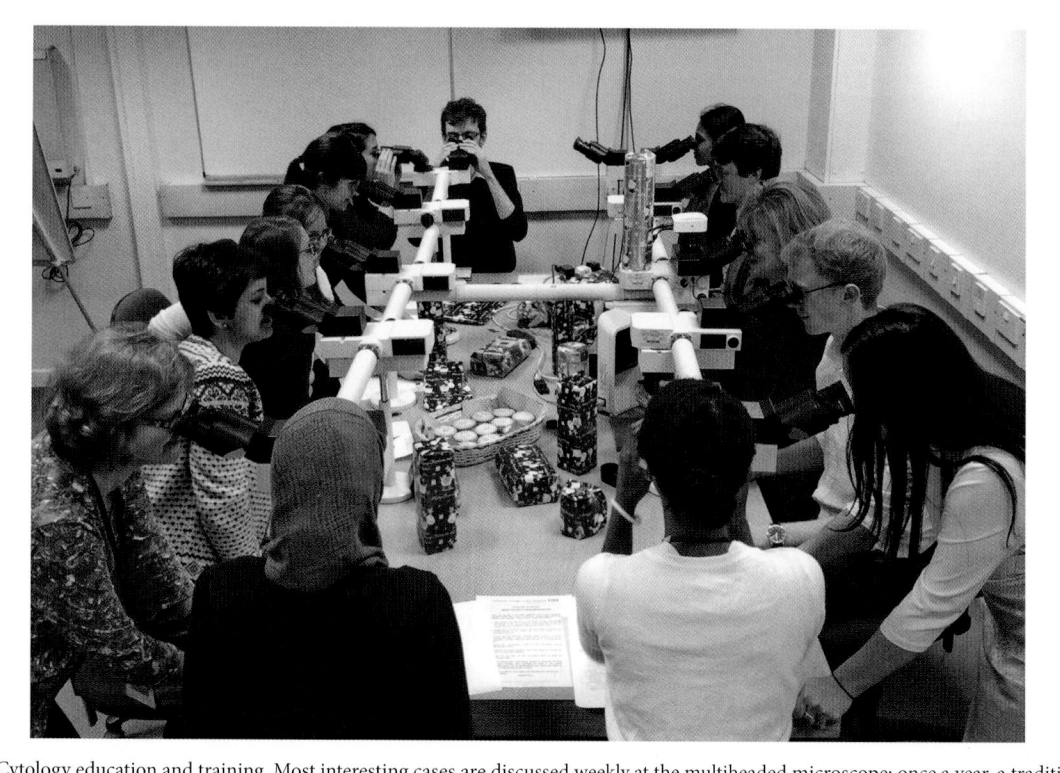

Figure 1.10 Cytology education and training. Most interesting cases are discussed weekly at the multiheaded microscope; once a year, a traditional Christmas quiz, in addition to the seasonal jollity, provides a reminder of the most difficult cases.

References

1. Daraei P, Moore CE. Racial Disparity Among the Head and Neck Cancer Population. *J Cancer Educ.* 2015 Sep; **30**(3): 546–51.

2. Zumsteg ZS, Cook-Wiens G, Yoshida E, Shiao SL, Lee NY, Mita A, Jeon C, Goodman MT, Ho AS. Incidence of Oropharyngeal Cancer Among Elderly Patients in the United States. *JAMA Oncol.* 2016 Jul 14. doi: 10.1001/jamaoncol.2016.1804. [Epub ahead of print]

3. Kocjan G, Ramsay A, Beale T, O'Flynn P. HN cancer in the UK: what is expected of cytopathology? *Cytopathology* 2009 Apr; **20**(2): 69–77.

4. Howlett DC, Harper B, Quante M, Berresford A, Morley M, Grant J, Ramesar K, Barnes S. Diagnostic adequacy and accuracy of fine needle aspiration cytology in neck lump assessment: results from a regional cancer network over a one year period. *J Laryngol Otol.* 2007 Jun; **121**(6): 571–9.

5. Oyafuso MS, Longatto Filho A, Ikeda MK. The role of fine needle aspiration cytology in the diagnosis of lesions of the HN excluding the thyroid and salivary glands. *Tumori* 1992; **78**(2): 134–6.

6. Ono T, Kawai F, Nakamura M et al. Ultrasound-guided fine-needle aspiration cytology for neck lesions. *Rinsho Byori* 1999; **47**(12): 1173–6.

7. Witcher TP, Williams MD, Howlett DC. "One-stop" clinics in the investigation and diagnosis of head and neck lumps. *Br J Oral Maxillofac Surg.* 2007 Jan; **45**(1): 19–22.

8. Tandon S, Shahab R, Benton JI, Ghosh SK, Sheard J, Jones TM. Fine-needle aspiration cytology in a regional head and neck cancer center: comparison with a systematic review and meta-analysis. *Head Neck.* 2008 Sep; **30**(9):1246–52.

9. Schelkun PM, Grundy WG. Fine-needle aspiration biopsy of HN lesions. *J Oral Maxillofac Surg* 1991; **49**(3): 262–7.

10. Patt BS, Schaefer SD, Vuitch F. Role of fine-needle aspiration in the evaluation of neck masses. *Med Clin North Am* 1993; **77**(3): 611–23.

11. Wilson JA, McIntyre MA, Tan J, Maran AG. The diagnostic value of fine needle aspiration cytology in the HN. *J R Coll Surg Edinb* 1985; **30**(6): 375–9.

12. van den Brekel MW, Castelijns JA, Stel HV et al. Occult metastatic neck disease: detection with US and US-guided fine-needle aspiration cytology [published erratum appears in *Radiology* 1992 Jan; 182(1): 288]. *Radiology* 1991; **180**(2): 457–61.

13. Lin CK. Fine needle aspiration biopsy cytology of HN masses: a personal experience in Republic of China. *Chung Hua I Hsueh Tsa Chih* 1988; **42**(4): 255–60.

14. Oyafuso MS, Ikeda MK, Longatto Filho A. Fine needle aspiration cytology in the diagnosis of HN tumors (published erratum appears in *Rev Paul Med* 1991 May–Jun; 109(3): 140). *Rev Paul Med* 1990; **108**(4): 162–4.

15. Fulciniti F, Califano L, Zupi A, Vetrani A. Accuracy of fine needle aspiration biopsy in HN tumors. *J Oral Maxillofac Surg* 1997; **55**(10): 1094–7.

16. Slack RW, Croft CB, Crome LP. Fine needle aspiration cytology in the management of HN masses. *Clin Otolaryngol* 1985; **10**(2): 93–6.

17. Carroll CM, Nazeer U, Timon CI. The accuracy of fine-needle aspiration biopsy in the diagnosis of HN masses. *Ir J Med Sci* 1998; **167**(3): 149–51.

18. Makowska W, Bogacka-Zatorska E, Waloryszak B. Fine needle aspiration biopsy in the diagnosis of HN tumors. *Otolaryngol Pol* 1992; **46**(3): 268–72.

19. McLean NR, Harrop-Griffiths K, Shaw HJ, Trott PA. Fine needle aspiration cytology in the HN region. *Br J Plast Surg* 1989; **42**(4): 447–51.

20. Donahue BJ, Cruickshank JC, Bishop JW. The diagnostic value of fine needle aspiration biopsy of HN masses. *Ear Nose Throat J* 1995; **74**(7): 483–6.

21. Flynn MB, Wolfson SE, Thomas S, Kuhns JG. Fine needle aspiration biopsy in clinical management of HN tumors. *J Surg Oncol* 1990; **44**(4): 214–7.

22. Raju G, Kakar PK, Das DK et al. Role of fine needle aspiration biopsy in HN tumours. *J Laryngol Otol* 1988; **102**(3): 248–51.

23. Mondal A, Gupta S. The role of peroral fine needle aspiration cytology (FNAC) in the diagnosis of parapharyngeal lesions – a study of 51 cases. *Indian J Pathol Microbiol* 1993; **36**(3): 253–9.

24. Layfield LJ. Fine-needle aspiration in the diagnosis of HN lesions: a review and discussion of problems in differential diagnosis. *Diagn Cytopathol* 2007; **35**: 798–805.

25. Amedee RG, Dhurandhar NR. Fine-needle aspiration biopsy. *Laryngoscope* 2001; **111**: 1551–7.

26. Carroll CM, Nazeer U, Timon CI. The accuracy of fineneedle aspiration biopsy in the diagnosis of HN masses. *Ir J Med Sci* 1998; **167**: 149–51.

27. Bahar G, Dudkiewicz M, Feinmesser R et al. Acute parotitis as a complication of fine-needle aspiration in Warthin's tumor. A unique finding of a 3-year experience with parotid tumor aspiration. *Otolaryngol Head Neck Surg* 2006; **134**: 646–9.

28. National Institute of Clinical Excellence. Improving Outcomes in HN Cancers. Available at: www.nice.org.uk/guidance/csghn/guidance/pdf/English, 2004.

29. Layfield LJ. Fine-needle aspiration of the HN. *Pathology (Phila)* 1996; **4**(2): 409–38.

30. Knappe M, Louw M, Gregor RT. Ultrasonography-guided fine-needle aspiration for the assessment of cervical metastases. *Arch Otolaryngol Head Neck Surg* 2000; **126**: 1091–6.

31. British Association of Otorhinolaryngologists HN Surgeons. Effective HN Cancer Management Third Consensus Document. London: British Association of Otorhinolaryngologists HN Surgeons, Royal College of Surgeons, Document 6; 2002.

32. Kraft M, Laeng H, Schmuziger N, Arnoux A, Gurtler N. Comparison of ultrasound-guided core-needle biopsy and fine-needle aspiration in the assessment of HN lesions. *Head Neck* 2008; **30**: 1457–63.

33. Khalid AN, Quraishi SA, Hollenbeak CS, Stack BC Jr. Fine-needle aspiration biopsy versus ultrasound-guided fine-needle aspiration biopsy: cost-effectiveness as a frontline diagnostic modality for solitary thyroid nodules. *Head Neck* 2008 Aug; **30**(8): 1035–9.

34. Chng CL, Beale T, Adjei-Gyamfi Y et al. The role of the cytopathologist's interpretation in achieving diagnostic adequacy of head and neck fine needle aspirates. *Cytopathology.* 2014 Aug; **26**(4): 224–230.

35. Bartels S, Talbot JM, DiTomasso J et al. The relative value of fine-needle aspiration and imaging in the preoperative evaluation of parotid masses. *Head Neck* 2000; **22**: 781–6.

36. Wu M. A comparative study of 200 head and neck FNAs performed by a cytopathologist with versus without ultrasound guidance: evidence for improved diagnostic value with ultrasound guidance. *Diagn Cytopathol* 2011; **39**(10): 743–51.

37. Kocjan G, Chandra A, Cross P, Denton K, Giles T, Herbert A, Smith P, Remedios D, Wilson P. BSCC Code of Practice–fine needle aspiration cytology. *Cytopathology.* 2009 Oct; **20**(5): 283–96.

38. Chng CL, Beale T, Adjei-Gyamfi Y, Gupta Y, Kocjan G. The role of the cytopathologist's interpretation in achieving diagnostic adequacy of HN fine needle aspirates. *Cytopathology* 2014 Aug 11; doi: 10.1111/cyt.12175. [Epub ahead of print].

39. Eisendrath P, Ibrahim M. How good is fine needle aspiration? What results should you expect? *Endosc Ultrasound* 2014; **3**: 3–11.

40. Kocjan G. Evaluation of the cost effectiveness of establishing a fine needle aspiration cytology clinic in a hospital out-patient department. *Cytopathology* 1991; **2**(1): 13–8.

41. Cajulis RS, Gokaslan ST, Yu GH, Frias-Hidvegi D. Fine needle aspiration biopsy of the salivary glands. A five-year experience with emphasis on diagnostic pitfalls. *Acta Cytol* 1997; **41**(5): 1412–20.

42. Jandu M, Webster K. The role of operator experience in fine needle aspiration cytology of HN masses. *Int J Oral Maxillofac Surg* 1999; **28**(6): 441–4.

43. Yu X, Zhang C, Huang S. Study on measures to increase diagnostic accuracy of FNAC of breast masses. *Chung Hua Ping Li Hsueh Tsa Chih* 1997; **26**(6): 334–6.

44. Wu M, Burstein DE, Yuan S, Nurse LA, Szporn AH, Zhang D, et al. A comparative study of 200 fine needle aspiration biopsies performed by clinicians and cytopathologists. *Laryngoscope* 2006; **116**(7): 1212–5.

45. Lieu D. Cytopathologist-performed ultrasound-guided fine-needle aspiration and core-needle biopsy: a prospective study of 500 consecutive cases. *Diagn Cytopathol* 2008; **36**(5): 317–24.

46. Ganguly A, Burnside G, Nixon P. A systematic review of ultrasound guided FNAC. *Brit J Radiol* 2014; **87**(1044): 20130571.

47. Witt BL, Schmidt RL. Rapid onsite evaluation improves the adequacy offline-needle aspiration for thyroid lesions: a systematic review and meta-analysis. *Thyroid.* 2013 Apr;**23**(4): 428–35

48. Keshtgar MR, Barker SG, Ell PJ. Needle-free vehicle for administration of radionuclide for sentinel-node biopsy [letter]. *Lancet* 1999; **353**(9162): 1410–1.

49. Dey P, Ray R. Comparison of fine needle sampling by capillary action and fine needle aspiration. *Cytopathology* 1993; **4**(5): 299–303.

50. Hamaker RA, Moriarty AT, Hamaker RC. Fine-needle biopsy techniques of aspiration versus capillary in HN masses. *Laryngoscope* 1995; **105** (12 Pt 1): 1311–4.

51. Kate MS, Kamal MM, Bobhate SK, Kher AV. Evaluation of fine needle capillary sampling in superficial and deep- seated lesions. An analysis of 670 cases. *Acta Cytol* 1998; **42**(3): 679–84.

52. Song H, Wei C, Li D, Hua K, Song J, Maskey N, Fang L. Comparison of Fine Needle Aspiration and Fine Needle Nonaspiration Cytology of Thyroid Nodules: A Meta-Analysis. *Biomed Res Int.* 2015; 2015: 796120. doi: 10.1155/2015/796120. Epub 2015 Sep 29.

53. Yue XH, Zheng SF. Cytologic diagnosis by transthoracic fine needle sampling without aspiration. *Acta Cytol* 1989; **33**(6): 805–8.

54. Srikanth S, Anandam G, Kashif MM. A comparative study of fine-needle aspiration and fine-needle non-aspiration techniques in head and neck swellings. *Indian J Cancer* 2014; **51**(2): 98–9.

55. Herbert A. Cell blocks are not a substitute for cytology: why pathologists should understand cytopathology particularly in their chosen speciality. *Cytopathology* 2014 Dec; **25**(6): 351–5.

56. Keyhani-Rofahga S, O'Toole RV, Leming M. The role of cell block in fine-needle aspiration cytology. *Acta Cytol* 1984; **28**: 630–1.

57. Fetsch PA, Simsir A, Brosky K, Abati A. Comparison of three commonly used cytologic preparations in effusion immunocytochemistry. *Diagn Cytopathol* 2002; **26**: 61–6.

58. Billah S, Stewart J, Staerkel G et al. EGFR and KRAS mutations in lung carcinoma: molecular testing by using cytology specimens. *Cancer Cytopathol* 2011; **119**: 111–17.

59. Young NA, Naryshkin S, Katz SM. Diagnostic value of electron microscopy on paraffin-embedded cytologic material. *Diagn Cytopathol* 1993; **9**: 282–90.

60. Jain D, Mathur SR, Iyer VK. Cell blocks in cytopathology: a review of preparative methods, utility in diagnosis and role in ancillary studies. *Cytopathology* 2014 Dec; **25**(6): 356–71.

61. Mayall F, Darlington A. The poor man's cell block. *J Clin Pathology* 2010; **63**(9): 837–838.

62. Morton KD. Fine needle aspiration cytology of lesions of the HN and factors affecting outcome. *Scott Med J* 1989; **34**(5): 523–5.

CHAPTER 2

Salivary gland

Chapter contents

2.1 Introduction, 9
  2.1.1 Ultrasound guided FNAC, 10
  2.1.2 Diagnostic accuracy, 10
  2.1.3 Diagnostic pitfalls, 11
  2.1.4 Ultrasound versus other imaging modalities, 12
  2.1.5 FNAC versus frozen section and core biopsy, 12
  2.1.6 Cost effectiveness, 12
2.2 Diagnostic imaging of salivary glands, 13
  2.2.1 Normal Ultrasound appearance of salivary gland, 13
  2.2.2 Imaging Pitfalls and scanning issues, 13
    2.2.2.1 Parotid gland, 13
    2.2.2.2 US appearance of Submandibular gland, 14
2.3 Cytology of the salivary gland, 14
  2.3.1 Normal salivary gland cytology, 14
  2.3.2 Sialadenosis, 14
  2.3.3 Salivary gland cysts, 17
  2.3.4 Sialadenitis, 21
    2.3.4.1 Ultrasound, 21
    2.3.4.2 Submandibular ductal system scanning technique, 21
    2.3.4.3 Chronic sialadenitis (Kuttner's tumour), 22
    2.3.4.4 Granulomatous sialadenitis, 23
  2.3.5 Lymphoid proliferations of the salivary gland, 23
    2.3.5.1 Reactive lymphoid proliferations, 23
    2.3.5.2 Neoplastic lymphoid proliferations, 23
2.4 Salivary gland tumours, 29
  2.4.1 Pleomorphic adenoma, 29
  2.4.2 Adenolymphoma (Warthin's tumour), 35
  2.4.3 Basal cell adenoma, 37
  2.4.4 Oncocytoma, 39
  2.4.5 Rare benign tumours, 40
    2.4.5.1 Sclerosing polycystic adenosis, 40
    2.4.5.2 Myoepithelioma, 40
    2.4.5.3 Intraductal papilloma, 41

2.5 Malignant tumours of the salivary gland, 42
  2.5.1 Acinic cell carcinoma, 42
  2.5.2 Mucoepidermoid carcinoma, 44
  2.5.3 Adenoid cystic carcinoma, 48
  2.5.4 Polymorphous low grade adenocarcinoma, 51
  2.5.5 Epithelial myoepithelial carcinoma, 52
  2.5.6 Basal cell adenocarcinoma, 53
  2.5.7 Papillary cystadenocarcinoma, 54
  2.5.8 Mucinous adenocarcinoma, 54
  2.5.9 Oncocytic carcinoma, 54
  2.5.10 Salivary duct carcinoma, 55
  2.5.11 Adenocarcinoma (not otherwise specified), 57
  2.5.12 Carcinoma ex PLA, 57
  2.5.13 Primary squamous cell carcinoma of the salivary gland, 58
  2.5.14 Small cell carcinoma, 58
  2.5.15 Undifferentiated carcinoma of the salivary gland, 59
2.6 Miscellaneous tumours, 59
  2.6.1 Lymphoepithelial carcinoma, 59
  2.6.2 Mammary analogue secretory carcinoma, 59
  2.6.3 Cribriform adenocarcinoma of minor salivary gland, 60
  2.6.4 Soft tissue lesions, 61
    2.6.4.1 Benign neurilemmoma, 61
    2.6.4.2 Nodular fasciitis, 61
    2.6.4.3 Rhabdomyosarcoma, 61
    2.6.4.4 Maligant haemangiopericytoma, 61
    2.6.4.5 Leiomyosarcoma, 61
  2.6.5 Granulocytic sarcoma, 61
  2.6.6 Paediatric lesions, 61
  2.6.7 Lymphomas, 61
  2.6.8 Primitive neuroectodermal tumour, 62
  2.6.9 Metastatic tumours in salivary gland, 63
2.7 Clinical management of salivary gland lesions, 64
References, 65

2.1 Introduction

Most salivary pathology presents with a lump, swelling, pain or a dry mouth or a combination of these symptoms. All salivary lumps (apart from normal lymph nodes in the parotid) should be taken seriously. Indeed, the adage 'the smaller the salivary gland the more likely a malignancy' is a good one. In general, ultrasound cannot reliably distinguish benign from malignant lesions, however, benign lesions tend to have well defined margins with no infiltration and malignant lesions tend to have ill-defined, infiltrating margins into the normal parotid parenchyma. Nevertheless, it is important to appreciate that some malignant tumours have well defined margins and on ultrasound alone cannot be distinguished from malignant. Because there is overlap in their sonographic features, tissue diagnosis by means of Fine Needle Aspiration cytology (FNAC) plays an

important role in management. Ultrasound and FNAC cytology can provide accurate, diagnosis for salivary pathology [1–4].

Cytological diagnosis of salivary gland lesions is becoming one of the most sought after requests in the preoperative clinical management of patients. Therefore, a cytopathologist has to be familiar with the best approach to diagnosis. This involves, in the first instance, assessing the anatomical site. If it is within the area of major and minor salivary glands, it is important to establish if the lesion involves salivary gland or has arisen in adjacent tissues such as lymph nodes or skin (Fig. 2.1). In most cases, it is important to decide if the lesion is neoplastic or not. In many series, non-neoplastic lesions make for over 50% of the FNAC requests and fewer than 10% of these had subsequent surgery [5]. Approximately 44% of patients can be spared surgical intervention through diagnosis of a non-neoplastic process. The presence of a cytopathologist in the

Cytopathology of the Head and Neck: Ultrasound Guided FNAC, Second Edition. Gabrijela Kocjan.
© 2017 John Wiley & Sons Ltd. Published 2017 by John Wiley & Sons Ltd.
Companion website: www.wiley.com/go/kocjan/clinical_cytopathology_head_neck2e

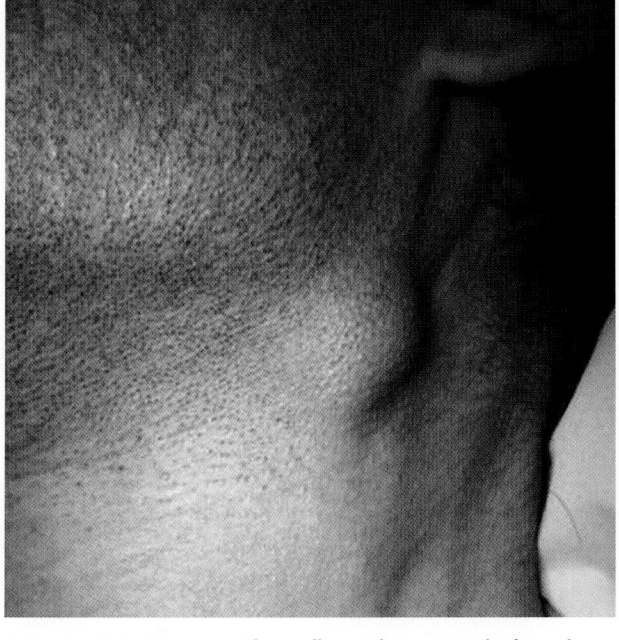

Figure 2.1 Patient presents with a swelling at the upper neck of 4 weeks duration. Clinically it was thought to be a Warthin's tumour. FNAC was requested to establish the anatomy and nature of the lesion. FNAC showed a granulomatous lymphadenitis consistent with TB. Culture was sent and patient treated appropriately.

clinic increases the likelihood of obtaining a diagnostic sample (Figs 1.2 and 1.3) [6]. If the lesion is neoplastic, the cytopathologist has to decide whether it is benign or malignant (low or high grade). The distinction is desirable for the appropriate management. Cytological diagnosis, apart from morphology, relies on clinical and radiological correlation [7]. FNAC is a safe diagnostic tool that has a reliable sensitivity and specificity for the assessment of salivary gland pathology [8]. It is applicable particularly in the initial assessment of parotid masses, and can play an important role in treatment planning [9] and in the conservative management of non-neoplastic lesions, and it may be useful for the accurate confirmation of tumour recurrence [10, 11].

2.1.1 Ultrasound guided FNAC (Simon Morley)

Ultrasound (US) is a useful technique for the assessment of superficial masses of the parotid and submandibular glands [12], and is increasingly becoming the method of choice for initial evaluation of the salivary glands (Figs 2.2 and 2.3). It is cheap, widely available and safe, and can be used to delineate superficial salivary gland lesions as precisely as CT and MRI [13]. It can also correctly differentiate malignant lesions from benign ones in 90% of cases, distinguish glandular from extraglandular masses with an accuracy of 98%, and confirm the clinical suspicion of a mass. Wu et al. describe the sensitivity, specificity, positive predictive value, negative predictive value and accuracy of ultrasound for the diagnosis of parotid gland masses to be 38.9, 90.1, 29.2, 93.3 and 85.2%, respectively, and accuracy for malignant masses was 20% [14]. Neoplasms are usually hypoechoic to normal glandular tissue and US has been reported to completely delineate 95% of major salivary gland lesions [12]. US cannot directly visualise the facial nerve, but can suggest its position by accurate identification of intraglandular vessels within the parotid, and therefore show whether lesions are superficial or deep lobe. High-frequency US provides excellent resolution and characterisation of tissue without the inherent danger of

radiation. It allows for the sampling of solid regions of complex masses and improves diagnostic yield while avoiding neighbouring structures.

In most instances, FNAC is performed in a standard manner, preferably using a non-aspiration technique (Fig 1.5) [15–21] and using a 25G needle. Local anaesthetic is usually not given, except in cases where patient is needle-phobic or the area is tender (Fig 1.4). One or two passes with a needle usually produce sufficient material. Material is spread onto the slides or collected in the liquid preservative. Needle washings are taken where appropriate for special stains. Slides are either air-dried or alcohol fixed. Rapid staining in the clinic usually establishes the cellularity and gives an indication of the type of the lesion so that, where necessary, extra material can be obtained (Fig 1.4). In many cases, diagnosis may be made immediately. Some centres use liquid based cytology preparations for analysis of salivary FNAC samples. In this case, material is ejected into a liquid medium and processed according to manufacturers' instructions [22, 23].

Ultrasound gels can be associated with a significant artefact in FNAC specimens. To eliminate this artefact, which may alter the adequacy, diagnosis or cytological appearance, Royer et al. advocate a specific gel type that is useful for ultrasound-guided FNAC [24].

FNAC of salivary gland is a safe procedure with no sinister complications. Patients often experience discomfort, particularly at FNAC of non-neoplastic conditions. However, the main concern is whether the needle interference will eventually lead to a higher recurrence rate in some tumours. Provided the standard FNAC technique is applied and standard calibre needle (<21 G, preferably 23 or 25 G) is used, there is no evidence, in many long term follow-up studies of patients with preoperative FNAC, that it influences recurrence of tumours. Occasionally, haemorrhage is encountered. In the case of submandibular gland, this results sometimes in bleeding through the salivary duct in the mouth. Although the effect appears dramatic, it is at the same time reassuring in terms of patency of the main duct.

Some reports suggest histological changes associated with preoperative FNAC of benign parotid lesions and the features that distinguish these changes from malignant neoplasms. A spectrum of histological alterations was observed, including squamous cell metaplasia, infarction and necrosis, subepithelial stromal hyalinisation, acute and chronic haemorrhage and inflammation with multinucleated giant cells, granulation tissue with subsequent fibrosis, cholesterol cleft formation, pseudoxanthomatous reaction, pseudocapsular invasion and microcystic degeneration. In cases with exuberant squamous metaplasia, necrosis or subepithelial stromal hyalinisation, a diagnosis of squamous cell carcinoma or low-grade mucoepidermoid carcinoma has to be seriously considered. The knowledge of a previous FNAC procedure and awareness of its effects on histology of the subsequent parotidectomy specimens are necessary to avoid potential misdiagnosis [25, 26].

2.1.2 Diagnostic accuracy

Retrospective studies have reported overall accuracy rates of FNAC for parotid masses ranging from 90 to 98% [27–29, 29a], well within the range of 81–98% established earlier [5, 10, 11, 27–29, 30, 31, 32, 43]. In a 10-year retrospective study of salivary gland FNAC by Kechiagas et al., sensitivity, specificity, diagnostic accuracy, PPV and NPV were 90% (28/31), 98% (54/55), 95.1% (82/86), 96% and 94% respectively [44, 44a]. Our own audit for the 8 year period showed the sensitivity and specificity of FNAC for a malignant outcome was 89% (33/37) and 97% (130/134) respectively. False negative and false positive

Table 2.1 Audit of salivary gland FNAC at University College Hospitals, London between 2005 and 2012. [44a]

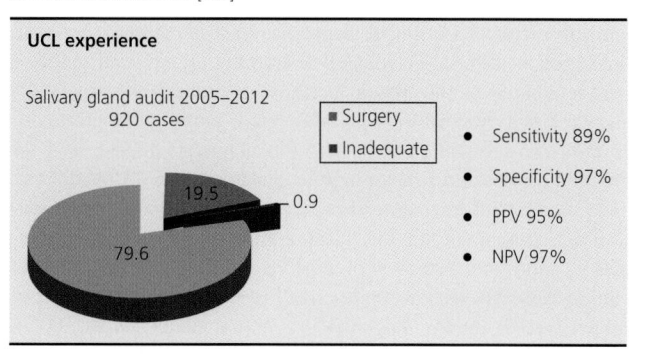

UCL experience

Salivary gland audit 2005–2012
920 cases

- Surgery
- Inadequate

19.5
0.9
79.6

- Sensitivity 89%
- Specificity 97%
- PPV 95%
- NPV 97%

diagnoses are described in most series and reach up to 5% each. As these series have shown, cytological interpretation of salivary gland cytology does not have a 100% sensitivity and specificity (Table 2.1). However, if type specific diagnoses are made only when all diagnostic criteria are present and any uncertainty clearly conveyed to the clinician, FNAC is a safe and accurate tool in the investigation of salivary gland lesions [5, 45].

The immunohistochemical evaluation of diagnostic and prognostic value of the proliferating cell nuclear antigen (PCNA) and Ki-67 showed that the values of MIB-1 parameters increased progressively in benign lesions in comparison with the normal and in malignant neoplasms in comparison with non-neoplastic and benign lesions. A high Ki67 index remains the most useful marker to predict adverse outcome in salivary carcinoma [46]. PCNA and MIB-1 indices may be one of the markers for discriminating between benign and malignant tumours of the parotid gland. The new developments in the molecular pathogenesis of head and neck tumours, in particular the tumour-specific chromosomal rearrangements important in tumourigenesis of various uncommon malignancies, such as mucoepidermoid carcinoma (MEC) and adenoid cystic carcinoma (AdCC), have been described (See Table 2.5, p42.) [46, 47]. These markers are being proposed as complementary to the current grading systems in the respective malignancies [48].

Flow cytometry has been shown to be useful in the diagnosis of lymphoproliferative lesions of salivary glands [49].

2.1.3 Diagnostic pitfalls

Salivary gland tumours are composed of epithelial cells, myoepithelial cells and stroma in various proportions. Cytological smears lack the architecture, which is particularly important in differentiating some of the tumours. Some tumours are rare so that a practising cytopathologist may not have come across the entity before either during training or in practice. Most frequently misdiagnosed lesions are pleomorphic adenoma (PLA), MEC, chronic sialadenitis and malignant lymphoma. Problems may also be encountered in differentiating hematopoietic from non-hematopoietic lesions and interpretation of spindle cell neoplasms, acinic cell carcinoma, AdCC, lymphoproliferative disorders and postirradiation changes [7].

Wide spectrum of benign and malignant tumours as well as the heterogeneiety of many tumours poses a formidable task for a cytopathologist with an ambition for a good histological correlation of their findings. The original series of salivary gland tumours described by Zajicek and co-workers at the Karolinska hospital in the 1960s and 1970s described the tumour types known at the time [15]. Since that time, many new entities have been described. The most recent WHO classification of salivary gland tumours now includes 9

benign tumours (adenomas) and 18 malignant (carcinomas), with the added non-epithelial tumours, malignant lymphoma, tumour-like lesions and metastatic tumours (Table 2.2) [36, 50].

There is sometimes overlap between different conditions showing similar appearances. The main problem areas in FNAC of salivary gland lesions are the following: cystic lesions (neoplastic and non neoplastic), atypical cells in PLA, cellular smears with epithelial cells and no stroma, squamous or 'squamoid' differentiation, tumours with a 'clear cell' pattern, hyaline stromal globules and prominent lymphoid component in some lesions [5, 37–40]. These present potential pitfalls, of which the cytopathologist needs to be aware and, if necessary, include differential diagnosis as part of the final report [51]. In a series by MacLeod and Frable, diagnostic pitfalls present only a minority (21 out of 582 in 17 years) and therefore should not distract from the fact that most salivary gland lesions can be confidently diagnosed as benign or malignant on cytological material [52]. Despite the relative rarity of salivary gland tumours, if established diagnostic criteria are present and strictly observed, the great majority of the common variants of the non-neoplastic and both benign and malignant salivary gland tumours can be diagnosed with a high level of accuracy [53]. The pitfalls in cytological interpretation can be avoided with increased practice.

Table 2.2 Revised WHO classification of salivary gland tumours and tumour-like conditions. [50]

1 Adenomas

1.1	Pleomorphic adenoma
1.2	Myoepithelioma (myoepithelial adenoma)
1.3	Basal cell adenoma
1.4	Warthin tumour (adenolymphoma)
1.5	Oncocytoma (oncocytic adenoma)
1.6	Info Canalicular adenoma
1.7	Sebaceous adenoma
1.8	Ductal papilloma - 1.8.1 Inverted ductal papilloma
	1.8.2 Intraductal papilloma
	1.8.3 Sialadenoma papilliferum
1.9	Cystadenoma - 1.9.1 Papillary cystadenoma
	1.9.2 Mucinous cystadenoma

2 Carcinomas

2.1	Acinic cell carcinoma
2.2	Mucoepidermoid carcinoma
2.3	Adenoid cystic carcinoma
2.4	Polymorphous low grade adenocarcinoma (terminal duct adenocarcinoma)
2.5	Epithelial-myoepithelial carcinoma
2.6	Basal cell adenocarcinoma
2.7	Sebaceous carcinoma
2.8	Papillary cystadenocarcinoma
2.9	Mucinous adenocarcinoma
2.10	Oncocytic carcinoma
2.11	Salivary duct carcinoma
2.12	Adenocarcinorna (not otherwise specified)
2.13	Malignant myoepithelioma (myoepithelial carcinoma)
2.14	Carcinoma in pleomorphic adenoma
2.15	Squamous cell carcinoma
2.16	Small cell carcinoma
2.17	Undifferentiated carcinoma
2.18	Other carcinomas

3 Non-epithelial tumours
4 Malignant lymphomas
5 Secondary tumours
6 Unclassified tumours

Tumour-like lesions

7.1	Sialadenosis
7.2	Oncocytosis
7.3	Necrotising sialometaplasia (salivary gland infarction)
7.4	Benign lymphoepithelial lesion
7.5	Salivary gland cysts
7.6	Chronic sclerosing sialadenitis of submandibular gland (Kuttner tumour)
7.7	Cystic lymphoid hyperplasia in AIDS

Special training is required to become proficient in both obtaining and interpreting aspirated material. It is not sufficient for pathologists to apply personal experience from tissue pathology to the diagnosis of cytological specimens [46]. Instead, a specialist training and skill are required for performing the aspiration and evaluating the cytological material. The pathologist's technique, interest and experience are important variables that influence FNAC results and likely account for the variance between the results of sensitivity and specificity. In most institutions, the rate of non-diagnostic smears is high because FNAC cannot be performed and immediately examined by an experienced on-site cytopathologist. A multidisciplinary approach and audit of result is an essential ingredient of a successful FNAC service [46a].

2.1.4 Ultrasound versus other imaging modalities

US is usually the first choice both for assessing superficial parotid and submandibular gland lesions and to guide cell/tissue examination for histological or cytological analysis. Wu et al. found the sensitivity, specificity, positive predictive value, negative predictive value and accuracy of ultrasound for the diagnosis of parotid gland masses were 38.9, 90.1, 29.2, 93.3 and 85.2%, respectively, and accuracy for malignant masses was 20% [14]. MRI can characterise locally invasive lesions, assess the extent of large lesions and identify nodal disease. When compared with FNAC, ultrasound and MRI have lower positive predictive value for preoperative diagnosis of malignant salivary gland tumours [54]. CT is principally used in thoracic staging of malignant disease and is a second line method in stone disease. Digital subtraction sialography, although invasive, is the most sensitive method for identifying ductal stones. Future advances are likely to include the more widespread use of new MR sequences for higher resolution imaging of the extracranial facial nerve along with the use of diffusion-weighted (DWI) MR techniques and nuclear medicine/PET in the characterisation of salivary gland lesions [55]. Inohara found the sensitivity/specificity/accuracy of combined FNAC and MRI were 90/95/94% and 81/92/89%, respectively. Either FNAC or MRI served equally to predict the malignant nature of parotid mass lesions. Interestingly, they found that the combination of FNAC and MRI yielded no diagnostic advantage over either modality alone [56]. Sonoelastography is a novel imaging technique that has been employed in the research setting in the evaluation of tissues including breast, thyroid, prostate and the salivary glands. More recently, it has been used as a diagnostic adjunct in the sonographic evaluation of major salivary gland lesions [57].

2.1.5 FNAC versus frozen section and core biopsy

The minimal recommended surgical approach to parotid tumours is partial parotidectomy with resection of the superficial lobe of the gland. Histological diagnosis prior to surgery is not possible, as incisional biopsies are contraindicated due to the possibility of facial nerve injury or incomplete tumour resection. Thus, if performed at all, the biopsies tend to be perioperative [58]. When comparing the outcomes of 171 salivary gland FNACs with subsequent histology, Layfield found that the false positive rate of FNAC in this series was 3.5% and false negative 4.7%. Corresponding frozen sections in 38 cases showed an exact histological correlation in 58% of cases, with no false positives but with 11% false negatives [59]. A comparison of the cytological diagnosis and frozen section made by Chan et al. showed that the overall diagnostic accuracy of FNAC for diagnosis of malignant and benign salivary gland tumours was 95% and frozen section was 91% [31]. The accuracy in diagnosing

the exact category of neoplastic disease was 70 and 77%, respectively. The diagnostic sensitivity for malignant disease was 86 and 70%, and specificity 99 and 100%, respectively. Frozen section, however, did supplement the FNAC diagnosis in some cases. Carvalho found that sensitivity of the frozen sections for malignancy was 61.5% and specificity was 98% [58]. Collela et al. found cytological concordance with histology to be 80% for malignant disease, 96% for benign tumours and 94% for non neoplastic disease [8]. Wade et al. have shown that the diagnostic accuracy of FNAC and frozen section are comparable for the interpretation of salivary gland neoplasms, and the accuracy of both is increased when used in conjunction. The diagnostic accuracy of FNAC is close to that of frozen section for the diagnosis of salivary gland neoplasms (78 versus 89%) and carcinomas (52 versus 67%). These findings support, as suggested by other authors, the combined use of intraoperative frozen section with FNAC in the evaluation of salivary gland neoplasms.

In recent years, percutaneous image-guided core needle biopsy (CNB) has gained widespread popularity for tissue sampling particularly of deep-seated masses throughout the body. CNB can be performed without the attendance of a pathologist under real-time US-guidance using a freehand technique [60]. A spring-loaded semi-automatic biopsy gun can be used with side-notch needles (length 100 mm; diameters 12 gauge (2.05 mm), 14 gauge (1.63 mm), 16 gauge (1.29 mm) and 18 gauge and a variable needle throw (forward feed, 15 or 22 mm) depending on the dimension of the target. Using this technique Pfeiffer et al. achieved sensitivity 94%; specificity 100%; accuracy 96%; positive predictive value 100%; negative predictive value 90% [61]. The main advantage of CNB over FNAC is that the material is processed as a histological sample and is therefore more familiar for interpretation in a non specialist centre. Immunocytochemistry and molecular investigations may be successfully performed on both, CNB and FNAC cell block samples. Histological grading and prognostic biomarkers in salivary gland tumours are best performed on the surgically excised tissue speciamen [48].

The problems with the use of CNB for the assessment of salivary gland lesions have been recorded, mainly facial nerve injury and tumour seeding, which may be the reasons for the small number of studies on this issue. The facial nerve cannot be visualised with sonography, but damage to it during CNB has not been reported. It has been proposed that facial nerve injury can be avoided under real-time ultrasound guidance because its position can be inferred, as the nerve passes in a plane immediately superficial to the retromandibular vein, which is well visualised with sonography [61].

2.1.6 Cost effectiveness

FNAC is a quick, safe and inexpensive method for obtaining material for pathological diagnosis. It is most useful in the diagnosis of a malignant tumour but it is probably most cost effective in avoiding surgery [62]. Sharma et al. found that 40% of patients were spared surgical intervention on the basis of findings from US-guided FNAC of salivary glands [1]. In an audit of 920 salivary gland FNAC, we found that only 20% of patients have undergone surgery [44a] (Table 2.1).

The speed with which FNAC can provide a diagnosis has been utilised in the so-called One Stop Clinics [63]. The aspirates are immediately reported by a cytopathologist and the reports conveyed to the surgeon during the same clinic visit. FNAC results are then compared with histology in those patients who undergo surgery and with the clinical course of the disease at subsequent clinic visits in patients where surgery was not performed. In the series of 92 patients, Roland et al. found that the cytological

diagnosis was incorrect in five cases, one of which was a false negative result. There were no false positive results. The sensitivity was 90.9% and the specificity 100%. This rapid report system of FNAC has been found to be safe, free of complications, and helpful in the planning of treatment [64].

2.2 Diagnostic imaging of salivary glands (Simon Morley)

US is the investigation of choice for major salivary gland disease, reserving other techniques for further assessment in the minority of cases.

Sialopathies can be quickly classified on US appearances into sialectasis, multiglandular parenchymal disease, uniglandular parenchymal disease, intraglandular lymphadenopathy and cystic orsolid masses, thereby generating a manageable differential diagnosis. This can be further refined with aknowledge of the clinical history but there should be alow threshold to performing FNAC. Sialography remains the gold standard for the assessment of suspected ductal calculi or strictures. Contrast enhanced CT is useful indefiying acute infection and MRI is essential for the assessment of deep lobe parotid tumours and any salivary gland malignancy.

Parotid gland: The parotid is assessed with a high frequency ~12 MHz linear probe in longitudinal and transverse planes.

2.2.1 Normal Ultrasound appearance of salivary gland

The normal parotid gland US shows homogenous echotexture and appears hyperechoic relative to the nearby masseter muscle. Dual screen views are useful for comparing the echogenicity – in order to demonstrate generalised salivary parenchymal abnormalities (Fig 2.2).

The parotid parenchyma thickness varies between individuals. There is also quite a wide range in the extent to which the parotid tissue extends anteriorly over the patient's cheek – the accessory lobe. If this is accessory parotid tissue is asymmetrical it may be detected as a lump in the patient's cheek. The main parotid duct runs through the centre of this accessory parotid tissue. Scanning

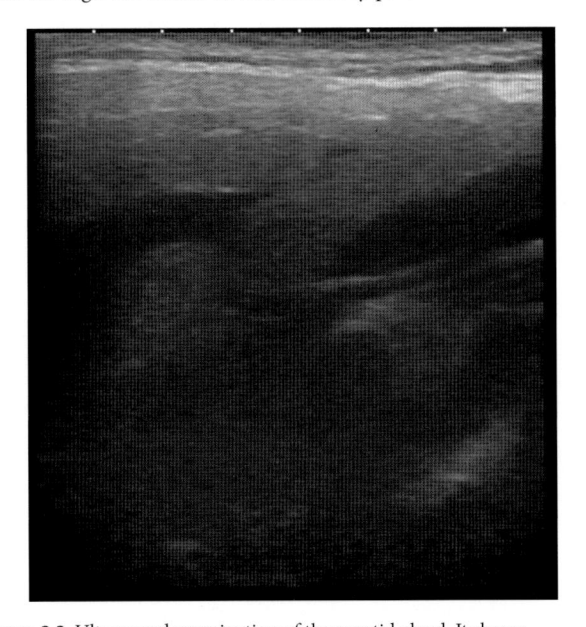

Figure 2.2 Ultrasound examination of the parotid gland. It shows homogeneous echogenicity and is increased in echoenicity compared to the nearby muscles. The normal retromandbular vein courses through the gland. Normal lymph nodes can be found within the parotid.

the accessory parotid tissue in a longitudinal plane allows even the normal parotid duct to be identified as a small round low echogenicity focus and followed anteriorly to the cheek. The normal parotid duct measures up to 1 mm.

The downstream duct at the ductal orifice can be difficult to identify as it passes over the buccal fat pad (a mobile hypoechoic, triangular area seen just anterior to masseter and sometimes wrongly interpreted as a mass). Identification of the parotid duct as it passes towards the buccal mucosa can be aided by asking the patient to puff out their cheeks – this shows the buccal mucosa as a crisp linear echogenic interface. Without this is easy to misinterpret teeth abutting the buccal mucosa as large calculi!

Compared with the other salivary glands the parotid glands are unique in that they may contain normal lymph nodes within. Frequently these are of no diagnostic challenge – if they are large enough – displaying ellipsoid shape and echogenic hila with central vascularity – however, sometimes the typical reactive features are absent. A relatively frequent presentation is when the patient is able to feel a small subcutaneous nodule within the most superficial aspect of the parotid. If the typical ultrasound features of a reactive node are not present on ultrasound, then it can be difficult to determine on morphological features whether the nodule represents a small primary salivary lesion or an incidental reactive lymph node. We would recommend an US FNAC in these circumstances to clarify.

If a lesion is identified in the parotid gland it is important to determine where the lesion lies in relation to the main branches of the facial nerve. This is an important consideration for a surgeon as a lesion centred in or extending into the deep lobe will necessitate a different surgical approach (and careful preservation of the facial nerve) compared to a lesion only in the superficial lobe.

The anatomical concept deep and superficial lobes was developed in order help surgeons guide management. In fact, there is no clear anatomical boundary between the deep and superficial lobes. Furthermore, the facial nerve itself it not actually visible on any imaging modality and so the division into deep and superficial lobes depends on visualisation of other structures that act as surrogate markers for the anatomical boundaries.

In most patients the facial nerve lies just lateral to the ECA and RMV and so on ultrasound these are used as 'rough' markers of the facial nerve location. From a practical point of view many radiologists fall back on MRI as being more reliable than ultrasound and will recommend MRI if a lesion is nearby the RMV or ECA without obviously passing deep to them.

2.2.2 Imaging Pitfalls and scanning issues (Simon Morley)

2.2.2.1 Parotid gland

Some patients with pathology in the parotid tail (most commonly, a Warthin's tumour) present with swelling or a lump in the upper neck. Ultrasound readily identifies the lump but it is well recognised that a lesion at the most inferior parotid tail may not be completely surrounded by normal parotid parenchyma. A diagnostic challenge therefore arises as to whether the lesion lies in the parotid tail or alternatively represents an enlarged lymph node in the upper deep cervical chain. Ultimately, an ultrasound guided FNAC may be needed to clarify but there are some ultrasound features that can be helpful in the assessment.

1 Relationship to the posterior belly of digastric muscle.
2 The presence of a normal upper deep cervical chain lymph node in addition to the palpable lesion suggests it most likely represents a parotid tail lesion
3 A recognition that it can be difficult and highlighting this uncertainty to the referring clinician and cytologist.

The parotid glands are normally more echogenic and absorb more of the ultrasound beam than the submandibular salivary glands. This is due to the higher fat content within normal parotid tissue. This makes ultrasound of the deep lobe of the parotid challenging because of the poor penetration of the ultrasound beam into the deep lobe. We have first-hand experience of deep lobe of parotid lesions that are simply not possible to visualise with the linear probe for this reason. In view of this, we recommend that the complete examination of the parotid should include using a curvilear 7 MHz probe. This allows examination of the deep aspect of the gland albeit with reduced spatial resolution.

2.2.2.2 US appearance of Submandibular gland

The submandibular salivary glands lie inferomedial to the posterior body of the mandible. They may be isoechoic or hypoechoic with reference to the parotid glands. The size of the submandibular glands varies between individuals and in some patients (with generally large salivary glands) the submandibular glands and the parotid tails may abut one another in the upper neck.

The submandibular salivary gland lies at the posterior, free margin of the mylohyoid muscle (Fig. 2.3). Some of the gland extends anteriorly between the mylohyoid muscle and the hyoglossus muscle – along the course of the submandibular duct. Normal vessels also pass alongside the normal duct and it can be difficult otodistinguish the submandibular duct from these vessels on grayscale ultrasound images. The use of colour Doppler can help discriminate. Additionally, vessels can be seen to branch, whereas the normal submandibular duct does not branch. The submandibular duct can be seen (when dilated) running anteriorly in the sublingual space anteriorly to the floor of mouth. The duct is difficult to identify anteriorly at the floor of mouth as it lies quite deep to the probe at this position.

The vessels within the submandibular gland parenchyma appear prominent and it is sometimes tempting to assume that they represent dilated intraglandular ducts. This can be easily assessed with colour flow Doppler.

When looking for submandibular calculi, the superior horn of the hyoid bone lies close to the inferior aspect of the submandibular gland and can on occasion mimic a submandibular calculus (in reality if this is the case then the angle of the ultrasound probe is too inferior – the duct lies more superiorly in the sublingual space).

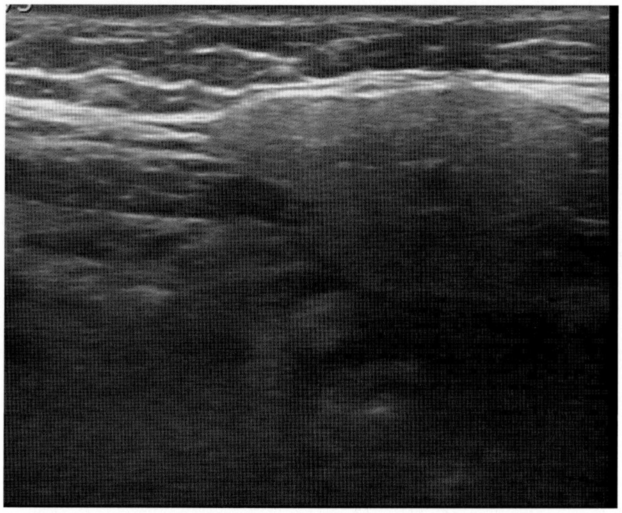

Figure 2.3 The submandibular salivary gland shows homogenous echogenicity and is increased in echogenicity compared to the nearby muscles.

The submandibular gland (unlike the parotid) does not contain any lymph nodes. Normal lymph nodes do lie in the submandibular region and on occasion it can be difficult to determine whether a lesion is a lymph node abutting the submandibular gland or a lesion extending to the margin of a submandibular gland.

2.3 Cytology of the salivary gland

2.3.1 Normal salivary gland cytology

FNAC from normal salivary glands are usually performed when there is a dilemma as to the nature of the swelling (lymph node, salivary gland, other?). Procedure is usually unduly painful and the material poorly cellular. Smears consist of acinar cells, occasional ductal cells and fat cells (Fig. 2.4). Acinar cells usually present in cohesive, branching aggregates with rounded edges. Serous acinar cell has eccentric small round nuclei with inconspicuous nucleoli and abundant vacuolated cytoplasm. Mucinous acinar cells, which are present abundantly in the submandibular gland, have intracytoplasmic mucin. Ductal cells are usually closely associated with acinar cells but may lie separately. They are arranged in flat, honeycomb sheets of small, cuboidal, tightly cohesive cells, with centrally placed, relatively large nuclei and inconspicuous nucleoli.

Normal salivary gland cells may show degenerative and regenerative changes due to inflammation, cyst formation, radiotherapy and chemotherapy. Acinar cell nuclei may present as bare nuclei surrounding the aggregates, sometimes in large numbers. They should not be mistaken for lymphocytes. The latter have a well-defined rim of cytoplasm and, apart from having a different chromatin pattern, are usually oval rather than round. Ductal cells may undergo squamous metaplasia (Fig. 2.5).

2.3.2 Sialadenosis

Sialadenosis refers to a non-inflammatory, painless, non-neoplastic, often recurrent enlargement of salivary glands, usually associated with an underlying systemic disorder. Bilateral and symmetric, it usually affects parotid and occasionally submandibular gland or minor salivary glands [65]. It is seen in alcoholism, malnutrition, diabetes, anorexia nervosa, bulimia and some other disorders. There is no sex predilection, and the peak age incidence is between 30 and 70 years of age. The common underlying pathogenesis for this seemingly disparate group of patients is a peripheral autonomic neuropathy, seen as a demyelinating polyneuropathy. This seems to be which is responsible for disordered metabolism and secretion, resulting in acinar enlargement [66–69]. Histologically, salivary glands show enlargement of the acini and increased granulation of serous cells; in chronic disease there is acinar atrophy and fatty replacement of the salivary gland.

FNAC is performed on painless diffuse parotid swellings (Fig. 2.6). FNAC smears reveal relatively cellular aspirates containing clusters of enlarged acini and numerous naked nuclei of acinar origin in the background (Fig. 2.7). There is absence of inflammatory cells. In the chronic phase, degeneration of acini and replacement of epithelium with fat cells is seen. Gupta et al. performed morphometric measurements, which showed a significant increase in mean acinar diameter in a sialadenotic gland as compared to a normal gland (76.03 μm vs. 53.79 μm). Cytomorphological features of sialadenosis are distinctive enough to enable a diagnosis consistent with sialadenosis [70].

Recognising sialadenosis is important because it may point to the unsuspected presence of underlying systemic disease [71]. It also excludes other causes of diffuse painless enlargement of the salivary gland, for example lymphoepithelial lesions. It is important to be

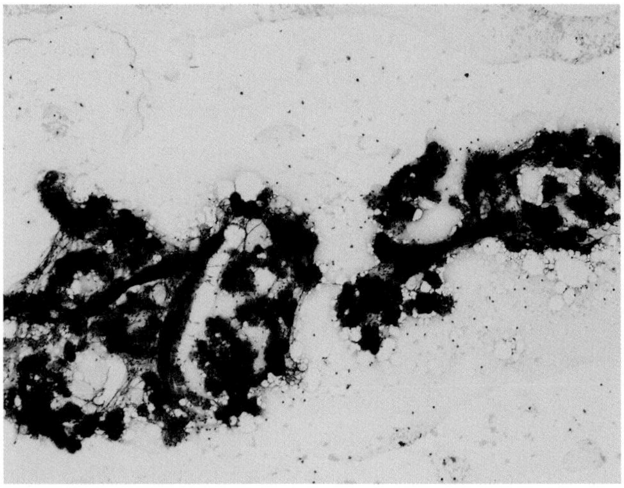

(A)

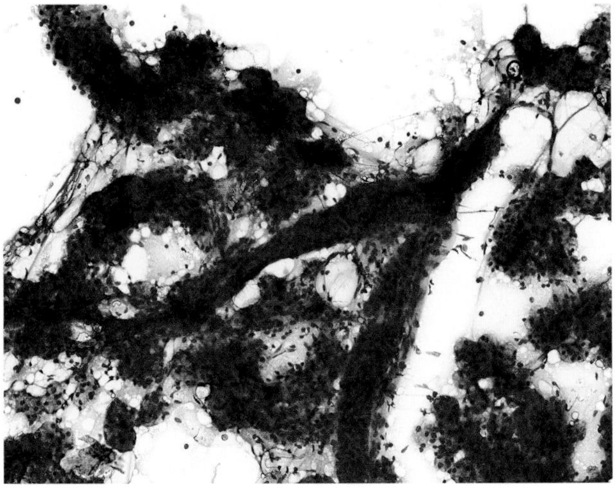

(B)

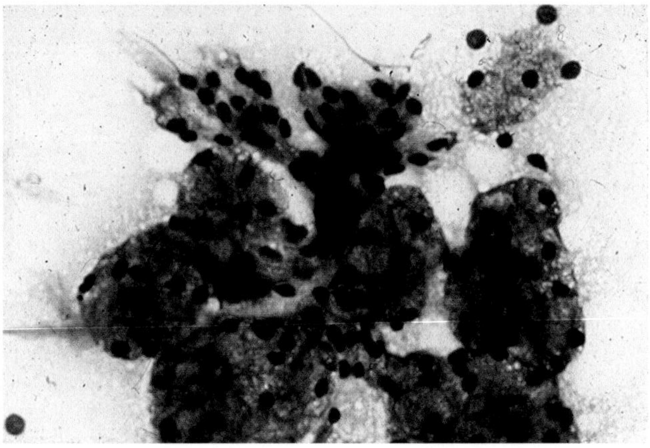

(C)

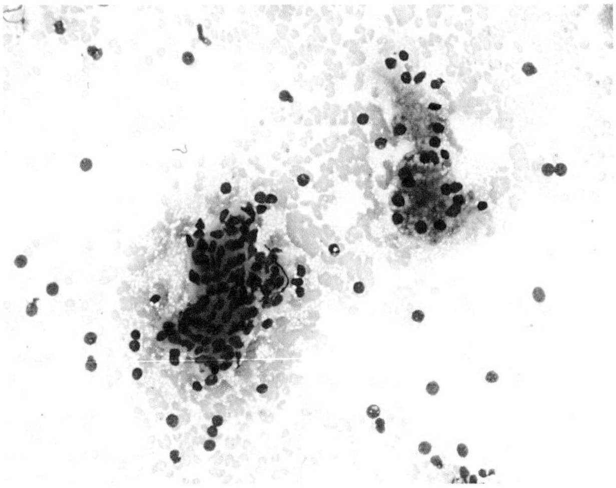

(D)

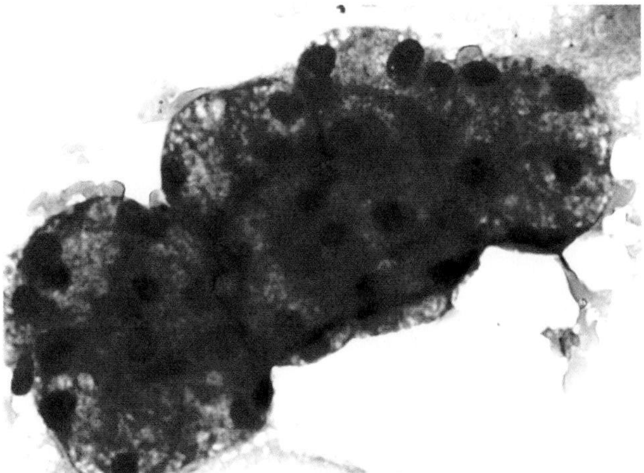

(E)

Figure 2.4 Normal salivary gland cytology. (A) A low power view reveals numerous tightly cohesive round aggregates held together as a bunch of grapes by capillaries and ducts. (MGG, ×100). (B) Same case, higher power acinar cells in aggregates, only a few naked nuclei in the background. Capillaries and small fat vacuoles are frequently seen. (MGG ×200). (C) Similar features are shown on this alcohol fixed smear. Well outlined acini, duct and fat cells (Papanicolaou ×200). (D) Ducts and acini often in close proximity (MGG ×600, oil immersion). (E) Acinar cells have eccentric, relatively small nuclei and inconspicuous nucleoli. Cytoplasm is vacuolated, abundant and well outlined in well preserved cells. There are, however, often bare nuclei of acinar cells in the background. These should not be confused with lymphocytes.

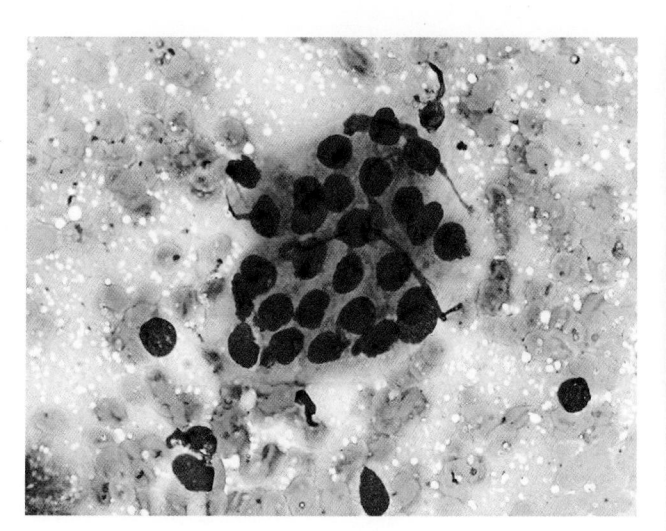

Figure 2.5 Ductal cells. Ductal epithelium of the normal salivary gland are usually closely associated with acinar cells but may lie separately. They are arranged in flat, honeycomb sheets of small cuboidal cells (×600 MGG).

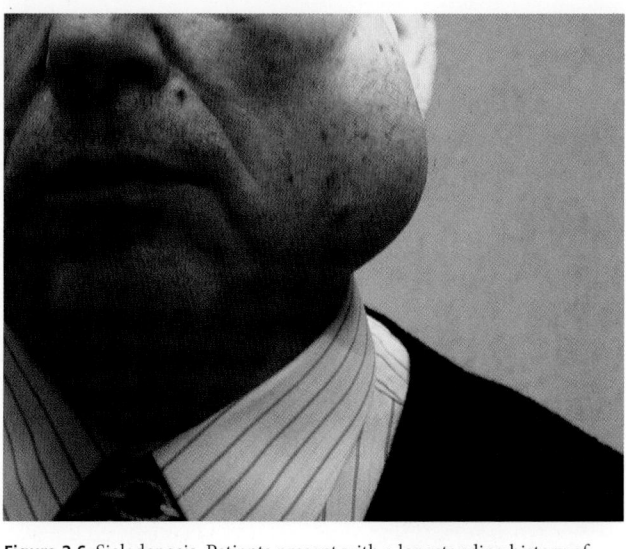

Figure 2.6 Sialadenosis. Patients present with a longstanding history of diffuse painless swelling. Lesion is soft, not clearly demarcated but mobile. FNAC produces fatty material.

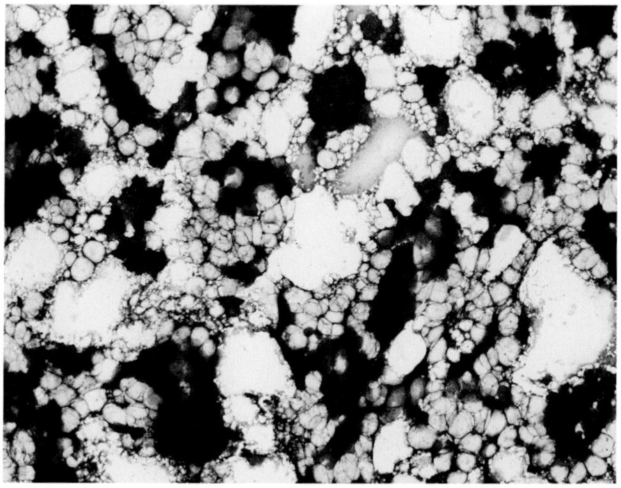

(A)

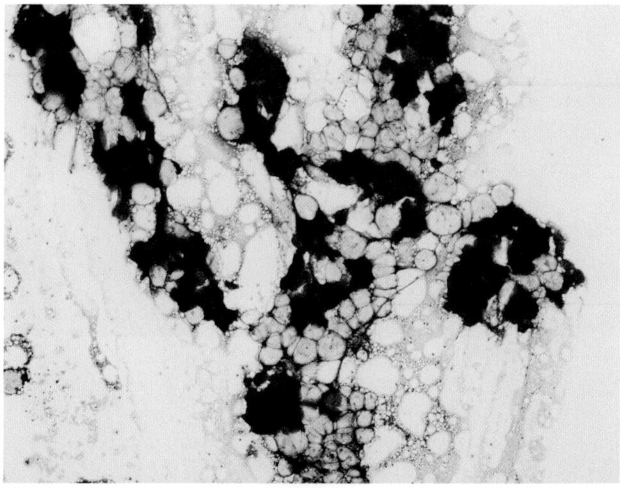

(B)

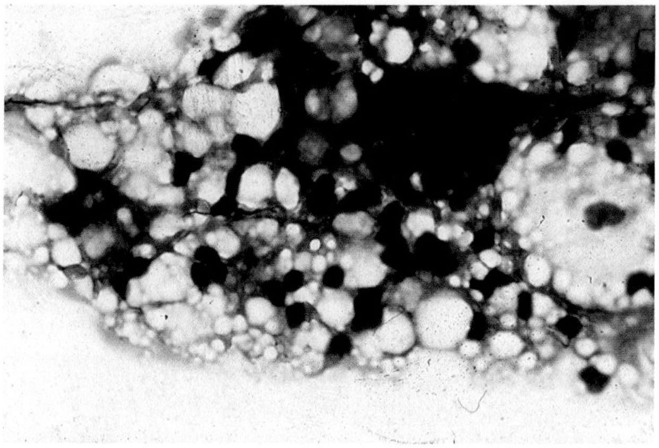

(C)

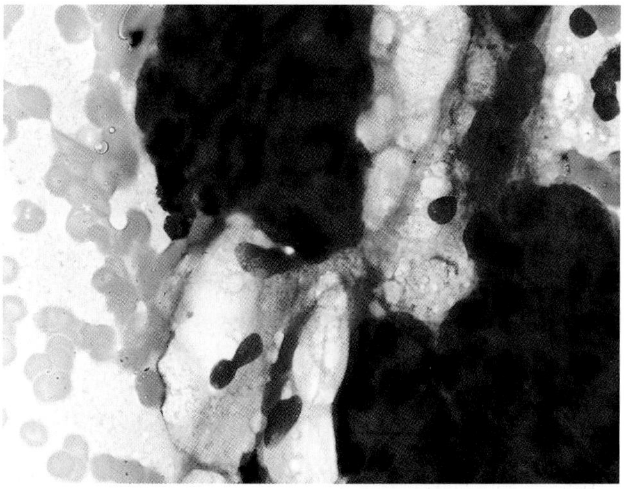

(D)

Figure 2.7 FNAC of sialadenosis. (A) Smears contain enlarged acini interspersed with fat cells. (B) High power view, same case MGG ×400. (C) Increased granulation of the acinar cells MGG ×600. (D) In the chronic phase, there is acinar atrophy and fatty replacement of the salivary gland. (MGG ×400).

aware of this entity, as most cases do not require surgical intervention [72]. Management of sialadenosis depends upon identification of the underlying cause, which must then be corrected. In bulimia, the swellings may be refractory to standard treatment modalities and parotidectomy may be considered as a last resort to improve the unacceptable aesthetics.

2.3.3 Salivary gland cysts

Mucocoele is a painless, soft, diffuse swelling of the salivary gland due to extravasation of saliva/mucus. It is rare in submandibular glands. Clinically it may be mistaken for tumours (Fig. 2.8) [72a]. It may occur as a sequel of surgery for benign tumours.

FNAC findings are those of a dense mucinous background (PAS-D positive) with foamy macrophages (Fig. 2.9). Absence of inflammation

or epithelium is significant in excluding other pathology. Treatment is surgical excision (Table 2.3).

A *retention cyst* is a salivary gland swelling due to obstruction. Content of the cyst is usually turbid fluid.

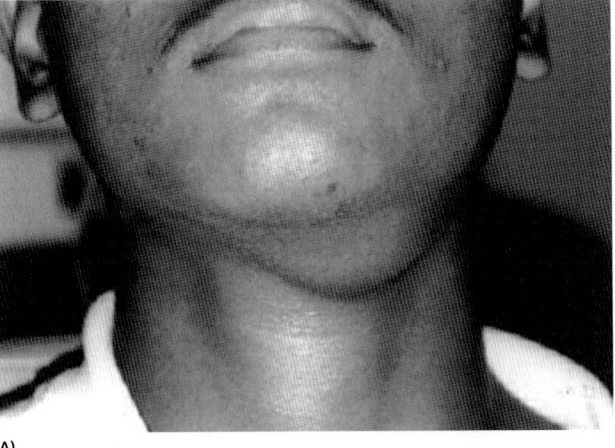

(A)

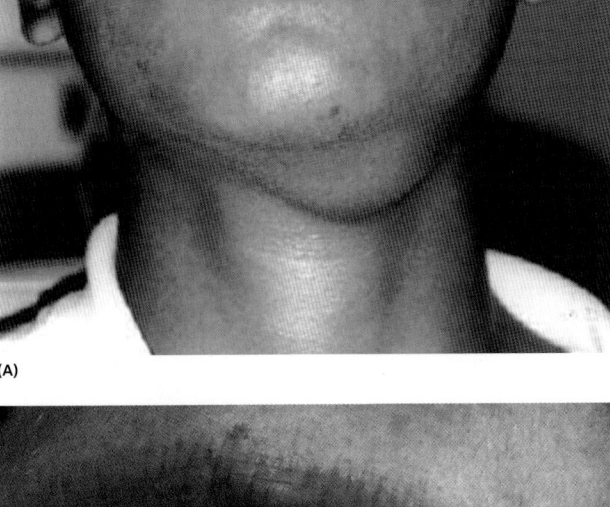

(B)

Figure 2.8 (A) A left submandibular swelling in a young patient extending from the left submandibular triangle and crossing the midline anteriorly. Figure from Anastassov G.E. [72a] (B) A young patient with a painless soft palate swelling which proved to be a mucocoele.

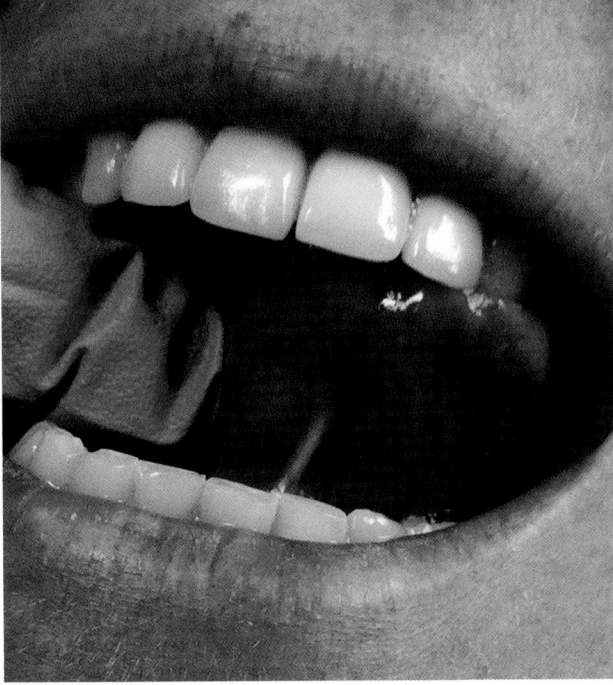

(A)

(B)

(C)

Figure 2.9 Mucocoele. (A) Mucocoele FNAC smears contains macrophages against a mucinous background. (B) MGG shows macrophages. (C) PAS diastase shows background mucin. No epithelium is seen.

Table 2.3a Cystic lesions of the salivary gland and their FNAC findings [139].

Lesion	cytological features
Mucocele/mucus retention reaction	Abundant mucus without an epithelial component. Small numbers of inflammatory cells especially histiocytes may be present.
Polycystic disease of the parotid gland	Clean or bloody background in which are scattered small clusters of bland cuboidal or polygonal cells. Cells have moderate amounts of nongranular cytoplasm.
Benign lymphoepithelial cyst	Cellular smears with a mixed population of lymphocytes. Rare squamous, cuboidal, or columnar cells may be present. Tingible-body giant cells are often present.
Warthin's tumor	Mixed population of lymphocytes with a small number of oncocytic epithelial cells lying in a "dirty" protein-rich background.
Low-grade mucoepideromid carcinoma	Mucin-rich background with a variable number of large mucin-filled epithelial cells (often with a vacuolated appearance), along with intermediate cells and rare epidermoid cells.
Cystadenoma	Watery proteinaceous background in which are distributed a moderate number of bland epithelial cells occasionally forming papillary fragments. Atypical squamous elements may be present.
Cystadenocarcinoma	Watery or mucoid background containing papillary clusters of atypical columnar and cuboidal cells. Nuclear atypia is easily recognized. Some smears will contain only single atypical epithelial cells.

Table 2.3b Algorithm for cytological analysis of cystic salivary gland lesions [139].

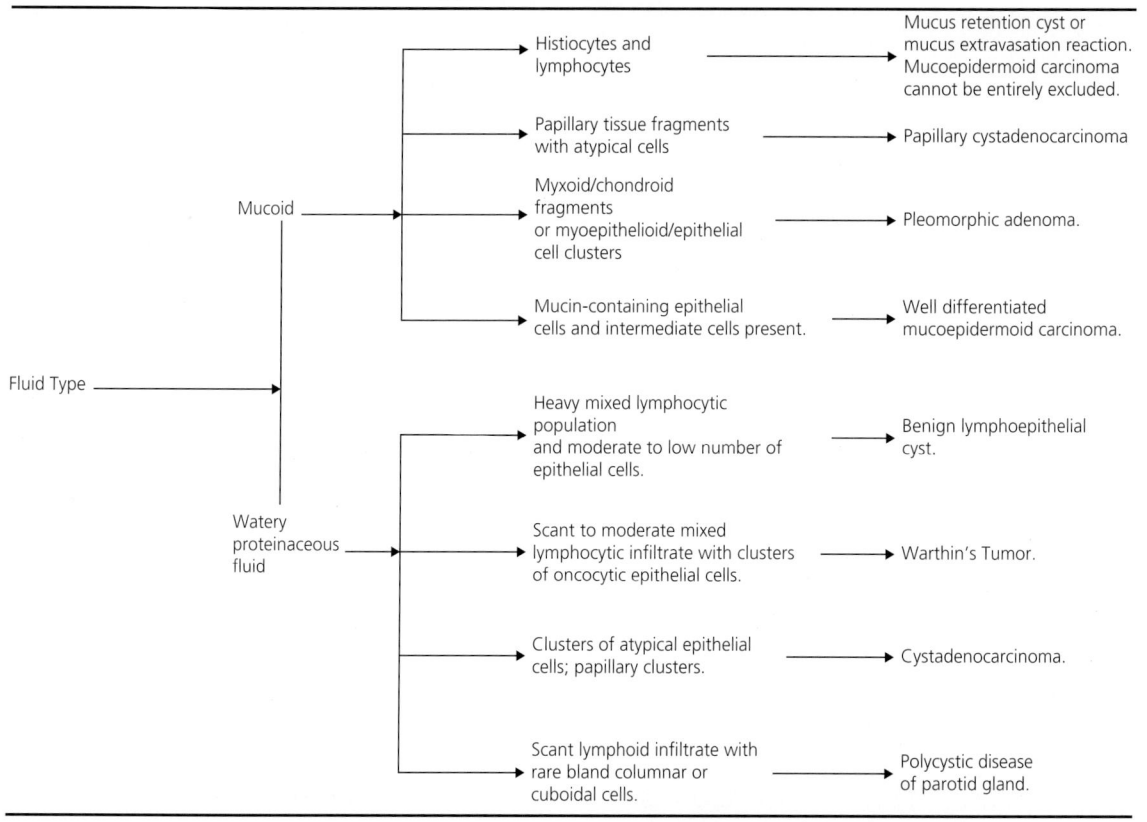

FNAC findings in retention cyst show a dense proteinaceous background, debris, macrophages, some epithelial cells (columnar or squamous) and variable degree of inflammation (Fig. 2.10). Differential diagnosis of squamous cells in FNAC of salivary gland lesions includes chronic sialadenitis, lymphoepithelial cyst, branchial cleft cyst, PLA, Warthin's tumour, MEC and squamous cell carcinoma. The squamous cells may be a defining feature of the lesion, or an occasional and thus unexpected finding, with a consequent potential for misdiagnosis [73, 74].

Lymphoepitelial cyst of salivary gland has been known for nearly 100 years but was uncommon until the last decade. It is seen more frequently in association with HIV infection. Patients present with non tender, gradually increasing over 6 months, diffuse swellings in either or both of the parotid glands (Fig. 2.11).

Salivary gland is a frequent site of pathology in HIV positive patients. Although lymphoepitelial lesions are the most common (74.8%), inflammatory processes (13.6%) and neoplasms (5.8%) may also be seen. The latter includes malignant lymphomas and metastatic carcinoma [75]. Malignancies are rare and since FNAC is reliable, most benign lesions can be managed conservatively.

FNAC is an appropriate tool for diagnosing these lesions and may sometimes be the first indication of an underlying retroviral infection. Histologically, cysts are lined by squamous epithelium, have cystic areas and lymphoid cells including lymphoid follicles with germinal centres. FNAC yields 2–5 ml of yellow to brown, non-viscous fluid. Smears show dense proteinaceous background with small and large lymphocytes, occasional

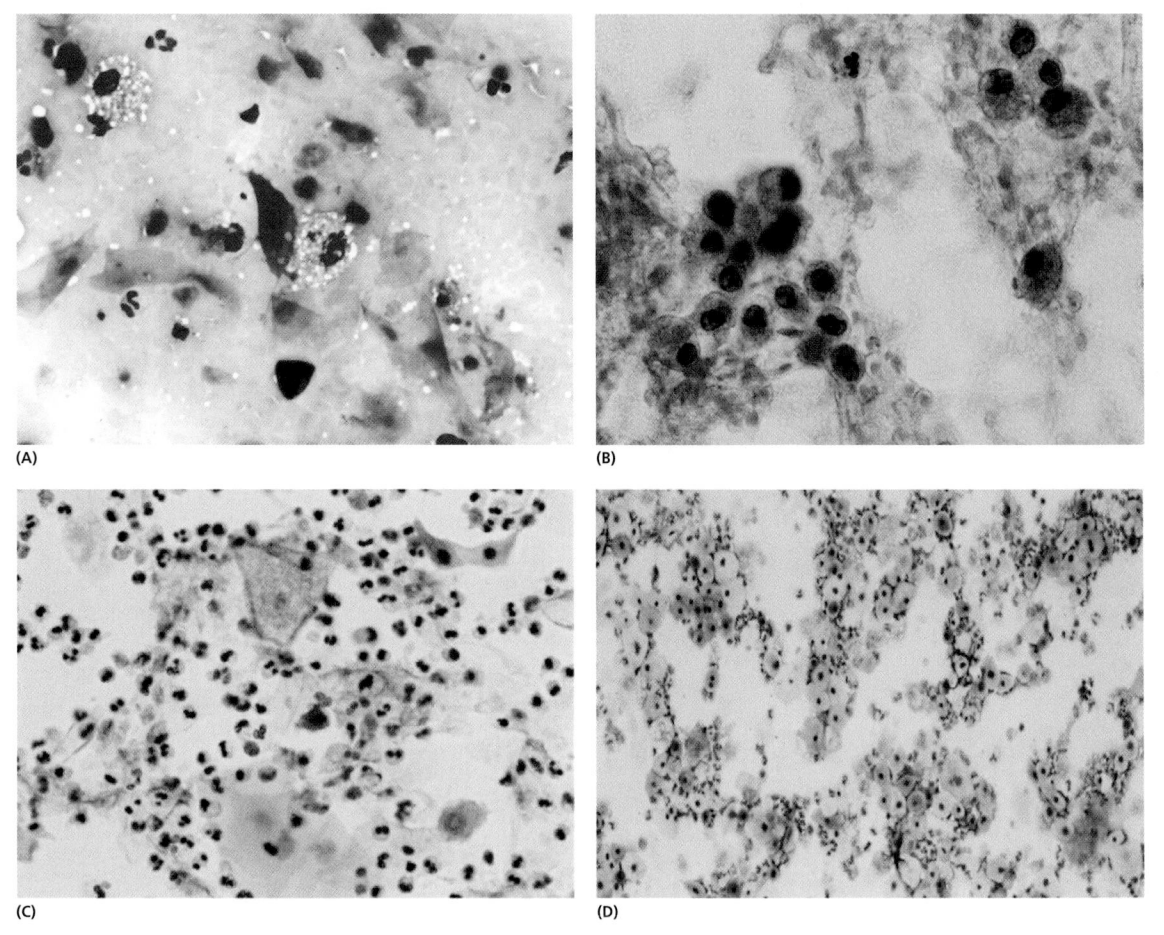

Figure 2.10 (A) Retention cyst and branchial cleft cyst. Low power view reveals many inflammatory cells, macrophages, debris and degenerate epithelial cells (PAP ×200). (B) Same case. Numerous macrophages, fresh and haemolised blood (PAP ×400). (C) Branchial cleft cyst. This contains many mature squamous cells, anucleate squamous cells and inflammatory cells. Macrophages are comparatively sparse (PAP ×400). (D) Branchial cleft cyst in an air dried preparatio shows cholesterol crystals, mature sqyamous cells and inflammatory cells (MGG ×400).

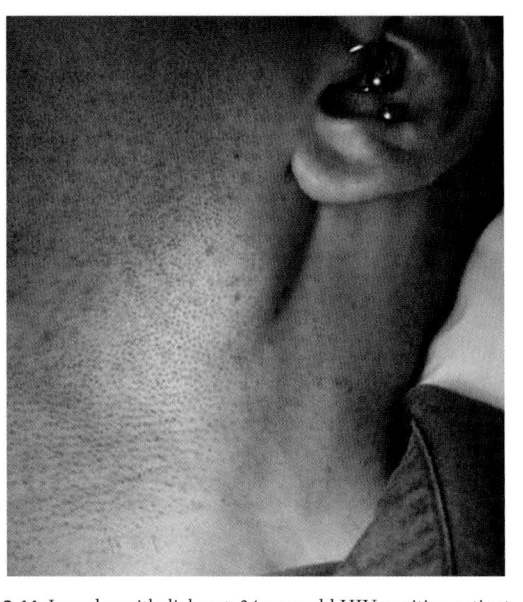

Figure 2.11 Lymphoepithelial cyst. 34-year-old HIV positive patient presented with a 6-month history of painless, diffuse soft swelling at the angle of mandible. FNAC yielded bloodstained fluid.

lymphoid aggregates (residual follicle centre cell fragments) (Fig. 2.12). Small and polygonal non-keratinised squamous cells are dispersed in this material and are, in our experience, invariably sparse and show degenerate changes. Macrophages, siderophages and multinucleate giant cells are also seen [76]. These show p24 (HIV-1) protein positivity, which can be useful diagnostic marker, particularly in cases, which lack epithelial component. Amylase crystalloids, described in sialadenitis may also be present [77].

Differential diagnosis of cystic lesions, cytologically, includes epidermoid cyst, dermoid cyst, low-grade MEC, Warthin's tumour, cystic benign lymphoepithelial lesion and non-Hodgkin's lymphoma (Tables 2.3 and 2.4). In epidermoid and dermoid cysts, there is absence of lymphoid cells. Cystic low-grade MEC may produce mucin with a few lymphocytes, mucin producing cells and a few squamous cells with minimal nuclear atypia. MEC lacks the polymorphic population of lymphoid cells [78]. Warthin's tumour showing squamous metaplasia and secondary inflammation is also a potential source of error. Oncocytes and mast cells need to be present for a confident diagnosis of Warthin's tumour.

Lymphoid cells from a lymphoepithelial cyst, particularly in HIV positive patients, may come from hyperplastic germinal centres that is reflected in a large number of centroblasts in the FNAC material.

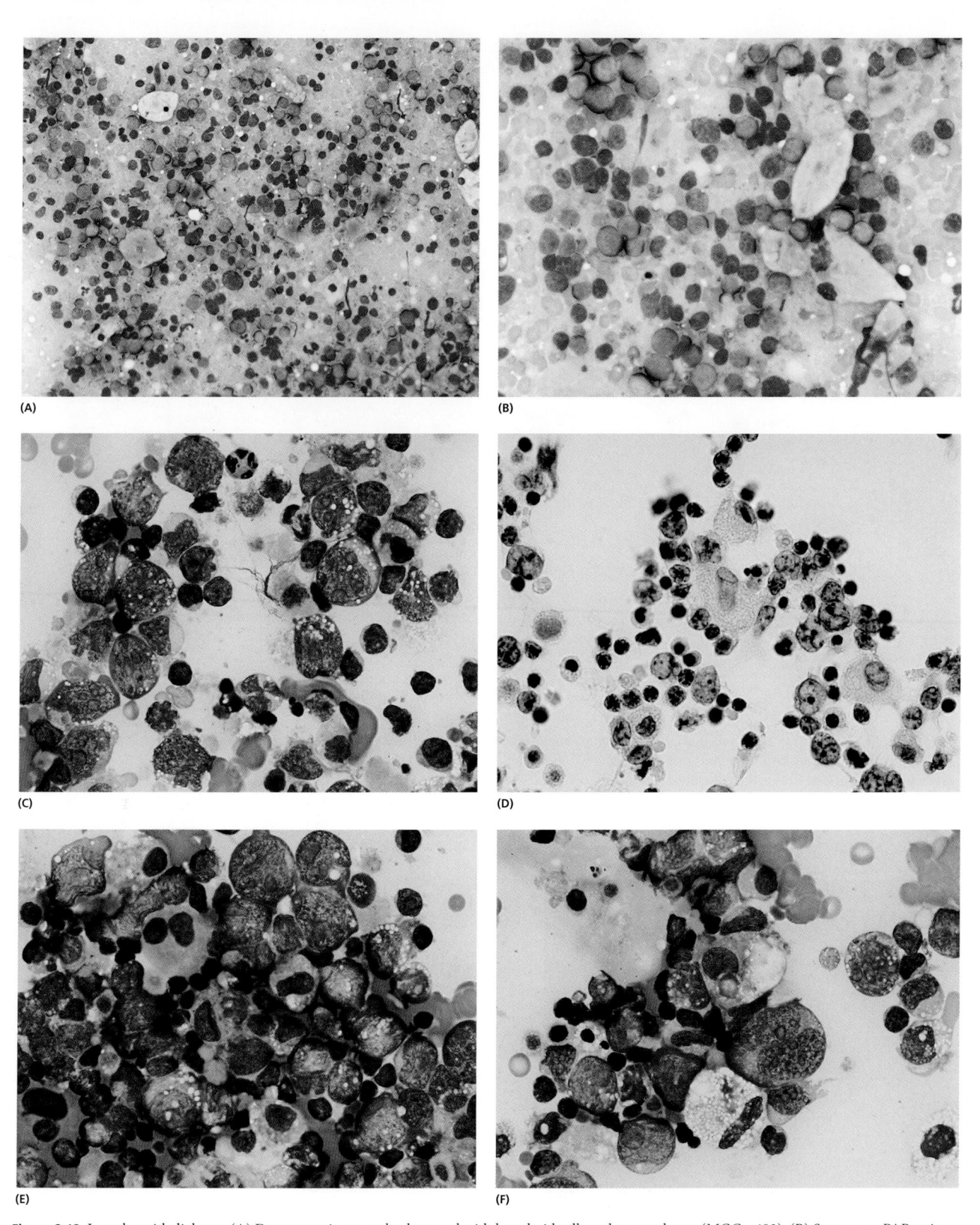

(A)

(B)

(C)

(D)

(E)

(F)

Figure 2.12 Lymphoepithelial cyst. (A) Dense proteinaceous background with lymphoid cells and macrophages (MGG ×400). (B) Same case. PAP stain reveals anucleate squamous cells and background debris (PAP ×400). (C) Only rarely are large epithelial fragments seen (PAP ×200). (D) Lymphoid cells include variety of follicle centre cells (MGG ×600 oil). (E) Sometimes centroblasts are numerous and may be misleading the diagnosis (MGG ×600). (F) High power view of the blasts may wrongly be assumed to be a lymphoma. (G) Secondary infection may cause a mixed inflammatory exudate (MGG ×400). (H) HIV sialadenitis with multinucleate giant cells (MGG ×400).

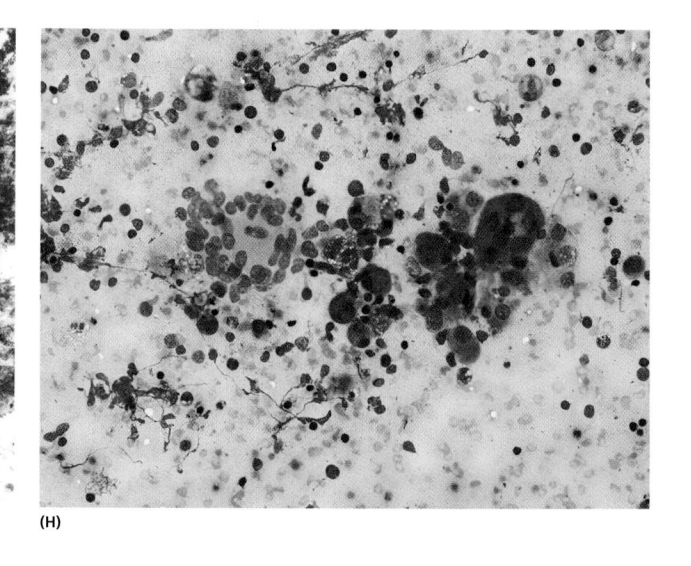

(G)

(H)

Figure 2.12 (*Continued*)

Table 2.4 Lymphoid rich FNAC of parotid lesions (Modified from Young JA. [7]).

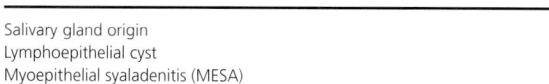

Salivary gland origin
Lymphoepithelial cyst
Myoepithelial syaladenitis (MESA)
Sjogren's syndrome
Chronic sialadenitis
Warthin's tumour
Malignant lymphoma
Mucoepidermoid carcinoma
Acinic cell carcinoma

Lymph node origin
Reactive lymph node hyperplasia
Malignant lymphoma of nodal origin

Lymphoid cells may give the impression of non-Hodgkin's lymphoma. The presence of epithelium and polymorphous nature of lymphoid cells may be helpful.

Rare cysts are the *odontogenic keratocyst, dermoid cyst, multiple oncocytic cysts* and have been described as occurring in salivary glands [79–81].

2.3.4 Sialadenitis

Inflammation of the salivary gland is most commonly caused by obstruction. Patients present with a short history of a painful swelling that may fluctuate in size and may be associated with eating/production of saliva (Figs 2.13 and 2.14). Most commonly, obstruction is caused by sialolithiasis, a salivary stone.

Salivary stone disease results from the formation of salivary crystals within the ductal system. This can occur either as a primary phenomenon or related to previous infective disease resulting in salivary ductal strictures, salivary stasis and stone formation. Most salivary calculi occur in the submandibular glands and this is thought to be due to the antigravitational drainage of the submandidular system in humans, which tends to salivary stasis.

The presenting complaint of intermittent facial swelling associated with eating food is strongly suggestive of salivary stone disease and should alert the radiologist to this possibility.

2.3.4.1 Ultrasound

US scanning for calculi is related to identifying three main features:

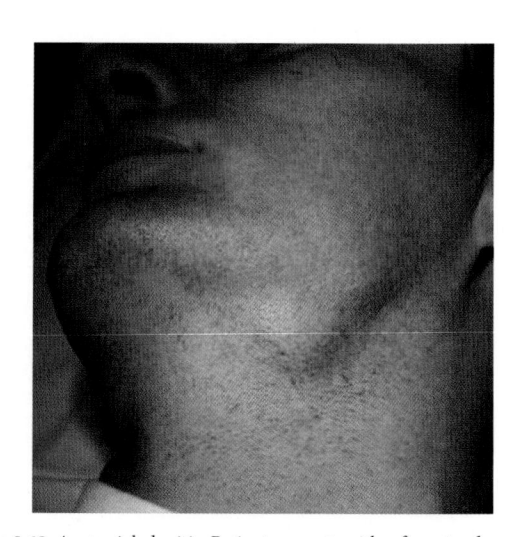

Figure 2.13 Acute sialadenitis. Patient presents with a firm, tender swelling in the submandibular area of several weeks duration.

1 Ductal dilatation (intra or extraglandular, transition point)
2 The actual stone(s)
3 Any obstructive sialadenitis.

Identifying ductal dilatation necessitates a knowledge of the normal anatomy of the main salivary ductal systems in the parotid and submandibular salivary glands (Figs 2.2 and 2.3). These ductal systems are then assessed carefully for evidence of ducatal dilatation. The normal main salivary ducts measure approximately 0.5–1 mm and the normal duct is frequently difficult to identify. Sialogogues such as lemon juice can be routinely administered to the patient to stimulate salivary flow and potentiate the appearances of a salivary obstruction if overt ductal obstruction is not present at the time of initial scanning.

2.3.4.2 Submandibular ductal system scanning technique

Identifying a normal or minimally dialated submandibular duct can be technically difficult. The US probe is held in a longitudinal plane along the submandibular region. Two key muscles are identified – mylohyoid and hyoglossus – providing readily identifiable landmarks through which the submandibular duct passes (Fig 2.3). The duct can be mistaken from nearby vascular structures (lingual

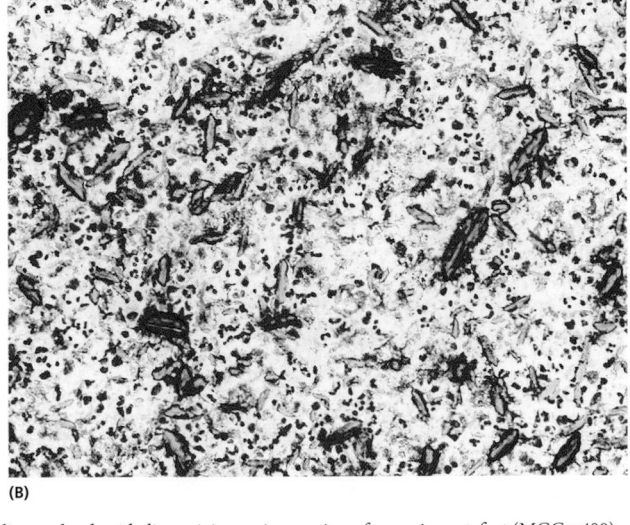

Figure 2.14 Acute syaladenitis. (A) Numerous polymorphs surround degenerate salivary gland epithelium giving an impression of smearing artefact (MGG ×400). (B) Numerous crystals may be seen in acute and chronic sialadenitis (MGG ×200).

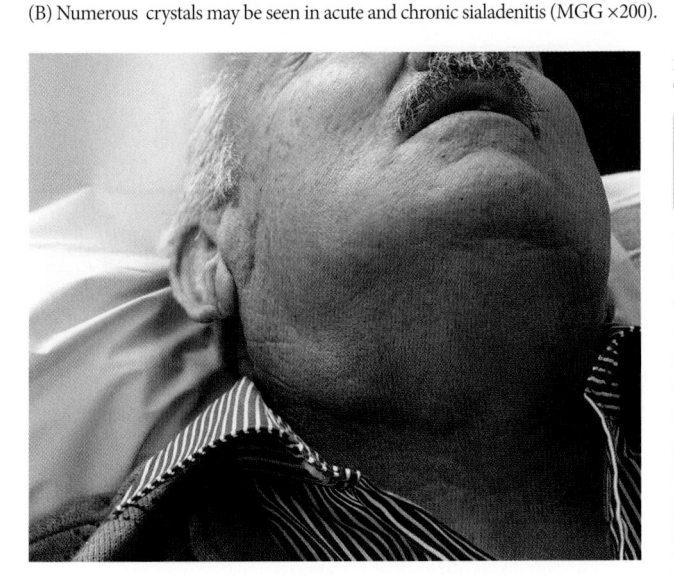

Figure 2.15 Sialadenitis. Patient presented with several months' history of diffuse tender swelling, which fluctuates in size.

vein and artery) but colour flow Doppler and the presence of branches in the vascular structures can be used to discriminate. The downstream duct close to the ductal orifice can be difficult to identify as it runs deep in the sublingual space. The probe may need to be angled anteriorly in the coronal plane under the patients chin to demonstrate calculi in the commonest site at the ductal orifice.

Calculi are identified as echogenic foci casting acoustic shadows. It is important to document to size and position of calculi as this is useful for treatment planning and determining whether calculi may be amenable to retrieval with interventional salivary techniques.

2.3.4.3 Chronic sialadenitis (Kuttner's tumour)
Chronic non-specific sialadenitis of the parotid gland is an insidious inflammatory disorder, which is characterised by intermittent, often painful, swelling of the gland (Figs 2.15 and 2.16). The disease tends to progress and may lead to the formation of a fibrous mass, which may be clinically mistaken for a tumour. Patients may have temporary facial nerve weakness and temporary paraesthesia of the cheek [82]. Histology shows marked atrophy of acinar epithelium, increased

fibrous connective tissue and an intense lymphocytic infiltration (See Table 2.4).

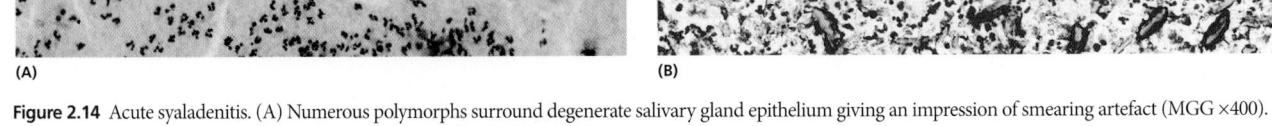

[See BOX 2.1. Summary of ultrasound features: **Chronic sclerosing sialadenitis** on www.wiley.com/go/kocjan/clinical_cytopathology_head_neck2e]

Depending on the stage of disease, FNAC contains variable amount of inflammatory cells, but most frequently sparse duct epithelium and very few degenerate or no acinar cells (Fig. 2.17). Duct epithelium can sometimes show squamous metaplasia and may mimic squamous cell carcinoma (Fig. 2.17D, E). This is particularly the case with patients with history of neck irradiation for previous head and neck malignancy. These patients often present with a firm submandibular swelling which is clinically indistinguishable from lymph nodes and requires investigation prior to the possible radical neck dissection of lymph nodes [36]. Squamous metaplasia is known to occur in benign salivary gland lesions, such as PLA and Warthin's tumours, as well as in salivary duct cysts and necrotising sialometaplasia [72]. A case of parotid duct carcinoma arising from chronic obstructive sialadenitis has been described [83].

In some patients with sialadentis, crystalloids of salivary alpha-amylase can be identified by May-Grunwald-Giemsa and Papanicolaou stains (Fig. 2.14.B and 2.18) [84]. These appear as numerous non birefringent crystalloids of varying sizes and shapes: rectangles, needles, squares and rods mixed with neutrophils and rare multinucleated giant cells. No salivary gland components need be seen, and all special staining with alcian blue, mucicarmine, Von Kossa and congo red are negative [85]. In the salivary gland, several kinds of crystals or crystalloids can be found: cholesterol crystals, calcium oxalate crystals, tyrosine-rich crystalloids. Apart from sialolithiasis and sialadenitis, crystalline structures are seen in neoplasms: Warthin's tumour, oncocytic papillary cystadenoma and pleomorphic adenoma (PLA). Tyrosine-rich crystalloids are rarely found in salivary gland tumours. However, when present they support the diagnosis of PLA. Non-tyrosine crystalloids are found in highest concentrations in cystic spaces lined with oncocytic metaplastic cells and are possibly a product of oncocytic cell secretion [86]. Conservative management of patients with parotid masses that contain nontyrosine crystalloids is indicated [87].

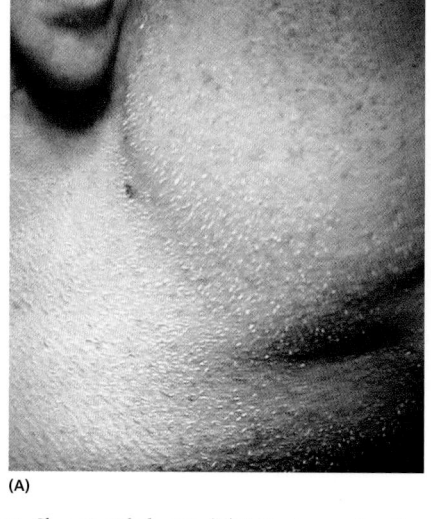
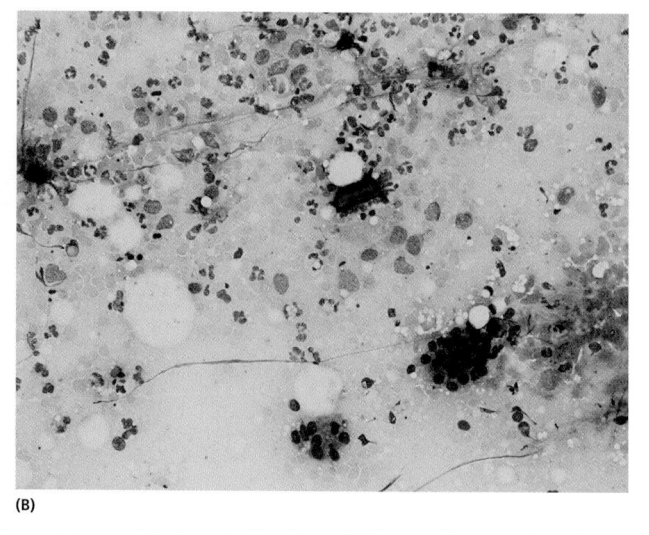

(A)   (B)

Figure 2.16 Chronic sialadenitis. (A) Patient presents with a firm, painless, mobile lump in the submandibular area that may clinically mimic tumour (Kuttner tumour). (B) Cytological features show inflammatory cells and sparse ductal epithelium in tightly cohesive aggregates (MGG ×400).

2.3.4.4 Granulomatous sialadenitis

Granulomatous lesions of the salivary gland are rare. It is most often a response to liberated ductal contents, particularly mucin, in various degrees of obstructive sialadenopathy, often a calculous duct obstruction [88]. Far less often is a granulomatous sialadenitis the result of specific infective granulomata or systemic granuloma-forming diseases. In these instances, the salivary parenchymal involvement is usually secondary to disease localisation in regional lymph nodes. Other causes of granulomatous sialadenitis are tuberculosis, sarcoidosis, carcinomatous duct obstruction and may be undetermined [89]. The tuberculous glands show caseation in the majority of cases but may consist predominantly of discrete granulomas with minimal necrosis. The sarcoid granulomas are typically non-caseating (Fig. 2.19 and 2.20). The specific cytological features include histiocytes of both epithelioid and giant multinucleated types, without background necrosis [90]. Calculous and carcinomatous duct obstruction contains single to multiple small granulomas, which contain mucin and are related to ruptured ducts. It is suggested that the frequency of calculi and the mixture of serous and mucous acini in the submandibular gland account for the distribution of obstructive granulomata. Granulomatous reactions can be seen in rare cases of Marginal Zone B-cell lymphoma (MZCL) of the parotid gland. However, the cytological features of the lymphoid infiltrate can suggest the possibility of MZCL in the clinical setting of FNAC performed from an extranodal location, such as the parotid gland [89].

Rare infections: in patients with immune deficiency, cytomegalovirus (CMV) sialadenitis can be diagnosed from FNAC. Characteristic viral intranuclear inclusions are best appreciated on Papanicolaou stain [90]. The same applies to salivary gland mycoses. Histoplasmosis and candida infections have been described and diagnosed on FNAC [91].

2.3.5 Lymphoid proliferations of the salivary gland

Lymphoid proliferations of the salivary glands can be either reactive or neoplastic. The two are difficult to separate, both clinically and morphologically, and are both included in this section for purpose of closer comparison (Table 2.4). Further details on neoplastic lymphoid proliferations may be found in Chapter 4.

2.3.5.1 Reactive lymphoid proliferations

These include the following: **cystic lymphoid hyperplasia** – a multicystic ductal proliferation with reactive germinal centres, seen most often in intravenous drug users infected with HIV – and the **lymphoepithelial sialadenitis of Sjogren's syndrome** (so-called benign lymphoepithelial lesion [BLEL] or myoepithelial sialadenitis [MESA]). In some cases, it is preceded by a chronic sialectatic parotitis [92] or can be associated with Hepatitis-C liver disease [93]. The lymphoid proliferation involves infiltration of ductal epithelium by lymphocytes of marginal zone or monocytoid B-cell type, forming lymphoepithelial lesions (epimyoepithelial islands). There is a high prevalence of monoclonality in the lymphoepithelial lesions of the major salivary glands [94].

2.3.5.2 Neoplastic lymphoid proliferations

Patients with lymphoepithelial sialadenitis have a 44-fold increased risk of developing salivary gland or extrasalivary lymphoma, of which 80% are marginal zone/mucosa associated lymphoid tissue (MALT) type. These lymphomas arise from sites normally devoid of lymphoid tissue, but are preceded by chronic inflammatory, usually autoimmune, disorders that result in the accumulation of lymphoid tissue [95–100]. Broad strands of marginal zone or monocytoid B-cells around lymphoepithelial lesions and monotypic immunoglobulin detection by immunohistochemistry are considered diagnostic of MALT lymphoma. Different B-cell clones may dominate during the course of MALT lymphoma [101]. B-cell clones are detected in over 50% of cases of MESA by molecular genetic methods. 'Nodal' type B-cell lymphomas of the salivary glands are either follicular lymphoma (35%), which may arise in intra-salivary gland lymph nodes and behave similarly to follicular lymphoma in other sites, or Diffuse Large B-cell lymphoma (30%), which may arise *de novo* or secondary to either MALT or follicular lymphomas [102]. A simultaneous occurrence of both, follicular and MALT lymphoma, phenotypically distinct but clonally identical, in a patient with Sjogren's syndrome has been described [103].

The criteria for distinguishing BLEL from low grade B-cell lymphomas of MALT type in salivary glands and the significance of genotypically documented clonality in this setting are controversial. In addition, the clinical implications of a neoplastic diagnosis

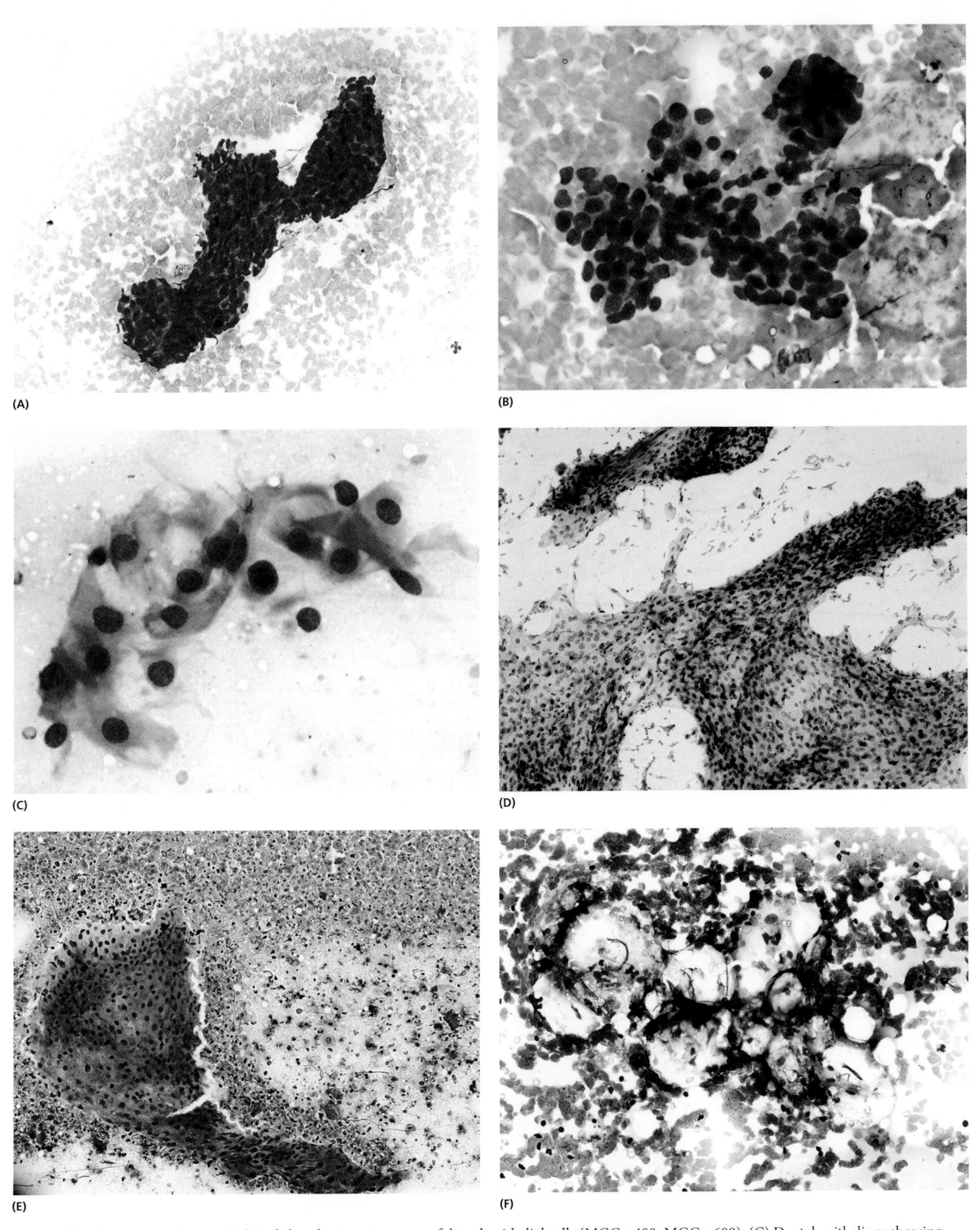

Figure 2.17 Chronic syaladenitis. (AB) Tightly cohesive aggregates of ductal epithelial cells (MGG ×400, MGG ×600). (C) Ductal epithelium showing squamous metaplasia (MGG ×600 oil). (D) Squamous metaplasia may be mistaken for squamous cell carcinoma (MGG ×600 oil). (E) Same case as (D): Histology of the salivary duct showing squamous metaplasia in chronic syaladenitis (H&E ×200). (F) Acinar collapse seen sometimes in chronic sialadenitis usually contains ductal epithelium only (MGG ×400).

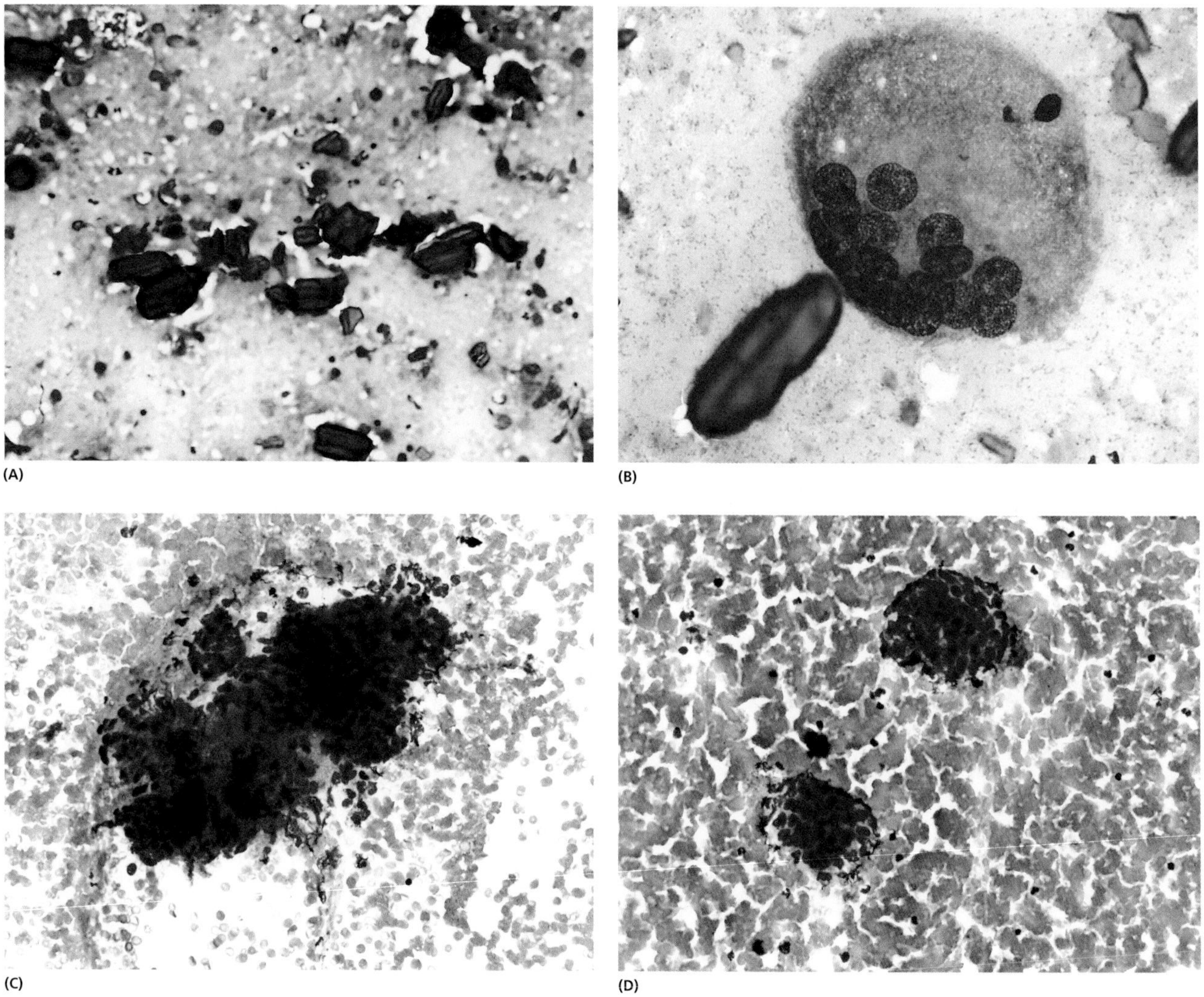

(A)

(B)

(C)

(D)

Figure 2.18 Syaladenitis with crystalloids. (A) Crystalloids are non-birefringent, of varying sizes and shapes, rectangles, needles, squares and rods mixed with neutrophils and occasional multinucleate giant cells (MGG ×400). (B) Multinucleate giant cell in chronic sialadenitis with crystalloids (MGG ×600). (C,D) Sparse fragments of ductal epithelium, often tightly cohesive and three dimensional (MGG ×400, MGG ×600)

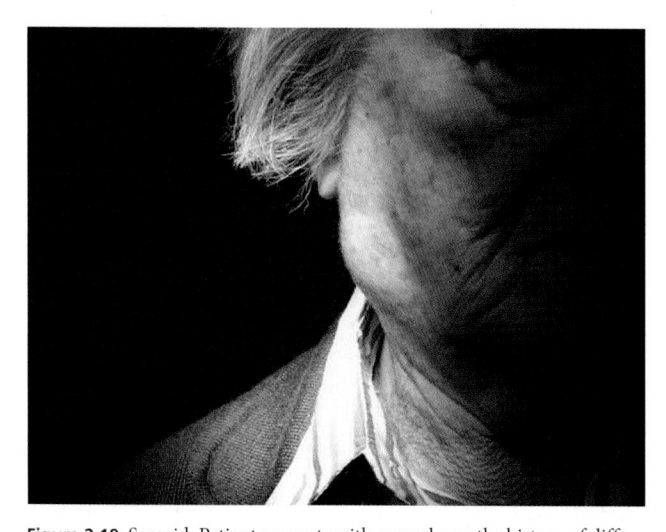

Figure 2.19 Sarcoid. Patient presents with several months history of diffuse firm swelling clinically mimicking tumour.

are unclear [104]. Patients have a history of long lasting recurrent indolent swelling of one or both parotid glands (Fig. 2.21). Raised ESR, hypergammaglobulinaemia and persistent swelling, despite the immunosupresssive therapy, clinically suggest lymphoma [105].

Clinically, reactive intraparotid lymph nodes and lymphomas present as diffuse parotid enlargements that are clinically indistinguishable from PLAs. FNAC is the only method of establishing a preoperative diagnosis of lymphoproliferative condition in these patients (Fig. 2.21).

[See BOX 2.2 Summary of ultrasound features: Parotid lymphoma on www.wiley.com/go/kocjan/clinical_cytopathology_head_neck2e]

FNAC features of MESA, a benign lymphoepithelial lesion, may be difficult to differentiate from lymphoma. In benign lymphoepithelial lesions, a cellular aspirate is obtained. Smears should be examined on low to medium power for presence of epimyoepithelial islands. Lymphocytes, centrocytes, centroblasts, plasma cells,

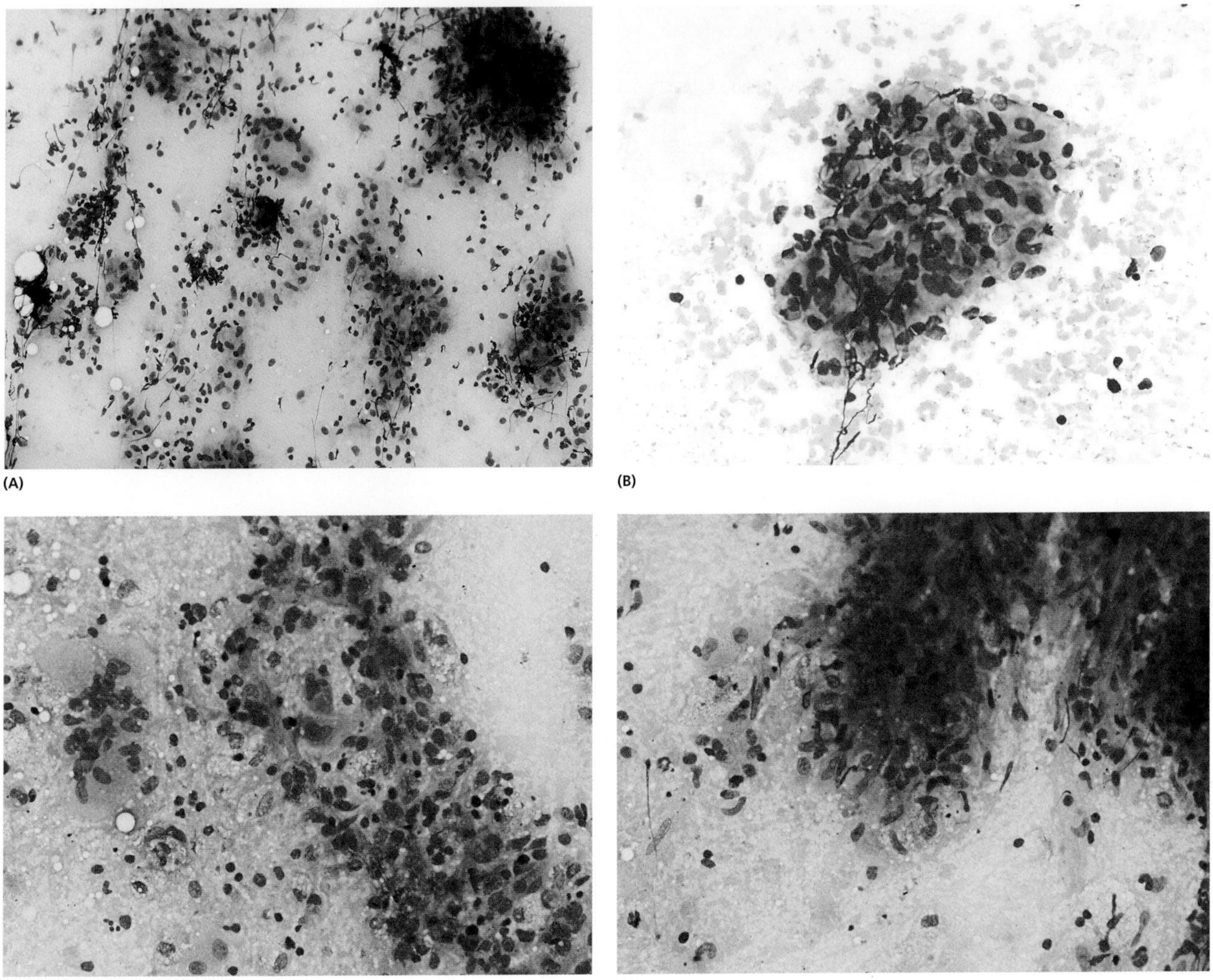

(A)

(B)

(C)

(D)

Figure 2.20 Granulomatous sialadenitis. (A) Sarcoid affecting salivary gland. Numerous aggregates of epithelioid cells almost totally replacing salivary gland epithelium (MGG ×400). (B) Epithelioid cells forming granulomata appear as a 'shoal of fish', superimposed on each other without a clear cytoplasmic definition and with typical twisted sausage-like appearance of the nucleus (MGG ×600 oil). (C) Multinucleate giant cell in the case of granulomatous sialadenitis due to tuberculosis (MGG ×600 oil). (D) Epithelioid cells in tuberculous sialadenitis (MGG ×600).

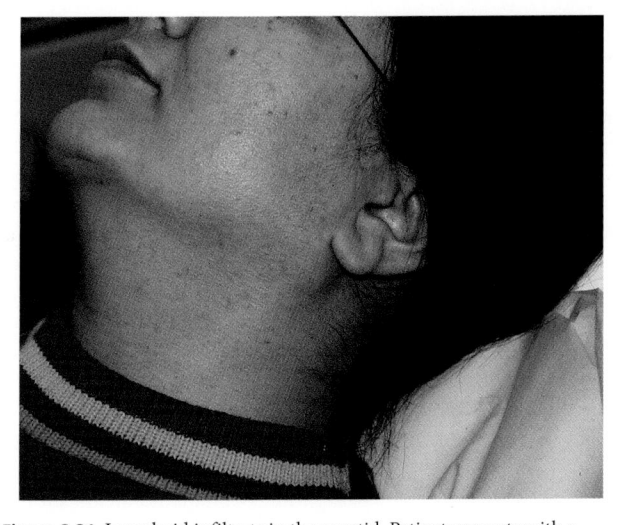

Figure 2.21 Lymphoid infiltrate in the parotid. Patient presents with a 2-year history of a diffuse swelling at the angle of mandible. Swelling did not change in size and is painless.

tingible body macrophages and occasional clusters of salivary gland cells are a common finding (Fig. 2.22). Clusters of myoepithelial cells may be present but they are not always identifiable on FNAC. Aspirates from intraparotid lymph nodes and some other salivary gland lesions such as lymphocoele, may also result in 'lymphoid rich' cytological preparations (Fig. 2.23) (Table 2.4). Given the difficulty in distinguishing the condition from a MALT lymphoma, the possibility of lymphoma should be raised.

FNAC findings of MALT lymphoma show intermediate size lymphocytes with a round to irregular nuclear outline and distinct pale cytoplasm intermixed with small mature lymphocytes (Fig. 2.24). The chromatin is slightly paler and less clumped than in small mature lymphocytes. A small inconspicuous nucleolus is seen in most of the cells. These centrocyte-like cells may be seen to infiltrate epithelial island and form lymphoepithelial lesions (Fig. 2.25). The persistent and often prominent follicle centre fragments in FNAC smears, may create an impression of 'follicular 'pattern and be mistaken for a follicular hyperplasia of an intraparotid node. The cytomorphology coupled with the immunophenotyping study in this clinical context suggest the diagnosis of low-grade B-cell

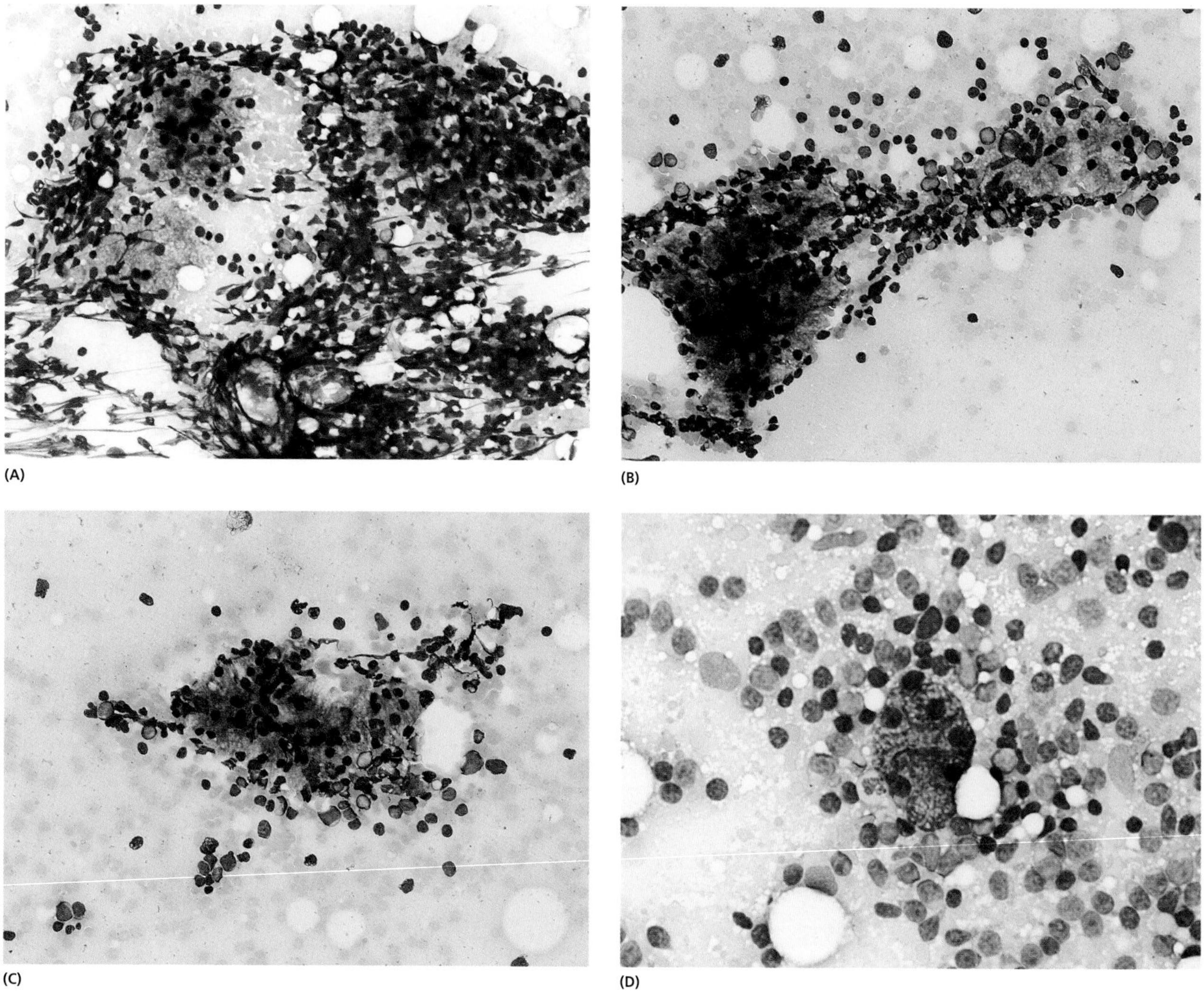

Figure 2.22 Lymphoepithelial sialadenitis: (A) Low power view of a lymphoid infultrate in the parotid. Numerous small to medium size lymphoid cells including follicle centre cells and salivary glandepithelium. (MGG ×200). (B) lymphoid cells are admixed with epithelium of the salivary gland. (C) lymphoid cells are a mixture of small lymphocytes and follicle centre cells. (D) A high power view of lymphoid cells surrounding an intact salivary gland acinus. A diagnosis of lymphoid infiltrate is made. Patient undergoes biopsy to exclude MALT lymphoma. Myoepithelial sialadenitis is diagnosed.

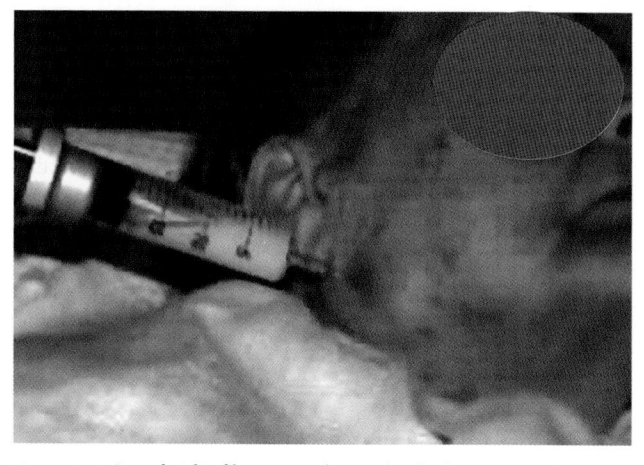

Figure 2.23 Lymphoid infiltrates in salivary gland. This 83-year-old patient presented with a parotid swelling. FNAC yielded white milky fluid. Microscopy revealed numerous small lymphocytes in the absence of any other features. Lesion was considered benign, probably a lymphocoele/lymphoepithelial cyst.

lymphoma of MALT [106]. Different MALT lymphomas show a tendency for diverse cytological expressions, such as: small lymphocytes in the lung, monocytoid cells in salivary glands and plasmacytic cells in the thyroid and skin [107].

Delineation of low-grade B-cell lymphoma from benign lymphoid lesions of myoepithelial sialadenitis (MESA) may be very difficult by means of cytomorphological criteria alone. As in tissue material, monoclonal bands which may be demonstrated on PCR or flow cytometry [106] from FNAC, although more commonly found in MALT may nevertheless be present in MESA [108]. When evaluating the effectiveness of FNAC in the diagnosis of primary lymphoid processes of the salivary gland, MacCallum et al. reviewed 35 patients who underwent FNAC of the salivary gland and had a diagnosis of a primary lymphoid process. Most presented with palpable parotid (28 patients) or submandibular (4 patients) swellings. Sixteen cases of reactive hyperplasia and nine cases of malignant lymphoma diagnosed by FNAC were confirmed by subsequent histopathological examination. Lymphoma was confirmed in six of eight cases diagnosed as suspicious for lymphoma by FNAC. In all cases, the FNAC diagnosis of either a reactive or malignant

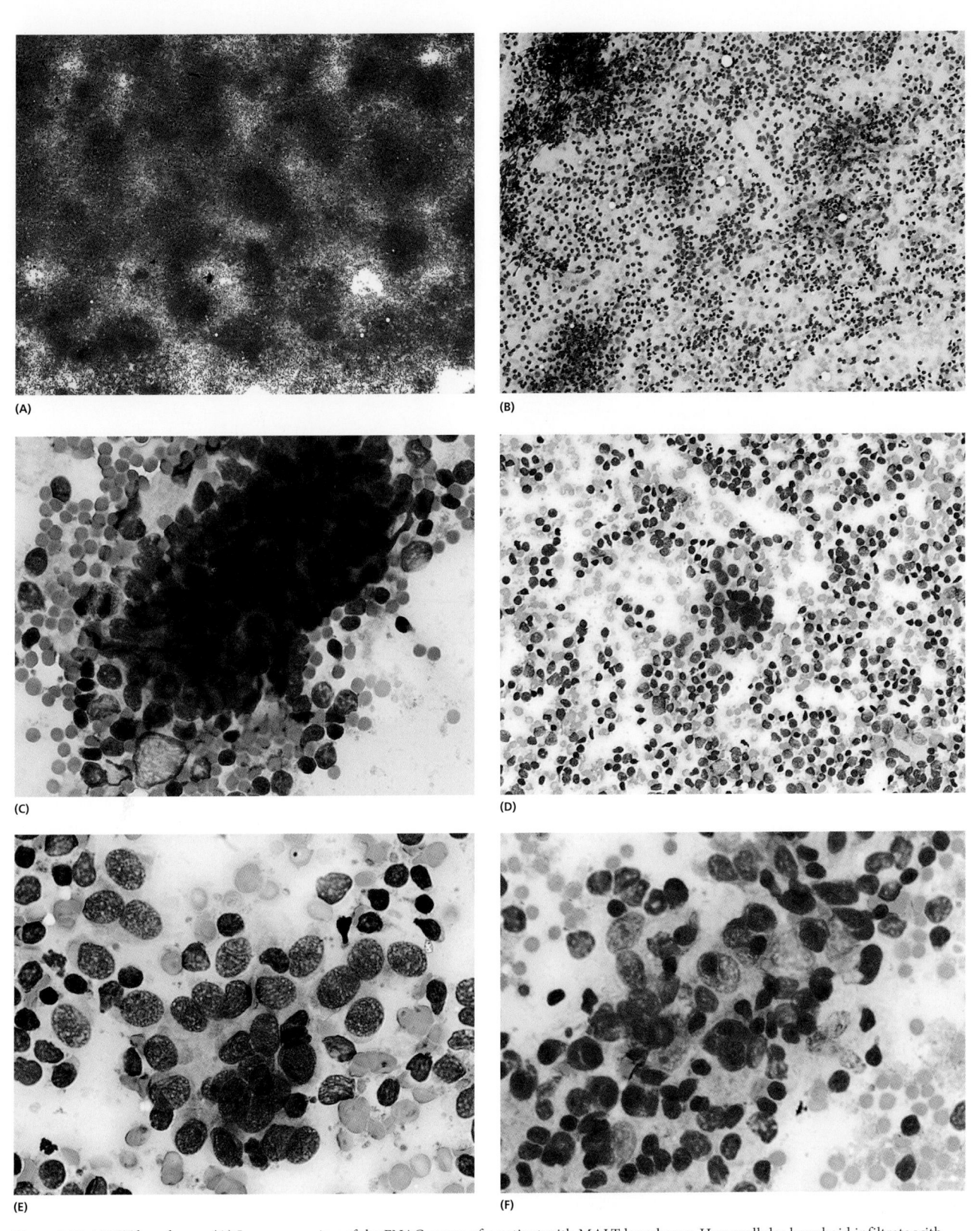

(A)

(B)

(C)

(D)

(E)

(F)

Figure 2.24 MALT lymphoma. (A) Low power view of the FNAC smear of a patient with MALT lymphoma. Hypercellular lymphoid infiltrate with monotonous pattern and no definite evidence of salivary gland epithelium (MGG ×100). (B, C) The number of follicular dendritic cells may be increased in MALT giving the infiltrate a 'follicular'/reactive pattern. See also (F). (D) When found, salivary gland epithelium appears surrounded by pale staining lymphocytes (MGG ×200). (E) High power view of the same duct, which seems to be covered with lymphocytes (MGG ×600 oil). (D) High power view of the lymphoid cells infiltrating the epithelium (MGG ×1000 oil). In other areas, it is more difficult to establish the presence of any epithelium that has disappeared under the lymphoid infiltrate and follicular dendritic cells. (F) Lymphoid infiltrate is composed of centrocyte like cells and small lymphocytes.(MGG ×600). (G) Centrocyte like cells may be difficult to recognise as neoplastic (MGG ×1000). (H) Tumour cells show light chain restriction for kappa chain.

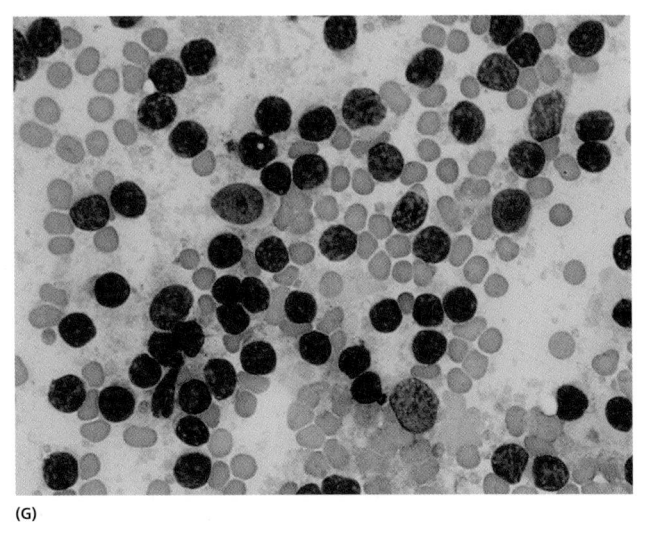

(G)

(H)

Figure 2.24 (*Continued*)

lymphoid process was unexpected and influenced the patient's management. For patients with a preoperative FNAC diagnosis of lymphoma, a more limited biopsy could be performed, thereby reducing the operative risk to the patient and plans to process the tissue according to the institution's lymphoma protocol could be made [109]. Clinicians and pathologists should be aware of the possibility that MALT lesions including MALT lymphoma may be present in children who have AIDS [110].

2.4 Salivary gland tumours

Salivary gland tumours are uncommon, and most swellings are due to inflammation or non-neoplastic disease. Less than 3% of tumours of the head and neck arise in the salivary glands. Most tumours are seen in the parotid gland; the ratio is approximately 100 parotid tumours to 10 submandibular tumours to 10 minor salivary gland tumours to one sublingual gland tumour [111]. Approximately one in six parotid tumours are malignant, one in three submandibular tumours are malignant and three in four tumours in minor salivary glands are malignant. The average annual age-adjusted incidence rate per 100 000 is 4.7 for benign tumours and 0.9 for malignant tumours. Incidence rates for both benign and malignant tumours increase with age until ages around 65 to 74 years and then decline. Benign mixed tumours occurr more frequently in female patients, whereas Warthin's tumours and malignant tumours occurr more frequently in male patients (P < 0.05). Warthin's tumour is rare in black patients. Salivary gland tumours are an uncommon but epidemiologically diverse group of tumours. Histologically they are classified according to the 2005 WHO classification (Table 2.2 [50]).

The ratio of benign to malignant tumours is 4:1. Histological distribution shows a frequency of 54% PLAs, 28% adenolymphomas and 18% other tumours. The greatest number (85%) arise in the parotid. There is an average 3% recurrence rate, most frequently in PLA [112]. The revised WHO Histological classification of benign tumours lists benign salivary gland into nine categories [50].

It is challenging to use US for differentiating between benign and malignant parotid gland masses. To make a definite diagnosis, US-guided FNAC or core biopsy is advocated [113].

The sonographic characteristics of parotid masses including shape, margin, echogenicity, echotexture and vascularisation between benign and malignant lesions had no significant difference, which indicates that it is hard to distinguish malignant parotid masses from benign masses using sonography [114–120].

The sensitivity, specificity, positive predictive value, negative predictive value and accuracy of US for the diagnosis of parotid gland masses were 38.9, 90.1, 29.2, 93.3 and 85.2%, respectively, and accuracy for malignant masses was 20%. Wu et al. conclude that the sonographic characteristics of parotid masses between benign and malignant lesions had no significant differences [113].

2.4.1 Pleomorphic adenoma

Pleomorphic adenoma (PLA) is the commonest benign tumour seen in the parotid. It represents up to 80% of salivary tumours and most commonly presents as a painless lump. Typically, it arises in the tail of parotid gland and is slow growing. When resected, the vast majority are 2–6 cm in size, with exceptions up to 26 cm in diameter (giant PLA) [121]. Patients (average age 40–45, female predominance) present with a painless, well-defined, mobile, firm nodule of some months or years duration (Fig. 2.26). Rarely, it may be bilateral, synchronous or familial [122]. Most unusually, a benign tumour, it sometimes gives rise to distant metastases [123].

The most common US appearance is of a well defined hypoechoic lump, containing homogeneous internal echogenicity and minimal or absent internal vascularity. These lesions can also have a lobulated outline. Rarer but recognised appearances include cystic change and foci of increased echogenicity from calcification. Some PLA display ill-defined margins (1–2%).

[See BOX 2.3. Summary of ultrasound features: PLEOMORPHIC ADENOMA on www.wiley.com/go/kocjan/clinical_cytopathology_head_neck2e]

Performing an FNAC on a PLA using standard technique produces adequate material for cytological diagnosis. Typically, the material obtained appears rather waxy and can spread quite thickly on the glass slide. On occasion the material in the lesion is so thick that it can be difficult to obtain it with usual capillary technique and aspiration is needed (Figs 1.5 and 1.6).

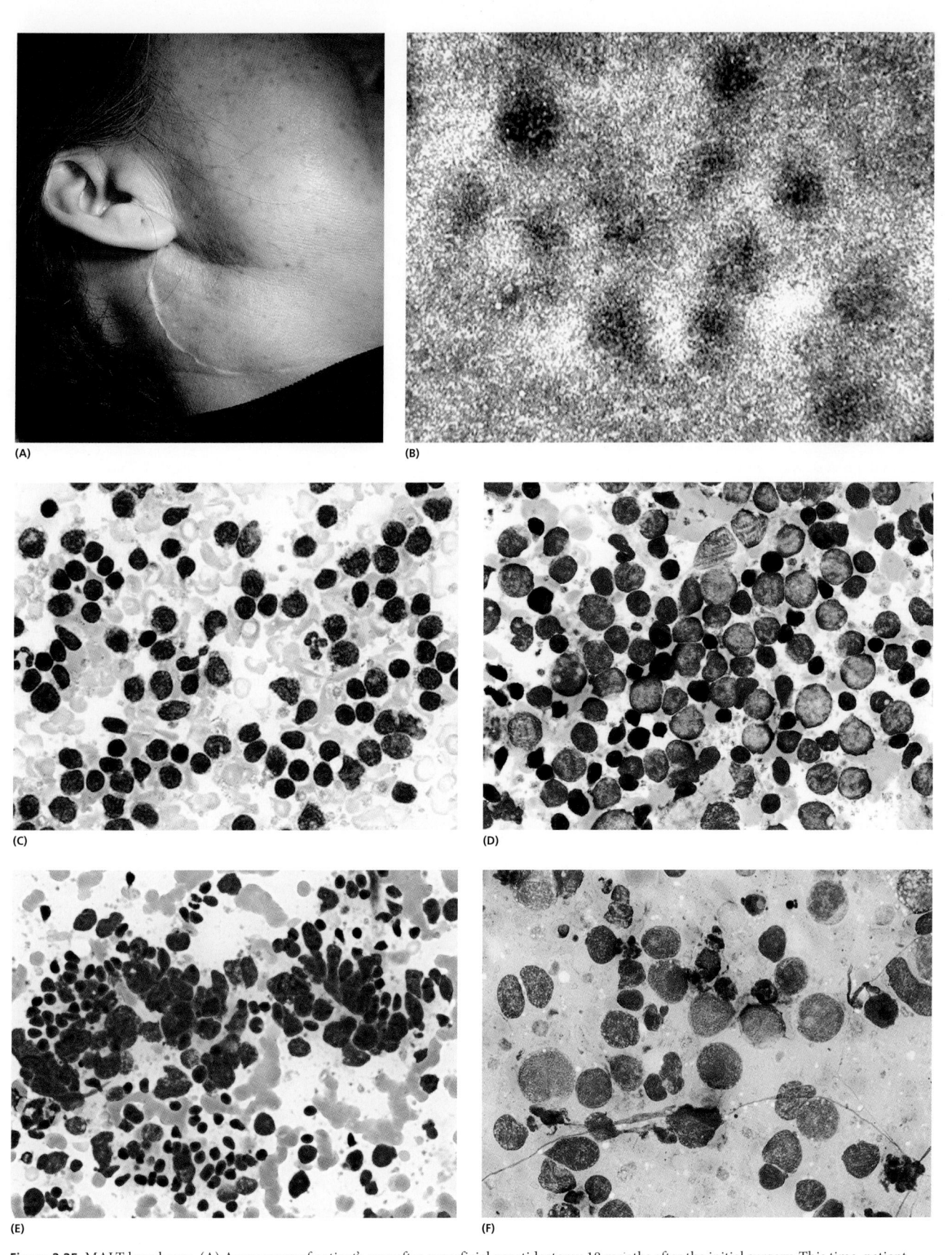

Figure 2.25 MALT lymphoma. (A) Appearance of patient's scar after superficial parotidectomy 18 months after the initial surgery. This time, patient presented with a swelling on the contralateral side. (B) FNAC showed dense lymphoid population with apparent residual follicle centre fragments overrun with small centrocyte like cells which may give the impression of lymph node hyperplasia. (MGG ×100). (C) Higher power shows intermediate size lymphocytes with a round to irregular nuclear outline guided distinct pale cytoplasm intermixed with small mature lymphocytes. (D) The chromatin is slightly paler and less clumped than in small mature lymphocytes. A small inconspicuous nucleolus is seen in most of the cells. (E) Areas of blastic proliferation within the MALT. (F) Lymphoblasts and apoptotic debris may raise a suspicion of a high grade lymphoma.

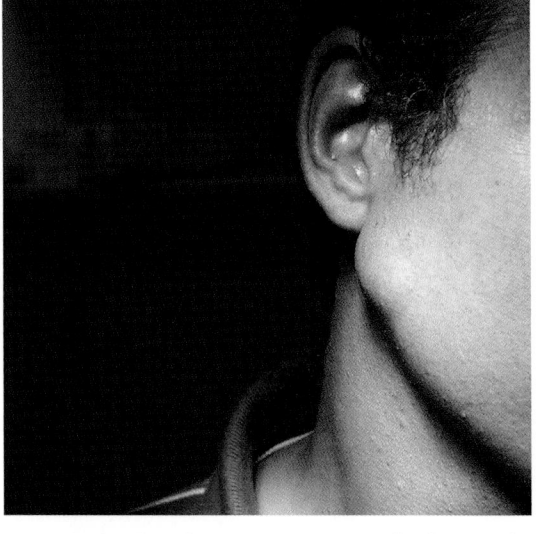

Figure 2.26 Pleomorphic adenoma. Patient presented with a typical, well-defined, firm, mobile lump at the angle of mandible. FNAC yielded dense, transparent material with particles. Microscopy was typical of pleomorphic adenoma.

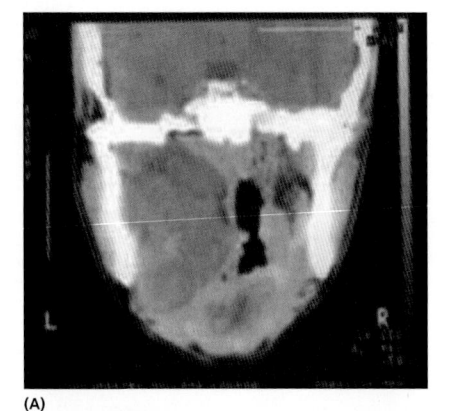

(A)

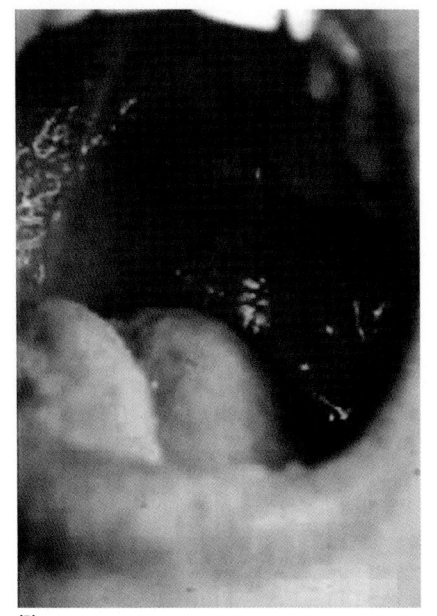

(B)

The aim of surgery for PLA is to obtain a complete resection with clear histopathological margins while carefully preserving the surrounding structures, such as the facial nerve and their function (Fig 2.27). On occasion, sometimes in the context of an incomplete primary resection but sometimes when the histopathological margins appear entirely clear, PLA can recur.

FNAC is a recognised method for preoperative diagnosis. With appropriate sampling, high degree of accuracy can be achieved [124]. The sensitivity and specificity of the cytological diagnosis of PLA is around 93 and 98%, respectively [125]. Klijanienko et al. analysed 412 preoperatively diagnosed PLAs and found 95% concordance with postoperative histology. This particularly applies to chondromyxoid histological type (cellular, myoepitehlial and metaplastic achieved 82% concordance) [126]. Cytopathologists must be aware that the importance of preoperative diagnosis is in order to achieve complete resection. Incompletely resected tumours have a high recurrence rate [127].

Cytological features classically present no difficulty in diagnosis of PLA. They include variable cellularity, an extracellular myxoid stroma with uniform, cytologically bland epithelial cells arranged in cohesive clusters, individually or in a tubular arrangement (Figs 2.28 and 2.29). The epithelial cells have plasmacytoid or spindle cell appearance. Peripherally located spindle shaped myoepitehlial cells mingle imperceptibly with the myxoid stroma giving the epitehlium the 'sunburst' appearance [128]. Cytological features reflect considerable histological variation of the cellular composition within the same tumour, composed of different proportions of epithelial and myoepitehlial cells and stroma. Klijanienko classifies tumours into chondromyxoid type (70% of cases) and cellular type (26.9%) (Fig. 2.30A–C) with minority cases classified as myoepitehlial or metaplastic [126].

Minor variations in cytological presentation of PLA consist of duct metaplasia: mucinous, squamous (Figs 2.30, 2.31 and 2.32), oxyphilic (Figs 2.33 and 2.34) and sebaceous, variable stromal cellularity, tyrosine and collagenous crystalloid deposition and intranuclear cytoplasmic inclusions. In most cases, these changes are found in material otherwise typical of PLA. Major cytological variations are represented by cellular atypia, cystic transformation and the presence of a cylindromatous pattern resembling adenoid cystic carcinoma (AdCC) (Fig. 2.32D). These must be considered in order to avoid important errors in the preoperative management of and surgical approach to salivary gland lesions [124].

Apart from PLA, cystic change can be seen in low-grade mucoepidermoid carcinoma (MEC), Warthin's tumour, acinic cell carcinoma, cystadenoma, cystadenocarcinoma, metastatic squamous cell carcinoma and benign, non-neoplastic lesions such as mucocoele and salivary gland retention cyst (Table 2.3). PLA should be suspected when epithelial and stromal elements are seen within the mucinous material.

Differential diagnosis of cellular PLA is wide: MEC, AdCC, acinic cell carcinoma, basal cell adenoma, myoepithelioma, spindle cell neoplasm and malignant myoepithelioma [129, 130].

The excess of mesenchymal mucinous stroma can be misinterpreted as mucin and PA may be mistaken for cyst fluid of low-grade MEC. For diagnosis of MEC, the presence of squamous, intermediate

Figure 2.27 Pleomorphic adenoma. (A) CT scan of the oropharynx in a 27-year-old patient with a large parapharyngeal mass. Tumour was of unusual size and presented at a young age. Clinically, a malignant tumour was suspected. (B) Same patient, mass viewed from the mouth. FNAC was performed from the inside of the mouth. Smears were typical of pleomorphic adenoma. Investigation allowed careful preoperative planning in order to achieve complete excision.

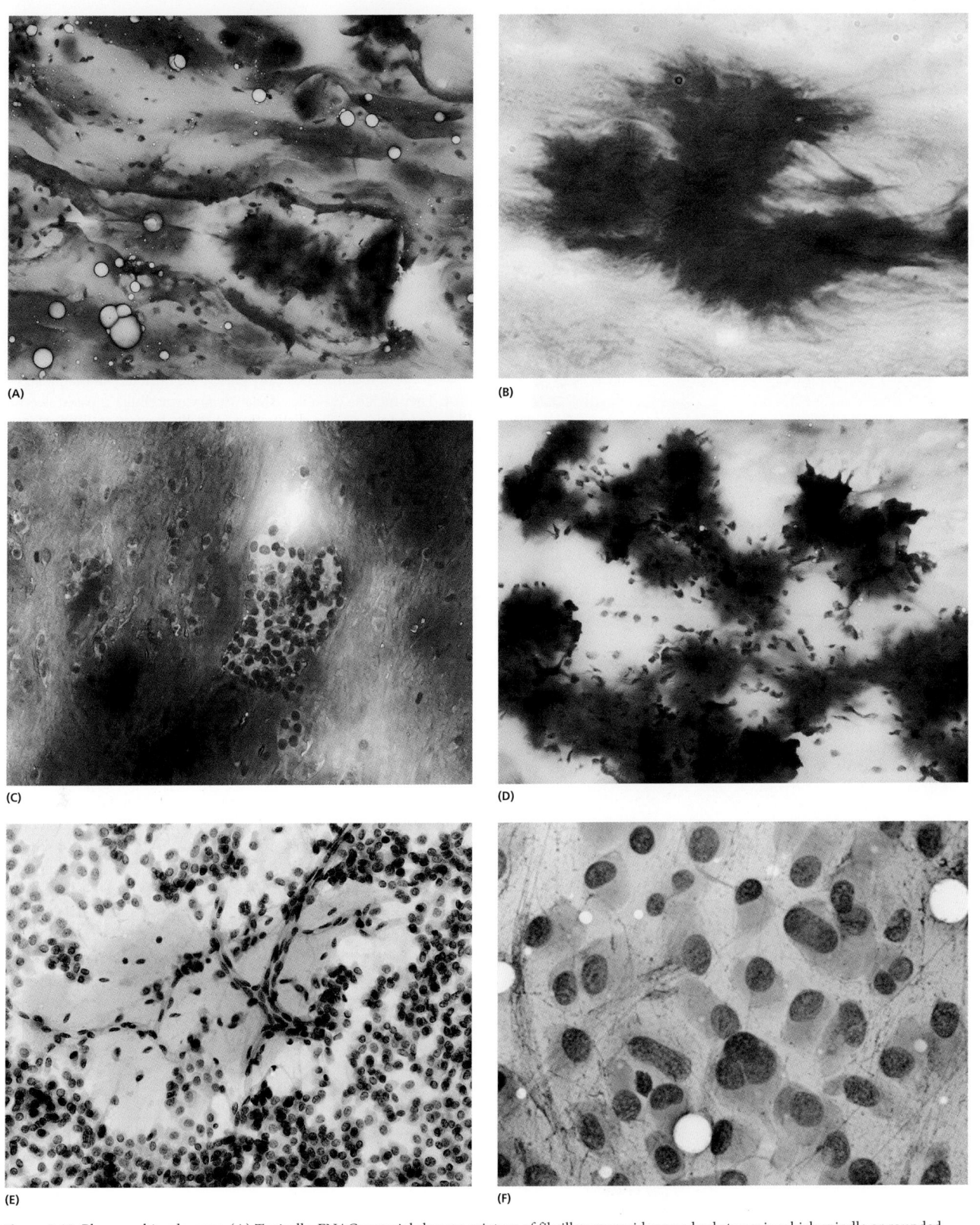

(A)

(B)

(C)

(D)

(E)

(F)

Figure 2.28 Pleomorphic adenoma. (A) Typically, FNAC material shows a mixture of fibrillary myxoid ground substance in which spindle or rounded cells are found either in clusters or lying free (MGG ×200). (B, C) Same case. Cells are often immersed within the chondromyxoid stroma and may appear poorly stained because of the reduced stain penetration (MGG ×400). (D) Clusters of epithelial cells with 'sunburst' appearance imparted by the peripheral epithelial cells streaming into the fibrillary material (MGG ×400, ×600). (E) Papanicolaou staining of PLA shows a less noticeable myxoid stroma but shows sppindle and round cells corresponding to epithelium and myoepithelium (PAP, ×400). (F) High power view of the myoepithelial cells shows bland, round, eccentric nuclei and dense, poorly outlined cytoplasm (PAP, ×600).

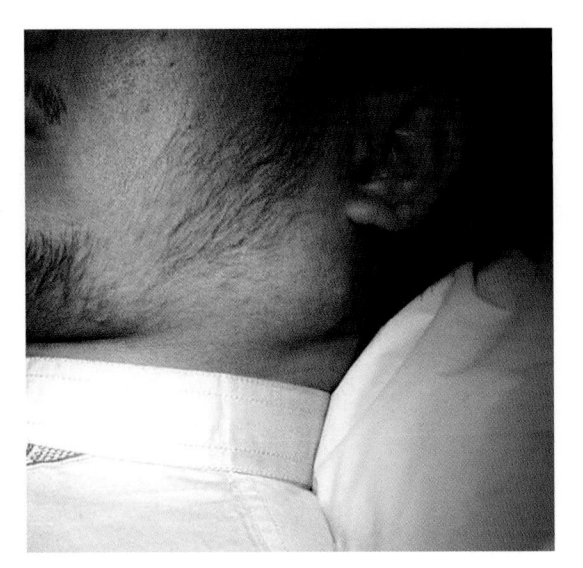

Figure 2.29 Pleomorphic adenoma. A 27-year-old patient presented with a solid, mobile, painless swelling at the angle of mandible.

and vacuolated cells is necessary. PLA with cylindromatous pattern should not be mistaken for AdCC. In AdCC, cells are usually smaller and hyperchromatic. Stroma may be present but is usually homogenous as opposed to fibrillary stroma of PLA. Although there are cytological features common to both tumours, each has a unique relationship of epithelial cells to stroma. Aspirates in PLA show cell clusters with a 'sunburst' appearance caused by peripheral spindled cells streaming into a fibrillary myxoid stroma. In AdCC, well-delineated, tightly cohesive, basaloid cells surround mucoid/hyaline globules or clear spaces in a honeycomb pattern are seen. The cytological distinction between PLA and acinic cell carcinoma is sometimes difficult, particularly if the epithelial cells of PLA show 'plasmacytoid' appearance and are scattered singly and in clusters. These cells have eccentrically placed, oval to round nuclei with finely granular chromatin, inconspicuous nucleoli and dense cytoplasm, sometimes containing hyaline globules [128].

Benign primary neoplasms of the salivary gland such as monomorphic adenoma and myoepithelioma can be easily mistaken for PLA on cytology. The distinction is of little practical importance since the treatment is the same. The similarity of PLA with benign

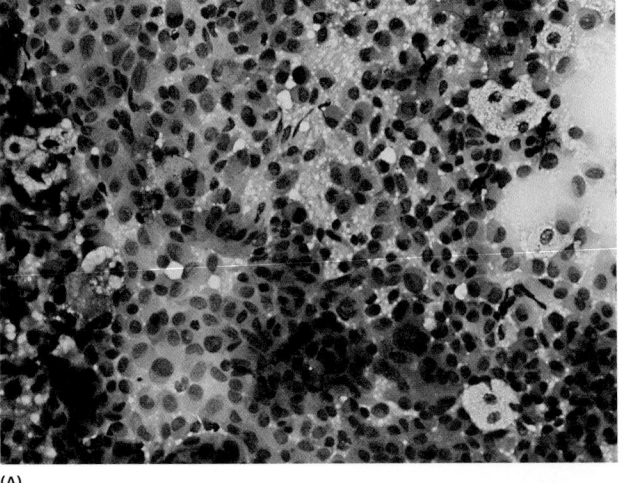

(A)

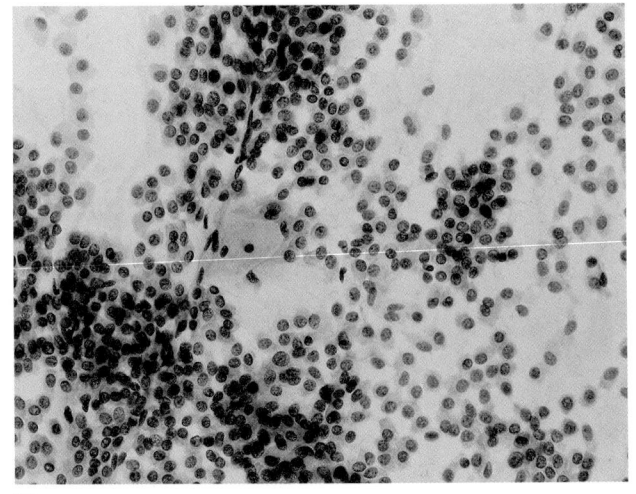

(B)

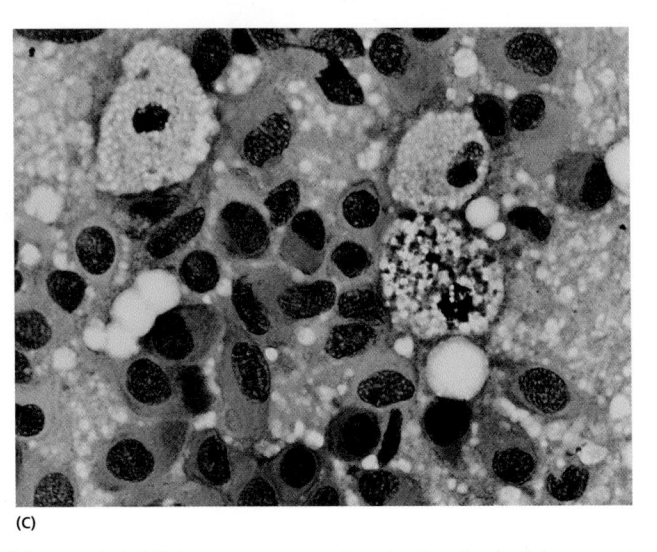

(C)

Figure 2.30 Pleomorphic adenoma, cellular type. (A) Cellular smears composed predominantly of cellular material with discrete myxoid stroma (MGG ×400). (B) Myoepithelial cells have bland, plasmacytoid appearance with oval or round nuclei, fine chromatin, inconspicuous nucleoli (MGG ×600, oil). (C) High power view of myoepithelial cells and macrophages indicating cystic change (MGG, ×600).

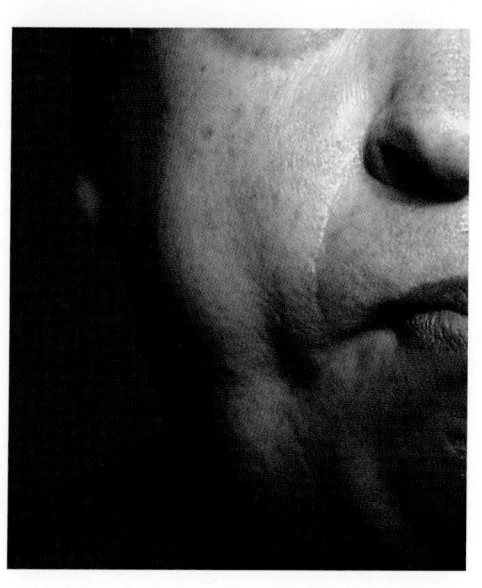

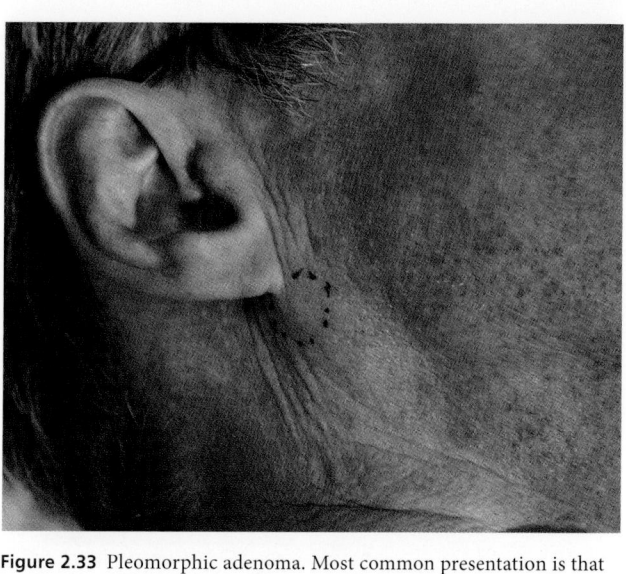

Figure 2.31 Pleomorphic adenoma. Patient presented with a swelling within the cheek, most prominent when muscles were tense. Pleomorphic adenoma of the accessory parotid was found on FNAC.

Figure 2.33 Pleomorphic adenoma. Most common presentation is that of a discrete swelling at the angle of mandible, barely visible but readily palpable. Patients often say that they have had the lump for many years. Only rarely they appear to have noticed it recently. In both instances, the lesion warrants investigation.

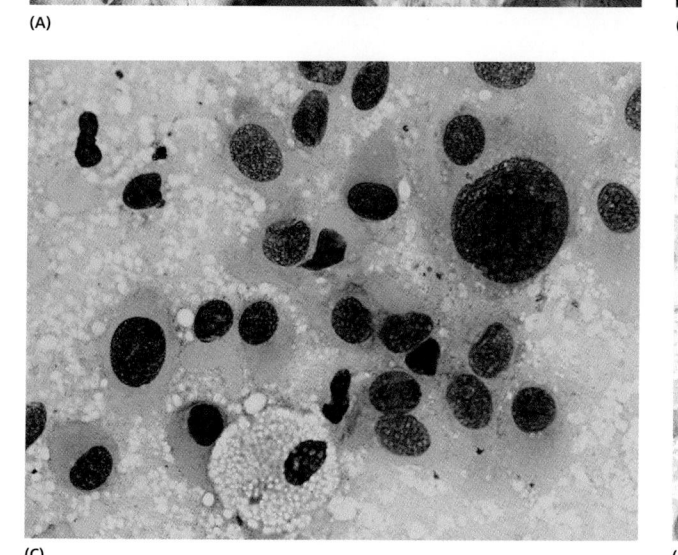

(A)

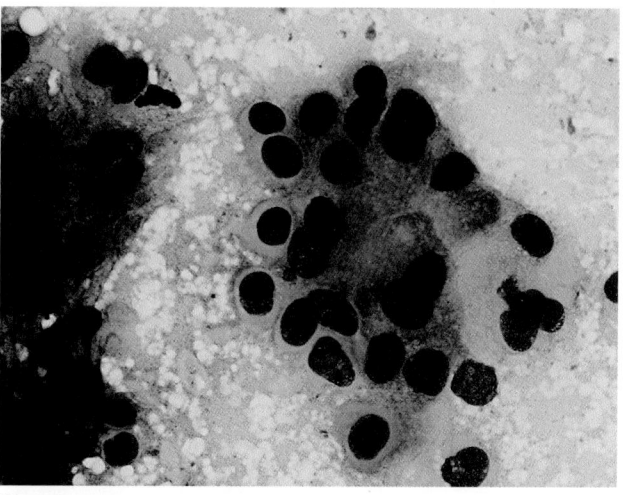

(B)

(C)

(D)

Figure 2.32 Pleomorphic adenoma: pitfalls in diagnosis. (A) Chondromyxoid material may show chondroid differentiation and very little epithelium. (B) Squamous metaplasia within a pleomorphic adenoma. Keratinisation may be misleading into diagnosis of squamous or mucoepidermoid carcinoma. (C) Anisonucleosis and mild cytological atypia can be seen in PLA. (D) Cylindromatous pattern. Spherical balls of stromal material are surrounded by epithelial cells. Note the presence of cytoplasm and bland nuclei of epithelial cells.

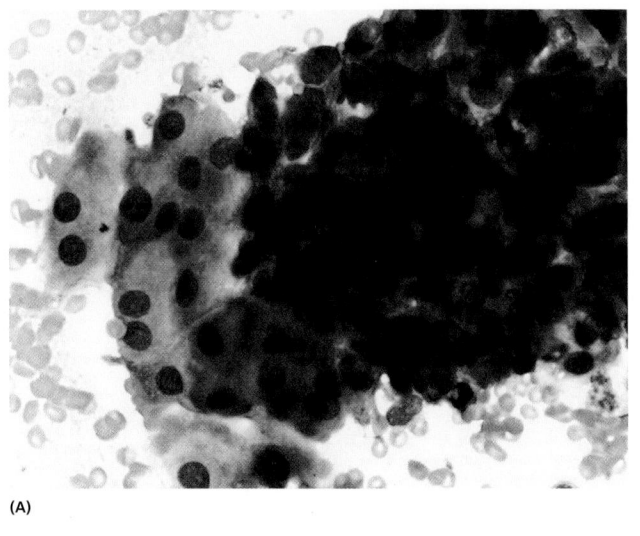 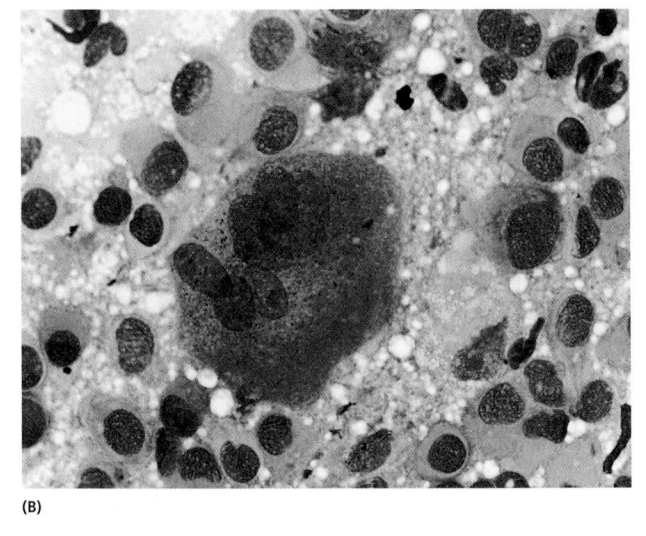

(A)   (B)

Figure 2.34 Pitfalls in pleomorphic adenoma. (A) Metaplastic changes in PLA. Predominantly oncocytic cells may be mistaken for Warthin's tumour or oncocytoma. (B) Cellular atypia and occasional giant cells can be seen. This should not be overinterpreted as malignant.

neurilemmomma is particularly prominent in the spindle type PLA. Intranuclear cytoplasmic inclusions are relatively common and nuclear grooves have been described. Diagnosis should not be confused with papillary carcinoma of the thyroid. Intravenous pyogenic granuloma is a rare, benign lesion occurring usually as a subcutaneous mass in the neck or upper extremity. Cytologically it may mimic PLA [126]. Nodular fasciitis may on occasions mimic the appearances of PLA [126a]. In all cases where morphological diagnosis is difficult on FNAC, case should be discussed at a multidisciplinary meeting.

Rare cases of benign salivary gland PLAs metastatic to bone (benign-metastasising PLAs and not carcinoma-ex-PLA or carcinosarcoma) diagnosed by FNAC have been described [132]. The metastatic lesions contained benign epithelial, myoepithelial, and stromal components. No evidence of malignancy was observed on cytological smears or histological sections in any of the cases. The differential diagnosis is primary bone tumours. Clinically, metastasising PLAs may represent unrecognised malignancy, because the biological course of tumours may lead to fatal outcomes [133].

2.4.2 Adenolymphoma (Warthin's tumour)

This is the second most common benign salivary gland tumour. It represents approximately 5–6% of salivary gland lesions, arises most commonly within the parotid gland, grows slowly and is typically detected around 55 years of age (Fig. 2.35). There is a male predominance. Histologically, tumour consists of double layer of oncocytic epithelium with lymphoid stroma containing lymphoid follicles and cystic spaces containing inflammatory/necrotic material.

[See BOX 2.4. Summary of ultrasound features: WARTHIN'S TUMOUR on www.wiley.com/go/kocjan/clinical_cytopathology_head_neck2e]

Cytological features include three distinct components: oncocytic cells in flat sheets or papillary structures, lymphoid stroma and contents of the cystic spaces with inflammation/necrosis (Figs 2.36 and 2.37). Oncocytic cells are round or polyhedral with centrally placed nuclei and dense, well-outlined cytoplasmic borders. Nucleoli are usually not prominent but may be conspicuous. Epithelial cells are characteristically associated with mast cells that

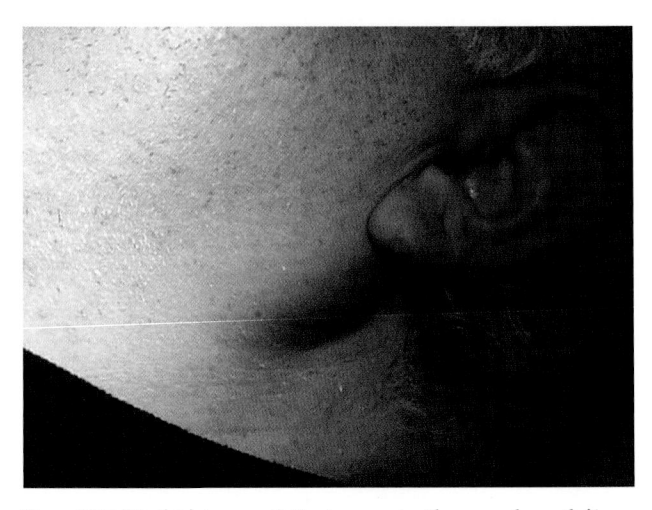

Figure 2.35 Warthin's tumour. Patients present with a several months'/years' history of a soft swelling that does not vary in size. FNAC may yield turbid fluid. In this case it is advisable to sample the wall of the lesion to avoid sampling errors.

may be detected on the MGG stain [134, 135]. Lymphoid cells represent follicle centre cells and range from mature lymphocytes to blasts and plasma cells. Cystic debris contains macrophages, may contain polymorphs and crystals [75]. All three components are present in about 28% of cases, two components in 55% (oncocytes and necrosis or oncocytes and lymphocytes) and 17% show one component only [136]. Diagnosis of Warthin's tumour is easily made when all three components are present, or even two components, since the oncocytes are in most cases obvious. If a smear shows a single component, diagnosis is more difficult and differential diagnosis should include oncocytoma, intraparotid lymphadenitis, salivary gland cyst or low-grade MEC. Careful attention should be directed at identifying the extracellular fluid components present (mucoid vs watery proteinaceous) as well as the predominant cellular component (e.g. lymphocytes, histiocytes, epithelial cells and oncocytes). It is important to recognise, however, that occasionally epithelial cells may not be detected on FNAC of cystic salivary gland lesions, as a result of either cellular dilution by cyst fluid or

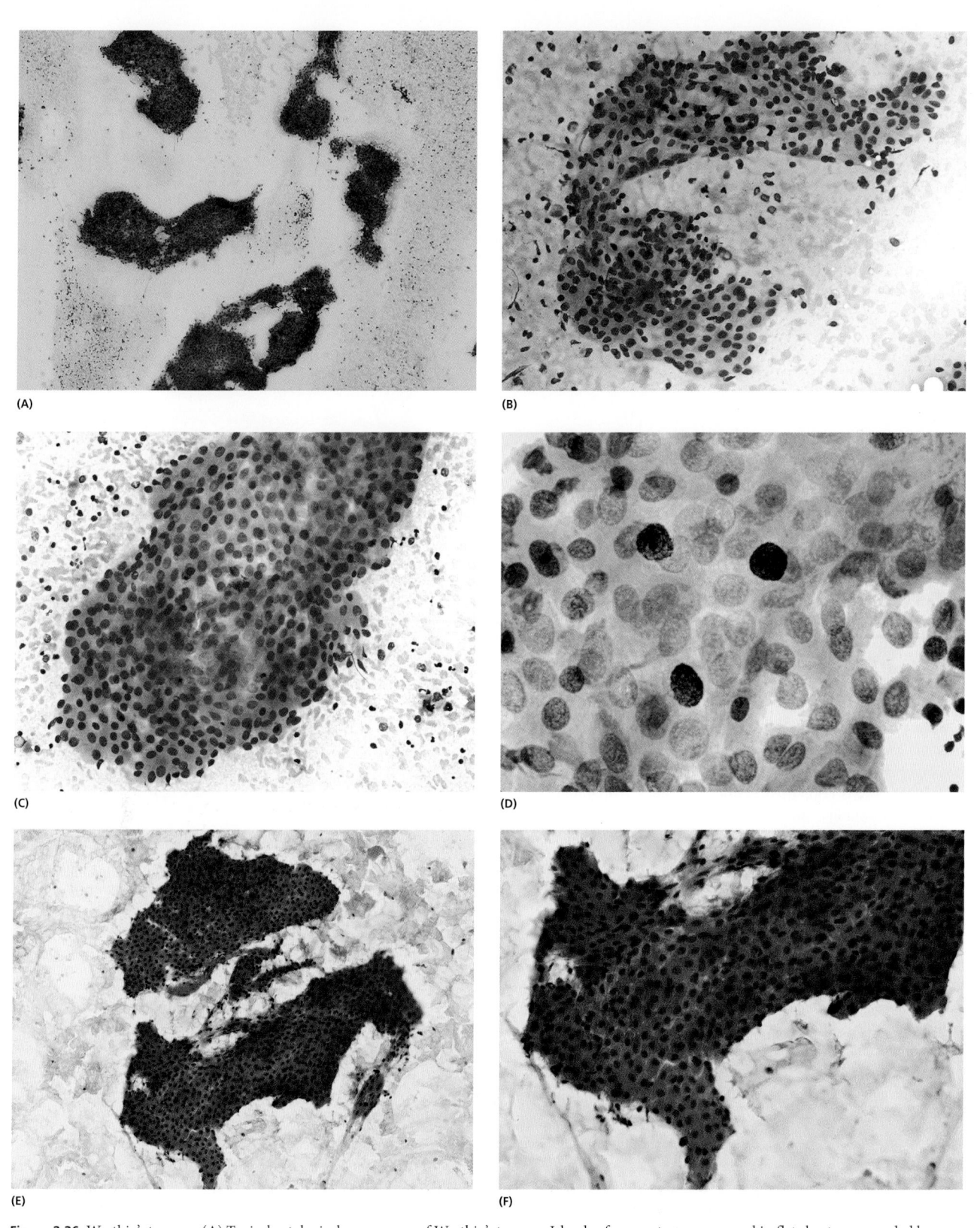

(A)

(B)

(C)

(D)

(E)

(F)

Figure 2.36 Warthin's tumour. (A) Typical cytological appearance of Warthin's tumour. Islands of oncocytes are arranged in flat sheets surrounded by lymphoid cells. (B) Same case. Oncocytic epithelium has centrally placed nuclei and dense eosinophilic cytoplasm. (C) Oncocytic epithelium may be sparse or, as in this case, may dominate the FNAC. Differential diagnosis is oncocytoma (MGG ×200). (D) Oncocytes in air dried smears are often associated with mast cells. This may be helpful in distiguishing this tumour from other oncocyte containing tumours (MGG ×600 oil). (E) Low power features of Warrthin's tumour in alcohol fixed slides (PAP stain) may show intracytoplasmic granules in oncocytic epithelium. (F) Uniformly arranged benign oncocytic epithelium should not be mistaken for a lymph node metastasis.

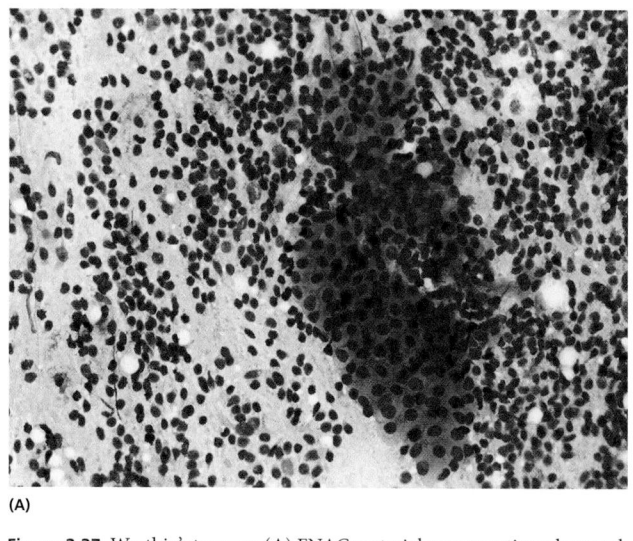 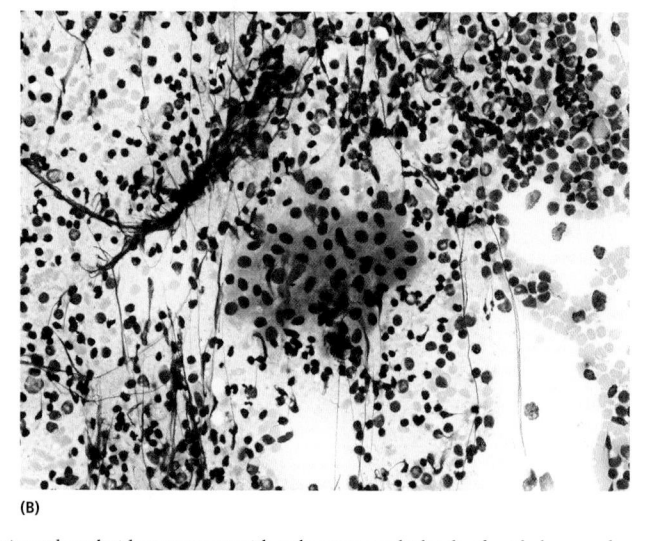

(A)　　　　　　　　　　　　　　　　　　　　　　　　　　(B)

Figure 2.37 Warthin's tumour. (A) FNAC material can sometimes have a dominant lymphoid component with only occasional islands of epithelium and be mistaken for a lymphoepithelial lesion. (B) Oncocytic epithelium may show squamous metaplasia and is a significant cause of false positive diagnosis of a metastasis of a squamous cell carcinoma. This is particularly true of the metaplastic (or infarcted) variant of Warthin's tumour.

inadequate sampling. In these cases, the referring clinician should be informed that a low grade MEC cannot be ruled out [137]. Mucus retention cysts, lymphoepithelial cysts, cystadenomas, Warthin's tumours, cystic PLAs, low-grade MECs, cystadenocarcinomas and examples of polycystic disease of the parotid gland all may appear cystic (Table 2.3). The cellular component within the fluid obtained from these lesions may be exceedingly scant or absent, making cytological diagnosis difficult and, at times, impossible.

Diagnostic errors may be caused by a lack of typical features and the presence of individual atypical squamous cells in a necrotic background mimicking carcinoma, particularly in cases where there is squamous metaplasia and mucinous content of the cystic space [138]. In this case, a low-grade MEC should be considered. However, further caution is needed, since Layfield describes the presence of atypical squamous metaplasia in oncocytic lesions as a significant cause of false-positive diagnoses of carcinoma (7% of cases) [139]. This is particularly true of the metaplastic (or infarcted) variant of Warthin's tumour. It is characterised by replacement of much of the original oncocytic epithelium by metaplastic squamous cells, along with areas of extensive necrosis, fibrosis and inflammatory change. The pathogenesis is unknown, but it is most likely to be vascular in origin. An association with a previous FNAC (1–4 months pre surgery) has been suggested [25]. Another possible association with the previously performed FNAC of Warthin's tumour is the finding of multiple sarcoid like granulomas with multinucleate giant cells on tissue sections. These are probably caused by the exposure of lymphoid tissue to the contents of cystic spaces [140]. In addition to Warthin's tumour, a spectrum of neoplastic and non-neoplastic lesions of the salivary glands may contain squamous cells. These include chronic sialadenitis, lymphoepithelial cyst, PLA, MEC and squamous cell carcinoma [71]. It is therefore important to recognise metaplastic Warthin's tumour, because the differential diagnoses of this benign neoplasm include MEC and squamous carcinoma, both primary and metastatic.

Oncocytic change, so typically a part of Warthin's tumour, may be seen in other tumours. Oncocytes are large, apparently swollen epithelial cells with cytoplasm densely filled with eosinophilic granules scattered amongst the ductal and acinar cells of the salivary gland cells. The name originates from the Greek word ονκοσ, meaning 'to swell' or 'gain in size'. Hürthle first described them in

1894 [141]. They are mitochondria rich epithelial cells characterised by the presence of granules in the cytoplasm. The granules sometimes coalesce so that the cytoplasm appears homogeneous. The cell of origin is thought to be the multipotential cell of intercalated ducts, as evidenced by the transition of small basophilic cuboidal cells into swollen acidophilic granular cells.

Oncocytes are not typically a prominent feature of MEC of the salivary glands, and only five such cases have been reported [60, 142].Because most salivary gland lesions with oncocytic change are benign, it is important to distinguish MEC from other entities that may show prominent oncocytic change.

Recently described phenomena of electrocautery induced oncocytic change deserve the attention of histopathologists. These are believed to occur as a consequence of the electrothermal discharge [143]. Oncocytic change can also be seen in multifocal oncocytic adenomatous hyperplasia [144].

Lymphoid cells within Warthin's tumour may be mistaken for an intraparotid lymph node or for a lymphoma (Fig. 2.37) (Table 2.4) [8]. Follicle centre non-Hodgkin lymphoma (NHL) and Warthin's tumour involving the same site have been described [145]. The localised NHL described suggests that the NHL initially arose in the lymph node involved by Warthin's tumour, and, thus, the Warthin's tumour may have provided a source of long-term antigenic stimulation from which a monoclonal B-cell population subsequently arose. These findings support the hypothesis that Warthin's tumour arises from heterotopic salivary gland ducts within lymph nodes.

Malignant transformation of Warthin's tumour is a rare event and very few cases of MEC arising in Warthin's tumour in the parotid gland have been described [146, 147]. Extraparotid Warthin's occasionally arise in the cervical region [148] or in the larynx [94]. Awareness of this may prevent diagnostic difficulties.

2.4.3 Basal cell adenoma

Basal cell adenoma (BCA) is an uncommon salivary gland tumour and makes up approximately 1.2% of all salivary gland tumours. Histologically, basal cell adenomas are subdivided into solid, tubular, trabecular and membranous variants. Monomorphic adenomas are rare benign tumours that do not recur or metastasise,

hence they should be recognised and separated from other tumours. They have unique morphologic features, some of which can be recognised on FNAC, helping in further clinical management.

It is difficult to make an unequivocal diagnosis of BCA based on FNAC alone. This is due to its rarity and overlapping of its cytological features with some benign and malignant entities [149]. The classical appearances are those of uniform small basaloid epithelial cells with round or oval nuclei, inconspicuous nucleoli and scant cytoplasm. The basaloid cells surround acellular, dense, homogenous material or are surrounded by acellular or paucicellular dense homogeneous material possibly containing bland spindle cells. The basaloid cells are present in variably sized three-dimensional clusters, acini, or sheets with variable cohesion. The dense homogenous material surrounded by basaloid cells may be interconnected. High power magnification reveals the homogeneous material to have a fibrillary texture. The edges of dense homogenous materials are well-demarcated (Fig. 2.38). **Trabecular** variant contains hyaline globules and **membranous** variant contains membranous material around the cell groups. **Solid** variant contains very little apart from basaloid cells. A focal squamous metaplasia may be seen in some BCA,

but it is rare to see extensive squamous metaplasia, especially with cellular atypia [150].

Differential diagnosis of BCA on FNAC material is: PLA, basal cell adenocarcinoma, AdCC and metastatic basal cell carcinoma. The cells of PLA tend to be less cohesive, with cell aggregates appearing to fall apart at the edges. The cells of BCA tend to adhere to sheets of basement membrane. Basal cell adenocarcinomas are similar to BCA but usually contain some cell pleomorphism, occasional mitoses and/or focal necrosis (Figs 2.50 and 2.51). Reviews of six major studies encompassing 10 cases of basal cell adenocarcinoma diagnosed on FNAC show cumulatively 100% sensitivity and specificity [151].

Cytological features of the cell-stroma interface are useful in distinguishing between monomorphic adenomas of the basal cell type and AdCC. In BCA, the collagenous stroma interdigitates with adjacent cells, whereas in AdCC, the two are separated by a sharp smooth border. Furthermore, the stroma of BCA can contain rare spindle cells or capillaries, but the cylinders of AdCC are acellular. Occasionally, however, AdCC shows the small blue cell pattern and cell-stroma interface features of BCA and does not contain smooth-bordered cylinders typical of AdCC. These may be

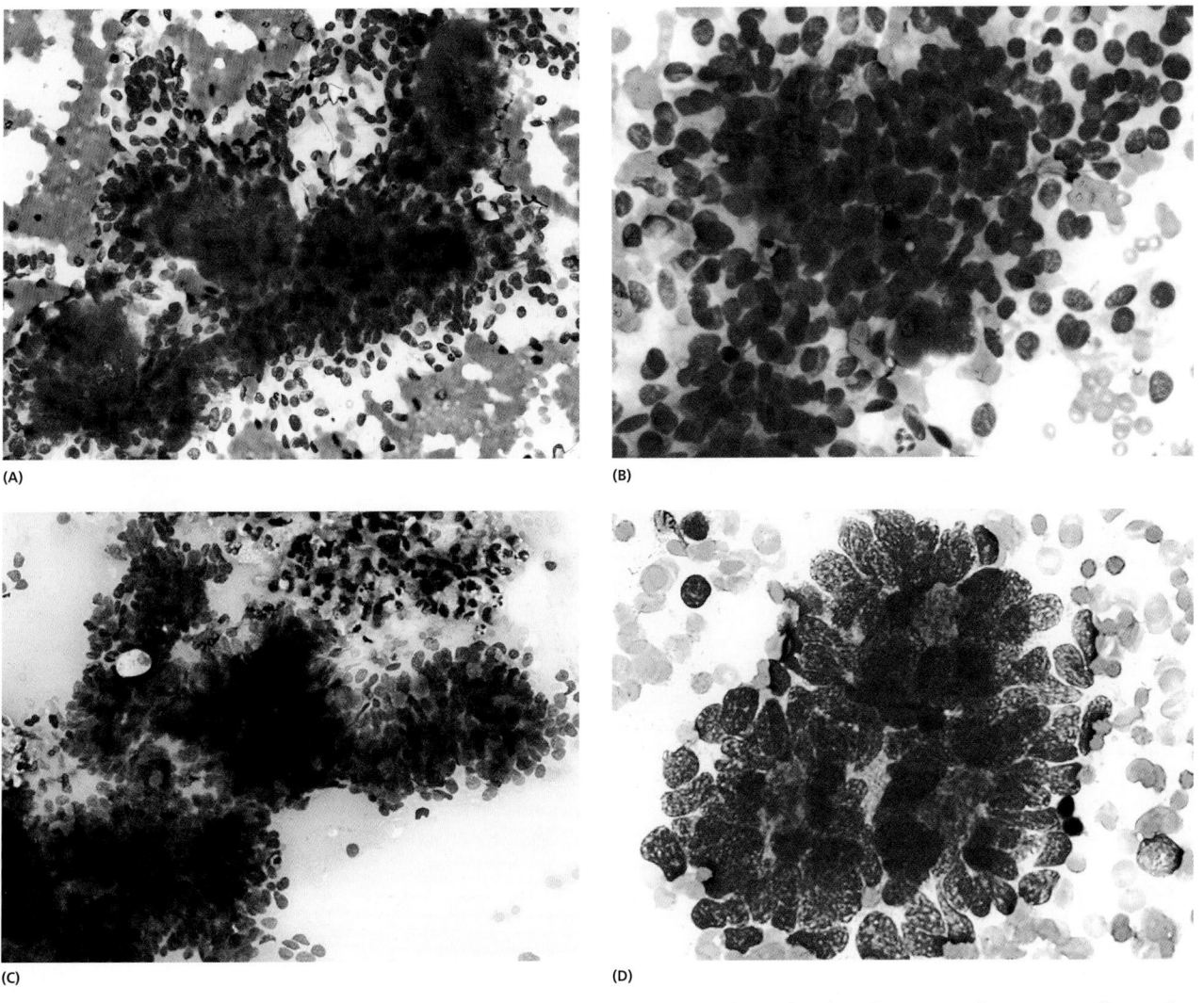

(A)

(B)

(C)

(D)

Figure 2.38 Basal cell adenoma. (A) Tightly cohesive clusters of small uniform cells with round or oval nuclei and scanty cytoplasm seem to adhere to the basement membrane material (MGG ×200). (B) Sparse homogenous background material (MGG ×600, oil). (C) Low power view showing numerous well defined globules of eosinophilic material. An erroneous diagnosis of Adenoid Cystic carcinoma was made. (D) High power view of the same case as in (C) shows collagenous stroma interdigitating with basaloid cells which have fine granular nuclei.

incorrectly interpreted as benign at the time of FNAC. Stanley et al. suggest that the stroma aspirated from solid AdCC represents desmoplastic tumour stroma that mimics the pattern of BCA in smear material. Occasionally, hyaline globules in trabecular and canalicular types of BCA may be misinterpreted as AdCC (Fig 2.38) [152]. Close attention should be paid to the appearance of the epithelial nuclei. These are bland with a finely granular and no or inconspicuous nucleoli in BCA and hyperchromatic and coarse in AdCC. Distinction between BCA and AdCC (particularly the solid type) at the time of FNAC remains a difficult problem [152]. Squamous metaplastic cells with hyperchromatic, enlarged, bizarre and pleomorphic nuclei can be seen on FNAC smears of BCA [150].

2.4.4 Oncocytoma

Oncocytomas are rare benign salivary gland neoplasms that represent approximately 1.5% of all salivary gland tumours. Parotid gland is most commonly involved; the submandibular gland is very rarely the site of this tumour. Males and females are equally affected and the age range is 21–88 years. Clinically, the tumours are generally asymptomatic, well circumscribed masses that increase in size over a period ranging from several weeks to 20 years and are occasionally associated with pain. Histologically, the tumours are characterised by large epithelial cells with eosinophilic, granular cytoplasm. The cytoplasm stains positively with stains used to demonstrate mitochondria (phosphotungstic acid-hematoxylin-PTAH, Novelli, Cresyl violet V, and Kluver–Barrera Luxol fast blue stains). Immunohistochemical reactions demonstrate an epithelial origin (keratin and epithelial membrane antigen), whereas markers for myoepitehlial derivation (S-100 protein, actin and glial fibrillary acidic protein-GFAP) are not identified [153]. Surgical resection is the only treatment.

Cytological features include cohesive multilayered sheets of oncocytic cells with small regular round nuclei and abundant well-outlined cytoplasm. There is absence of cystic change, lymphoid cells and debris (Fig. 2.39).

Differential diagnosis of oncocytoma includes Warthin's tumour and other salivary gland tumours in which cells resemble oncocytes, for example oncocytic carcinoma (see Fig 2.53), acinic cell carcinoma (see Fig 2.41a,b), intermediate grade MEC and adenocarcinoma cells all have these appearances occasionally (see 'Differential

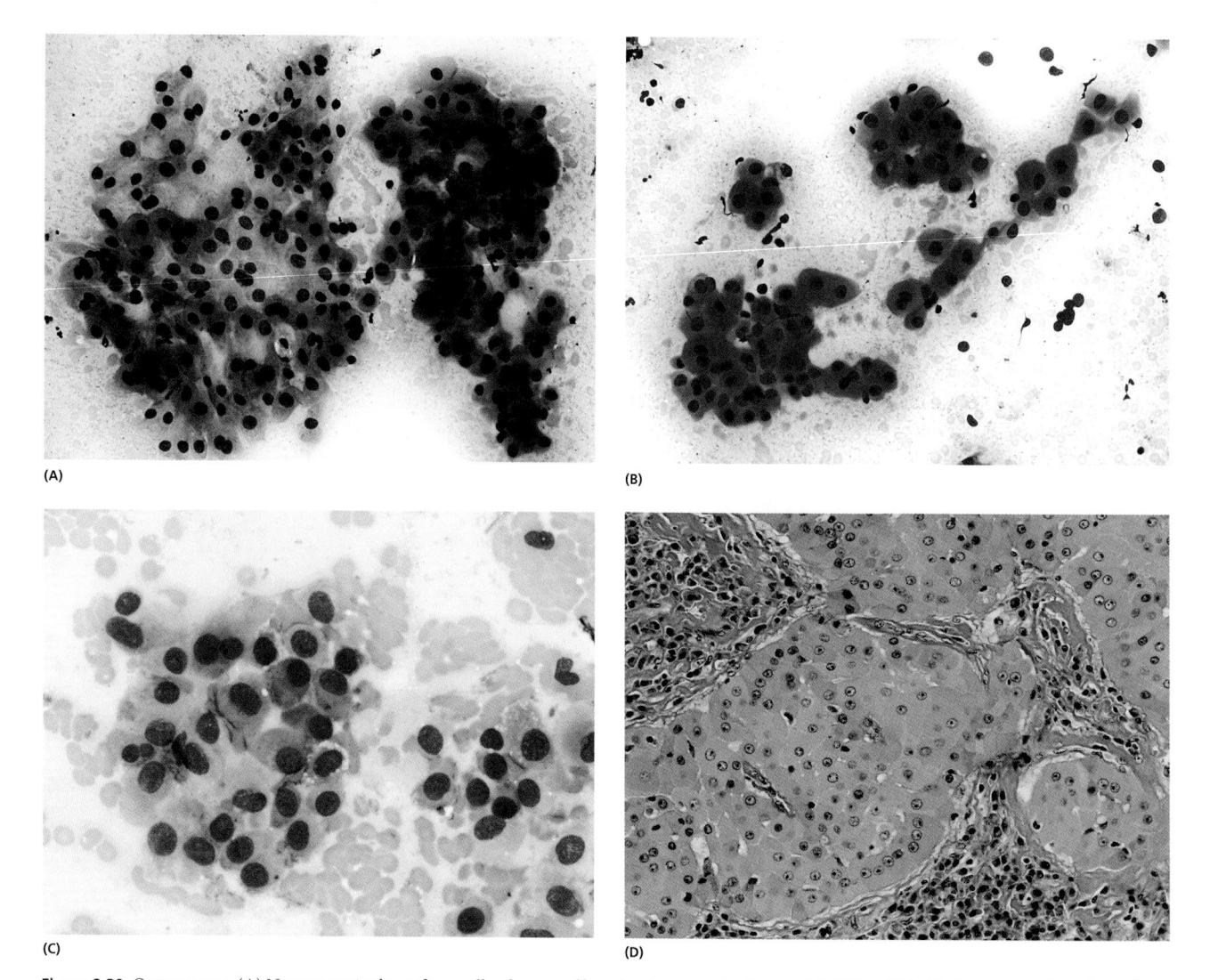

(A)

(B)

(C)

(D)

Figure 2.39 Oncocytoma. (A) Numerous single uniform cells, absence of lymphoid or cystic background (MGG, ×400). (B) Oncocytic cells with small, regular, round nuclei and abundant, well-outlined cytoplasm (MGG, ×400). (C) Cells are occasionally arranged in multilayered sheets (MGG, ×600). (D) Histology of oncocytic adenoma (H&E, ×400).

Diagnosis of Mucoepidermoid Carcinoma', Section 2.5.2). Oncocytic cells in Warthin's tumour are usually monolayered and in oncocytoma multilayered.

Cases of benign parotid gland oncocytoma with pseudomalignant change that mimics acinic cell carcinoma have been described. In histological sections, there are clusters of pigmented cells with PAS-positive foamy to finely granular cytoplasm similar to those seen in salivary gland acinic cell carcinomas. This is a diagnostic pitfall that may be observed in histological tissue specimens removed after FNAC of oncocytic tumours [154]. Malignant oncocytoma of the parotid has been described (Fig. 2.53) [155].

2.4.5 Rare benign tumours

2.4.5.1 Sclerosing polycystic adenosis

Sclerosing polycystic adenosis (SPA) is a recently described, rare, reactive/neoplastic, process of the major or minor salivary glands that is similar to fibrocystic changes, sclerosing adenosis and adenosis tumours of the breast [156]. Both have cystic components with a prominent lobular or multilobular arrangement often with

small, proliferating, closely packed ductal structures, surrounded by a peripheral myoepithelial layer. Similar to breast, the salivary gland tumours may be associated with ductal epithelial hyperplasia and atypia, ranging from mild dysplasia to severe dysplasia/carcinoma in situ.

FNAC appearances are characterised by the tightly cohesive, sharply outlined clusters of hyperplastic ductal epithelium with no inflammation or acinar cells in the background (Fig. 2.40). Ductal epithelium is associated with smaller darker myoepithelial cells lying on a different plane. Some sheets of ductal epithelium show mild architectural atypia, such as loss of polarity, and occasional mitoses.

2.4.5.2 Myoepithelioma

Of all salivary gland tumours, myoepithelioma accounts for less than 1%. Myoepitehlial tumours affect patients of both sexes equally. The mean age of the patients is 54 years. It involves parotid but also submandibular gland. Rare cases have been found to involve the sinonasal tract, lacrymal gland and larynx. Myoepitheliomas

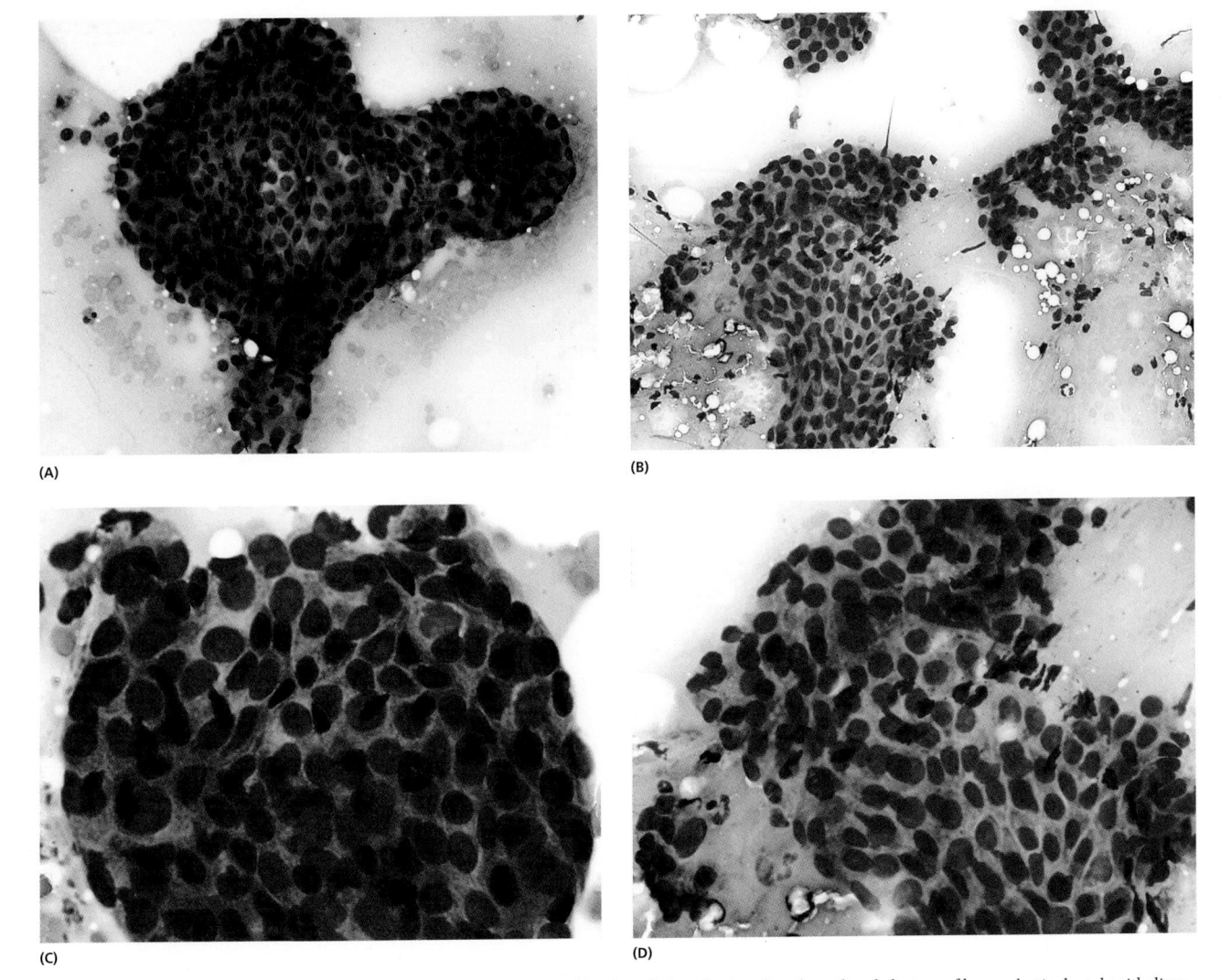

(A)

(B)

(C)

(D)

Figure 2.40 Scllerosing polycystic adenosis. (A) Smears are characterised by the tightly cohesive, sharply outlined clusters of hyperplastic ductal epithelium (MGG, ×400). (B) Low power view does not show any inflammation or acinar cells in the background (MGG, ×200). (C) Ductal epithelium is associated with smaller darker myoepithelial cells lying on a different plane (MGG, ×600). (D) Some sheets of ductal epithelium show mild architectural atypia, such as loss of polarity, and occasional mitoses (MGG, ×600).

also occur in breast. Myoepithelioma is benign and has a good prognosis. Conservative surgical management is curative [157–159]. Malignant variant of the tumour (malignant myoepithelioma) usually develops in a pre-existing salivary gland tumour, usually PLA but also myoepithelioma [160, 161].

Histologically, myoepitehlial tumours are composed of epithelioid, plasmacytoid, spindle or clear cell types, and they show a solid or a myxoid pattern of growth.

Cytological features show a uniform population of small, spindle cells with elongated oval nuclei with evenly distributed, homogenous chromatin, inconspicuous nucleoli with cytoplasm which forms thin bipolar wispy processes (Fig. 2.41). Occasionally cells have a plasmacytoid appearance, similar to plasmacytoid cells of PLA [162, 163]. The diagnosis can be confirmed by ultrastructural and immunohistochemical analysis demonstrating myofilaments aggregation pattern and positive staining for S100-protein, vimentin and keratin antibodies. Glial fibrillary acidic protein is positive in 53%, and muscle-specific actin and smooth-muscle actin are positive in only 20% of cases. Desmin is negative in both benign and malignant tumours.

Myoepithelioma composed of bland spindle cells is difficult to distinguish from soft tissue lesions, for example nodular fasciitis, leiomyoma, nerve sheath tumour or haemangiopericytoma (see Fig. 2.61) [126a, 164].

Given the relative rarity of the tumour, most cytopathologists will not be familiar with the entity and will report a 'spindle cell neoplasm', which needs excision.

2.4.5.3 Intraductal papilloma

Intraductal papilloma of the salivary gland is an extremely rare benign salivary gland tumour that occurs most commonly in the minor salivary glands. They are cystic, solitary neoplasms that arise from ductal epithelium and produce painless swellings from which fluid is usually aspirated. Excision is curative and recurrences rare.

Cytological features of intraductal papilloma are three-dimensional epithelial clusters, some with a papillary configuration and histiocytes.

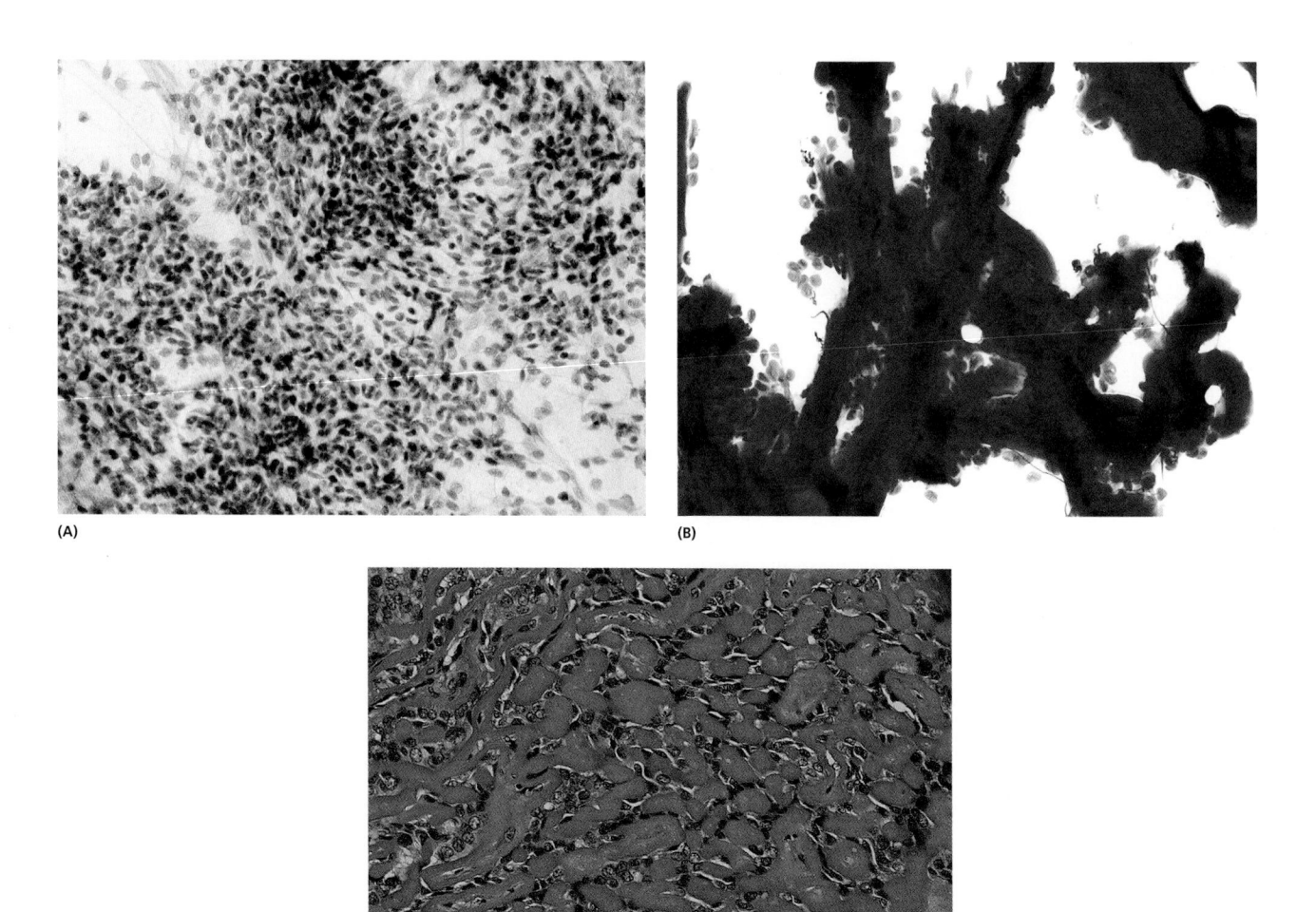

(A) (B) (C)

Figure 2.41 Myoepithelioma. (A) FNAC yields cellular smears composed of interconnected aggregates and single cells spindle cells immersed in the background mesenchymal material (PAP, ×400). (B) Basement membrane material may dominate in some cases of myoepithelioma, making distinction from adenoid cystic carcinoma difficult. The plump nuclei of myoepithelioma may be mistaken for leiomyoma or nerve sheath tumour (MGG, ×400). (C) Histology of myoepithelioma case in the previous figure (H&E, ×400).

The majority of cells show oncocytic differentiation; however, benign-appearing ductal cells in honeycomb sheets can also be present [165]. Sebaceous differentiation may be seen [166].

Other *salivary gland tumours with papillary components* include other benign entities such as inverted duct papilloma, sialadenoma papilliferum, papillary cystadenoma and Warthin's tumour. Polymorphous low grade adenocarcinoma, cystic MEC and papillary variant of acinic cell carcinoma can all have papillary structures [166]. Papillary oncocytic cystadenoma has been reported mainly in the minor salivary glands and occasionally in the parotid glands [167]. In cases with extensive necrotic debris and metaplastic squamous cells, branchial cyst and cystic metastatic squamous carcinoma may also need to be considered (see Table 2.3).

A malignant counterpart of intraductal papilloma, intraductal papillary adenocarcinoma, has only recently been described [168]. It is architecturally similar to intraductal papilloma with the addition of cytological atypia, intraductal extension, microinvasion, and lymph node metastases. Cytological assessment of any papillary salivary gland lesions must be made with the appreciation of the wide spectrum of the differential diagnoses.

2.5 Malignant tumours of the salivary gland

Currently, salivary gland malignancies are classified according to the 2005 WHO classification [50] (see Table 2.2). The most important developments since the WHO classification of 2005 is the identification of specific translocations which is revolutionising the way salivary tumours are considered and will have a major impact on future diagnostic practice. This is true so far in four malignancies: mammary analogue secretory (MASC), MEC, AdCC, and hyalinising clear cell (HCCC) carcinomas. In each, the gene rearrangement is found in 80% or more of cases [169] (see Table 2.5).

Malignant parotid tumours are uncommon and present a significant management challenge. Cytology can correctly diagnose malignancy with 88–100% sensitivity [170]. More precise tumour typing, together with other prognostic factors (age, sex, grading, TNM and pTNM, facial nerve involvement) means that a radical parotidectomy is required in a proportion of patients, the rest undergoing superficial parotidectomy [171]. The crude 5- and 10-year survival rates are 68–75% and 49–67% respectively while

the loco-regional control rate at 10 years of 79% [170, 172]. Radical surgery with appropriate reconstruction followed by planned postoperative adjuvant radiotherapy gives effective control of malignant parotid tumours.

Radiological appearances of malignant salivary gland tumours include an ill-defined margin, irregular shape, increased vascularity with a peripheral distribution and the presence of malignant lymphadenopathy either within the parotid itself or in the deep cervical chain.

Unfortunately, none of these imaging features in isolation or in combination are specific enough to be able to discriminate 100% benign from malignant salivary lesions. It is well recognised that some malignant salivary tumours (such as low grade MEC) may have no typically malignant imaging characteristics and therefore FNAC is mandatory in all salivary lumps to establish a full cytological diagnosis. Nevertheless, most malignant lesions will display some or all of the typical malignant features on imaging and so, on the whole, US findings are helpful in forewarning that a lesion is likely to be malignant.

FNAC allows distinction between neoplastic and non-neoplastic salivary gland lesions Within the neoplasms, if established diagnostic criteria are present, it can separate benign from malignant tumours with a high level of accuracy [64].

In an attempt to find a useful ancillary technique to help distinguish benign and malignant neoplasms, p53, PC10 and Ki-67 (MIB1) and flow cytometry may be useful markers (Table 2.5) [173–175].

2.5.1 Acinic cell carcinoma

Acinic cell carcinoma (ACC) is considered the third most common primary salivary gland carcinoma after AdCC and MEC with incidence ranging from 2–19%. It arises mainly in major salivary glands, can be bilateral [176], shows preponderance of females, age range 10–84. Familial occurrence has been described [177]. Tumour size ranges from 1–8 cm, although giant acinic cell carcinomas have been reported [178]. In the majority of cases patients present with a painful swelling as a main symptom [179]. It is locally recurrent in 18–42% of cases with 5% local lymph node metastases [179]. The interval between the primary and recurrent cancer ranges between 17–24 years [180]. It is currently considered as a low-grade malignancy with unpredictable local recurrences and lymph node metastases. Management of ACC is based on reports of small numbers of cases accrued over several decades. The National Cancer Data Base

Table 2.5 Salivary carcinomas and molecular abnormalities.

	Tumour	Translocation	Genes involved	Approx %
Well-established abnormalities in relatively common carcinomas	MASC	t(12;15)(p13;q25)	*ETV6-NTRK3*	Translocation 80 % ETV6 break 99%
	MEC	t(11;19)(q21;p13) t(11;15)(q21;q26)	*CRTC1-MAML2* *CRTC3-MAML2*	60–80% 6% or less
	AdCC	t(6;9)(q22-23;p23-24)	*MYB-NFIB*	80–90%
	HCCC	t(12;22)(q13;q12)	*EWSR1- ATF1*	80%
Rare salivary malignancies	DSRCT	t(11;22)(p13;q12)	*EWS-WT1*	Up to 97%
	NUT carcinoma	t(15;19)(q14, p13.1) t(9;15)(q34.2;q14) t(15;?)(q14;unknown)	*BRD4-NUT* *BRD3-NUT* *NUT-variant*	approx. 67% } remaining third of cases
Few studies, so not yet well-established	CATS	t(1;14)(p36.11;q12) t(X;14)(p11.4;q12)	*AR1D1A-PRKD1* DDX3X-PRKD1 Other abnormalities of *PRKD2* and *PRKD3*	} possibly as many as 80%.
	EMC	No translocations, but a mutation	*HRAS* exon 3, codon 61	27% in one small series

Source: Simpson RH, Skálová A, Di Palma S, Leivo I. Recent advances in the diagnostic pathology of salivary carcinomas. *Virchows Arch* 2014; 465(4): 371–84 [169].

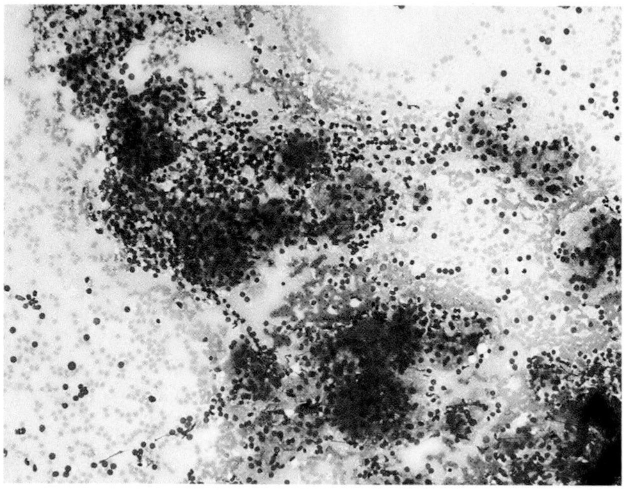

(A)

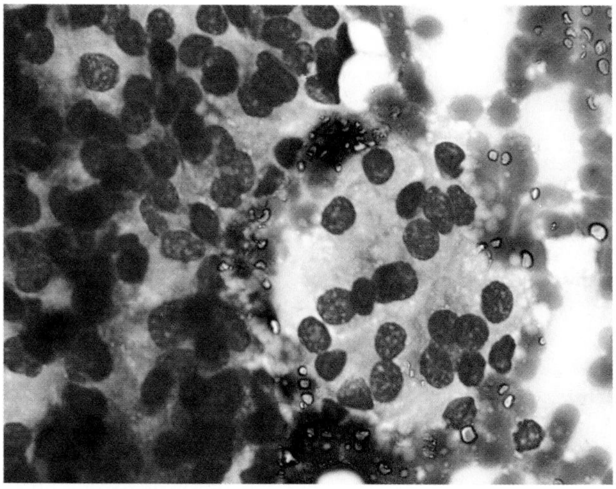

(B)

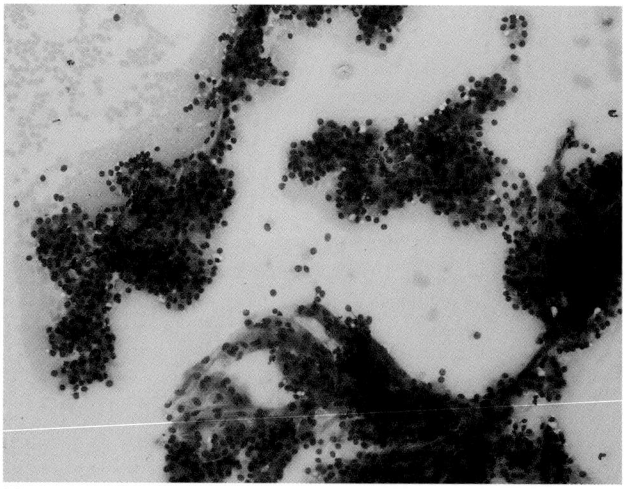

(C)

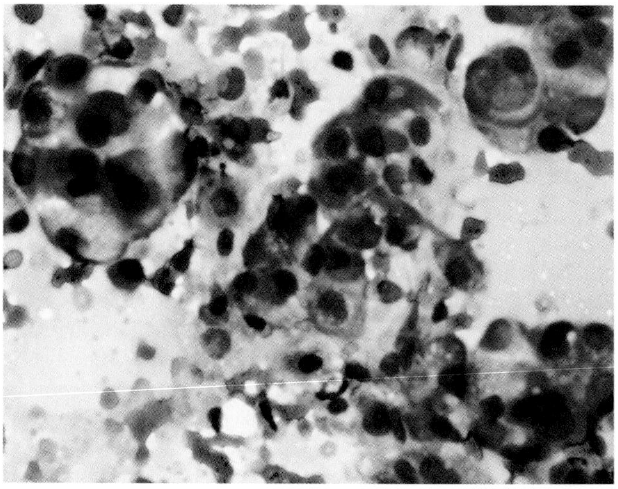

(D)

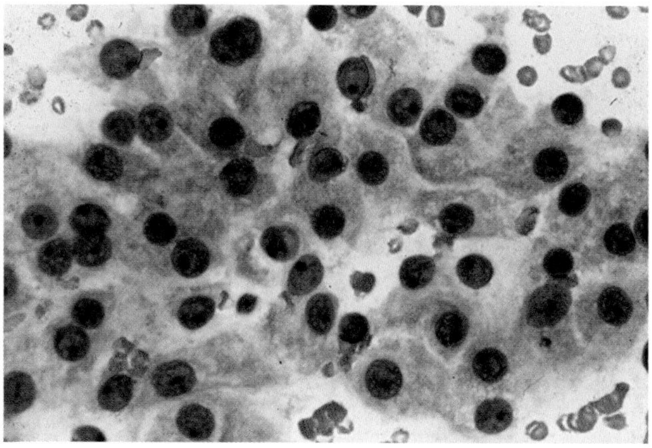

(E)

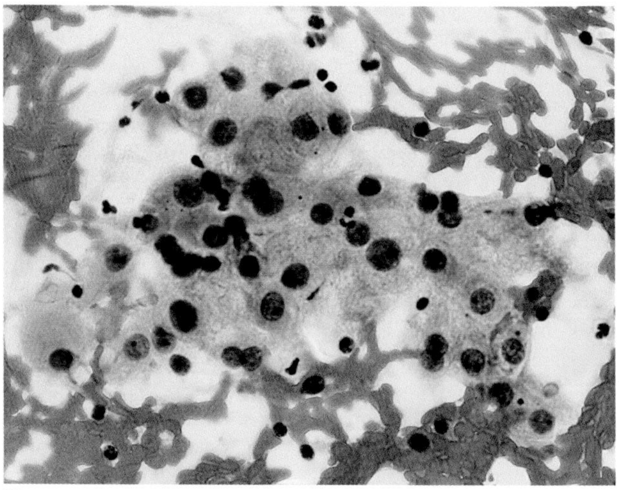

(F)

Figure 2.42 Acinic cell carcinoma. (A) Well-differentiated ACC. Abundant cohesive cell clusters with cells mimicking normal salivary gland cells. Nuclei are small and regular, cytoplasm fragile, relatively abundant and finely vacuolated (oncocyte-like) containing granules. However, the smears are more cellular than normal salivary gland, nuclei larger and less evenly distributed and the nuclear/cytoplasmic ratio is higher. No ductal epithelium is seen. (B) Resemblance of ACC cells to oncocytes can cause difficulty in distinguishing them from oncocytoma and Warthin's tumour, particularly if there is a prominent lymphoid cell infiltrate in some of the ACCs (MGG ×600 oil, courtesy of Dr A Rubin). (C) Fairly uniform cells in aggregates. (D) Abundant, sometimes vacuolated cytoplasm may be confused with mucoepidermoid carcinoma or adenocarcinoma. ACC lacks the cell pleomorphism of adenocarcinoma and variability of MEC. (E) Intracytoplasmic purple granules may be barely visible or marked as in this case. (F) Pap staining shows better nuclear detail, with prominent nucleoli and granules in the cytoplasm.

identified 1353 cases of ACC [181]. Five-year survival was 83.3% (observed) and 91.4% (disease specific). Worse survival was associated with high grade, age greater or equal to 30 years and the presence of metastatic disease. An aggressive subset of ACC which is characterised by high grade and advanced stage rarely occurs in patients younger than 30 years old. Although better outcome was not statistically demonstrated for combined therapy, surgery with irradiation is the most common management in the United States for cases with regional metastases, high grade and microscopic positive margins [181].

Histologically, ACC can be solid, microcystic, papillary cystic and follicular. According to cell morphology, they can also be classified as well differentiated, composed predominantly of acinic cells, moderately differentiated, containing duct-like, vacuolated or clear cells and poorly differentiated, showing undifferentiated cells. About a half of acinic cell carcinomas exhibit more than one cell pattern. The grade of differentiation influences prognosis. Well-differentiated acinic cell carcinoma is the most common histological type and also has better prognosis (2 years overall survival, 100%; 5 years overall survival, 83%; 10 years overall survival, 50%) than poorly differentiated tumours (2 years overall survival, 70%; 5 years overall survival, 50%; 10 years overall survival, 30%) [182].

Cytological features of a well-differentiated ACC show a characteristically bland picture of cohesive clusters of cells with abundant, fragile, finely vacuolated or granular cytoplasm and an acinar architectural pattern (Fig. 2.42). The cells are similar to acinar cells of normal salivary gland. Cytoplasmic granules are purple with Papanicolaou staining, red with MGG, stain with alcian blue and are PAS positive. Many bare nuclei are often seen in the background. In addition to these diagnostic clue cells, other types of neoplastic cells including vacuolated cells, clear cells, cells resembling oncocytes and non-specific glandular cells may be encountered. A pronounced lymphocytic reaction is a hallmark in some ACCs [182]. Macrophages and debris may be seen in papillary cystic type. Both, the varieties of tumour cell differentiation and the pronounced lymphocytic reaction observed in ACC, might result in confusion with other salivary gland lesions (See Tables 2.3 and 2.4).

The differential diagnosis of ACC encompasses normal salivary gland, epithelial myoepitehlial carcinoma, adenocarcinoma, AdCC, clear cell MEC, cellular PLA, oncocytic neoplasms, sebaceous adenoma and metastatic renal and hepatocellular cell carcinoma [182, 183]. Differentiation from normal salivary gland and acinic cell hyperplasia is by the abundance of acinic cells and the absence of adipocytes, ductal epithelium and the presence of numerous naked nuclei. In the presence of vacuolated/clear acinic cells, epithelial myoepithelial carcinoma (EMC) presents main differential diagnosis. In EMC there is a bimodal population of large 'clear' myoepitehlial cells and clusters of small cuboidal epithelial cells. ACC with duct like glandular structures may resemble adenocarcinoma. In poorly differentiated carcinomas, only a diagnosis of malignancy can be made. Cytoplasmic granules of ACC may help to distinguish the two tumours of different prognosis. Although these are prominent in some tumours, they are not always seen. Small, purple (MGG) intracytoplasmic granules can also be seen in cellular PLA and MEC. Differentiation from the clear cell variant of MEC can be achieved by confirming the intra and extracellular mucin in the former. Differentiation from oncocytic type neoplasm, including Warthin's, can be made through analysis of cell borders, which are not as sharp in ACC, by the cell arrangement in acinar structures rather than in flat sheets and by the absence of amorphous debris

in ACC. Cystic variants of ACC have to be differentiated from other tumours with cystic components; Warthin's, PLA, intraduct papilloma and MEC.

2.5.2 Mucoepidermoid carcinoma

Mucoepidermoid carcinoma (MEC) is a malignant glandular epithelial neoplasm characterised by mucous, intermediate and epidermoid cells, with columnar, clear cell and oncocytoid features [40]. It is the commonest primary salivary carcinoma worldwide, and as such, its usual histological features are well-known [39].

However, the proportion of the different cell types and their architectural configuration (including cyst formation) vary between cases and sometimes within any individual neoplasm, and this may lead to difficulty in identification. Mucous cells are cuboidal, columnar or goblet-like and form solid masses or line cysts in one or more layers. Mucus-filled cysts may rupture and elicit an inflammatory response. Epidermoid cells usually have intercellular bridges, but keratinisation in definite cases of MEC is exceptionally rare. Intermediate cells are usually small with dark-staining nuclei but can be larger with a clear cytoplasm. There are several relatively uncommon histological variants: a clear cytoplasm may be seen in either the squamous or intermediate cells, and MEC may thus take the form of a clear cell tumour. Similarly, oncocytes can be plentiful and even bland spindle cells have been reported. A sclerosing variant has been described, with some examples containing numerous IgG4-positive plasma cells; none of these patients had systemic IgG4-related sclerosing disease [184]. Histological grading is agreed to be prognostically useful, but there is no consensus as to the best scheme [185].

Other techniques of prognostic value include the Ki-67 index [186]. and the differential expression of membrane-bound mucins, MUC4 and MUC1 [187].

Molecular genetics: Most cases of MEC harbour one of two recurrent translocations, either t(11;19)(q21;p13) resulting in a fusion of the genes, CRTC1 (also known as MECT1, TORC1 or WAMP1) to MAML2 or in a small number of mutually exclusive cases t(11;15)(q21;q26) leading to a CRTC3- MAML2 fusion these appear to be specific to MEC and are not seen in, for example, metaplastic Warthin's tumour [188, 189]. The median survival of 'fusion-positive' patients appears to be better than those without it, but at present, molecular assessment should not supplant histological grading as a prognostic marker [190, 191].

The therapy of choice is a radical ablative surgery of the primary tumour and resection of the related lymphatic system in patients suspected of having metastases of the regional lymph nodes. The prognosis is excellent in patients with a localised manifestation of the disease only. Patients who die for reasons of tumour metastases had all been classified as stage III or IV at the time of initial diagnosis. Distant metastases are rarely found even decades after surgical therapy, therefore a long-term follow-up is recommended [192].

It is useful to have an appreciation of the **US appearances** of MEC. Although a malignant tumour, it can show features that suggest it is benign – such as well-defined margins – however, the feature that may lead to misdiagnosis is the presence of cystic change. This can both complicate interpretation – the appearance is similar to a sialocele or benign salivary cyst – and FNAC may not be helpful either – particularly if mainly the cystic area is sampled. In this case the cytopathologist may only have scanty material and can be misled by the ultrasound impression that the lesion is benign (See Table 2.3, a and b).

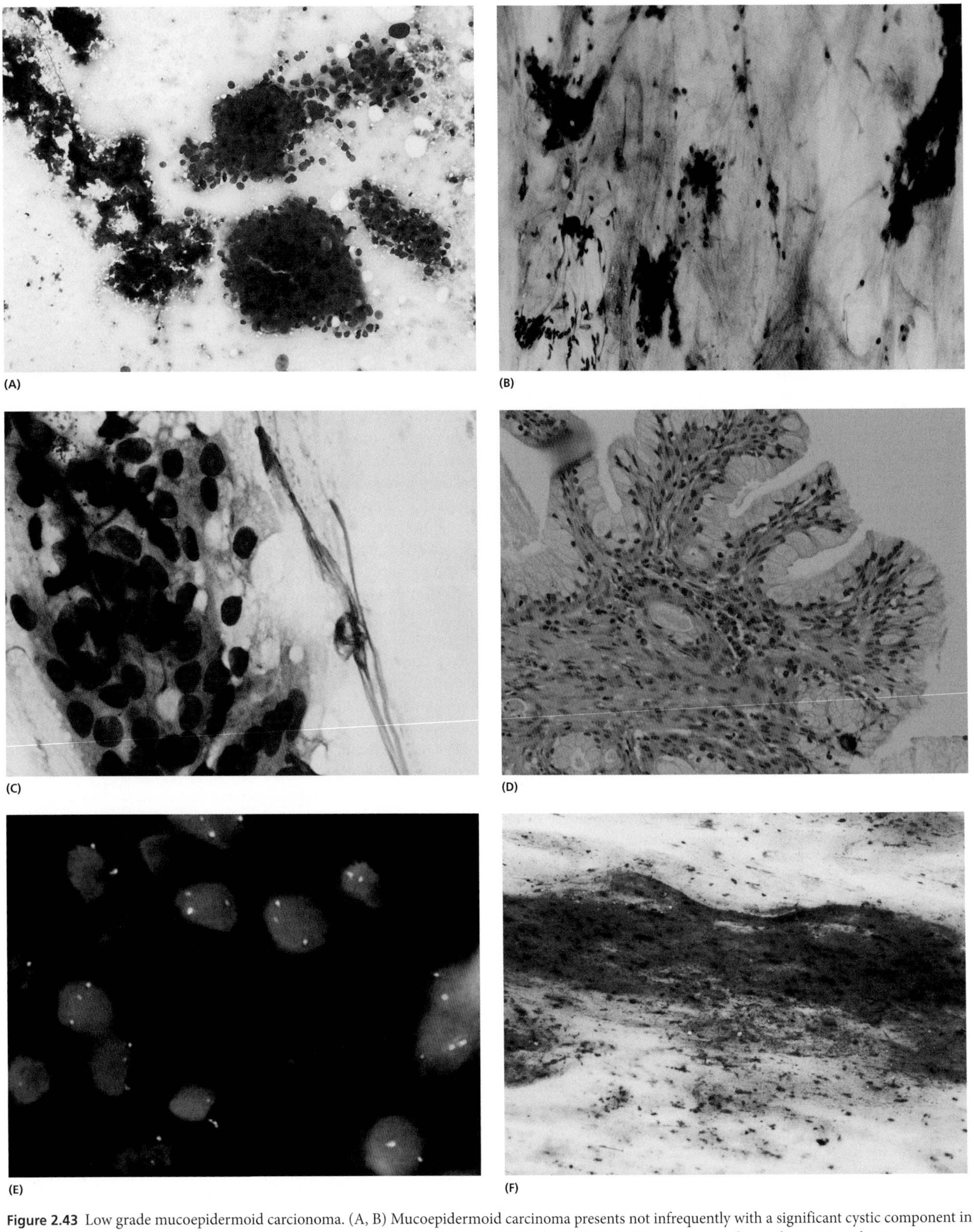

(A)

(B)

(C)

(D)

(E)

(F)

Figure 2.43 Low grade mucoepidermoid carcionoma. (A, B) Mucoepidermoid carcinoma presents not infrequently with a significant cystic component in which debris, macrophages, cholesterol crystals are seen as well the epithelium. (C) The epithelial cells are sparse and may show minimal or no atypia. Intracytoplasmic vacuoles may be seen and are helpful in making a diagnosis. (D) histological section of this tumour shows mucoepidermoid carcinoma with cyst lining epithelium appearing very bland, mucin secreting. (E) Mucoepidermoid carcinoma: FISH analysis using break apart rearrangement probe, VysisZytoLight SPEC MAML2 DualColor Break Apart Probe (11q21) nuclei with one fusion (yellow), one orange and one green (split) signal pattern indicative of arrangement of one copy of the MAML2 gene region. (Source: Simpson RHW et al. [169]). (F) MEC case that was misdiagnosed as a non specific cystic lesion because it contained only necrotic debris and mucinous background. Cases with an apparently unexplained mucinous and necrotic background should be discussed at multidisciplinary meetings.

Cytological features. Of the common salivary gland tumours, MEC is probably the most difficult to diagnose accurately by FNAC. Different cell types and degrees of differentiation make for a variety of cytological presentations with a result that there are no specific diagnostic features of MEC but rather a combination of cellular and background features that may lead to a correct diagnosis. A combination of squamous and mucin secreting epithelium is thought to be diagnostic of MEC. However, this may sometimes be difficult to prove, especially in cystic lesions. Cohen et al. used three cytological features as most predictive of MEC. These were: intermediate cells, squamous cells and overlapping epithelial groups. Using these three features together, they achieved the sensitivity and specificity of accurately diagnosing MEC of 97% and 100%, respectively [193]. Other reports differentiate between the sensitivity of FNACs diagnosis for high and intermediate grade (87 and 85%, respectively) and low grade tumours where sensitivity is lower (68%) [194].

The presence of intermediate, squamous and vacuolated, mucin producing cells in flat sheets or clusters against a background of mucus and debris is usually found in low-grade tumours (Fig. 2.43). Cells may look bland and if there is predominance of intermediate (metaplastic) cells they may look rather oncocytic, therefore the features may be mistaken for a benign cystic lesion, for example Warthin's tumour. High-grade tumours have more obvious features of malignancy with overlapping, crowding and prominent nucleoli but may be difficult to type (Fig. 2.44). Cells are variably squamoid, vacuolated or have clear cytoplasm, probably due to glycogen. Intermediate cells from tissue sections correspond to the metaplastic looking cells in smears.

Wade et al. tried to identify morphological features that may be useful in the FNAC diagnosis of MEC [60]. They assessed for percentage cystic component, extracellular mucin, mucous and intermediate cells, oncocytes, cells with foamy/clear cytoplasm, keratinised cells and lymphocytes. On FNAC 12/23 (52%) cases were diagnosed as consistent with or suggestive of MEC; 6/23 (26%) as salivary gland neoplasm and 5/23 (22%) as no tumour seen. The cystic component was >/=50% in 18/23 (78%) and <50% in 5 cases. The features prevalent in FNAC and histology were: mucous cells (96 and 91%), extracellular mucin (91% both), intermediate cells (100 and 83%), lymphocytes (96 and 78%) and cells with foamy/clear cytoplasm (74% both). (see Table 2.5) Oncocytes were seen in 43 and 22% and keratinised cells in 48 and 13% cases. Cases with oncocytes and lymphocytes were interpreted as favouring Warthin's tumour on FNAC. Presence of mucous cells, cells with foamy/clear cytoplasm, intermediate cells and lymphocytes in a mucinous background are diagnostic indicators of MEC; presence of oncocytes should not refrain from diagnosing MEC in FNAC specimens. The most helpful features in differentiating MEC containing oncocytic cells from other salivary gland lesions in FNAC specimens is the presence of extracellular mucin, mucous cells and pseudogoblet/clear cells [60].

Differential diagnosis of MEC includes other squamous lesions, oncocytic tumours, ACC and other cystic tumours. High-grade tumours are difficult to distinguish from other poorly differentiated primary or metastatic tumours. The nuclei of salivary duct carcinoma have abundant, dense, eosinophilic cytoplasm, which can be mistaken for squamous differentiation. Cystic MEC may resemble benign lesions eg mucus retention cysts, inflammatory processes with squamous metaplasia, mucus and debris, lymphoepithelial cysts, cystadenomas, Warthin's tumours, cystic PLAs, cystadenocarcinomas and polycystic disease of the parotid gland.

Careful attention to the cellular elements present often allowed definitive cytological diagnosis, with an overall accuracy rate of 84%(see Table 2.3a, b and Table 2.6) [139]. Aspirates of low-grade MEC may contain no epithelial cells and result in false-negative diagnoses (1 case, 2%) [139]. Lymphocytic infiltrate may be prominent within MEC making distinction from benign conditions difficult. Oncocytic change within the MEC is rare and only a few cases have been reported [60, 142, 195]. Oncocytic change is not typically a prominent feature of MEC of the salivary glands. Because most salivary gland lesions with oncocytic change are benign, it is important to distinguish MEC from other entities that may show prominent oncocytic change. MEC arising in Warthin's tumour has been described [146]. Since oncocytic change is said to be occasionally a consequence of previous FNAC and/or electrocautery, caution in interpreting the oncocytic change in an inappropriate background is needed [23, 143]. Mammary analog secretory carcinoma (MASC) should be included in the differential diagnosis of mucinous salivary lesions with cystic changes on FNAC. Immunohistochemistry for mammaglobin and S-100 helps in excluding morphologic mimics. FISH helps to confirm the diagnosis. (See Table 2.5) Age alone should not be a deterrent in diagnosing a carcinoma [196].

MEC ex PLA may cytologically present as non-specific high-grade malignancy and consist of highly malignant cells, in clusters or isolated, rarely associated with intracellular and extracellular mucin. A background of cellular and stromal elements consistent with PLA can be identified. Although it is nearly impossible cytologically to distinguish these lesions from other high grade primary or metastatic carcinomas (such as poorly differentiated squamous cell carcinomas, adenosquamous carcinomas, and salivary duct carcinomas), this limitation is not dramatic. Cytological diagnosis of high grade malignancy per se allows for proper preoperative patient management [197].

Prognostic features: Clinical features associated with metastasis or death are: more advanced age, tumour size and preoperative symptoms. Histopathological features that correlate with poor outcome are: cystic component less than 20%, four or more mitotic figures per 10 high-power fields, neural involvement, necrosis, and anaplasia. Patients with tumours of equal histopathological grade have a better prognosis when their tumours are in the parotid gland than when their tumours are in the submandibular gland. Molecular prognostic factors have been discussed earlier under the 'molecular genetics' section.

Although the role of cytopathologist in the primary diagnosis may be difficult, the knowledge of the possible pitfalls may prevent missing a neoplasm in the first instance, particularly in the low-grade tumours. In the cases of diagnostic staging or recurrence, FNAC diagnosis should not pose any problems. It can offer a valuable service ensuring that these relatively indolent tumours are cured.

Table 2.6 Key morphological featurs of mucoepidermoid carcinoma observed in histology and FNA specimens.

Cell type observed	% in Histology	% in FNA
Mucous (pseudogoblet) cells	(22/23) 96%	(21/23) 91%
Lymphocytes	(22/23) 96%	(18/23) 78%
Clear cells	(17/23) 74%	(17/23) 74%
Intermediate cells	(23/23) 100%	(19/23) 83%
Keratinized squamous cells	(11/23) 48%	(3/23) 13%
Oncocytes	(10/23) 43%	(5/23) 22%

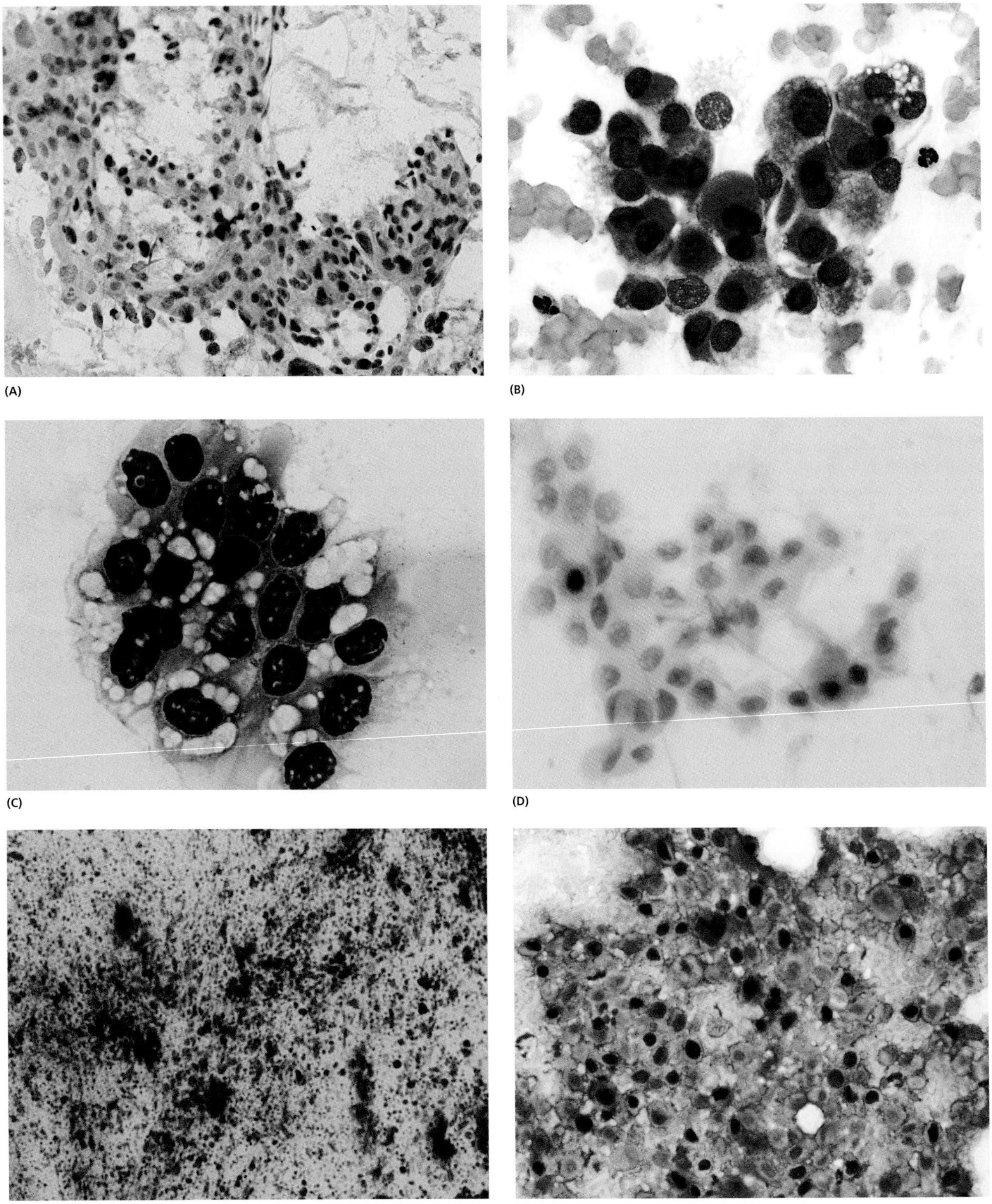

(A)

(B)

(C)

(D)

(E)

(F)

Figure 2.44 High grade mucoepidermoid carcinoma. (A) Low power view shows obvious features of malignancy, pleomorphism, overlapping and crowding. (B, C, D) High power view shows intermediate, vacuolated cells and squamoid cells, with features of malignancy. Mucin secreting vacuolated cells are a useful pointer to the diagnosis in some cases. (E, F) Background is often composed of necrosis and apoptotic cell debris.

2.5.3 Adenoid cystic carcinoma

Adenoid cystic carcinoma (AdCC) is defined as 'a basaloid tumour consisting of epithelial and myoepithelial cells in variable morphological configurations, including *tubular, cribriform and solid patterns*. It has a relentless clinical course and usually a fatal outcome [198]. A system of three histological grades has been shown to be of prognostic value; this is based on the relative proportions of tubular, cribriform and solid patterns, particularly the latter; grade 3 is defined as when the solid component exceeds 30–50% of the tumour. Nevertheless, clinical stage still appears to be a better predictor than grade [169].

The incidence of lymph node metastases is low, ranging 5–15% of cases. Patients may present with facial nerve paresis since tumour often involves nerves.

[See BOX 2.5. Summary of ultrasound features: Adenoid Cystic Carcinoma on www.wiley.com/go/kocjan/clinical_cytopathology_head_neck2e]

US features of AdCC can vary according to the grade of the neoplasm, from indolent to aggressive. The former has more benign features whereas the latter is often diffusely infiltrating throughout the salivary gland – often with a markedly hypoechoic echogenicity – sometimes extending to the skin. AdCC is often associated with perineural spread and features of nerve involvement may be seen clinically or at US at the time of presentation. In the parotid this involves a facial nerve palsy and in the submandibular region atrophy of the anterior belly of digastrics and mylohyoid muscles may be seen.

Despite the variability in its consistency, one noticeable feature at US FNAC is that these tumours are often woody hard to pass the needle, which can make it difficult to obtain a cellular specimen (Fig. 2.45). On occasion, a core biopsy may be needed to establish the diagnosis. In addition, these tumours are often quite painful.

Cytological features of AdCC are most characteristically seen as large hyaline globules of extracellular matrix (basement membrane

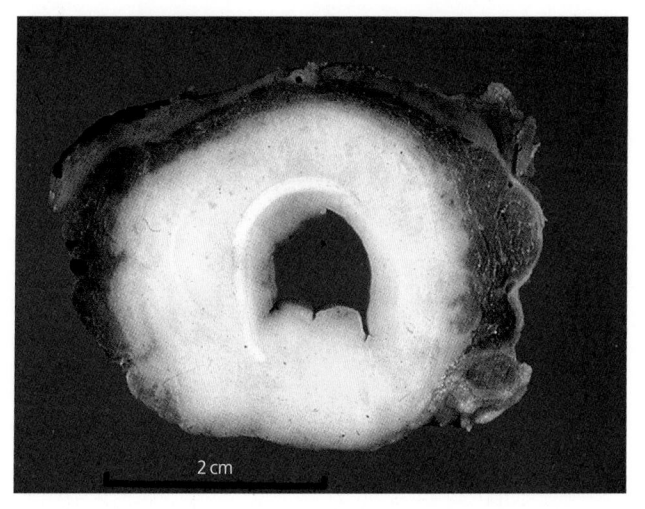

Figure 2.45 Section of larynx showing adenoid cystic carcinoma in a 27-year-old woman. CT scan was suggesting an unusual infiltrate in the larynx (?soft tissue?amyloid). FNAC was performed transcutaneously tangential to trachea. Diagnosis of adenoid cystic carcinoma was made. Patient underwent laryngectomy with the intent of surgical cure.

material), staining red/magenta (MGG) or green (Papanicolaou), partially surrounded by basaloid tumour cells (Fig. 2.46). The hyaline globules may vary considerably in size. Basement membrane material, as well as in hyaline globules, is seen in finger-like structures with naked nuclei. Cylindrical structures containing naked nuclei, closely cohesive in the middle of the cylinder and dissociated at each end are thought to be characteristic (Fig. 2.46D) [199]. Basaloid cells are tightly cohesive or single, with uniform oval or round nuclei, coarse chromatin and very scanty or absent cytoplasm. Nuclei may be hyperchromatic with prominent nucleoli, particularly in the poorly differentiated tumours without hyaline globules. When hyaline globules are present in large numbers, a diagnosis of AdCC can confidently be made [200]. However, hyaline globules are not always present, particularly in the solid type (Fig. 2.47). Hyaline globules are not pathognomonic for AdCC. They can be seen in basal cell adenoma, epithelial myoepitehlial carcinoma and polymorphous low-grade carcinoma. In FNACs with predominance of basaloid tumour cells, but lacking characteristic globules, all other benign and malignant salivary gland tumours of epithelial-myoepithelial differentiation should be considered in the cytological diagnosis [201].

Pleomorphic adenoma (PLA) is the tumour most frequently confused with AdCC. The best way to distinguish AdCC from PLA is the much higher Ki-67 proliferation index in the former [202] Morphological differentiation between AdCC and PLA could be attempted by observing the amount of cytoplasm of individual tumour cells. Plasmacytoid appearance is a reliable finding for PLA, and it enables to rule out AdCC [26]. In contrast with PLA, most AdCCs show little cytoplasm. Hyaline spherical globules are specific but not sensitive for diagnosis of AdCC. They are found in 80% of AdCCs but only rarely in PLA [199]. Fibrillary chondromyxoid ground substance and a mixture of epithelial cells with stroma are found in the majority of the PLAs. The pattern of cell clusters is helpful to differentiate PLA from AdCC. Large, loose clusters with a spindle cell core suggest PLA. Small, dense trabeculae with a smooth margin and dense clusters containing clear, round spaces are more suggestive of AdCC. Overall cellularity, proportion of isolated cells, orientation of cellular clusters and degree of cellular overlapping give almost no help in making the distinction between the lesions.

Distinction from rare neoplasms of salivary glands with epithelial-myoepithelial cell differentiation, including basal-cell adenoma and carcinoma, epithelial-myoepithelial carcinoma, and polymorphous low-grade adenocarcinoma, as well as some non-salivary gland neoplasms presenting an adenoid cystic pattern, for example dermal sweat gland tumours such as pilomatrixoma, must be considered in differential diagnosis of AdCC. Distinction from basal cell adenoma may be difficult and includes cell arrangement and the features of the background. Hyaline globules can be present in both tumours (trabecular type of basal cell adenoma) [203]. Differentiation from an EMC is made on the basis of characteristic appearance of EMC with three-dimensional cellular aggregates of basaloid cells, which are clear at the periphery. Given the ultrastructural similarities between the EMC and AdCC (both tumours produce excess basal lamina at the margins of cellular nests and widened intercellular spaces contain reduplicated basal lamina and accumulations of glycosaminoglycans) as well as not infrequent histomorphological 'hybrid' tumours; the distinction may be difficult on cytology alone [204]. Distinction from polymorphous low-grade carcinoma may be difficult since the

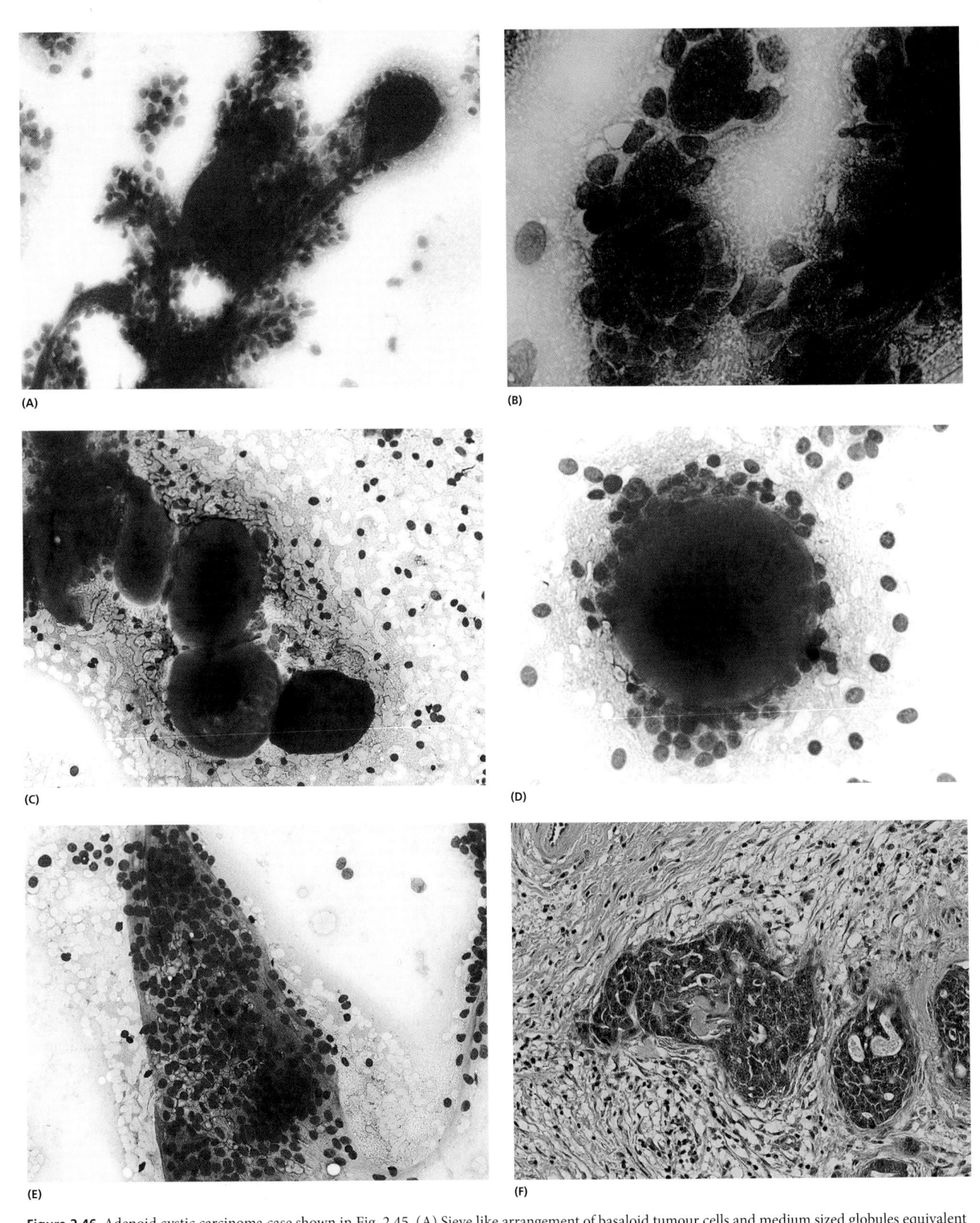

(A)

(B)

(C)

(D)

(E)

(F)

Figure 2.46 Adenoid cystic carcinoma case shown in Fig. 2.45. (A) Sieve like arrangement of basaloid tumour cells and medium sized globules equivalent to the cribriform histological pattern. (B) Basaloid tumour cells arranged in rosette-like formations surrounding small homogenous globules (MGG ×100). (C) Globules of hyaline material of various size presenting as a matrix structure. (D) Another case. Cylindrical structures with concentrations of nuclei at either end representing stromal fragments partially surrounded and containing basaloid tumour cells. (E) Finger-like reddish structures with low concentration of naked nuclei. (F) Histology of adenoid cystic carcinoma.

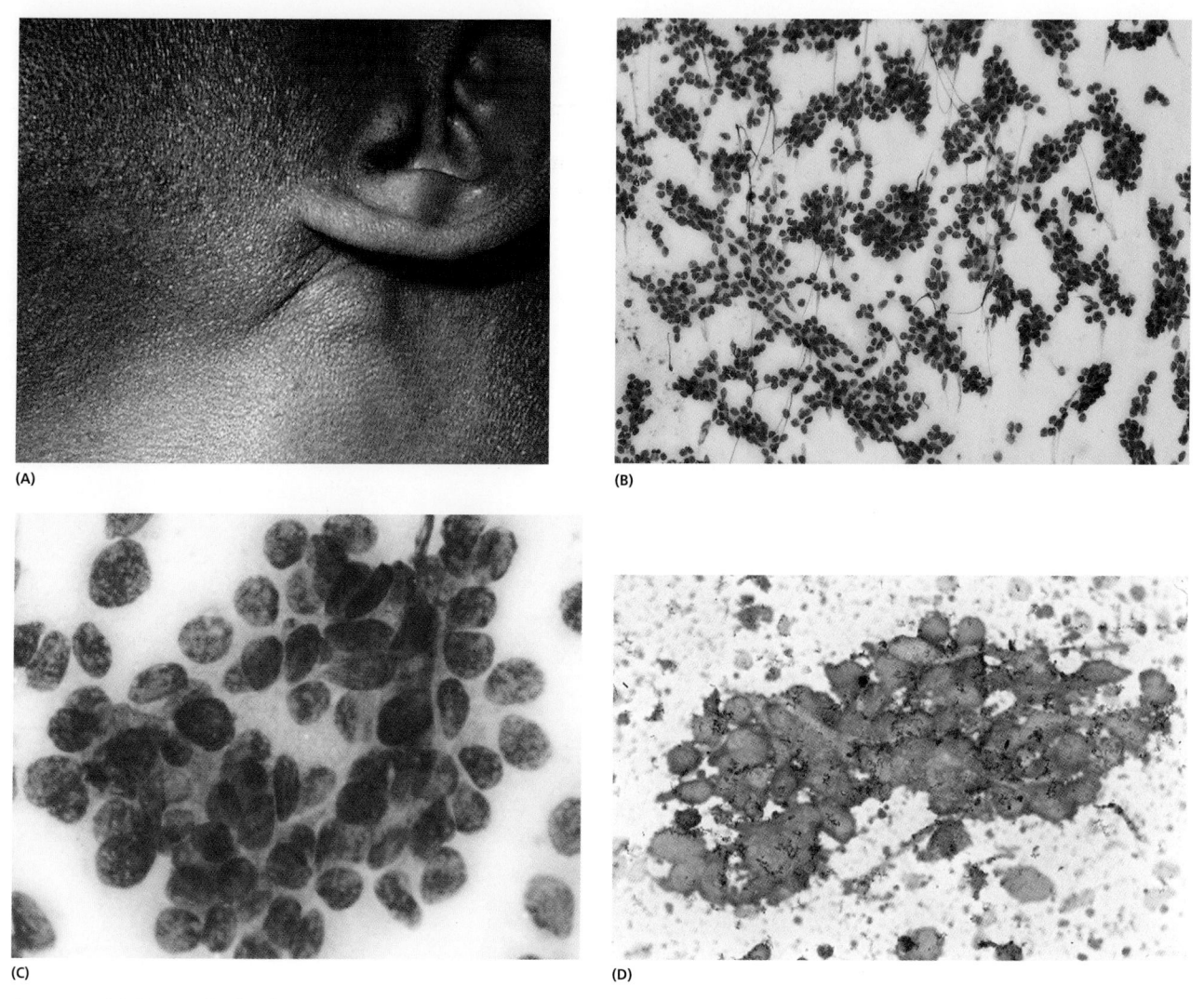

Figure 2.47 (A) Salivary gland malignant tumour. Patient with a 4-month history of swelling at the left angle of mandible. Mass was adherent to surrounding tissues with skin pulling. Facial nerve paralysis was present. (B) FNAC showed features of adenoid cystic carcinoma: Basaloid tumour cells with no globules or hyaline stroma (MGG ×400). Clinical features were helpful in diagnosing malignancy. (C) Basal cells show overlapping and crowding and irregular chromatin pattern but these features are subtle and may be difficult to distinguish from other tumours containing basal cells (see text) (MGG ×600, oil). (D) Laminin positivity for basement membrane material is helpful but non specific. Smooth muscle and calponin may be helpful.

tumour has small to medium-sized, regular cells without nuclear atypia. It occurs more frequently in the palate. Although both tumours are malignant, AdCC has a more aggressive behaviour. Immunocytochemistry for smooth muscle and calponin markers may be helpful in distinguishing the two. Poorly differentiated AdCC can be mistaken for anaplastic carcinoma and metastatic carcinoma.

Immunocytochemistry using three novel smooth muscle-specific proteins, alpha-smooth muscle actin, smooth muscle myosin heavy chains and calponin, may be helpful in cases where myoepitehlial differentiation needs to be established. In benign and malignant salivary gland tumours. In AdCCs and epithelial-myoepithelial carcinomas, all three markers exclusively highlight the myoepithelial cell components and the epithelial cells are entirely negative. No immunostaining is detected in canalicular adenomas, oncocytomas, Warthin tumours, ACC, MEC, squamous cell carcinomas, and polymorphous low-grade adenocarcinomas. Salivary duct carcinomas and adenocarcinomas, not otherwise specified, have a distinctive pattern of uniform periductal staining of reactive myofibroblastic cells, and in salivary duct carcinomas some ducts retain a peripheral immunoreactive myoepithelial cell layer.

Immunoreactivity for these three smooth muscle-specific proteins confirms the known neoplastic myoepithelial component of AdCCs and EMC. The consistently positive staining pattern in AdCCs may be diagnostically useful in discriminating histologically and cytologically similar but consistently negative polymorphous low-grade adenocarcinomas. Periductal linear staining in adenocarcinoma, not otherwise specified and salivary duct carcinomas is distinctive and appears to represent a tight cuff of myofibroblasts associated with the infiltrating glands [205].

More recently, Stenman and others have shown a recurrent translocation t(6;9)(q22–23;p23–24) in at least 80– 90 % of cases of AdCC [206]. This consistently results in a fusion of the MYB oncogene to the transcription factor NFIB, leading to overexpression of MYB-NFIB fusion proteins. The importance of this is that MYB plays an important role in the control of cell proliferation, apoptosis and differentiation. In contrast, the MYB-NFIB fusion has not been found in any carcinomas of the salivary glands other than AdCC, confirming the high specificity of the MYB-NFIB fusion for AdCC [207] and its possible use as a diagnostic bio-marker in distant metastases (Table 2.5) [208].

Diagnostic accuracy of FNAC of AdCC, as analysed in several large studies, is 84% with 13.7% of tumours diagnosed as benign [209].

2.5.4 Polymorphous low grade adenocarcinoma

Polymorphous low-grade adenocarcinoma of the salivary glands is a low grade neoplasm that occurs almost exclusively in the oral cavity [210]. In this site it is amenable to biopsy and histological diagnosis. However, experience with FNAC findings in these tumours is limited. Although they are well circumscribed and appear clinically benign, they lack capsule and show local invasion [211]. The rate of local invasion and lymph node metastases is 17% and 9%, respectively [212]. Histologically, polymorphous low-grade carcinoma is composed of variety of morphological patterns, including tubular, solid, fascicular and cribriform areas [213]. Tumour cells are regular with small cuboidal and short spindle cells and exhibit variation of both, cellular nature and architecture between and within the tumours.

Cytological features, originally described as terminal duct carcinoma, show hypercellular smears with branching papillae,

sheets and clusters composed of bland uniform cells with round-to-oval nuclei, dispersed chromatin, and absent or inconspicuous nucleoli. The cells have a scant-to-moderate amount of eosinophilic cytoplasm. Mitoses and nuclear pleomorphism are absent (Fig. 2.48). These cells form tubular structures containing hyaline globules and often a dispersed myxohyaline stroma. Bare nuclei also frequently appeared in the background [214, 215]. In addition, short, spindle shaped myoepithelial-like cells with ill-defined cell borders may be present. Stromal fragments may be present. Cytological diagnosis of malignancy can be established in 83% of cases [215]. Tyrosine-rich crystalloids may be seen [216].

Differential diagnosis includes PLA and myoepithelioma. The cellular variant of PLA is the one that is most difficult to distinguish from polymorphous low-grade carcinoma. Both tumours have cuboidal and spindle shaped cells with various amounts of myxoid but not chondromatous material. The nuclear atypia of cellular PLA may be the same or greater than in polymorphous low-grade carcinoma. The finding of pallisading short spindle cells around myxoid material may be pointing towards polymorphous low grade

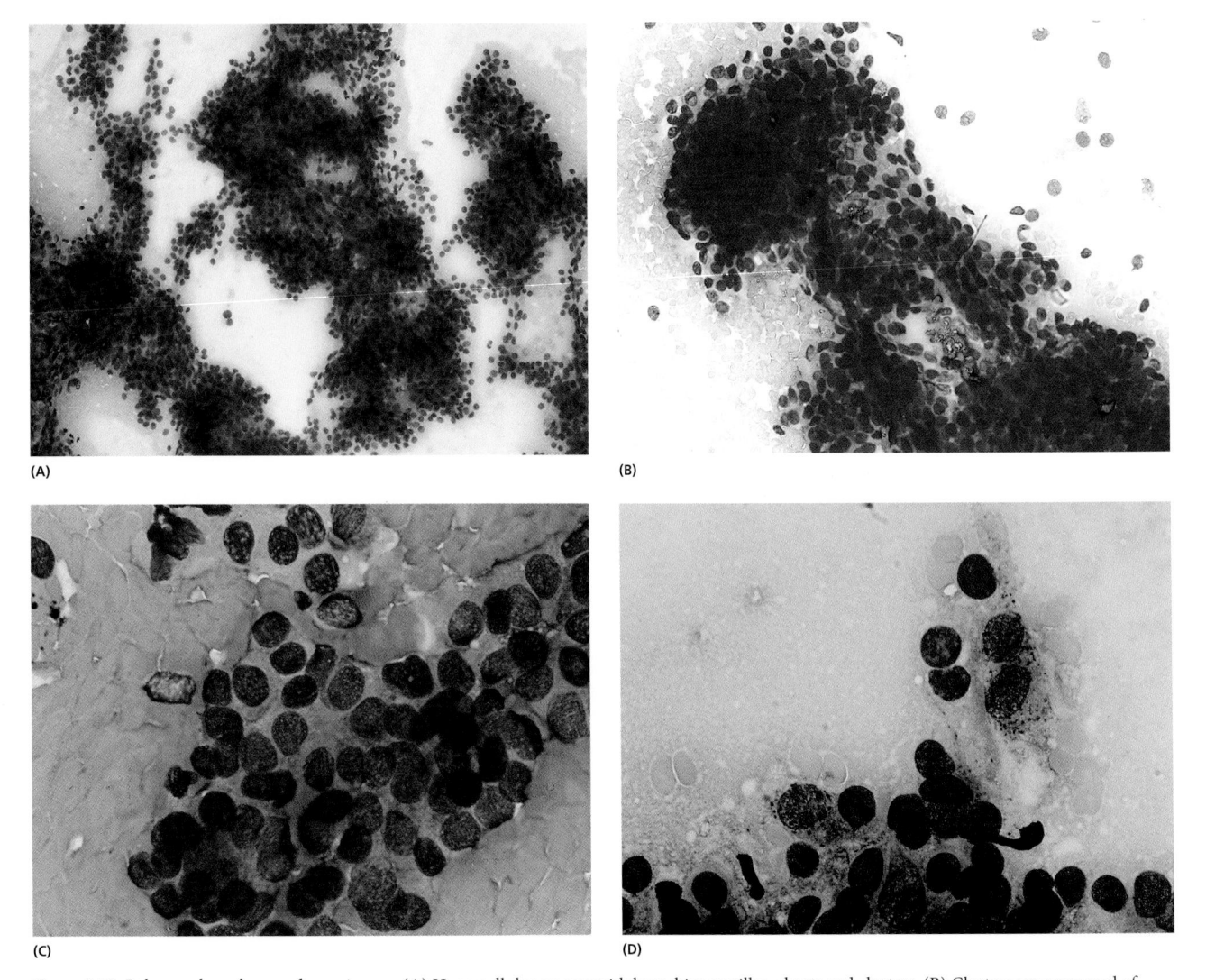

(A)　　(B)　　(C)　　(D)

Figure 2.48 Polymorphous low grade carcinoma. (A) Hypercellular smears with branching papillae, sheets and clusters. (B) Clusters are composed of bland uniform cells with round-to-oval nuclei, dispersed chromatin, and absent or inconspicuous nucleoli. (C) The cells have a scant-to-moderate amount of eosinophilic cytoplasm. Mitoses and nuclear pleomorphism are absent. These cells form tubular structures containing hyaline globules and often a dispersed myxohyaline stroma. (D) Bare nuclei also frequently appeared in the background.

carcinoma because the myxoid material of PLA is conventionally present around the cell clusters or intimately intermingled with the tumour, sometimes as hyaline globules [217]. Myoepithelioma is composed mainly of spindle and plasmacytoid cells. The nuclei of myoepithelioma are more elongated and smaller than those in polymorphous low-grade carcinoma. Clusters of cuboidal cells are not seen in myoepithelioma.

2.5.5 Epithelial myoepithelial carcinoma

Epithelial-myoepithelial carcinoma (EMC) is a rare low-grade salivary gland neoplasm, with an incidence of less than 1%, that occurs in both major and minor salivary glands. The majority of these tumours arise in the parotid in women with a peak incidence from the sixth to the eighth decade [218]. There is preponderance of females. Although they are thought to be of low-grade malignancy, epithelial myoepitehlial carcinomas are locally aggressive, with recurrence rate of 37% and fatal courses have been described [219, 221].

Histologically, EMC shows a high degree of differentiation. It typically has a multinodular growth pattern with islands of tumour separated by dense fibrous connective tissue. These tumour masses are composed of well-defined tubules lined by two layers of cells: outer cells are large clear with variable amount of glycogen, inner cells are small, cuboidal and eosinophilic. Perineural invasion and necrosis are occasionally seen. In some cases, this biphasic pattern is less apparent with solid masses of clear cells. Electron microscopic and immunohistochemical studies confirm the epithelial and myoepithelial differentiation [221]. Immunoreactivity of smooth muscle-specific proteins, alpha-smooth muscle actin, smooth muscle myosin heavy chains and calponin, to assess myoepithelial differentiation show that in AdCC and EMC, all three markers exclusively highlight the myoepithelial cell components and the epithelial cells are entirely negative. No immunostaining is detected in canalicular adenomas, oncocytomas, Warthin tumours, ACCs, MECs, squamous cell carcinomas and polymorphous low-grade adenocarcinomas. Salivary duct carcinomas and adenocarcinomas, not otherwise specified, had a distinctive pattern of uniform periductal staining of reactive myofibroblastic cells [205].

Cytological features: The usual type of EMC is characterised by bimodal population dominated by large 'clear' myoepithelial cells and clusters of small cuboidal ductal cells (Fig. 2.49). The

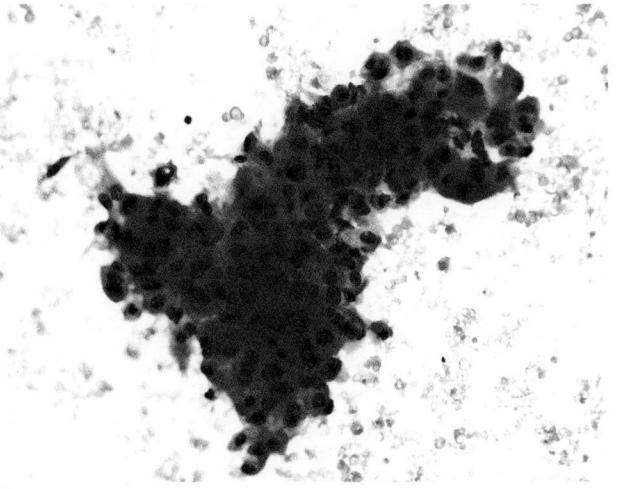

(A)

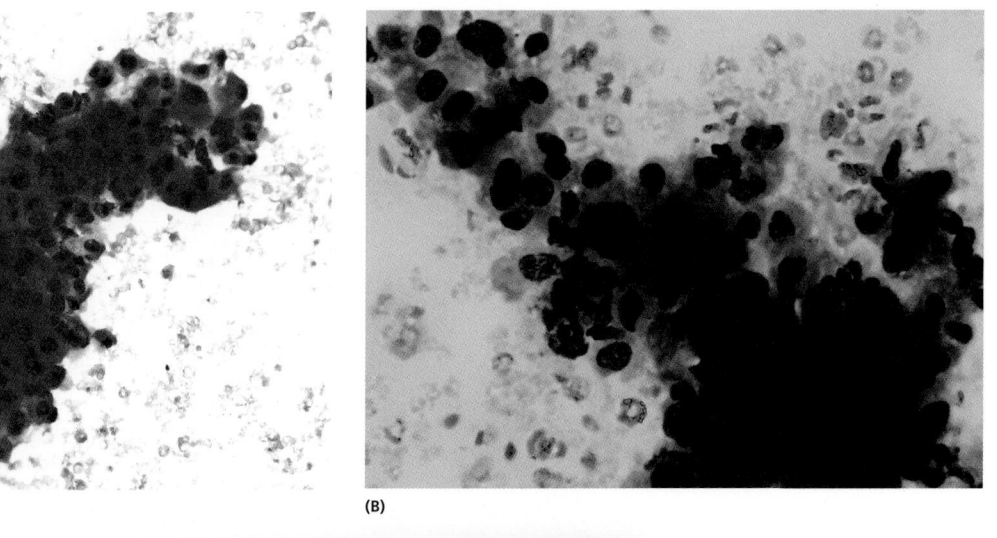

(B)

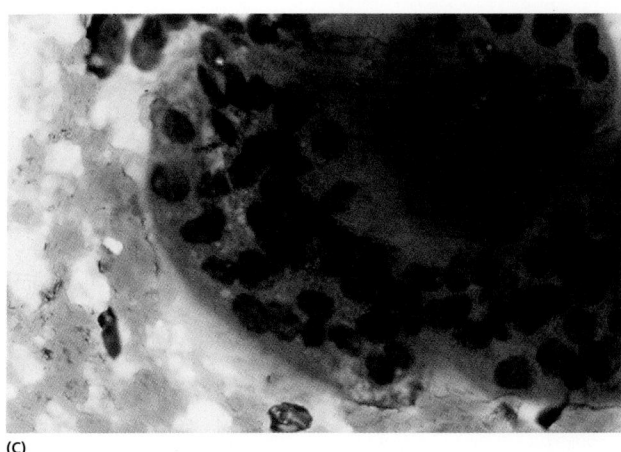

(C)

Figure 2.49 Epithelial myoepithelial carcinoma. (A) Ductal cells showing oncocytic change, tend to form tubules among background sheets of clear myoepithelial cells. (B) Bimodal population dominated by large 'clear' myoepithelial cells and clusters of small cuboidal ductal cells. (C) Tubules are lined by outer cells that are large and contain variable amount of glycogen and inner cells which are cuboidal and eosinophilic. Hyaline, pale homogeneous acellular material surrounding cell clusters is another diagnostic clue. The case was reported on FNAC as pleomorphic adenoma and reviewed after the histological diagnosis was made on the resection specimen. [225]

myoepithelial cells have small, uniform nuclei, ample, clear cytoplasm and distinct cell borders. Ductal cells tend to form tubules among background sheets of clear myoepithelial cells. This feature, if present, was an important diagnostic clue [222]. Hyaline, pale homogeneous acellular material surrounding cell clusters is another diagnostic clue [223]. Focal AdCC-like areas with hyaline globules are commonly present. Immunocytochemistry positivity for S100 would confirm the nature of 'clear' cells. Recently, the cytological features of *ductal-predominant-type* EMC have been described [224]. Depending on the ratio of ductal to myoepithelial cell components, EMC has different cytological presentations.

The differential diagnosis includes PLA, AdCC, and 'clear cell' tumours of the salivary gland: ACC, clear cell oncocytoma, sebaceous carcinoma, MEC, primary clear cell carcinoma, basal cell adenoma and metastatic renal cell carcinoma [5, 40].

EMC is a tumour of low-grade malignancy of duct origin, which should be differentiated from salivary duct carcinoma. While the cytological appearances may closely mimic that of other salivary gland tumours, certain peculiar cytological features may allow a distinction to be made on FNAC [225].

2.5.6 Basal cell adenocarcinoma

Basal cell adenocarcinoma was first introduced as an entity in the second edition of WHO's 'Histological Typing of Salivary Gland Tumours' in 1991. Basal cell adenocarcinoma accounts for about 2.9% of all salivary gland malignancies. More than 90% of the tumours are situated in the parotid gland. Intraoral manifestations are known from case reports only. Tumours of the palate have been mentioned in three cases [226]. Basal cell adenocarcinoma of the parotid gland is a low-grade malignant neoplasm. It has cytological features of basal cell adenoma and a histologically infiltrative growth pattern of malignant tumours with perineural and vascular invasion. Histologically this tumour can be easily confused with basal cell adenoma and the solid basaloid subtype of AdCC (Fig. 2.50).

Cytological features are those of cohesive, focally papillary and filiform groups of neoplastic cells, which are highly reminiscent of basal cell adenoma on low power examination (Figs 2.50, 2.51) [227]. Higher power reveals significant cytological atypia and

mitotic activity. No single cytological feature is thought to unequivocally distinguish this lesion from basal cell adenoma and/or solid variant of AdCC (Figs 2.38, 2.48). Therefore, for diagnostic purposes, Moroz et al. group all three lesions under the term basal cell tumours [228]. Other differential diagnoses include epithelial rich PLA, myoepithelial lesions, small cell undifferentiated carcinoma and metastatic carcinoma. Evaluation of DNA content of tumour cells reveals diploid histograms in both cytological material and paraffin-embedded tissue. Infiltrative tumour nests, the histological basis for differentiating basal cell adenocarcinoma from adenoma, showed the same diploid pattern. Though DNA quantitation may not discriminate basal cell adenoma from basal cell adenocarcinoma, it may prove useful in separating them from AdCC, which is considered to be a tumour with high malignant potential [228].

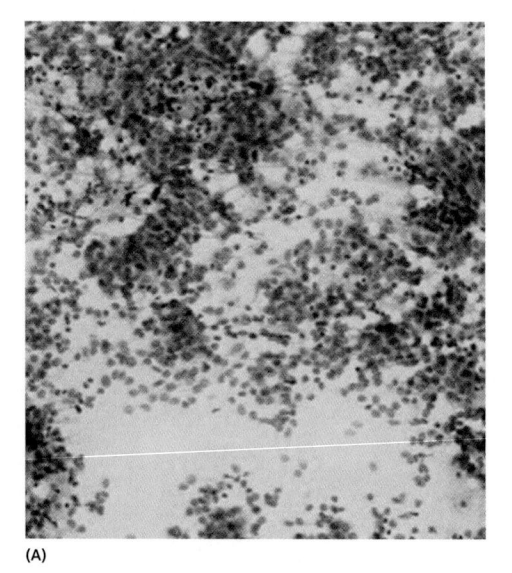

(A)

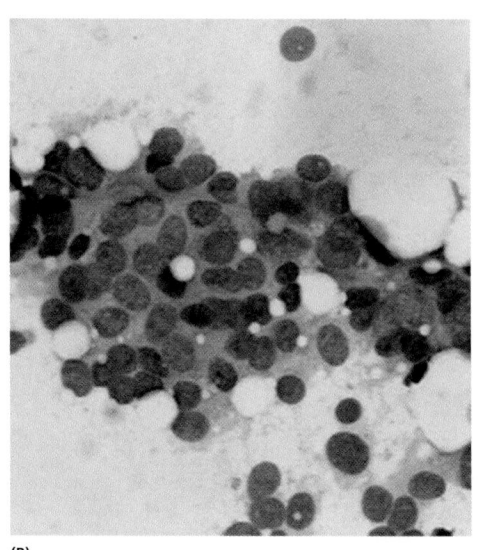

(B)

Figure 2.51 Basal cell carcinoma. (A) Cohesive, focally papillary and filiform groups of neoplastic cells, which are highly reminiscent of basal cell adenoma on low power examination. (B) High power view shows tubular structures with peripheral pallisading. No single cytological feature is thought to unequivocally distinguish this lesion from basal cell adenoma and/or solid variant of AdCC.

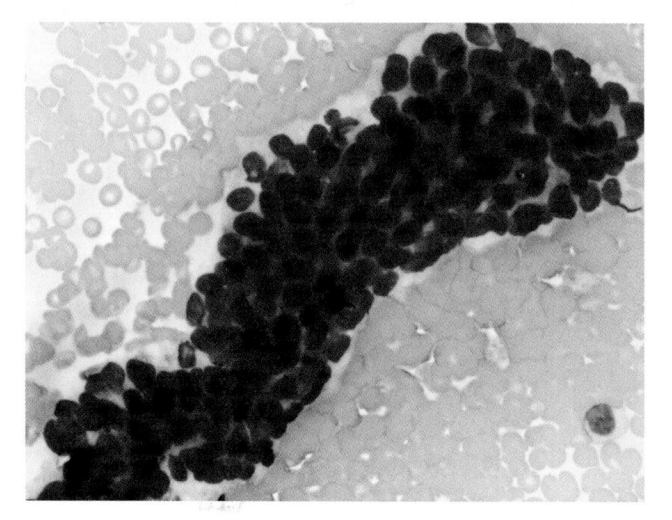

Figure 2.50 Basal cell carcinoma. Local spread of a known basal cell carcinoma helped the diagnosis in this case of FNAC parotid gland where aggregates of small oval cells showed peripheral pallisading.

2.5.7 Papillary cystadenocarcinoma

Salivary gland cystadenocarcinomas represent a distinct group of malignancies that have an indolent biological behaviour [229]. Current classification schemes for salivary gland neoplasms categorise cystadenocarcinomas on the basis of a recurring morphological pattern of cystic, and often, papillary growth without features of other specific types of salivary gland tumours. The tumour affects patients aged 20 to 86 years, and patients aged over 50 years-old account for 71% of cases [230]. Majority of tumours occurs in major salivary glands. Grossly, the lesions are cystic or multicystic masses that range in size from 0.4 to 6.0 cm. Histologically, tumours demonstrate an invasive, cystic growth pattern, and have a conspicuous papillary component. The predominant cell type varies among tumours and includes small cuboidal cells, large cuboidal cells, and tall columnar cells (Fig. 2.52). Cytologically, it may resemble other cystic lesions (see Table 2.3a,b) [139]. Ruptured cysts with haemorrhage and granulation tissue are common. Tumour may recur locally or rarely metastasise to regional lymph nodes.

2.5.8 Mucinous adenocarcinoma

Mucinous adenocarcinoma rarely arises as a primary tumour within the parotid gland, and only one case report of cytological features has been described [231]. Tumour was cystic on computed tomography. FNAC yielded monomorphic, moderately atypical cells, both single and clustered, associated with abundant mucoid material and focal necrosis. Tumour cells had eccentric nuclei, prominent nucleoli and occasional cytoplasmic vacuolisation. A few binucleated and multinucleated tumour cells were present. Histological sections of the resected gland showed mucinous adenocarcinoma. The differential diagnoses on cytology included other primary tumours of the parotid gland producing mucin or a mucoid matrix and metastatic mucinous adenocarcinomas.

2.5.9 Oncocytic carcinoma

Malignant oncocytoma is exceedingly rare salivary gland tumour [232]. Oncocytes are large, apparently swollen epithelial cells with cytoplasm densely filled with eosinophilic granules (see Section 2.3.2). Oncocytic carcinomas appear to arise from benign

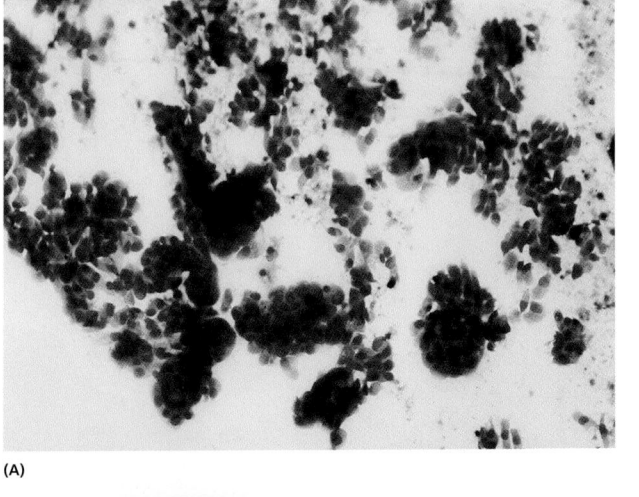

(A)

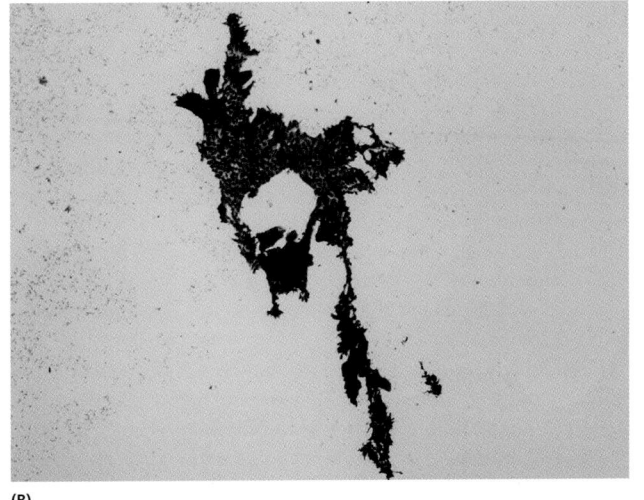

(B)

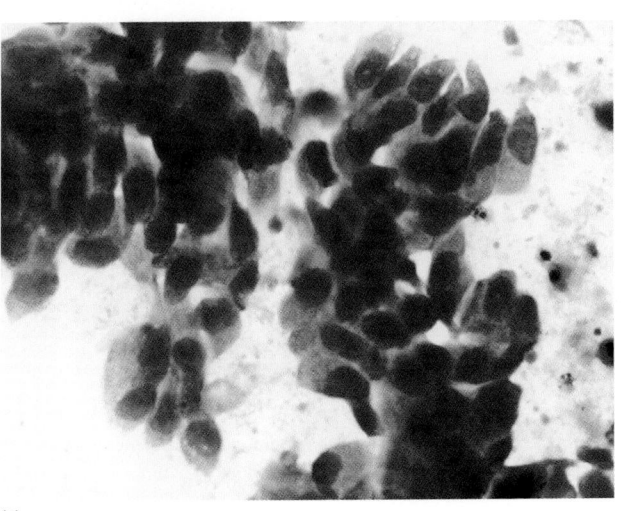

(C)

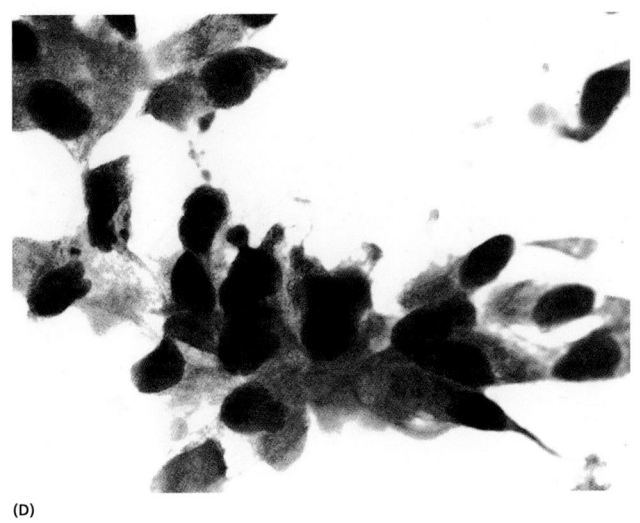

(D)

Figure 2.52 Papillary cystadenocarcinoma. (A) low power view reflects cystic background with epithelial clusters. (B, C, D) Same case. Epithelial cells may appear cuboidal, distinctly columnar or plump rounded (MGG ×400, ×600 oil). Although it is a low grade tumour, malignancy can usually be diagnosed on FNAC.

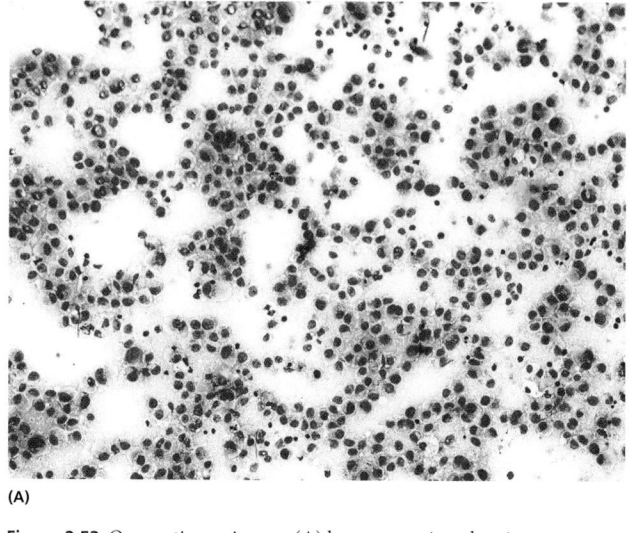

(A)   **(B)**

Figure 2.53 Oncocytic carcinoma. (A) low power view showing numerous single cells, similar to that in oncocytoma (see Fig. 2.39A) (PAP x200). (B) Low power view revels oncocytic cells with characteristic eccentric nuclei and dense cytoplasm (MGG ×200).

oncocytomas, or may also arise *de novo*. In oncocytic carcinoma of the head and neck, the presence of distant, rather than local lymph node metastasis is the most important prognostic indicator [233].

Cytological features show numerous, predominantly dissociated cells with nuclear enlargement and anisonucleosis, prominent nucleoli, multinucleation and abundant homogeneous cytoplasm (Fig. 2.53). This is in contrast with benign oncocytoma in which cells occur in cohesive clusters with well-defined cell borders, small nuclei, bland chromatin pattern and inconspicuous nucleoli (Fig. 2.39).

In the FNAC of oncocytoma, *differential diagnosis* includes Warthin's tumour and malignant oncocytoma. The morphological difficulty in oncocytic lesions is distinguishing between benign and malignant tumours. In a review of literature to include 34 malignant or locally aggressive oncocytomas, Gray set the histological criteria for malignancy as: cellular pleomorphism, frequent mitoses, local lymph node metastases and distant metastases [234].

2.5.10 Salivary duct carcinoma

Salivary duct carcinoma (SDC) is an aggressive adenocarcinoma which microscopically resembles high-grade breast ductal carcinoma, both *in situ* and invasive. It accounts for 4–6% of all salivary carcinomas, most often occurring in parotid glands of males >50 years. More than half develop from a pre-existing PLA. In addition to the usual type, a few uncommon morphological variants have been reported: *papillary, micropapillary, mucin-rich, sarcomatoid and oncocytic.* Unlike most breast cancers, staining for ERa is almost always negative in SDC, but about 80% express androgen receptors (AR), and 15–20% are positive for HER-2 by either immunohistochemistry or FISH. Based on this, SDC can be classified into three molecular subtypes analogous to breast cancer: luminal ARþ; HER2þ (HER2 immunohistochemical expression 3þ, HER2/neu gene amplified); and basal phenotype (AR –, HER2 –, CK5/6þ). SDC is one of the most aggressive salivary malignancies, has a tendency for early metastases leading to death in 60–80% of patients, usually within 5 years [235]. Standard treatment at present is complete surgical excision with radical neck dissection followed by radiotherapy and possibly chemotherapy. The implications of the molecular classification are yet to be realised, but early results show that some ARþ patients respond to anti-androgen therapy and HER2þ tumours to drugs such as trastuzumab [236].

Cytological features can be observed in highly cellular samples. Typically, cells are arranged in clusters or flat sheets with a cribriform pattern and eccentric, round hyperchromatic nuclei, abundant finely granular cytoplasm and necrosis in the smear background (Fig 2.54) [237, 238]. They are similar to comedo type breast carcinoma but may also have predominantly oncocytic features. Cribriform and papillary pattern with necrosis and cystic change are often present. The cytoplasm of well-preserved cells is polygonal, well outlined, basophilic and may contain vacuoles. Oncocytic type cells have ill defined eosinophilic cytoplasm and usually do not show necrosis. Nucleoli may be prominent [239]. The recently described variant of '*low grade salivary duct carcinoma*' shows cells arranged in individual papillary clusters or in complex branching papillae. Cells are medium sized and show minimal cytological atypia. The tumour, in contrast to the salivary duct carcinoma seems biologically indolent.

Differential diagnosis includes high-grade MEC with necrotic background and vacuolated cells, squamous cell carcinoma, metastatic breast carcinoma and oncocytic carcinoma. FNAC can exclude solid type of AdCC, carcinoma ex PLA, undifferentiated carcinoma, myoepitehlial carcinoma and adenosquamous carcinoma [240]. Squamous cell carcinoma with much keratinisation excludes both salivary duct carcinoma and MEC. Oncocytic carcinoma, apart from being very rare, usually does not exhibit such nuclear atypia as salivary duct carcinoma. Salivary duct carcinoma arising on the basis of PLA has been described [241].

Immunocytochemistry of salivary duct carcinoma shows diffuse positivity for epithelial membrane antigen (100%), keratin (AE1/AE3) (88%), Ber-EP4, alpha-lactalbumin (88%), GCDFP-15 (76%), and carcinoembryonic antigen (72%); S-100 protein was rarely detected (4%). Stains for estrogen receptor were uniformly negative [242]. Overexpression of c-ERB B-2 is absent and <5% show immunoreactivity for p53 [243]. Prasad et al. used alpha-smooth muscle actin, smooth muscle myosin heavy chains, and calponin, to assess myoepithelial differentiation. They found periductal linear staining in adenocarcinoma, not otherwise specified and salivary duct carcinomas, which is distinctive and appears to represent a tight cuff of myofibroblasts associated with the infiltrating glands (see epithelial myoepitehlial carcinoma) [205].

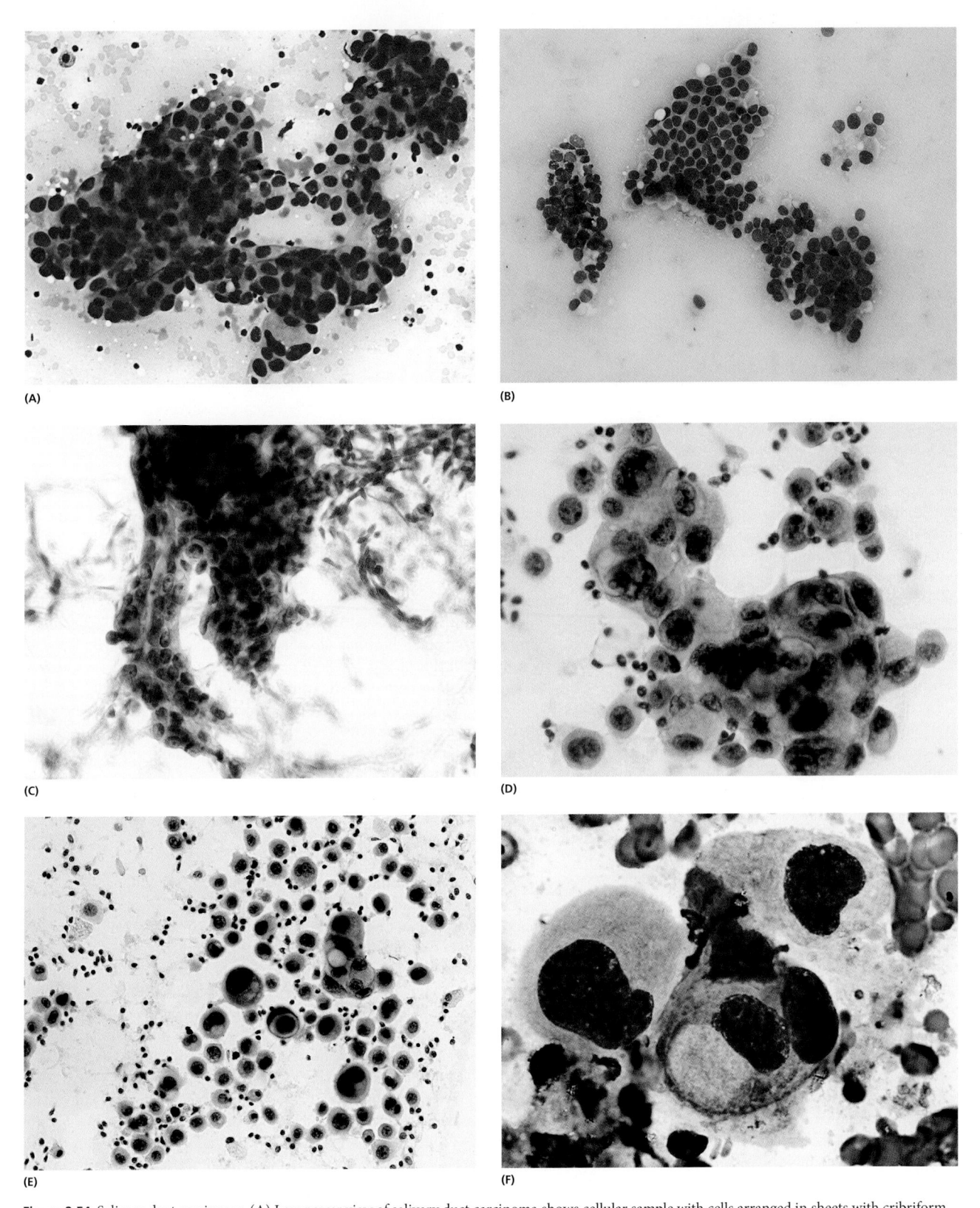

Figure 2.54 Salivary duct carcinoma. (A) Low power view of salivary duct carcinoma shows cellular sample with cells arranged in sheets with cribriform pattern (PAP ×200). (B, C) Cells have round, oval irregular nuclei and may have abundant granular cytoplasm (PAP ×600, oil). (D, E, F) Cytoplasm of the cells may contain vacuoles making the distinction from mucoepidermoid carcinoma difficult (MGG ×600, oil).

Cerilli et al. made analysis of chromosome 9p21 deletion and p16 gene mutation in salivary gland carcinomas. Seven of nine salivary duct carcinomas showed loss of heterozigosity of one or more polymorphic markers. Loss of heterozygosity was found in one of 10 AdCCs and one of eight MECs and was absent in the remaining subtypes. No mutations in exon 1 or exon 2 or homozygous deletion of p16 were found in these two particular neoplasms with loss of heterzygosity. These results suggest that inactivation of p16 is important in the development or progression of at least some salivary duct carcinomas [244]. When studying prognostic markers, Felix et al. found that tumour size, distant metastasis, and C-erbB2 amplification are independent prognostic parameters in patients with salivary duct carcinoma [245]. Female sex is though to be a negative prognostic factor [242].

Although the cytological appearances may vary and sometimes be difficult in terms of tumour type, diagnosis of malignancy is rarely in doubt. Cumulative diagnostic accuracy of cytological diagnosis of salivary duct carcinoma as suspicious of malignancy or malignant, in the studies published up to date, is 94.3%. False negative rate is 6.7% (3 out of 40) [230]. The three false negative diagnoses were in the low-grade salivary duct carcinoma and in two other salivary duct carcinomas with low-grade areas. 'Low grade salivary duct carcinoma' is a new and challenging entity, as evidenced by the high rate of false negative cytological diagnoses [246].

2.5.11 Adenocarcinoma (not otherwise specified)

Adenocarcinoma includes several entities ranging from the relatively indolent polymorphous low-grade adenocarcinoma to the usually fatal salivary duct carcinoma. Cytologically, it is usually possible to diagnose malignancy and, in the absence of any specific features, to indicate the degree of differentiation (Fig. 2.55).

2.5.12 Carcinoma ex PLA

It is recognised that over the long term there is a potential for PLA to develop into a malignant tumour, usually a carcinoma. Ultrasound recognition that this has occured depends on eliciting a history of a longstanding lump (or known history of PLA) which has subsequently increased in size. The US features are generally of a malignant lesion (ill-defined margins and increased vascularity). The diagnosis is confirmed using FNAC.

Cytological features: Epithelial atypia within an otherwise typical PLA should not generally be interpreted as indicating malignancy. Enlarged, irregular, even bizarre nuclei of stromal cells are sometimes found in smears of benign tumours. The abnormal cells are most likely degenerative in nature (See Fig 2.32c). On the other hand, obviously atypical epithelial cells showing nuclear enlargement, hyperchromasia, nucleoli, found side by side with the usual PLA cells is suspicious of carcinoma ex PLA (Fig. 2.56). Definitive diagnosis is deferred because invasive growth is a necessary criterion. In an attempt to analyse which, if any, features might indicate a greater likelihood of malignant transformation of PLA (13.8%), Auclair et al. studied the atypical histological features of PLA: hypercellularity, capsule invasion, hyalinisation, necrosis and cellular anaplasia [247]. The mitotic rate was also analysed. Benign PLA that showed prominent zones of hyalinisation or at least moderate mitotic activity were more likely to develop

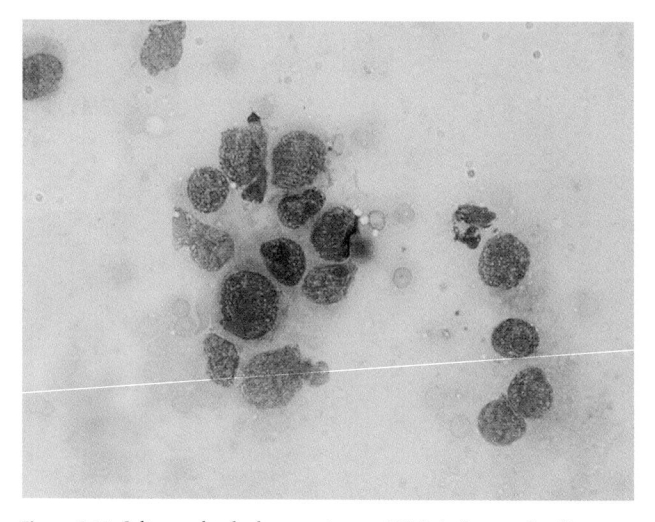

Figure 2.55 Salivary gland adenocarcinoma, NOS. A cluster of malignant cells forming a vague glandular structure are seen. Non-specific malignant features.

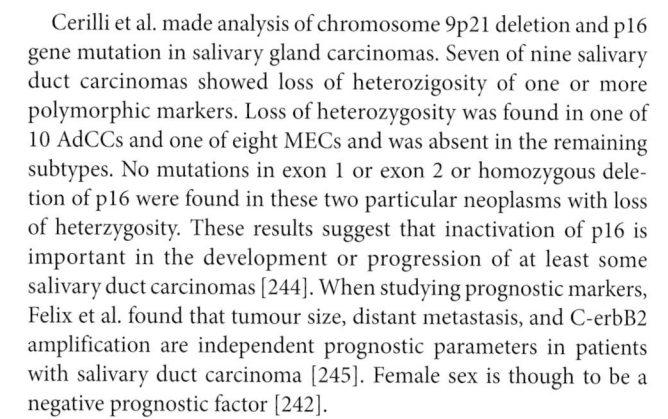

(A)

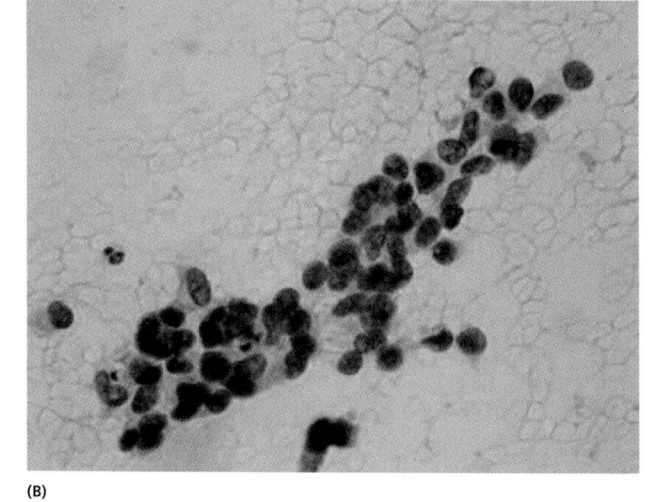

(B)

Figure 2.56 Carcinoma ex pleomorphic adenoma. (A) Large cellular clusters intermixed with myxoid stroma (MGG x400). (B) High power view reveals marked cytological atypia, overlapping and crowding.

carcinoma than those that did not. Clinical findings at the initial diagnosis that indicated a greater likelihood of malignant transformation were occurrence in the submandibular gland, older patient age and large tumour size [247]. Sudden increase in growth rate of a tumour that has been present for many years gives clinical support to the diagnosis [37].

Myoepitehlial carcinoma with predominance of plasmacytoid cells arising in a PLA of the parotid gland has been described [248].

2.5.13 Primary squamous cell carcinoma of the salivary gland

Primary squamous cell carcinoma (SCC) of the parotid is an uncommon, aggressive malignancy with a poor prognosis (Fig. 2.57). It repesents 2% of malignant salivary gland tumours [249] and is localised predominantly in the major salivary glands. Patients usually present in advanced stage and with facial nerve

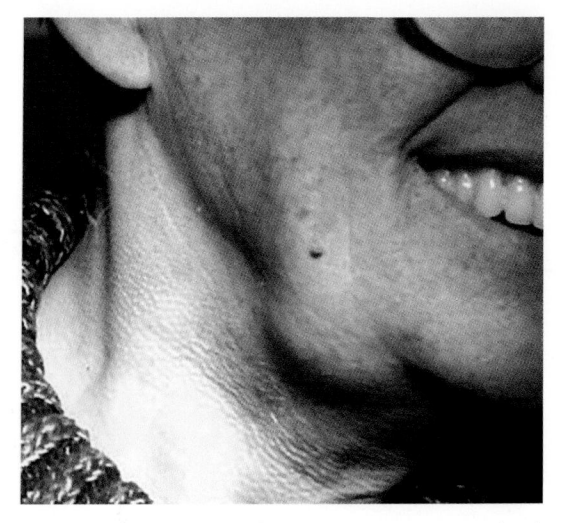

Figure 2.57 Primary squamous cell carcinoma. Patient presented with a 3-month history of painless, non-mobile, hard swelling in the submandibular area. There was no history of other regional or systemic disease.

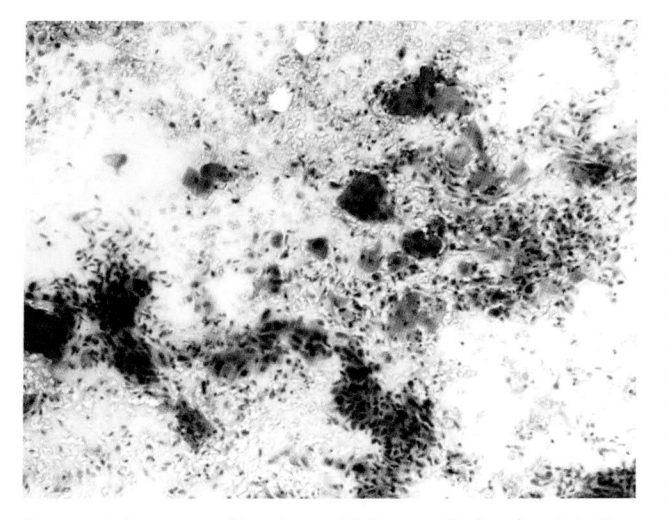

Figure 2.58 Squamous cell carcinoma. Malignant cells show keratinisation, surrounded by necrotic debris. Diagnosis of primary squamous cell carcinoma is made by exclusion of any other primary site in the head and neck or elsewhere.

involvement or cervical metastases. Prognosis is poor even with radical surgery and adjunctive radiotherapy.

The **US features** of SCC in the salivary gland are non specific and diagnosis is made with cytology rather than ultrasound. When this diagnosis is made it inevitably raises the issue as to whether the tumour has arisen primarily within the parotid or whether the lesion represents a metastatic deposit from a head and neck primary tumour or skin tumour. The usual outcome is that the patient undergoes a CTPET scan to assess for an alternative primary followed by an examination under anaesthesia with relevant biopsies (e.g. Tonsils). If these investigations are negative, then the primary is assumed to have arisen in the parotid gland.

FNAC of SCC is usually straightforward. However, there are some pitfalls that should be avoided: squamous cell metaplasia in non-tumourous diseases of the salivary gland (e.g. necrotising sialometaplasia) as well as in benign or malignant salivary gland tumours (e.g. metaplastic Warthin tumour), both of which can can simulate SCC. Other differential diagnostic problems are the structural variants of SCC which develop predominantly in the minor salivary glands, but not in the major salivary glands. Special types include, the very rare adenoid SCC with pseudoglandular structures as the result of acantholysis, the biphasic adenosquamous carcinoma with differentiation as SCC and adenocarcinoma, the biphasic basaloid squamous carcinoma with a structure as SCC, solid basaloid carcinoma (analogous to the solid type of adenoid-cystic carcinoma) and the poorly differentiated MEC (grade III) with biphasic structure of undifferentiated epidermoid and intermediate cells as well as inclusion of small groups of mucous-producing goblet cells [250].

Cytological features are similar to those of SCC elsewhere (Fig. 2.58). Cytological diagnosis of malignancy is possible in 95% of SCC [251]. A spectrum of neoplastic and non-neoplastic lesions of the salivary glands may contain squamous cells. These include chronic sialadenitis, lymphoepithelial cyst, PLA, Warthin's tumour, MEC and SCC. The squamous cells may be a defining feature of the lesion, or an occasional and thus unexpected finding, with a consequent potential for misdiagnosis. Clinical management of these lesions differs significantly and careful evaluation of the squamous elements, along with attention to other cellular and background components, facilitates accurate diagnosis [71].

2.5.14 Small cell carcinoma

Extrapulmonary small cell carcinomas are recognised as a clinico-pathologic entity distinct from small cell lung cancer. Such carcinomas as primary tumours have been described in several locations in the head and neck although most cases of metastatic tumour in the neck originate from a pulmonary primary. Review of the current literature shows that small cell carcinomas in the head and neck are extrapulmonary primary tumours [252]. Since histological criteria are the same, a pulmonary neoplasm has to be excluded in every case. The differentiation between a primary head and neck tumour and metastatic disease as well as the location and staging are essential criteria for therapy and prognosis [253].

Cytological features of small cell carcinoma show nuclear granularity and markedly angular nuclear moulding of numerous small cells that are usually present as large syncytia in an inflammatory background. Numerous mitotic figures are also present in this vascular lesion. Immunohistochemistry demonstrates positivity for neuroendocrine markers indicating a neuroendocrine derivation

for this neoplasm instead of the more usual origin of salivary gland undifferentiated carcinoma in ductal epithelial or myoepithelial tissue [254].

2.5.15 Undifferentiated carcinoma of the salivary gland

Undifferentiated carcinoma of the salivary gland is a rare, high-grade neoplasm which accounts for a very small number (1–5.5%) of salivary gland tumours [255]. It may occur in parotid and in small salivary glands. There is no known sex predilection and middle aged and elderly patients are most commonly affected. Grossly, large cell undifferentiated carcinoma is solid, poorly circumscribed, infiltrating with foci of necrosis and haemorrhage.

Undifferentiated carcinomas of salivary glands are those epithelial malignancies whose histopathological features are not sufficient to place them in other defined classes of carcinoma. They are ultrastructurally heterogeneous and can manifest neuroendocrine differentiation. With or without the latter, the carcinomas are biologically high-grade and rank with salivary duct and high-grade MECs in terms of morbidity and mortality [256].

Cytological features show isolated and loosely cohesive large cells with abundant cytoplasm and variably pleomorphic nuclei with prominent nucleoli. Multinucleated tumour giant cells and macrophage polykaryons may be seen. There is no evidence of squamous, myoepithelial or widespread mucinous differentiation by morphological, cytochemical or immunohistochemical analyses (focal rare mucin production identified on special stains occasionally).

The differential diagnosis is lengthy and consists of other high-grade primary salivary gland malignancies as well as metastatic adenocarcinoma, poorly differentiated squamous cell carcinoma, anaplastic lymphoma, high-grade sarcomas and metastatic melanoma. Differentiation from high-grade MEC may be difficult. In high-grade MEC, large cells of epidermoid differentiation are conspicuous in FNAC material and may resemble large cell undifferentiated carcinoma. However, MEC usually has an admixture of basaloid cells. A mixture of low and high-grade appearances, common in MEC, is usually not seen in large cell undifferentiated carcinoma. AdCC or adenocarcinoma not otherwise specified, may contain foci of anaplastic large cells as well as non-epithelial, osteoclast like giant cells. These, however, represent only a portion of tumour and should not be diagnosed as a large cell undifferentiated carcinoma. Distinction from salivary duct carcinoma may be difficult since the latter is also a high grade tumour and has same age (old) and site (parotid) predilection. Characteristic feature differentiating the two tumours is the presence of cribriform, complex glandular, architecture in salivary duct carcinoma. Malignant lymphoepithelial carcinoma (see 2.6.1) can present in cytological preparations as a high grade malignant tumour composed of syncitial islands of large malignant cells in a necrotic background [257]. A major clue as to its accurate diagnosis is the admixture of mature lymphocytes. Differentiation from oncocytic carcinoma may be difficult since the cells of large cell undifferentiated carcinoma may strongly resemble malignant oncocytes. Distinction from high grade non-Hodgkin lymphoma can usually be made on immunocytochemistry.

The pattern of immunohistochemical reactivity (positive keratin, negative S-100 and HMB-45 antigens), and lack of conspicuous mucin production or significant lymphoid infiltrate, are useful in establishing the correct diagnosis.

2.6 Miscellaneous tumours

2.6.1 Lymphoepithelial carcinoma

Lymphoepithelial carcinoma is a rare, undifferentiated epithelial malignancy with a predilection for Chinese and Eskimo populations, associated with Epstein–Barr virus. Most common is a rapidly growing nasopharyngeal neoplasm, it can arise in the salivary gland.

Cytological features show a highly malignant tumour in individual or cohesive clusters of medium to large polygonal and spindled cells with one or more prominent nucleoli intermingling with mature lymphocytes. These can be misinterpreted as lymphohistiocytic [258]. Sometimes much necrotic debris and only a few lymphocytes admixed with tumour cells are seen. Neither cytology nor histology of the cervical lymph nodes is conclusive in establishing the primary site of a metastatic lymphoepithelioma-like carcinoma. MLEL of the salivary glands must be included in the differential diagnosis (Fig. 4.68, Chapter 4) [257].

2.6.2 Mammary analogue secretory carcinoma

The mammary analogue secretory carcinoma (MASC) was first recognised in 2010 by Skálová et al. [259] and so called because of histomorphological, immunohistochemical and molecular features are almost identical to secretory carcinoma of the breast. It is now clear that MASC is not rare, most examples having previously been labelled as 'odd looking ACCs'. MASC occurs at any age (range 21–75 years; mean 46) and has a slight male predominance. The commonest location is the parotid, but significant numbers also arise in the submandibular and minor glands [260].

Histologically, MASC is usually circumscribed but not encapsulated, demonstrating a 'broad front' invasion into salivary and extra-glandular tissues. Perineural infiltration has been described but not lymphovascular invasion. The architecture consists of lobules composed of tubular, solid and cribriform structures with microcystic and glandular spaces as well as occasional larger cysts and even thyroid colloid-like areas [10]. Abundant eosinophilic homogenous bubbly secretion is present within the spaces, positive for PAS (±diastase) and mucicarmine. The tumour cells have low-grade vesicular nuclei with finely granular chromatin and centrally located small nucleoli, surroundedby pale pink granular or vacuolated cytoplasm; rarely, they can assume a hobnail shape. Cellular atypia is mild, and mitotic figures are generally rare. No PAS-diastase-positive serous acinar zymogen granules are seen, but focal intracytoplasmic mucin has been described [261]. MASC is also lipid-rich, as demonstrated with adipophilin [262].

Immunohistochemistry of MASC shows strong diffuse staining with cytokeratins and epithelial membrane antigen (EMA), but more usefully in practice, mammaglobin, vimentin and S-100 protein are also positive, whereas DOG-1 is largely negative [263]. There is moderate to strong immunoreactivity for c-kit in the majority of tumour cells. A rearrangement of the ETV6 gene on fluorescence in situ hybridisation has been documented.

Basal/myoepithelial cell markers, such as p63, calponin, CK5/6, CK14 and smooth muscle actin, are usually negative, although occasionally an incomplete basal layer has been demonstrated [264].

Proliferative activity is variable with Ki-67 indices ranging between 5 and 28%. MASC appears to be more aggressive than its

breast counterpart, as 4/13 patients in the original paper suffered local recurrences; two died, one of them due to multiple local recurrences and extensionto the temporal bone and another due to widespread metastatic dissemination [265].

Recently, three cases of MASC with genuine high-grade transformation have been reported, with the ETV6-NTRK3 translocation present in both usual and high-grade components [266].

FNAC cytology of MASC shows low to moderate cellularity featuring loosely cohesive small sheets and clusters of neoplastic cells with low-grade nuclear features forming vague acinar structures (Fig 2.59) [267]. The nuclei had mostly smooth contours with only focal nuclear membrane irregularities and finely dispersed chromatin with occasional minute nucleoli. The cytoplasm was moderately abundant with a slightly bubbly appearance and the cell borders were indistinct. Round to irregular elongated secretory ('colloid-like') material with variable staining intensity was intimately admixed with the tumour cells on the MGG-stained

smear. Differential diagnosis includes acinic cell carcinoma (papillary cystic, microcystic and follicular type), low-grade cribriform cystadenocarcinoma and low-grade mucoepidermoid carcinoma.

2.6.3 Cribriform adenocarcinoma of minor salivary gland

Cribriform adenocarcinoma of minor salivary gland (CAMSG) is a recently characterised low-grade salivary gland malignancy that most commonly presents as a mass in the base of the tongue, frequently with regional lymph node metastasis [268].

Given its relative rarity and overlapping cytomorphology, CAMSG may be confused with polymorphous low grade adenocarcinoma (PLGA) in minor salivary gland sites and papillary thyroid carcinoma (PTC) in cervical metastasis, in both FNAC and excisional specimens.

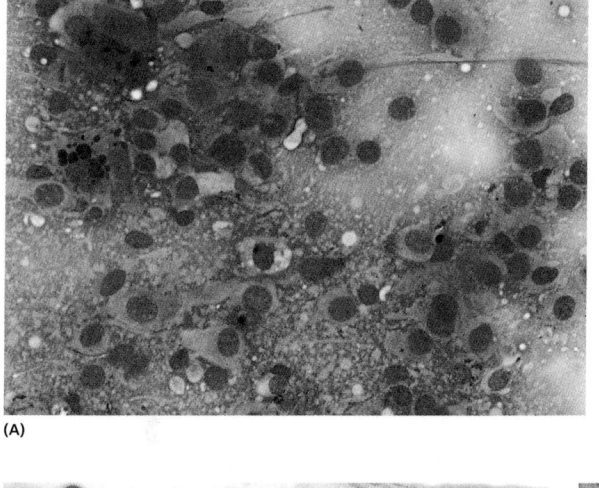

(A)

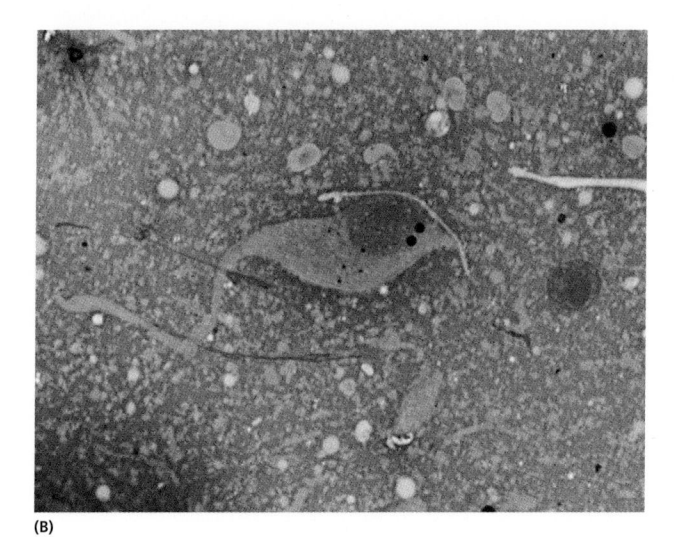

(B)

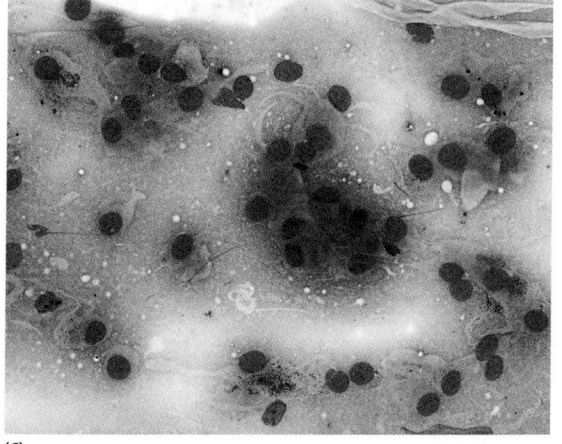

(C)

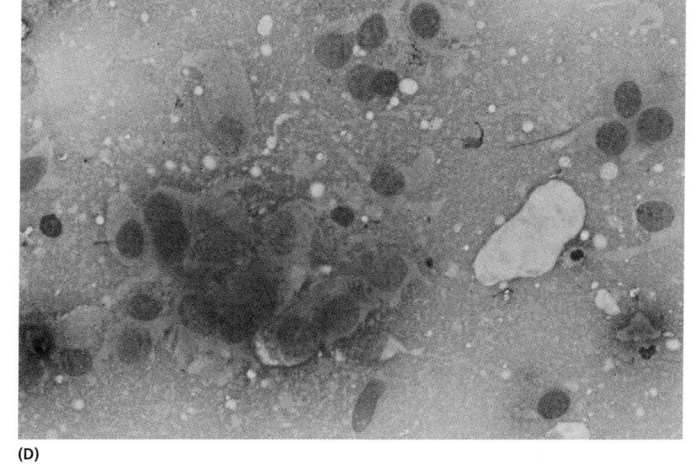

(D)

Figure 2.59 FNAC of MASC: (A) Smear shows low to moderate cellularity featuring loosely cohesive small sheets and clusters of isomorphic cells with bland nuclear features against a dense eosinophilic, proteinaceous background with bubbly secretions. Secretory material stains positive for periodic acid-Schiff (PAS) with and without diastase, mucicarmin and Alcian blue. Some cells contain round secretory ('colloidlike') material with variable staining intensity on the MGG-stained smear. Intracellular mucin positivity has been described. (B) The nuclei are eccentric, have smooth contours and finely dispersed chromatin with occasional central nucleoli. The cytoplasm is abundant, often elongated ('hobnail' shaped) with well defined cell borders and colloid like cytoplasmic secretions. (C, D) Dispersed and dissociated cells with cytoplasmic extensions and a dense, bubbly background. Many cells contain abundant cytoplasm with coarse granules.

FNAC of CAMSG contain polymorphic fragments of epithelial cells arranged in monolayer sheets, papillary fronds and tips and occasional cribriform configurations and metachromatic stromal fragments, which may be misinterpreted as colloid [268]. A background of myxoid/mucoid material also reminiscent of colloid was prominent. The nuclei can be essentially identical to those seen in cases of papillary thyroid carcinoma (PTC) with irregular nuclear contours, nuclear grooves and rare intranuclear inclusions. The key distinguishing features to differentiate CAMSG from PTC are the quality and character of the background. While PTC can occasionally be stroma-rich, aspirate smears of CAMSG have a much more 'salivary gland-type' background with frequent fragments of metachromatic stroma and flocculent pink myxoid/mucoid material that must be differentiated from colloid. A very important caveat is that on Pap stain this flocculent background material is washed away, making a specific diagnosis even more difficult.

By *immunohistochemistry*, the tumour cells react with AE1/AE3, CAM5.2, CK7 and CK8/18. They also highlight with basal and myoepithelial markers, including S-100 protein, p63, CK5/6 (variable), CK14, calponin and smooth muscle actin [269–271].

This co-expression of both epithelial and myoepithelial markers convinced early reporters that these cells were hybrid secretory-myoepithelial cells, which was supported by ultrastructure [269, 270]. While CK19, galectin-3 and HBME-1 may be positive, importantly, TTF-1 and thyroglobulin are negative. Epithelial membrane antigen, epidermal growth factor receptor, and HER-2/neu are also negative. 2 CD117 (c-kit) positivity is variably present in 42% of cases. Variable cyclin D1, p16 and p53 positivity is reported, but the significance is unknown. Of the 10 tumours studied by Skalova et al., only one was high risk HPV-positive [270].

No mutations of BRAF, KRAS, HRAS, RET, c-kit and PDGFRa have been detected. Laco et al. detected three separate polymorphisms in the RET proto-oncogene in three of five cases and the same polymorphism of HRAS in three separate cases [271].

2.6.4 Soft tissue lesions

2.6.4.1 Benign neurilemmoma
The benign nerve sheath tumour can be found in the salivary gland and erroneously reported as PLA or myoepithelioma [272, 273] (see Fig. 5.7, Chapter 5).

2.6.4.2 Nodular fasciitis
Nodular fasciitis (NF) is a benign, reactive lesion with a self-limiting process. Because NF is rare in the parotid gland and has many cytological similarities to other benign or malignant tumors, cytological misinterpretation is common (see Ch5, p178).

2.6.4.3 Rhabdomyosarcoma
The head and neck region is one of the most common locations of rhabdomyosarcoma. Salivary gland involvement is usually secondary to advanced disease and presentation as a primary salivary gland tumour is very rare. Patients are usually children and adolescents (although the tumour can occur in adults), presenting with parotid gland enlargement. Clinically, the enlargements appear to be inflammatory and they are treated unsuccessfully with antibiotics.

Cytological features vary from those of a small round cell tumour to a monomorphic population of spindle cells in a metachromatic stroma or spindle cells with moderate cellular pleomorphism (Fig. 5.13, Chapter 5). Immunohistochemical or ultrastructural studies confirm the diagnosis of rhabdomyosarcoma [274].

Synovial sarcoma is a distinctive neoplasm that usually arises in the extremities in the region of joints. Although synovial sarcomas arising in the head and neck region are well described, tumours actually originating in and around the major salivary glands are exceedingly rare (Fig. 2.60) [275].

2.6.4.4 Maligant haemangiopericytoma
The FNAC smear shows a spindle-cell neoplasm with capillaries and benign endothelial cells. The spindle cells posses pleomorphic, hyperchromatic elongated nuclei and a moderate amount of ill-defined cytoplasm. They show papillary arcades surrounded and encased by relatively small ovoid to short spindle cells [276]. Radiation induced angiosarcoma have been described [277].

2.6.4.5 Leiomyosarcoma
A primary leiomyosarcoma of the parotid gland has been reported only three times in English literature [278]. This type of tumour represents an extremely rare group of salivary gland neoplasm. A review of the literature reveals that primary leiomyosarcoma and other sarcomas of the major salivary glands may share similar histogenesis and biological behaviour with their soft tissue counterparts.

2.6.5 Granulocytic sarcoma

Granulocytic sarcoma can on occasions infiltrate the parotid gland without the evidence of acute myeloid leukaemia or chronic myeloproliferative disease at time of diagnosis. The myeloid nature of the tumour can be discovered with the aid of immunocytochemistry. Granulocytic sarcoma should be considered in the differential diagnosis of malignant tumours of the parotid gland, although it is rare [279].

2.6.6 Paediatric lesions

Although paediatric parotid masses are unusual, they can represent a variety of pathological diagnoses, including malignancy. Orvidas et al. had undertaken a survey of nearly 30 years experience with parotid masses in patients aged 18 years and younger that were evaluated and treated at the Mayo Clinic, Rochester, MI, USA. Parotid masses were identified in 118 children (60 boys and 58 girls) most of which had asymptomatic mass at presentation. Forty-three patients (36.4%) had infectious or inflammatory lesions, 56 (47.5%) had benign lesions, and 19 (16.1%) had malignant lesions. The most common benign lesions were PLA (22.9%) and hemangioma (10.2%) [280, 281]. The most common malignant lesions were MEC (6.8%) and acinic cell carcinoma (3.4%). The most common treatment was total parotidectomy (40.7%). PLA recurred in 4 (14.8%) of 28 patients and MEC in 3 (37.5%) of 8 patients. One patient with AdCC died of the tumour. The authors advocate prompt evaluation and treatment of these masses.

2.6.7 Lymphomas

Primary salivary gland lymphomas are rare. The low grade extranodal non-Hodgkin lymphomas of MALT type (marginal zone lymphoma) have been described earlier in this chapter (Fig. 2.24, 2.25). Nodal lymphomas can occur in the salivary gland and the morphology is the same as in other lymph nodes (see Chapter 4. Fig. 4.55) (Fig. 2.61). Concurrent presentation of follicular and MALT lymphoma in the same salivary gland has been described. High-grade non-Hodgkin's lymphoma presenting

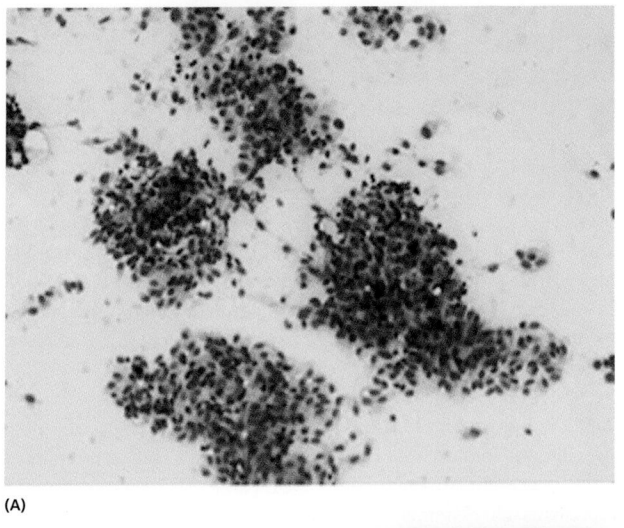

(A)

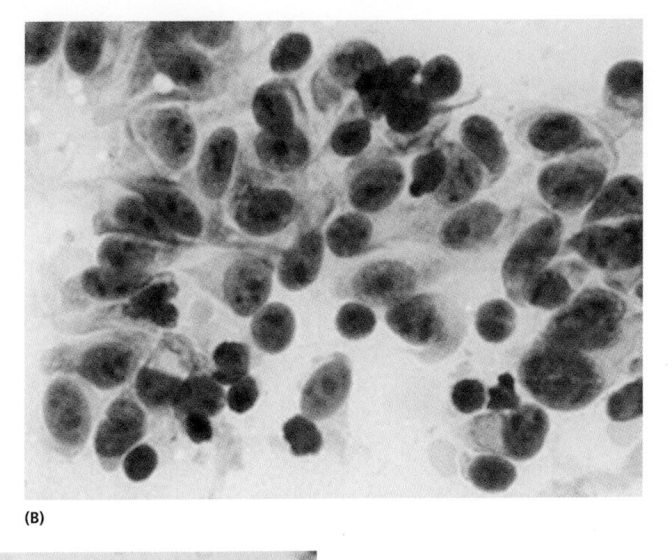

(B)

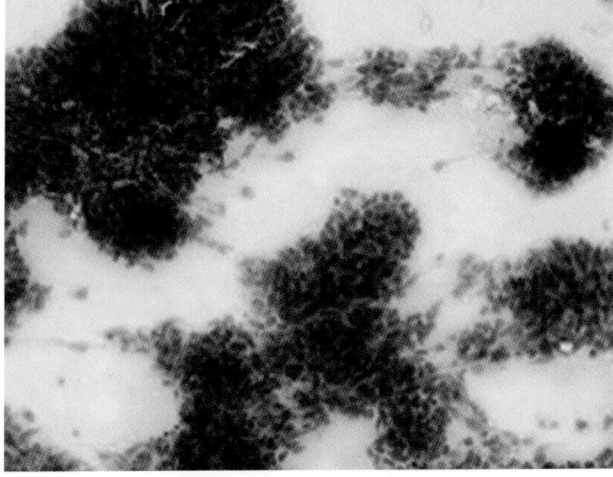

(C)

Figure 2.60 Synovial sarcoma. (A) Spindle cells with blunt nuclei in an aggregate. Cytoplasmic processes. Diagnosis of a mesenchymal tumour, probably malignant was made. Biopsy revealed synovial sarcoma (MGG ×600). (B) Individual cell of synovial sarcoma have oval or round nucleus and unipolar cytoplasm. Nucleoli are prominent. Features suggest malignancy but are not specific of synovial sarcoma (MGG ×1000). (C) Bcl2 as well as cytokeratin positivity combined are a characteristic marker for a spindle cell synovila sarcoma. Cytokeratin and CD99 are also used in detection of synovial sarcoma (Bcl2 ×400).

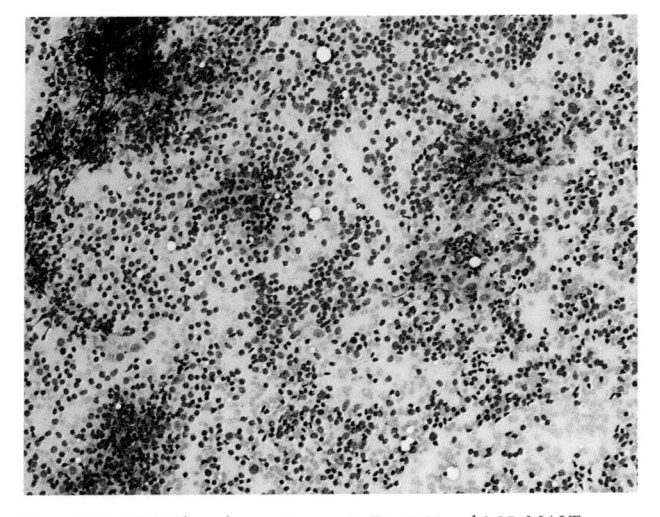

Figure 2.61 MALT lymphoma. As seen in Figs 2.24 and 2.25, MALT lymphoma may have a polymorphic cell population of small and medium size lymphocytes admixed with follicular dendritic cells. Lymphoepithelial lesions may be absent (MGG ×600).

in the salivary gland are managed in the similar way as elsewhere (Fig. 2.62, 2.63).

The *ultrasound appearances* of lymphoma as part of a generalised non-MALT lymphoma are of multiple rounded hypoechoic enlarged lymph nodes within the parotid and elsewhere in the neck (see Box 2.2).

[See BOX 2.2 Summary of ultrasound features: Parotid lymphoma on www.wiley.com/go/kocjan/clinical_cytopathology_head_neck2e]

Primary lymphoma arising in the submandibular salivary glands is recognised and presents as a malignant appearing hypoechoic mass that is otherwise non-specific. It cannot be distinguished from other salivary malignancies on US alone.

2.6.8 Primitive neuroectodermal tumour

The primitive neuroectodermal tumour (PNET) is a malignant, small, round cell tumour that exhibits neuroepithelial differentiation. Isolated cases of PNET have been reported in visceral sites such as the kidney, uterus, ovary, testis, urinary bladder and pancreas. Debb

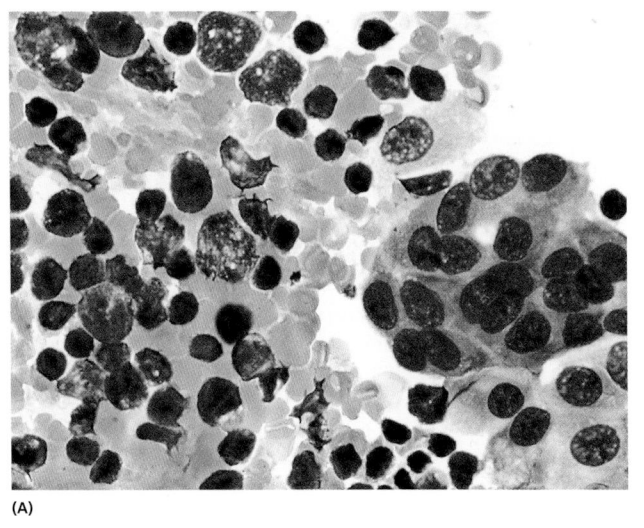

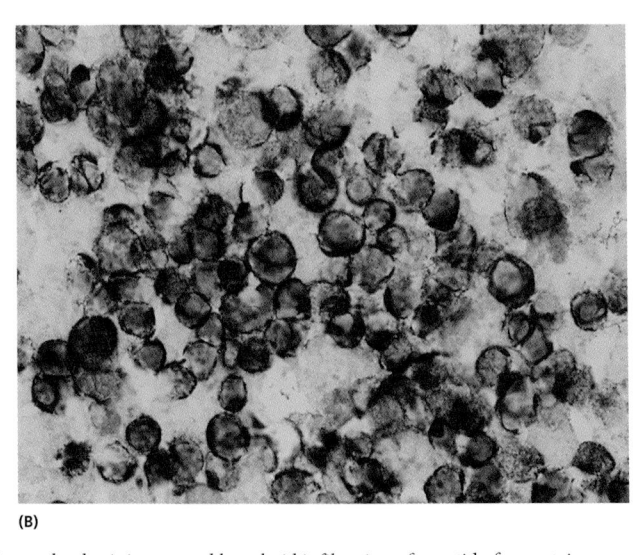

(A)   (B)

Figure 2.62 Parotid lymphoma. (A) Polymorphic lymphoid infiltrate and salivary gland acini suggested lymphoid infiltration of parotid of uncertain nature. Biopsy was advised. (B) CD3 positivity confirms a peripheral T-cell lymphoma.

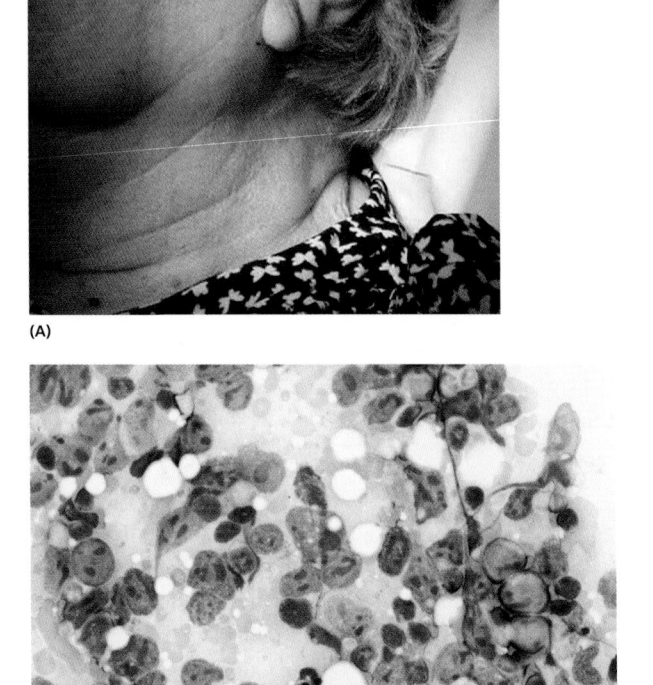

(A)

(B)

Figure 2.63 (A) A 65-year-old man presented with a 2-month history of diffuse painless parotid swelling. FNAC revealed a diffuse large B-cell lymphoma. (B) FNAC showed numerous large pleomorphic lymphoid cells. Immunocytochemistry confirmed a diffuse large B-cell lymphoma.

et al. were the first to report the tumour occurring in the parotid [282]. They postulate the origin to be from the facial nerve.

Cytological features show a highly cellular, poorly cohesive smear pattern exhibiting small round cells, with scanty cytoplasm forming occasional rosette-like structures (Fig. 5.14, Chapter 5). Numerous intact single cells with fragile cytoplasm, finely granular chromatin, and inconspicuous nucleoli are present together with single nuclei in the background [283].

2.6.9 Metastatic tumours in salivary gland

Salivary glands are not an infrequent site of metastases. Metastases or secondary deposits account for 16% of the malignant neoplasms involving the major salivary glands. A correct diagnosis of a secondary neoplasm is important for appropriate management to avoid unnecessary radical surgery and to guide further therapy.

US features of metastases: Lymph node metastases are fairly easy to recognise on US, usually showing multiple but occasionally solitary round to ovoid enlarged lymph nodes within the parotid. In advanced cases extranodal spread can occur and the lymph nodes develop ill-defined margins. Secondary lymph node metastatic disease involving the parotid are seen arising from a spectrum of tumours that are mainly either skin (scalp or pinna) tumours such as melanoma (Fig. 2.64) or SCC or head and neck primary tumours – such as nasopharyngeal carcinoma or SCC of the external auditory canal. Nodal involvement from oropharyngeal and laryngeal/hypopharyngeal tumours occurs rarely. Metastatic nodal involvement of the parotid may occur in isolation – as the presenting complaint or as part of more generalised lymphadenopathy in the neck. Particularly in the latter patients, it is important to highlight and prove nodal involvement (with FNAC if necessary) to the clinical team in order to ensure that this component of the disease is treated with radiotherapy. The parotid is normally otherwise spared from direct radiotherapy treatment in head and neck patients because of the dry mouth resulting. Very occasionally the parotid is the site of nodal involvement from a primary tumour outside the head and neck area. Prostate, breast, lung and colon cancer are all recognised as primary tumours in this instance but this usually occurs in the context of disseminated nodal disease and a known primary tumour.

The absence of lymph nodes within the submandibular salivary glands means that lymph node metastatic deposits are not possible however direct (non nodal) metastatic spread to the submandibular salivary glands can rarely be seen.

FNAC is non-invasive diagnostic tool for evaluating metastatic lesions. Zhang et al. reviewed 36 metastatic tumours in the salivary glands and found a mixture of adenocarcinomas, squamous cell carcinomas, undifferentiated carcinoma, cutaneous basal cell carcinoma cutaneous melanomas, osteosarcomas, non-Hodgkin lymphomas and multiple myelomas [284]. FNAC is a reliable tool to differentiate haematological malignant neoplasms and melanomas from other salivary gland neoplasms. Knowledge of clinical history, review of previous pathologic materials and, in some instances, the use of ancillary studies is crucial for recognising solid malignant neoplasms secondarily involving the salivary glands.

In their review of 20 cases of metastatic carcinoma Malata et al. found that most tumours originated from the head and neck region, the two main types being SCC and malignant melanoma [285]. All

20 presented with a parotid mass and 11/20 had associated lymphadenopathy. Patients underwent superficial, total or radical, parotidectomy, neck dissection and adjuvant postoperative radiotherapy. The cumulative 5-year survival rate was 51% [286]. Superficial parotidectomy is usually an adequate treatment for secondary parotid tumours (when disease is clinically limited to the superficial lobe). Patients in whom metastatic disease of the parotid gland is suspected do not require neck dissection if they have no palpable lymph nodes and MRI shows no evidence of spread. There seems to be no survival advantage in radical over modified neck dissection. Small cell lung carcinoma, adenocarcinoma from upper airways and digestive tracts, renal cell carcinoma, have all been described as occurring in the parotid [287–289].

2.7 Clinical management of salivary gland lesions

Although it is accepted that clinical and radiological assessment (including the two-phase helical CT) of parotid masses cannot distinguish reliably between benign and malignant lesions [290], the value of FNAC in the evaluation and management of salivary gland pathology has been controversial for a long time. The major reasons for this controversy are the difficulty in cytological evaluation and the fact that the extent of surgery can be easily defined based on clinical judgement, particularly at a cancer referral centre (where clinicians may be experienced at diagnosing parotid gland malignancies) [10, 46a]. However, a preoperative diagnosis is helpful in discussions with patients regarding the extent and type of surgery. Most centres using salivary gland FNAC do so selectively, in an attempt to obtain a preoperative diagnosis in order to distinguish between neoplasms and non-neoplastic conditions and thus avoid surgery in conditions, which clinically mimic neoplasm. A combination of MRI findings and cytology results is optimal for diagnosing malignancies of the parotid lesions (Table 2.7) [291].

Apart from the fact that FNAC can distinguish benign from malignant conditions, it is also very useful in distinguishing between salivary and other non-salivary pathology. Preoperative diagnosis of Warthin's tumour, lymphoma or benign lymphoepithelial disease is essential to the correct management of these patients [292]. With using FNAC in a multidisciplinary setting, surgical excision is often unnecessary and may be reduced to 20% [44a].

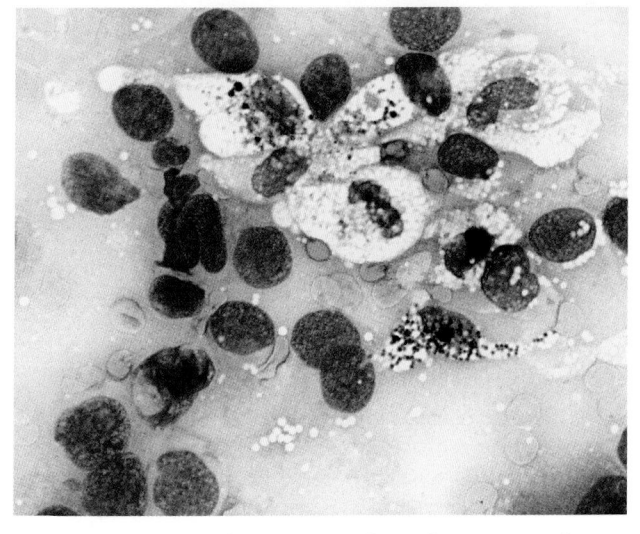

Figure 2.64 Metastatic melanoma. FNAC of parotid in a patient with no known history, reveals numerous single malignant cells with eccentric nuclei, well-outlined cytoplasm and prominent nucleoli. Pigment is seen in the macrophages.

Table 2.7 The role of salivary gland FNAC in clinical management.

Algorithm of clinical management following the FNAC diagnosis

Benign	Uncertain	Malignant
Sialadenitis PA Warthin's	Cystic lesions Oncocytic tumours	Mucoep Acinic / Adenoid cystic Adenoca NOS
	Ancillary	
Discharge 70–80% of cases	Follow up or Excision	Excision / Definitive excision

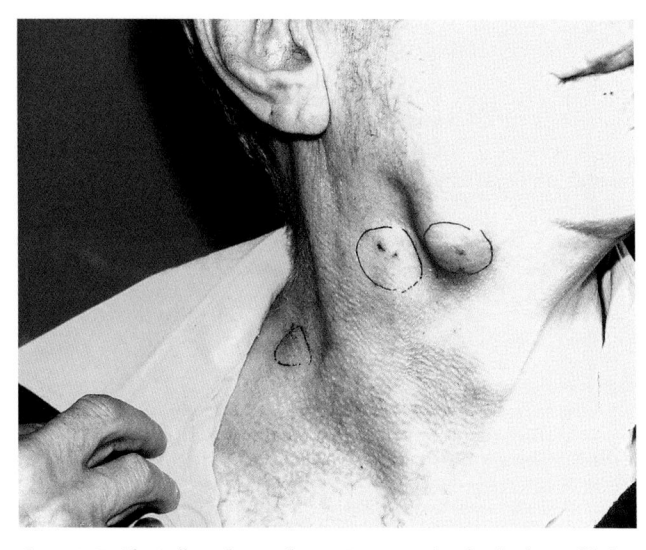

Figure 2.65 Clinically malignant lesion. Patient with a fixed submandibular mass and enlarged cervical nodes which have undergone FNAC. Cytology showed a salivary duct carcinoma with regional metastases. Patient underwent excision with a radical neck lymph node dissection.

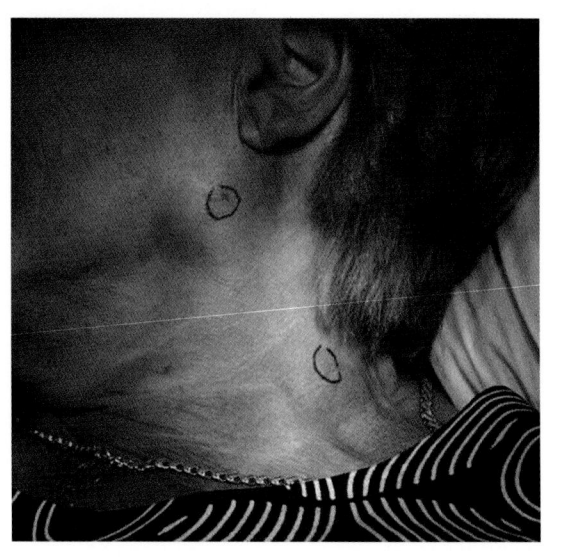

Figure 2.66 Clinically suspicious angle of mandible swelling and regional lymph node enlargement. FNAC showed pleomorphic adenoma and a reactive lymph node hyperplasia unrelated to the salivary pathology. Without the FNAC result, it would have been tempting to assume malignancy with regional spread.

This chapter also has online only material. Ultrasound Summary boxes, which have been cited throughout the chapter text as 'Summary of ultrasound features', are available on www.wiley.com/go/kocjan/clinical_cytopathology_head_neck2e for the following diseases:

Box 2.1 Summary of ultrasound features: Chronic sclerosing sialadenitis
Box 2.2 Summary of ultrasound features: Parotid lymphoma
Box 2.3 Summary of ultrasound features: Pleomorphic Adenoma
Box 2.4 Summary of ultrasound features: Warthin's tumour
Box 2.5 Summary of ultrasound features: Adenoid Cystic Carcinoma

When assessing the impact of FNAC of salivary gland masses in clinical decision-making, Heller et al. compared the clinician's initial clinical impression with the FNAC diagnosis and the final diagnosis in each case. Overall, FNAC resulted in a change in the clinical approach to 35% of the patients. As a result, they recommend the performance of FNAC in almost all patients with salivary masses [293] (Figs. 2.65, 2.66). FNAC provides accurate diagnosis of most salivary gland lesions and contributes to conservative management in many patients with non-neoplastic conditions [11]. By using FNAC, an operation was avoided in 70, 79% and 80% of patients with a non-neoplastic lesion and a metastasis, respectively [44a, 294]. FNAC plays an important role in the preoperative and postoperative assessment of parotid masses by aiding in the evaluation of tumours in poor surgical candidates and unresectable tumours, and by identifying metastases from other sites. Although definitive subclassification of some lesion types remains poor, FNAC is invaluable in patient triage. From the practical point, cytological subtyping of tumours is unnecessary since it rarely influences management. Although diagnosis in some common tumours is not difficult in most cases, sampling error may cause difficulties in interpretation.

References

1. Sharma G, Jung AS, Maceri DR et al. US-guided fine-needle aspiration of major salivary gland masses and adjacent lymph nodes: accuracy and impact on clinical decision making. *Radiology* 2011; **259**(2): 471–8.
2. Jung AS, Sharma G, Maceri D et al. Ultrasound-guided fine needle aspiration of major salivary gland masses and adjacent lymph nodes. *Ultrasound Q* 2011; **27**(2): 105–13.
3. Isa AY, Hilmi OJ. An evidence based approach to the management of salivary masses. *Clin Otolaryngol* 2009; **34**(5): 470–3.
4. Shekar K, Singh M, Godden D et al. Recent advances in the management of salivary gland disease. *Br J Oral Maxillofac Surg* 2009; **47**(8): 594–7.
5. Orell SR. Diagnostic difficulties in the interpretation of fine needle aspirates of salivary gland lesions: the problem revisited. *Cytopathology* 1995; **6**(5): 285–300.
6. Siewert B, Kruskal JB, Kelly D et al. Utility and safety of ultrasound-guided fine-needle aspiration of salivary gland masses including a cytologist's review. *J Ultrasound Med* 2004; **23**(6): 777–83.
7. Young JA. *Fine needle aspiration cytopathology.* Blackwell Scientific Publications, London, 1993.
8. Colella G, Cannavale R, Flamminio F, Foschini MP. Fine-needle aspiration cytology of salivary gland lesions: a systematic review. *J Oral Maxillofac Surg* 2010; **68**(9): 2146–53.
9. Al-Khafaji BM, Nestok BR, Katz RL. Fine-needle aspiration of 154 parotid masses with histologic correlation: ten-year experience at the University of Texas M. D. Anderson Cancer Center. *Cancer* 1998; **84**(3):1: 53–9.
10. Stewart CJ, MacKenzie K, McGarry GW, Mowat A. Fine-needle aspiration cytology of salivary gland: A review of 341 cases. *Diagn Cytopathol* 2000; **22**(3): 139–46.
11. Salgarelli AC, Cappare P, Bellini P, Collini M. Usefulness of fine-needle aspiration in parotid diagnostics. *Oral Maxillofac Surg* 2009; **13**(4): 185–90.
12. Gritzmann N. Sonography of the salivary glands. *AJR Am J Roentgenol* 1989; **153**(1): 161–6.
13. Kress E, Schulz HG, Neumann T. Diagnosis of diseases of the large salivary glands of the head by ultrasound, sialography and CT-sialography. A comparison of methods. *HNO* 1993; **41**(7): 345–51.
14. Wu S, Liu G, Chen R, Guan Y. Role of ultrasound in the assessment of benignity and malignancy of parotid masses. *Dentomaxillofac Radiol* 2011; **41**(2): 131–5.
15. Zajicek J. 1. Introduction to aspiration biopsy. *Monogr Clin Cytol* 1974; **4**: 1–211.
16. Dey P, Ray R. Comparison of fine needle sampling by capillary action and fine needle aspiration. *Cytopathology* 1993; **4**(5): 299–303.
17. Hamaker RA, Moriarty AT, Hamaker RC. Fine-needle biopsy techniques of aspiration versus capillary in head and neck masses. *Laryngoscope* 1995; **105**(12 Pt 1): 1311–4.
18. Mair S, Dunbar F, Becker PJ, Du Plessis W. Fine needle cytology – is aspiration suction necessary? A study of 100 masses in various sites [see comments]. *Acta Cytol* 1989; **33**(6): 809–13.
19. Santos JE, Leiman G. Nonaspiration fine needle cytology. Application of a new technique to nodular thyroid disease [see comments]. *Acta Cytol* 1988; **32**(3): 353–6.

47. Bhaijee F, Pepper DJ, Pitman KT, Bell D. New developments in the molecular pathogenesis of head and neck tumors: a review of tumor-specific fusion oncogenes in mucoepidermoid carcinoma, adenoid cystic carcinoma, and NUT midline carcinoma. Ann Diagn Pathol 2011; 15(1): 69-77.

48. Seethala RR. Histologic grading and prognostic biomarkers in salivary gland carcinomas. Adv Anat Pathol 2011; 18(1): 29-45.

49. Stacchini A, Aliberti S, Pacchioni D, et al. Flow cytometry significantly improves the diagnostic value of fine needle aspiration cytology of lymphoproliferative lesions of salivary glands. Cytopathology 2014; 25(4): 231-40.

50. Barnes L, Eveson JW, Reichart P, Sidransky D. World Health Organization tumors: Head and neck tumors. IARC Press, Lyon.

51. Hughes JH, Volk EE, Wilbur DC, et al. Pitfalls in salivary gland fine-needle aspiration cytology: lessons from the College of American Pathologists Interlaboratory Comparison Program in Nongynecologic Cytology. Arch Pathol Lab Med 2005; 129(1): 26-31.

52. MacLeod CB, Frable WJ. Fine-needle aspiration biopsy of the salivary gland: problem cases. Diagn Cytopathol 1993; 9(2): 216-24; discussion 224-5.

53. Boccato P, Altavilla G, Blandamura S. Fine needle aspiration biopsy of salivary gland lesions. A reappraisal of pitfalls and problems. Acta Cytol 1998; 42(4): 888-98.

54. de Ru JA, van Leeuwen MS, van Benthem PP, et al. Do magnetic resonance imaging and ultrasound add anything to the preoperative workup of parotid gland tumors? J Oral Maxillofac Surg 2007; 65(5): 945-52.

55. Burke CJ, Thomas RH, Howlett D. Imaging the major salivary glands. Br J Oral Maxillofac Surg 2011; 49(4): 261-9.

56. Inohara H, Akahani S, Yamamoto Y, et al. The role of fine-needle aspiration cytology and magnetic resonance imaging in the management of parotid mass lesions. Acta Otolaryngol 2008; 128(10): 1152-8.

57. Westerland O, Howlett D. Sonoelastography techniques in the evaluation and diagnosis of parotid neoplasms. Eur Radiol 2012; 22(5): 966-9. Epub 2012 Feb 26.

58. Carvalho MB, Soares JM, Rapoport A, et al. Perioperative frozen section examination in parotid gland tumors. Sao Paulo Med J 1999; 117(6): 233-237.

59. Layfield LJ, Tan P, Glasgow BJ. Fine-needle aspiration of salivary gland lesions. Comparison with frozen sections and histologic findings. Arch Pathol Lab Med 1987; 111(4): 346-53.

60. Haidar S, Mandala U, Skelton E, Chow V, Turner SS, Tighe D, Williams M, Howlett D. Diagnostic investigation of parotid neoplasms: a 16-year experience of freehand fine needle aspiration cytology and ultrasound-guided core needle biopsy. Int J Oral Maxillofac Surg 2015; 44: 151-157.

61. Pfeiffer J, Ridder GJ. Diagnostic value of ultrasound-guided core needle biopsy in patients with salivary gland masses. Int J Oral Maxillofac Surg 2012; 41(4): 437-43.

62. Zakowski MF. Fine-needle aspiration cytology of tumors: diagnostic accuracy and potential pitfalls. Cancer Invest 1994; 12(5): 505-15.

63. Rimm DL, Stastny JF, Rimm EB et al. Comparison of the costs of fine-needle aspiration and open surgical biopsy as methods for obtaining a pathologic diagnosis. Cancer 1997; 81(1): 51-6.

64. Roland NJ, Caslin AW, Smith PA et al. Fine aspiration cytology of salivary gland lesions reported immediately in a head and neck clinic. J Laryngol Otol 1993; 107(11): 1025-8.

65. Saleh HA, Ram B, Harmse JL et al. Lipomatosis of the minor salivary glands. J Laryngol Otol 1998; 112(9): 895-7.

66. Coleman H, Altini M, Nayler S, Richards A. Sialadenosis: a presenting sign in bulimia [see comments]. Head Neck 1998; 20(8): 758-62.

67. Kim D, Uy C, Mandel L. Sialosis of unknown origin. N Y State Dent J 1998; 64(7): 38-40.

68. Ascoli V, Albedi FM, De Blasiis R, Nardi F. Sialadenosis of the parotid gland: report of four cases diagnosed by fine-needle aspiration cytology. Diagn Cytopathol 1993; 9(2): 151-5.

69. Mandel L, Hamele-Bena D. Alcoholic parotid sialadenosis. J Am Dent Assoc 1997; 128(10): 1411-5.

70. Gupta S, Sodhani P. Sialadenosis of parotid gland: a cytomorphologic and morphometric study of four cases. Anal Quant Cytol Histol 1998; 20(3): 225-8.

71. Mooney EE, Dodd LG, Layfield LJ. Squamous cells in fine-needle aspiration biopsies of salivary gland lesions: potential pitfalls in cytological diagnosis. Diagn Cytopathol 1996; 15(5): 447-52.

72. Jayaram G, Pathmanathan R, Khanijow V. Cystic lesion of the parotid gland with squamous metaplasia mistaken for squamous cell carcinoma. A case report. Acta Cytol 1998; 42(6): 1468-72.

72a. Anastassov GE et al. Oral Surg Oral Med Oral Pathol Oral Radiol Endod 2000; 89: 159-63.

73. Chhieng DC, Argosino R, McKenna BJ, Cangiarella JF, Cohen JM. Utility of fine-needle aspiration in the diagnosis of salivary gland lesions in patients infected with human immunodeficiency virus. Diagn Cytopathol 1999; 21(4): 260-4.

74. Vicandi B, Jimenez-Heffernan JA, Lopez-Ferrer P et al. HIV-1 (p24)-positive multinucleated giant cells in HIV-associated lymphoepithelial lesion of the parotid gland. A report of two cases. Acta Cytol 1999; 43(2): 247-51.

4a. Ostović KT, Lukšić I, Virag M, Macan D, Manojlović S. The importance of team work of cytologist and surgeon in preoperative diagnosis of intraoral minor salivary gland tumours. Coll Antropol. 2012 Nov; 36 Suppl 2: 151-7.

46. Cheuk W, Chan JK. Advances in salivary gland pathology. Histopathology 2007; 51(1): 1-20.

45. Ashraf A, Shaikh AS, Kamal F et al. Diagnostic reliability of FNAC for salivary gland swellings: a comparative study. Diagn Cytopathol. 2010; 38(7): 499-504.

44a. Maiteriham P, Jay A, Beale T, Morley S, Vaz F, Kalavrezos N, Kocjan G. Salivary gland FNA cytology: role as a triage tool and an approach to pitfalls in cytomorphology. Cytopathology. 2016 Apr; 27(2): 91-6.

44. Kechagias N, Ntomouchtsis A, Valeri R et al. Fine-needle aspiration cytology of salivary gland tumours: a 10-year retrospective analysis. Oral Maxillofac Surg 2012; 16(1): 35-40.

43. Young JA, Smallman LA, Thompson H, Proops DW, Johnson AP. Fine needle aspiration cytology of salivary gland lesions. Cytopathology 1990; 1(1): 25-33.

42. Layfield LJ, Glasgow BJ. Aspiration cytology of clear-cell lesions of the parotid gland: morphologic features and differential diagnosis. Diagn Cytopathol 1993; 9(6): 705-11; discussion 711-12.

41. Murphy P, Laing MR, Palmer TT. Fine needle aspiration cytology of head and neck lesions: an early experience. J R Coll Surg Edinb 1997; 42(5): 341-6.

40. Gray W, Kocjan G. Diagnostic cytopathology. Elsevier Limited, 2010.

39. Young JA. Diagnostic problems in fine needle aspiration cytopathology of the salivary gland. J Clin Pathol 1994; 47(3): 193-8.

38. Shintani S, Matsuura H, Hasegawa Y. Fine needle aspiration of salivary gland tumors. Int J Oral Maxillofac Surg 1997; 26(4): 2 84-6.

37. Orell SR, Nettle NJ. Fine needle aspiration biopsy of salivary gland tumours. Problems and pitfalls. Pathology 1988; 20: 332-7.

36. Kocjan G, Nayagam M, Harris M. Fine needle aspiration cytology of salivary gland lesions: advantages and pitfalls. Cytopathology 1990; 1(5): 269-75.

35. Frable MA, Frable WJ. Fine-needle aspiration biopsy of salivary glands. Laryngoscope 1991; 101(3): 245-9.

34. Cajulis RS, Gokaslan ST, Yu GH, Frias-Hidvegi D. Fine needle aspiration biopsy of the salivary glands. A five-year experience with emphasis on diagnostic pitfalls. Acta Cytol 1997; 41(5): 1412-20.

33. Candel A, Gattuso P, Reddy V et al. Is fine needle aspiration biopsy of salivary gland masses really necessary? Ear Nose Throat J 1993; 72(7): 485-9.

32. Cristallini EG, Ascani S, Farabi R et al. Fine needle aspiration biopsy of salivary gland, 1985-1995. Acta Cytol 1997; 41(5): 1421-5.

31. Chan MK, McGuire LJ, King W et al. Cytodiagnosis of 112 salivary gland lesions. Correlation with histologic and frozen section diagnosis. Acta Cytol 1992; 36(3): 353-63.

30. Megerian CA, Maniglia AJ. Parotidectomy: a ten year experience with fine needle aspiration and frozen section biopsy correlation. Ear Nose Throat J 1994; 73(6): 377-80.

29a. Shetty A, Geethamani V. Role of fine-needle aspiration cytology in the diagnosis of major salivary gland tumors: A study with histological and clinical correlation. J Oral Maxillofac Pathol. 2016 May-Aug; 20(2): 224-9.

29. Bajaj Y, Singh S, Cozens N, Sharp J. Critical clinical appraisal of the role of ultrasound guided fine needle aspiration cytology in the management of parotid tumours. J Laryngol Otol 2005; 119(4): 289-92.

28. Das DK, Petkar MA, Al-Mane NM et al. Role of fine needle aspiration cytology in the diagnosis of swellings in the salivary gland regions: a study of 712 cases. Med Princ Pract 2004; 13(2): 95-106.

27. Seethala RR, LiVolsi VA, Baloch ZW. Relative accuracy of fine-needle aspiration and frozen section in the diagnosis of lesions of the parotid gland. Head Neck 2005; 27(3): 217-23.

26. Lee SS, Cho KJ, Jang JJ, Ham EK. Differential diagnosis of AdCC from PLA of the salivary gland on fine needle aspiration cytology. Acta Cytol 1996; 40(6): 1246-52.

25. Di Palma S, Simpson RH, Skalova A, Michal M. Metaplastic (infarcted) Warthin's tumour of the parotid gland: a possible consequence of fine needle aspiration biopsy. Histopathology 1999; 35(5): 432-8.

24. Royer MC, Davidson RK et al. Ultrasound gel causes fine needle aspiration artifact: A clear choice. Acta Cytol 2012; 56(2): 146-54.

23. Al-Khafaji BM, Afify AM. Salivary gland fine needle aspiration using the Thinprep technique: diagnostic accuracy, cytologic artifacts and pitfalls. Acta Cytol 2001; 45(4): 567-74.

22. Parfitt JR, McLachlin CM, Weir MM. Comparison of ThinPrep and conventional smears in salivary gland fine-needle aspiration biopsies. Cancer 2007; 111(2): 123-9.

21. Rajasekhar A, Sundaram C, Chowdhary T, Chaitanya M, Ratnakar KS. Diagnostic utility of fine-needle sampling without aspiration: a prospective study. Diagn Cytopathol 1991; 7(5): 473-6.

20. Yue XH, Zheng SF. Cytological diagnosis by transthoracic fine needle sampling without aspiration. Acta Cytol 1989; 33(6): 805-8.

75. Lopez-Rios F, Ballestin C, Martinez-Gonzalez MA, et al. Lymphoepithelial cyst with crystalloid formation. Cytological features of two cases. *Acta Cytol* 1999; **43**(2): 277–80.

76. Kavishwar VS, Rege JD, Naik LP. Fine needle aspiration diagnosis of lymphoepithelial cyst of the parotid gland [letter]. *Acta Cytol* 1999; **43**(5): 972–4.

77. Chaushu G, Buchner A, David R. Multiple oncocytic cysts with tyrosine-crystalloids in the parotid gland [see comments]. *Hum Pathol* 1999; **30**(2): 237–9.

78. Moody AB, Avery CM, Harrison JD. Dermoid cyst of the parotid gland. *Int J Oral Maxillofac Surg* 1998; **27**(6): 4 61–2.

79. Righi PD, Wells WA, Wagner JD, et al. Odontogenic keratocyst of the mandible: an unusual cause of a parotid mass. *Ann Plast Surg* 1998; **41**(1): 89–93.

80. Bhatty MA, Piggot TA, Soames JV, McLean NR. Chronic non-specific parotid sialadenitis. *Br J Plast Surg* 1998; **51**(7): 517–21.

81. Hogg RP, Ayshford C, Watkinson JC. Parotid duct carcinoma arising in bilateral chronic sialadenitis. *J Laryngol Otol* 1999; **113**(7): 686–8.

82. Boutonnat J, Ducros V, Pinel C, et al. Identification of amylase crystalloids in cystic lesions of the parotid gland. *Acta Cytol* 2000 Jan–Feb; **44**(1): 51–6.

83. Gupta RK, Green C, Fauck R, Lallu S, Naran S. Fine needle aspiration cytodiagnosis of sialadenitis with crystalloids. *Acta Cytol* 1999; **43**(3): 390–2.

84. Nasuti JF, Gupta PK, Fleisher SR, LiVolsi VA. Nontyrosine crystalloids in salivary gland lesions: report of seven cases with fine-needle aspiration cytology and follow-up surgical pathology. *Diagn Cytopathol* 2000; **22**(3): 167–71.

85. Granter SR, Renshaw AA, Cibas ES. Nontyrosine crystalloids in fine-needle aspiration specimens of the parotid gland: a report of two cases and review of the literature. *Diagn Cytopathol* 1999; **20**(1): 44–6.

86. Batsakis JG. Granulomatous sialadenitis. *Ann Otol Rhinol Laryngol* 1991; **100**(2): 166–9.

87. Van der Walt JD, Leake J. Granulomatous sialadenitis of the major salivary glands. A clinicopathological study of 57 cases. *Histopathology* 1987; **11**(2): 131–44.

88. Mair S, Leiman G, Levinsohn D. Fine needle aspiration cytology of parotid sarcoidosis. *Acta Cytol* 1989; 3 **3**(2): 169–72.

89. Vaillo A, Gutierrez-Martin A, Ballestín C, Ruiz-Liso JM. Marginal zone B-cell lymphoma of the parotid gland associated with epithelioid granulomas. Report of a case with fine needle aspiration. *Acta Cytol* 2004; **48**(3): 420–4.

90. Santiago K, Rivera A, Cabaniss D, et al. Fine-needle aspiration of cytomegalovirus sialadenitis in a patient with acquired immunodeficiency syndrome: pitfalls of diff-quik staining. *Diagn Cytopathol* 2000 Feb; **22**(2): 101–3.

91. Raab SS, Thomas PA, Cohen MB. Fine-needle aspiration biopsy of salivary gland mycoses. *Diagn Cytopathol* 1994; **11**(3): 286–90.

92. Ussmuller J, Donath K. Histopathogenesis of chronic sialectatic parotitis as precursor of myoepithelial sialadenitis lesion (Sjogren syndrome). *Laryngorhinootologie* 1998; **77**(12): 723–7.

93. Haddad J, Deny P, Munz-Gotheil C et al. Lymphocytic sialadenitis of Sjogren's syndrome associated with chronic hepatitis C virus liver disease [see comments]. *Lancet* 1992; **339**(8789): 321–3.

94. Jordan J, Babinski D, Sova J. Adenolymphoma (Warthin's tumor) of the larynx: coexistence with the bilateral laryngocele. Contribution to differential diagnosis with oncocytic papillary cystadenoma. *Otolaryngol Pol* 1999; **53**(2): 213–6.

95. Isaacson PG. Mucosa-associated lymphoid tissue lymphoma. *Semin Hematol* 1999; **36**(2): 139–47.

96. Isaacson PG. Gastrointestinal lymphomas of T- and B-cell types. *Mod Pathol* 1999; **12**(2): 151–8.

97. Klijanienko J, El-Naggar AK, Servois V, et al. MEC ex PLA: nonspecific preoperative cytological findings in six cases. *Cancer* 1998; **84**(4): 231–4.

98. Harris NL, Isaacson PG. What are the criteria for distinguishing MALT from non-MALT lymphoma at extranodal sites? *Am J Clin Pathol* 1999; **111**(1 Suppl 1): S126–32.

99. Banks PM, Isaacson PG. MALT lymphomas in 1997. Where do we stand? *Am J Clin Pathol* 1999; **111**(1 Suppl 1): S75–83.

100. Du MQ, Isaacson PG. Recent advances in our understanding of the biology and pathogenesis of gastric mucosa-associated lymphoid tissue (malt) lymphoma. *Forum (Genova)* 1998; **8**(2): 162–73.

101. Lasota J, Miettinen MM. Coexistence of different B-cell clones in consecutive lesions of low-grade MALT lymphoma of the salivary gland in Sjogren's disease. *Mod Pathol* 1997; **10**(9): 872–8.

102. Harris NL. Lymphoid proliferations of the salivary glands. *Am J Clin Pathol* 1999; **111**(1 Suppl 1): S94–103.

103. Aiello A, Du MQ, Diss TC, et al. Simultaneous phenotypically distinct but clonally identical mucosa- associated lymphoid tissue and follicular lymphoma in a patient with Sjogren's syndrome. *Blood* 1999; **94**(7): 2247–51

104. Quintana PG, Kapadia SB, Bahler DW, et al. Salivary gland lymphoid infiltrates associated with lymphoepithelial lesions: a clinicopathologic, immunophenotypic, and genotypic study [see comments]. *Hum Pathol* 1997; **28**(7): 850–61.

105. Klussmann JP, Guntinas-Lichius O, Heilig B, et al. Sjogren syndrome and bilateral MALT lymphoma of the parotid gland. *HNO* 1999; **47**(7): 637–41.

106. Cha I, Long SR, Ljung BM, Miller TR. Low-grade lymphoma of mucosa-associated tissue in the parotid gland: a case report of fine-needle aspiration cytology diagnosis using flow cytometric immunophenotyping. *Diagn Cytopathol* 1997; **16**(4): 345–9.

107. Burke JS. Are there site-specific differences among the MALT lymphomas – morphologic, clinical? *Am J Clin Pathol* 1999; **111**(1 Suppl 1): S133–43.

108. Ruschenburg I, Korabiowska M, Schlott T et al. The value of PCR technique in fine needle aspiration biopsy of salivary gland for diagnosis of low-grade B-cell lymphoma. *Int J Mol Med* 1998; **2**(3): 339–341.

109. MacCallum PL, Lampe HB, Cramer H, Matthews TW. Fine-needle aspiration cytology of lymphoid lesions of the salivary gland: a review of 35 cases. *J Otolaryngol* 1996; **25**(5): 300–4.

110. Joshi VV, Gagnon GA, Chadwick EG et al. The spectrum of mucosa-associated lymphoid tissue lesions in pediatric patients infected with HIV: A clinicopathologic study of six cases. *Am J Clin Pathol* 1997; **107**(5): 592–600.

111. Pinkston JA, Cole P. Incidence rates of salivary gland tumors: results from a population-based study. *Otolaryngol Head Neck Surg* 1999; **120**(6): 834–40.

112. Christensen NR, Charabi S, Sorensen WT, et al. Benign neoplasms in the parotid gland in the county of Copenhagen 1986–1995. *Ugeskr Laeger* 1998; **160**(42): 6066–9.

113. Wu S, Liu G, Chen R, Guan Y. Role of ultrasound in the assessment of benignity and malignancy of parotid masses. *Dentomaxillofac Radiol* 2012; **41**(2): 131–5.

114. Białek EJ, Jakubowski W, Karpin´ska G. Role of ultrasonographyin diagnosis and differentiation of PLAs. *Arch Otolaryngol Head Neck Surg* 2003; **129**: 929–933.

115. Kim J, Kim EK, Park CS et al. Characteristic sonographic findings of Warthin's tumor in the parotid gland. *J Clin Ultrasound* 2004; **32**: 78–81.

116. Howlett DC. High resolution ultrasound assessment of the parotid gland. *Br J Radiol* 2003; **76**: 271–277.

117. Yonetsu K, Ohki M, Kumazawa S et al. Parotid tumors: differentiation of benign and malignant tumors with quantitative sonographic analyses. *Ultrasound Med Biol* 2004; **30**: 567–574.

118. Yasumoto M, Yoshimura R, Sunaba K, Shibuya H. Sonographic appearances of malignant lymphoma of the salivary glands. *J Clin Ultrasound* 2001; **29**: 491–498.

119. Zacharia TT, Ittoop A, Perumpillichira JJ, Chavhan G. Sonographic appearance of a congenital parotid gland hemangiolymphangioma simulating malignancy in an infant. *J Clin Ultrasound* 2003; **31**: 493–496.

120. Eichhorn KW, Arapakis I, Ridder GJ. Malignant non-Hodgkin's lymphoma mimicking a benign parotid tumor: sonographic findings. *J Clin Ultrasound* 2002; **30**: 42–44.

121. Buenting JE, Smith TL, Holmes DK. Giant PLA of the parotid gland: case report and review of the literature. *Ear Nose Throat J* 1998; **77**(8): 634, 637–8, 640.

122. Ahn MS, Hayashi GM, Hilsinger RL, Jr, Lalwani AK. Familial mixed tumors of the parotid gland. *Head Neck* 1999; **21**(8): 772–5.

123. Klijanienko J, El-Naggar AK, Vielh P. Fine-needle sampling findings in 26 carcinoma ex PLAs: diagnostic pitfalls and clinical considerations. *Diagn Cytopathol* 1999; **21**(3): 163–6.

124. Viguer JM, Vicandi B, Jimenez-Heffernan JA, Lopez-Ferrer P, Limeres MA. Fine needle aspiration cytology of PLA. An analysis of 212 cases. *Acta Cytol* 1997; **41**(3): 786–94.

125. Verma K, Kapila K. Role of fine needle aspiration cytology in diagnosis of PLAs. *Cytopathology* 2002; **13**: 121–127.

126. Klijanienko J, Vielh P. Fine-needle sampling of salivary gland lesions. I. Cytology and histology correlation of 412 cases of PLA. *Diagn Cytopathol* 1996; **14**(3): 195–200.

126a. Silvanto AM, Melly L, Hannan SA, Kocjan G. FNAC of nodular fasciitis mimicking a pleomorphic adenoma: another diagnostic pitfall. *Cytopathology* 2010; **21**(4): 276–7.

127. Laskawi R, Schott T, Schroder M. Recurrent PLAs of the parotid gland: clinical evaluation and long-term follow-up. *Br J Oral Maxillofac Surg* 1998; **36**(1): 48–51.

128. Kapadia SB, Dusenbery D, Dekker A. Fine needle aspiration of PLA and AdCC of salivary gland origin. *Acta Cytol* 1997; **41**(2): 487–92.

129. Elsheikh TM, Bernacki EG. Fine needle aspiration cytology of cellular PLA. *Acta Cytol* 1996; **40**(6): 1165–75.

130. Pusztaszeri M, Braunschweig R, Mihaescu A. PLA with predominant plasmocytoid myoepithelial cells: a diagnostic pitfall in aspiration cytology. Case report and review of the literature. *Diagn Cytopathol.* 2009 Jan; **37**(1): 56–60.

131. Domanski HA. Intravenous pyogenic granuloma mimicking PLA in a fine needle aspirate. A case report. *Acta Cytol* 1999; **43**(3): 439–41.

132. Pitman MB, Thor AD, Goodman ML, Rosenberg AE. Benign metastasizing PLA of salivary gland: diagnosis of bone lesions by fine-needle aspiration biopsy. *Diagn Cytopathol* 1992; **8**(4): 384–7.

133. Klijanienko J, El-Naggar AK, Servois V et al. Clinically aggressive metastasizing PLA: report of two cases. *Head Neck* 1997; **19**(7): 629–33.

134. Bottles K, Lowhagen T, Miller TR. Mast cells in the aspiration cytology differential diagnosis of adenolymphoma. *Acta Cytol* 1985; **29**(4): 513–5.

135. Kobayashi TK, Ueda M, Nishino T et al. Association of mast cells with Warthin's tumor in fine needle aspirates of the salivary gland. *Acta Cytol* 1999; **43**(6): 1052–8.

136. Klijanienko J, Vielh P. Fine-needle sampling of salivary gland lesions. II. Cytology and histology correlation of 71 cases of Warthin's tumor (adenolymphoma). *Diagn Cytopathol* 1997; **16**(3): 221–5.

137. Edwards PC, Wasserman P. Evaluation of cystic salivary gland lesions by fine needle aspiration: an analysis of 21 cases. *Acta Cytol* 2005; **49**(5): 489–94.

138. Ballo MS, Shin HJ, Sneige N. Sources of diagnostic error in the fine-needle aspiration diagnosis of Warthin's tumor and clues to a correct diagnosis. *Diagn Cytopathol* 1997; **17**(3): 230–4.

139. Layfield LJ, Gopez EV. Cystic lesions of the salivary glands: cytologic features in fine-needle aspiration biopsies. *Diagn Cytopathol* 2002; **27**(4): 197–204.

140. Ryska A, Seifert G. Adenolymphoma (Warthin's tumor) with multiple sarcoid-like granulomas. *Pathol Res Pract* 1999; **195**(12): 835–9.

141. Hürthle K. Beitrage zur Kenntnis de Sekretions-vorganges in der Schilddruse. *Arch F D Ges Physiol* 1894; **56**: 1–44.

142. Jahan-Parwar B, Huberman RM, Donovan DT, et al. Oncocytic MEC of the salivary glands. *Am J Surg Pathol* 1999; **23**(5): 523–9.

143. Shick PC, Brannon RB. Oncocytoid artifact of the parotid gland: a newly reported artifact. *Oral Surg Oral Med Oral Pathol Oral Radiol Endod* 1998; **86**(6): 720–2.

144. Strassburger S, Hyckel P, Kosmehl H. Multifocal oncocytic adenomatous hyperplasia of the parotid gland. A case report. *Int J Oral Maxillofac Surg* 1999; **28**(6): 457–8.

145. Park CK, Manning JT, Jr, Battifora H, Medeiros LJ. Follicle center lymphoma and Warthin tumor involving the same anatomic site. Report of two cases and review of the literature. *Am J Clin Pathol* 2000 ; **113**(1): 113–9.

146. Nagao T, Sugano I, Ishida Y, et al. MEC arising in Warthin's tumour of the parotid gland: report of two cases with histopathological, ultrastructural and immunohistochemical studies. *Histopathology* 1998; **33**(4): 379–86.

147. Seifert G. Carcinoma in pre-existing Warthin tumors (cystadenolymphoma) of the parotid gland. Classification, pathogenesis and differential diagnosis. *Pathologe* 1997; **18**(5): 359–67.

148. Patterson JW, Wright ED, Camden S. Extraparotid Warthin's tumor. *J Am Acad Dermatol* 1999; **40**(3): 468–70.

149. Jurczyk M, Peevey JF, Vande Haar MA, Lin X. Pitfalls of fine-needle aspiration cytology of parotid membranous basal cell adenoma – A review of pitfalls in FNA cytology of salivary gland neoplasms with basaloid cell features. *Diagn Cytopathol* 2015; **43**(5): 432–7.

150. Paker I, Yilmazer D, Arikok AT et al. Basal cell adenoma with extensive squamous metaplasia and cellular atypia: a case report with cytohistopathological correlation and review of the literature. *Diagn Cytopathol* 2012; **40**(1): 48–55.

151. Klijanienko J, el-Naggar AK, Vielh P. Comparative cytological and histologic study of fifteen salivary basal- cell tumors: differential diagnostic considerations. *Diagn Cytopathol* 1999; **21**(1): 30–4.

152. Stanley MW, Horwitz CA, Rollins SD, et al. Basal cell (monomorphic) and minimally PLAs of the salivary glands. Distinction from the solid (anaplastic) type of AdCC in fine-needle aspiration. *Am J Clin Pathol* 1996; **106**(1): 35–41.

153. Thompson LD, Wenig BM, Ellis GL. Oncocytomas of the submandibular gland. A series of 22 cases and a review of the literature. *Cancer* 1996; **78**(11): 2281–7.

154. Skalova A, Starek I, Michal M, Leivo I. Malignancy-simulating change in parotid gland oncocytoma following fine needle aspiration. Report of 3 cases. *Pathol Res Pract* 1999; **195**(6): 399–405.

155. Rajan PB, Wadehra V, Hemming JD, Hawkesford JE. Fine needle aspiration cytology of malignant oncocytoma of the parotid gland – a case report [see comments]. *Cytopathology* 1994; **5**(2): 110–3.

156. Gnepp DR. Salivary gland tumor 'wishes' to add to the next WHO Tumor Classification: sclerosing polycystic adenosis, mammary analogue secretory carcinoma, cribriform adenocarcinoma of the tongue and other sites, and mucinous variant of myoepithelioma. *Head Neck Pathol* 2014; **8**(1): 42–9.

157. Vo-Ngoc H, Dellagi K, Marandas P, Micheau C. Myoepithelioma (or myoepithelial cell adenoma). Report of a case. *Ann Pathol* 1994; **14**(2): 112–5.

158. Tanimura A, Nakamura Y, Nagayama K, et al. Myoepithelioma of the parotid gland. Report of two cases with immunohistochemical technique for S-100 protein and electron microscopic observation. *Acta Pathol Jpn* 1985; **35**(2): 409–17.

159. Dodd LG, Caraway NP, Luna MA, Byers RM. Myoepithelioma of the parotid. Report of a case initially examined by fine needle aspiration biopsy. *Acta Cytol* 1994; **38**(3): 417–21.

160. Alos L, Cardesa A, Bombi JA et al. Myoepithelial tumors of salivary glands: a clinicopathologic, immunohistochemical, ultrastructural, and flow-cytometric study. *Semin Diagn Pathol* 1996; **13**(2): 138–47.

161. Sironi M, Taccagni G, Assi A. A cytological, immunocytochemical and ultrastructural study of a malignant parotid gland myoepithelioma. *Cytopathology* 1997; **8**(1): 53–62.

162. Kumar PV, Sobhani SA, Monabati A et al. Myoepithelioma of the salivary glands. Fine needle aspiration biopsy findings. *Acta Cytol* 2004; **48**(3): 302–8.

163. Orell SR, Nettle WJ. Fine needle aspiration biopsy of salivary gland tumours. Problems and pitfalls. *Pathology* 1988; **20**(4): 332–7.

164. Ramdall RB, Cai G, Levine PH et al. Fine-needle aspiration biopsy findings in epithelioid myoepithelioma of the parotid gland: a case report. *Diagn Cytopathol* 2006; **34**(11): 776–9.

165. King PH, Hill J. Intraduct papilloma of parotid gland. *J Clin Pathol* 1993; **46**(2): 175–6.

166. Soofer SB, Tabbara S. Intraductal papilloma of the salivary gland. A report of two cases with diagnosis by fine needle aspiration biopsy. *Acta Cytol* 1999; **43**(6): 1142–6.

167. Zhang S, Bao R, Abreo F. Papillary oncocytic cystadenoma of the parotid glands: a report of 2 cases with varied cytologic features. *Acta Cytol* 2009; **53**(4): 445–8.

168. Nagao T, Sugano I, Matsuzaki O, et al. Intraductal papillary tumors of the major salivary glands [In Process Citation]. *Arch Pathol Lab Med* 2000 Feb; **124**(2): 291–5.

169. Simpson RH, Skálová A, Di Palma S, Leivo I. Recent advances in the diagnostic pathology of salivary carcinomas. *Virchows Arch* 2014; **465**(4): 371–84.

170. Malata CM, Camilleri IG, McLean NR, et al. Malignant tumours of the parotid gland: a 12-year review. *Br J Plast Surg* 1997; **50**(8): 600–8.

171. Calearo C, Pastore A, Storchi OF, Polli G. Parotid gland carcinoma: analysis of prognostic factors. *Ann Otol Rhinol Laryngol* 1998; **107**(11 Pt 1): 969–73.

172. Leverstein H, van der Wal JE, Tiwari RM, et al. Malignant epithelial parotid gland tumours: analysis and results in 65 previously untreated patients. *Br J Surg* 1998; **85**(9): 1267–72.

173. Nordkvist A, Roijer E, Bang G, et al. Expression and mutation patterns of p53 in benign and malignant salivary gland tumors. *Int J Oncol* 2000 Mar; **16**(3): 477–83.

174. Zhu Q, Tipoe GL, White FH. Proliferative activity as detected by immunostaining with Ki-67 and proliferating cell nuclear antigen in benign and malignant epithelial lesions of the human parotid gland. *Anal Quant Cytol Histol* 1999; **21**(4): 336–42.

175. Pinto AE, Fonseca I, Soares J. The clinical relevance of ploidy and S-phase fraction determination in salivary gland tumors: a flow cytometric study of 97 cases. *Cancer* 1999; **85**(2): 273–81.

176. Betkowski A, Cyran-Rymarz A, Domka W. Bilateral acinar cell carcinoma of the parotid gland. *Otolaryngol Pol* 1998; **52**(1): 101–4.

177. Depowski PL, Setzen G, Chui A et al. Familial occurrence of acinic cell carcinoma of the parotid gland. *Arch Pathol Lab Med* 1999; **123**(11): 1118–20.

178. Angeles-Angeles A, Caballero-Mendoza E, Tapia-Rangel B et al. Giant acinic cell parotid gland adenocarcinoma of the papillary-cystic type. *Rev Invest Clin* 1998; **50**(3): 245–8.

179. Laskawi R, Rodel R, Zirk A, Arglebe C. Retrospective analysis of 35 patients with acinic cell carcinoma of the parotid gland. *J Oral Maxillofac Surg* 1998; **56**(4): 440–3.

180. Klijanienko J, Vielh P. Fine-needle sample of salivary gland lesions. V: Cytology of 22 cases of acinic cell carcinoma with histologic correlation. *Diagn Cytopathol* 1997; **17**(5): 347–52.

181. Hoffman HT, Karnell LH, Robinson RA et al. National Cancer Data Base report on cancer of the head and neck: acinic cell carcinoma. *Head Neck* 1999; **21**(4): 297–309.

182. Nagel H, Laskawi R, Buter JJ et al. Cytological diagnosis of acinic-cell carcinoma of salivary glands. *Diagn Cytopathol* 1997; **16**(5): 402–12.

183. Moore FR, Bergman S, Geisinger KR. Metastatic hepatocellular carcinoma mimicking acinic cell carcinoma of the parotid gland: a case report. *Acta Cytol* 2010; **54**(5 Suppl): 889–92.

184. Tian W, Yakirevich E, Matoso A, Gnepp DR (2012) IgG4+ plasma cells in sclerosing variant of MEC: a new and evolving concept. *Am J Surg Pathol* **36**: 973–979.

185. Seethala RR. An update on grading of salivary gland carcinomas. *Head Neck Pathol* 2009; **3**: 69–77.

186. Skálová A, Lehtonen H, von Boguslawsky K, Leivo I. Prognostic significance of cell proliferation in MEC of the salivary gland: clinicopathological study using MIB1 antibody in paraffin sections. *Hum Pathol* 1994; **25**: 929–935.

187. Alós L, Lujan B, Castillo M et al. Expression of membrane-bound mucins (MUC1 and MUC4) and secreted mucins (MUC2, MUC5AC, MUC5B, MUC6 and MUC7) in MECs of salivary glands. *Am J Surg Pathol* 2005; **29**: 806–813.

188. Tonon G, Modi S, Wu L, et al. t(11;19)(q21;p13) translocation in MEC creates a novel fusion product that disrupts a Notch signalling pathway. *Nat Genet* 2003; **33**: 208–213.

189. Nakayama T, Miyabe S, Okabe M et al. Clinicopathological significance of the CRTC3-MAML2 fusion transcript in MEC. *Modern Pathol* 2009; **22**: 1575–1581.

190. Okabe M, Miyabe S, Nagatsuka H et al. MECT1-MAML2 fusion transcript defines a favourable subset of MEC. *Clin Cancer Res* 2006; **12**: 3902–3907.

191. Jee KJ, Persson M, Heikinheimo K et al. Genomic profiles and CRTC1-MAML2 fusion distinguish different subtypes of MEC. *Modern Pathol* 2013; **26**: 213–222.

192. Plambeck K, Friedrich RE, Schmelzle R. MEC of salivary gland origin: classification, clinical-pathological correlation, treatment results and long-term follow-up in 55 patients. *J Craniomaxillofac Surg* 1996; **24**(3): 133–9.

193. Cohen MB, Fisher PE, Holly EA et al. Fine needle aspiration biopsy diagnosis of MEC. Statistical analysis. *Acta Cytol* 1990; **34**(1): 43–9.

194. Klijanienko J, Vielh P. Fine-needle sampling of salivary gland lesions. IV. Review of 50 cases of MEC with histologic correlation. *Diagn Cytopathol* 1997; **17**(2): 92–8.

195. Hamed G, Shmookler BM, Ellis GL, et al. Oncocytic MEC of the parotid gland. *Arch Pathol Lab Med* 1994; **118**(3): 313–4.

196. Bajaj J, Gimenez C, Slim F et al. Fine-needle aspiration cytology of mammary analog secretory carcinoma masquerading as low-grade MEC: case report with a review of the literature. *Acta Cytol.* 2014; **58**(5): 501–10

197. Jacobs JC. Low grade MEC ex PLA. A diagnostic problem in fine needle aspiration biopsy. *Acta Cytol* 1994; **38**(1): 93–7.

198. El-Naggar AK, Huvos AG. AdCC. Chapter 5, Tumours of the salivary glands. In: Barnes EL, Eveson JW, Reichart P, Sidransky D (eds) *World Health Organization classification of tumours: pathology and genetics of head and neck tumours.* IARC, Lyon, pp. 221–2, 2005.

199. Klijanienko J, Vielh P. Fine-needle sampling of salivary gland lesions. III. Cytological and histologic correlation of 75 cases of AdCC: review and experience at the Institut Curie with emphasis on cytological pitfalls. *Diagn Cytopathol* 1997; **17**(1): 36–41.

200. Orell SR Sterett GF, Walters MN et al. *Manual and atlas of fine needle aspiration cytology.* Churchill Livingstone, 1992.

201. Nagel H, Hotze HJ, Laskawi R et al. Cytological diagnosis of AdCC of salivary glands. *Diagn Cytopathol* 1999; **20**(6): 358–66.

202. Skálová A, Simpson RHW, Lehtonen H, Leivo I. Assessment of proliferative activity using the MIB1 antibody helps to distinguish polymorphous low grade adenocarcinoma from AdCC of salivary glands. *Pathol Res Pract* 1997; **193**: 695–703.

203. Layfield LJ. Fine needle aspiration cytology of a trabecular adenoma of the parotid gland. *Acta Cytol* 1985; **29**(6): 999–1002.

204. Grenko RT, Abendroth CS, Davis AT et al. Hybrid tumors or salivary gland tumors sharing common differentiation pathways? Reexamining adenoid cystic and epithelial-myoepithelial carcinomas. *Oral Surg Oral Med Oral Pathol Oral Radiol Endod* 1998; **86**(2): 188–95.

205. Prasad AR, Savera AT, Gown AM, Zarbo RJ. The myoepithelial immunophenotype in 135 benign and malignant salivary gland tumors other than PLA. *Arch Pathol Lab Med* 1999; **123**(9): 801–6.

206. Stenman G (2013) Fusion oncogenes in salivary gland tumors: molecular and clinical consequences. *Head Neck Pathol* 7: S12–S19.

207. Brill LB, Kanner WA, Fehr A et al. Analysis of MYB expression and MYB-NFIB gene fusions in AdCC and other salivary neoplasms. *Modern Pathol* 2011; **24**: 1169–1176.

208. Di Palma S, Fehr A, Danford M et al. Primary sinonasal AdCC presenting with skin metastases – genomic profile and expression of the MYB-NFIB fusion biomarker. *Histopathology* 2014; **64**: 453–455

209. Puxeddu R, Puxeddu P, Parodo G, Faa G. Polymorphous low-grade adenocarcinoma of the parotid gland. *Eur J Morphol* 1998; **36**(Suppl): 262–6.

210. Barak AP, Grobbel MA, Rabaja DR. Polymorphous low-grade adenocarcinoma of the parotid gland. *Am J Otolaryngol* 1998; **19**(5): 322–4.

211. Vincent SD, Hammond HL, Finkelstein MW. Clinical and therapeutic features of polymorphous low-grade adenocarcinoma. *Oral Surg Oral Med Oral Pathol* 1994; **77**(1): 41–7.

212. Simpson RH, Clarke TJ, Sarsfield PT et al. Polymorphous low-grade adenocarcinoma of the salivary glands: a clinicopathological comparison with AdCC [see comments]. *Histopathology* 1991; **19**(2): 121–9.

213. Gibbons D, Saboorian MH, Vuitch F et al. Fine-needle aspiration findings in patients with polymorphous low grade adenocarcinoma of the salivary glands. *Cancer* 1999; **87**(1): 31–6.

214. Frierson HF, Jr., Covell JL, Mills SE. Fine-needle aspiration cytology of terminal duct carcinoma of minor salivary gland. *Diagn Cytopathol* 1987; **3**(2): 159–62.

215. Klijanienko J, Vielh P. Salivary carcinomas with papillae: cytology and histology analysis of polymorphous low-grade adenocarcinoma and papillary cystadenocarcinoma. *Diagn Cytopathol* 1998; **19**(4): 244–9.

216. Cleveland DB, Cosgrove MM, Martin SE. Tyrosine-rich crystalloids in a fine needle aspirate of a polymorphous low grade adenocarcinoma of a minor salivary gland. A case report. *Acta Cytol* 1994; **38**(2): 247–51.

217. Watanabe K, Ono N, Saito K et al. Fine-needle aspiration cytology of polymorphous low-grade adenocarcinoma of the tongue. *Diagn Cytopathol* 1999; **20**(3): 167–9.

218. Thiebault S, Mogras A, Brun I et al. Epithelial-myoepithelial carcinoma of the salivary glands: report of a case. *Ann Pathol* 1999; **19**(1): 30–2.

219. Kasper HU, Mellin W, Kriegsmann J et al. Epithelial-myoepithelial carcinoma of the salivary gland – a low grade malignant neoplasm? Report of two cases and review of the literature. *Pathol Res Pract* 1999; **195**(3): 189–92.

220. Batsakis JG, el-Naggar AK, Luna MA. Epithelial-myoepithelial carcinoma of salivary glands. *Ann Otol Rhinol Laryngol* 1992; **101**(6): 540–2.

221. Brocheriou C, Auriol M, de Roquancourt A et al. Epithelial-myoepithelial carcinoma of the salivary glands. Study of 15 cases and review of the literature. *Ann Pathol* 1991; **11**(5–6): 316–25.

222. Ng WK, Choy C, Ip P et al. Fine needle aspiration cytology of epithelial-myoepithelial carcinoma of salivary glands. A report of three cases. *Acta Cytol* 1999; **43**(4): 675–80.

223. Carrillo R, Poblet E, Rocamora A, Rodriguez-Peralto JL. Epithelial-myoepithelial carcinoma of the salivary gland. Fine needle aspiration cytological findings. *Acta Cytol* 1990; **34**(2): 243–7.

224. Yang GC, Soslow RA. Epithelial-myoepithelial carcinoma of the parotid. A case of ductal- predominant presentation with cytological, histologic and ultrastructural correlations. *Acta Cytol* 1999; **43**(6): 1113–8.

225. Kocjan G, Milroy C, Fisher EW, Eveson JW. Cytological features of epithelial-myoepithelial carcinoma of salivary gland: potential pitfalls in diagnosis. *Cytopathology* 1993; **4**(3): 173–80.

226. Plath T, Dallenbach F. Basal cell adenocarcinoma of the minor salivary glands of the palate. Case report and review of the literature. *Mund Kiefer Gesichtschir* 1998; **2**(5): 275–8.

227. Pisharodi LR. Basal cell adenocarcinoma of the salivary gland. Diagnosis by fine-needle aspiration cytology. *Am J Clin Pathol* 1995; **103**(5): 603–8.

228. Moroz K, Ferreira C, Dhurandhar N. Fine needle aspiration of basal cell adenocarcinoma of the parotid gland. Report of a case with assessment of DNA ploidy in aspirates and tissue sections by image analysis. *Acta Cytol* 1996; **40**(4): 773–8.

229. Foss RD, Ellis GL, Auclair PL. Salivary gland cystadenocarcinomas. A clinicopathologic study of 57 cases. *Am J Surg Pathol* 1996; **20**(12): 1440–7.

230. Tambouret RH, Yantiss RK, Kirby R, Eichhorn JH. Mucinous adenocarcinoma of the parotid gland. Report of a case with fine needle aspiration findings and histologic correlation. *Acta Cytol* 1999; **43**(5):8 42–6.

231. Ardekian L, Manor R, Peled M, Laufer D. Malignant oncocytoma of the parotid gland: case report and analysis of the literature. *J Oral Maxillofac Surg* 1999; **57**(3): 325–8.

232. Nakada M, Nishizaki K, Akagi H et al. Oncocytic carcinoma of the submandibular gland: a case report and literature review. *J Oral Pathol Med* 1998; **27**(5): 225–8.

233. Gray SR, Cornog JL, Jr., Seo IS. Oncocytic neoplasms of salivary glands: a report of fifteen cases including two malignant oncocytomas. *Cancer* 1976; **38**(3): 1306–17.

234. Brandwein MS, Jagirdar J, Patil J et al. Salivary duct carcinoma (cribriform salivary carcinoma of excretory ducts). A clinicopathologic and immunohistochemical study of 12 cases. *Cancer* 1990; **65**(10): 2307–14.

235. Simpson RH. Salivary duct carcinoma: new developments – morphological variants including pure in situ high grade lesions; proposed molecular classification. *Head Neck Pathol* 2013 Jul; 7 Suppl 1: S48–58.

236. Fyrat P, Cramer H, Feczko JD et al. Fine-needle aspiration biopsy of salivary duct carcinoma: report of five cases. *Diagn Cytopathol* 1997; **16**(6): 526–30.

237. Gilcrease MZ, Guzman-Paz M, Froberg K, Pambuccian S. Salivary duct carcinoma. Is a specific diagnosis possible by fine needle aspiration cytology? *Acta Cytol* 1998; **42**(6): 1389–96.

238. Dee S, Masood S, Issacs JH, Jr., Hardy NM. Cytomorphologic features of salivary duct carcinoma on fine needle aspiration biopsy. A case report. *Acta Cytol* 1993; **37**(4): 539–42.

239. Klijanienko J, Vielh P. Cytological characteristics and histomorphologic correlations of 21 salivary duct carcinomas. *Diagn Cytopathol* 1998; **19**(5): 333–7.

240. Garcia-Bonafe M, Catala I, Tarragona J, Tallada N. Cytological diagnosis of salivary duct carcinoma: a review of seven cases. *Diagn Cytopathol* 1998; **19**(2): 120–3.

241. Ersoz C, Cetik F, Aydin O et al. Salivary duct carcinoma ex PLA: analysis of the findings in fine-needle aspiration cytology and histology. *Diagn Cytopathol* 1998; **19**(3): 201–4.

242. Lewis JE, McKinney BC, Weiland LH et al. Salivary duct carcinoma. Clinicopathologic and immunohistochemical review of 26 cases. *Cancer* 1996; **77**(2): 223–30.

243. Colecchia M, Frigo B, Leopardi OM. Salivary duct carcinoma of the parotid gland. Report of a case with cytological and immunocytochemical findings on fine needle aspiration biopsy. *Acta Cytol* 1997; **41**(2): 593–7.

244. Cerilli LA, Swartzbaugh JR, Saadut R et al. Analysis of chromosome 9p21 deletion and p16 gene mutation in salivary gland carcinomas. *Hum Pathol* 1999; **30**(10): 1242–6.

245. Felix A, El-Naggar AK, Press MF et al. Prognostic significance of biomarkers (c-erbB-2, p53, proliferating cell nuclear antigen, and DNA content) in salivary duct carcinoma. *Hum Pathol* 1996; **27**(6): 561–6.

246. Klijanienko J, Vielh P. Reply: cytology of salivary duct carcinoma. *Diagn Cytopathol* 2000 Feb; **22**(2): 135.

247. Auclair PL, Ellis GL. Atypical features in salivary gland mixed tumors: their relationship to malignant transformation. *Mod Pathol* 1996; **9**(6): 652–7.

248. Di Palma S, Guzzo M. Myoepithelial carcinoma with predominance of plasma-cytoid cells arising in a PLA of the parotid gland [letter; comment]. *Histopathology* 1998; **33**(5): 485.

249. Flynn MB, Maguire S, Martinez S, Tesmer T. Primary squamous cell carcinoma of the parotid gland: the importance of correct histological diagnosis. *Ann Surg Oncol* 1999; **6**(8): 768–70.

250. Seifert G, Donath K. Differential diagnosis of squamous epithelial carcinoma of the salivary glands. *Pathologe* 1998; **19**(3): 201–8.

251. Klijanienko J, Vielh P. Fine-needle sampling of salivary gland lesions. VI. Cytological review of 44 cases of primary salivary squamous-cell carcinoma with histological correlation. *Diagn Cytopathol* 1998; **18**(3): 174–8.

252. Franzen A, Schmid S, Pfaltz M. Primary small cell carcinomas and metastatic disease in the head and neck. *HNO* 1999; **47**(10): 912–7.

253. Vural C, Dogan O, Yavuz E et al. Small cell neuroendocrine carcinoma of the parotid gland. *Otolaryngol Head Neck Surg* 2000 Jan; **122**(1): 151–2.

254. Mair S, Phillips JI, Cohen R. Small cell undifferentiated carcinoma of the parotid gland. Cytological, histologic, immunohistochemical and ultrastructural features of a neuroendocrine variant. *Acta Cytol* 1989; **33**(2): 164–8.

255. Moore JG, Bocklage T. Fine-needle aspiration biopsy of large-cell undifferentiated carcinoma of the salivary glands: presentation of two cases, literature review, and differential cytodiagnosis of high-grade salivary gland malignancies. *Diagn Cytopathol* 1998; **19**(1): 44–50.

256. Batsakis JG, Luna MA. Undifferentiated carcinomas of salivary glands. *Ann Otol Rhinol Laryngol* 1991; **100**(1): 82–4.

257. Gunhan O, Celasun B, Safali M et al. Fine needle aspiration cytology of malignant lymphoepithelial lesion of the salivary gland. A report of two cases. *Acta Cytol* 1994; **38**(5): 751–4.

258. Safneck JR, Ravinsky E, Yazdi HM. Fine needle aspiration biopsy findings in lymphoepithelial carcinoma of salivary gland. *Acta Cytol* 1997; **41**(4): 1023–30.

259. Skálová A, Vanaček T, Sima R. Mammary analogue secretory carcinoma of salivary glands, containing the ETV6-NTRK3 fusion gene: a hitherto undescribed salivary gland tumor entity. *Am J Surg Pathol* 2010; **34**: 599–608.

260. Petersson F, Lian D, Chau YP, Yan B. Mammary analogue secretory carcinoma: the first submandibular case reported including findings on fine needle aspiration cytology. *Head Neck Pathol* 2012; **6**: 135–139.

261. Connor A, Perez-Ordoñez B, Shago M et al. Mammary analog secretory carcinoma of salivary gland origin with the ETV6 gene rearrangement by FISH: expanded morphologic and immunohistochemical spectrum of a recently described entity. *Am J Surg Pathol* 2012; **36**: 27–34.

262. Mariano FV, dos Santos HT, Azañero WD et al. Mammary analogue secretory carcinoma of salivary glands is a lipid-rich tumour, and adipophilin can be valuable in its identifica- tion. *Histopathology* 2013; **63**: 558–567.

263. Skálová A. Mammary analogue secretory carcinoma of salivary gland origin: an update and expanded morphologic and immunohistochemical spectrum of recently described entity. *Head Neck Pathol* 2013; 7: S30–S36.

264. Laco J, Švajdler M, Andrejs J et al. Mammary analog secretory carcinoma of salivary glands: a report of 2 cases with expression of basal/myoepithelial markers (calponin, CD10 and p63 protein). *Pathol Res Pract* 2013; **209**: 167–172.

265. Skálová A, Vanaček T, Sima R et al. Mammary analogue secre- tory carcinoma of salivary glands, containing the ETV6-NTRK3 fusion gene: a hitherto undescribed salivary gland tumor entity. *Am J Surg Pathol* 2010; **34**: 599–608.

266. Skálová A, Vaneček T, Majewska H et al. Mammary analogue secretory carcinoma of salivary glands with high grade transformation: report of three cases with the ETV6- NTRK3 gene fusion and analysis of TP53, beta-catenin, EGFR and CCND1 genes. *Am J Surg Pathol* 2014; **38**: 23–33.

267. Petersson F, Lian D, Chau YP, Yan B. Mammary analogue secretory carcinoma: the first submandibular case reported including findings on fine needle aspiration cytology. *Head Neck Pathol.* 2012 Mar; **6**(1): 135–9.

267a. Bishop JA, Yonescu R, Batista DA, Westra WH, Ali SZ. Cytopathologic features of mammary analogue secretory carcinoma. *Cancer Cytopathol.* 2013 May; **121**(5): 228–33.

268. Gailey MP, Bayon R, Robinson RA. Cribriform adenocarcinoma of minor salivary gland: a report of two cases with an emphasis on cytology. *Diagn Cytopathol* 2014; **42**(12): 1085–90.

269. Michal M, Skálová A, Simpson RH et al. Cribriform adenocarcinoma of the tongue: A hitherto unrecognized type of adenocarcinoma characteristically occurring in the tongue. *Histopathology* 1999; **35**: 495–501.

270. Skalova A, Sima R, Kaspirkova-Nemcova J et al. Cribriform adenocarcinoma of minor salivary gland origin principally affecting the tongue: Characterization of new entity. *Am J Surg Pathol* 2011; **35**: 1168–76.

271. Laco J, Kamardova K, Vitkova P et al. Cribriform adenocarcinoma of minor salivary glands may express galectin-3, cytokeratin 19, and HBME-1 and contains polymor-phisms of RET and H-RAS proto-oncogenes. *Virchows Arch* 2012; **461**: 531–540.

272. Kuczkowski J, Jagielski J. A case of schwannoma in the parotid gland. *Otolaryngol Pol* 1997; **51**(3): 324–7.

273. Mair S, Leiman G. Benign neurilemmoma (schwannoma) masquerading as a PLA of the submandibular salivary gland. *Acta Cytol* 1989; **33**(6): 907–10.

274. Gil-Benso R, Carda-Batalla C, Navarro-Fos S et al. Cytogenetic study of a spindle-cell rhabdomyosarcoma of the parotid gland. *Cancer* Genet Cytogenet 1999; **109**(2): 150–3.

275. Grayson W, Nayler SJ, Jena GP. Synovial sarcoma of the parotid gland. A case report with clinicopathological analysis and review of the literature. *S Afr J Surg* 1998; **36**(1): 32–4; discussion 34–5.

276. Shimizu K, Ogura S, Kobayashi TK et al. Fine-needle aspiration cytology of malignant hemangiopericytoma of the salivary gland: A case report. *Diagn Cytopathol* 1999; **21**(6): 398–401.

277. Perez del Rio MJ, Garcia-Garcia J, Diaz-Iglesias JM, Fresno MF. Radiation-associated angiosarcoma involving the parotid gland [letter]. *Histopathology* 1998; **33**(6): 586–7.

278. Kang J, Levinson JA, Hitti IF. Leiomyosarcoma of the parotid gland: a case report and review of the literature. *Head Neck* 1999; **21**(2): 168–71.

279. Gutierrez Triguero M, Escamilla Carpintero Y, Martinez Guirado T et al. Granulocytic sarcoma. A case with an unusual location. *Acta Otorrinolaringol Esp* 1998; **49**(8): 667–70.

280. Orvidas LJ, Kasperbauer JL, Lewis JE et al. Pediatric parotid masses. *Arch Otolaryngol Head Neck Surg* 2000 Feb; **126**(2): 177–84.

281. Roebuck DJ, Ahuja AT. Hemangioendothelioma of the parotid gland in infants: sonography and correlative MR imaging. *Ajnr Am J Neuroradiol* 2000 Jan; **21**(1): 219–23.

282. Debb RA, Desai SB, Amonkar PP et al. Primary primitive neuroectodermal tumour of the parotid gland [see comments]. *Histopathology* 1998; **33**(4): 375–8.

283. Helsel JC, Mrak RE, Hanna E et al. Peripheral primitive neuroectodermal tumor of the parotid gland region: report of a case with fine-needle aspiration findings. *Diagn Cytopathol* 2000; **22**(3): 161–6.

284. Zhang C, Cohen JM, Cangiarella JF et al. Fine-needle aspiration of secondary neoplasms involving the salivary glands. A report of 36 cases. *Am J Clin Pathol* 2000 Jan; **113**(1): 21–8.

285. Elshenawy Y, Youngberg G, Al-Abbadi MA. Unusual clinical presentation of cutaneous malignant melanoma metastatic to the parotid gland; initially dis-covered by fine needle aspiration: case report and review of literature. *Diagn Cytopathol* 2011; **39**(5): 373–6.

286. Malata CM, Camilleri IG, McLean NR et al. Metastatic tumours of the parotid gland. *Br J Oral Maxillofac Surg* 1998; **36**(3): 190–5.

287. Pisani P, Krengli M, Ramponi A et al. Metastases to parotid gland from cancers of the upper airway and digestive tract. *Br J Oral Maxillofac Surg* 1998; **36**(1): 54–7.

288. Gangopadhyay K, Abuzeid MO, Martin JM, Saleem M. Metastatic renal cell carcinoma of the parotid gland presenting as a neck mass. *Int J Clin Pract* 1998; **52**(3): 196–8.

289. Takatsugi K, Komuta K, Hosen N et al. Metastasis of small cell lung cancer to the parotid gland as the initial clinical manifestation, followed by metastases to the pituitary gland and lumber spinal cord. *Nihon Kokyuki Gakkai Zasshi* 1998; **36**(3): 246–50.

290. Choi DS, Na DG, Byun HS et al. Salivary gland tumors: evaluation with two-phase helical CT. *Radiology* 2000 Jan; **214**(1): 231–6.

291. Takashima S, Takayama F, Wang Q et al. Parotid gland lesions: diagnosis of malignancy with MRI and flow cytometric DNA analysis and cytology in fine-needle aspiration biopsy. *Head Neck* 1999; **21**(1): 43–51.

292. Shaha AR, Webber C, DiMaio T, Jaffe BM. Needle aspiration biopsy in salivary gland lesions. *Am J Surg* 1990; **160**(4): 373–6.

293. Heller KS, Dubner S, Chess Q, Attie JN. Value of fine needle aspiration biopsy of salivary gland masses in clinical decision-making. *Am J Surg* 1992; **164**(6): 667–70.

294. Raab SS, Sigman JD, Hoffman HT. The utility of parotid gland and level I and II neck fine-needle aspiration. *Arch Pathol Lab Med* 1998; **122**(9): 823–7.

CHAPTER 3

Thyroid

Chapter contents

3.1 Introduction, 71
    3.1.1 Ultrasound and FNAC procedure, 72
    3.1.2 FNAC reporting categories, 74
    3.1.3 Diagnostic accuracy, 74
        3.1.3.1 Ultrasound, 74
        3.1.3.2 FNAC, 76
    3.1.4 Diagnostic pitfalls, 76
    3.1.5 The role of FNAC thyroid in clinical management, 76
    3.1.6 FNAC versus frozen section and core biopsy histology, 77
    3.1.7 Ancillary techniques, 78
    3.1.8 Complications of FNAC, 78
3.2 Non-neoplastic and inflammatory conditions, 79
    3.2.1 Colloid goitre (non-toxic goitre, adenomatous hyperplasia, multinodular goitre), 79
    3.2.2 Cysts, 81
    3.2.3 Hyperactive goitre (toxic goitre, thyrotoxicosis, primary hyperthyroidism, Graves' disease), 83
    3.2.4 Thyroiditis, 85
        3.2.4.1 Acute, 85
        3.2.4.2 Subacute (granulomatous thyroiditis, De Quervain's thyroiditis), 85
        3.2.4.3 Lymphocytic (Hashimoto), 85
        3.2.4.4 Riedel's, 86
3.3 Indeterminate cytological findings: follicular lesions, 87
    3.3.1 Atypia of uncertain significance (AUS)/Follicular lesion of uncertain significance (FLUS) (TBSRTC III, UK Thy 3a), 87

3.3.2 'Follicular lesions' (TBSTRC IV: Follicular neoplasm or suspicious for a follicular neoplasm) (UK: Thy 3f), 90
    3.3.2.1 Follicular adenoma, 91
    3.3.2.2 Oncocytic (Hürthle) cell tumours, 92
    3.3.2.3 Hyalinising trabecular adenoma, 93
3.4 Malignant tumours, 94
    3.4.1 Papillary carcinoma, 94
        3.4.1.1 Follicular variant, 95
        3.4.1.2 Tall cell variant, 96
        3.4.1.3 Columnar cell variant, 97
        3.4.1.4 Oncocytic variant, 97
        3.4.1.5 Papillary Hürthle cell carcinoma with lymphoplasmacytic stroma, 98
        3.4.1.6 Cribriform-morular variant, 98
        3.4.1.7 Diffuse sclerosing variant, 99
        3.4.1.8 Papillary carcinoma with a nodular fasciitis like stroma, 99
        3.4.1.9 Immunohistochemical markers, 99
        3.4.1.10 Molecular markers, 99
        3.4.1.11 Differential diagnosis, 100
    3.4.2 Follicular carcinoma, 101
    3.4.3 Medullary carcinoma, 101
    3.4.4 Anaplastic carcinoma, 103
    3.4.5 Thyroid lymphoma, 103
    3.4.6 Metastatic tumours, 105
References, 106

3.1 Introduction

Thyroid nodules are extremely common, affecting from 4 to 7% of the population. In addition to clinically palpable nodules, the frequent causes of unexpected nodule detection are unrelated investigations. These have resulted in a dramatic increase in the prevalence of clinically non-apparent thyroid nodules (see Table 3.1) [1–4]. Since 1975, the incidence of thyroid cancer has nearly tripled, from 4.9 to 14.3 per 100 000 individuals [5]. Virtually the entire increase was attributable to papillary thyroid cancer: from 3.4 to 12.5 per 100 000. The absolute increase in thyroid cancer in women (from 6.5 to 21.4 = 14.9 per 100 000 women) is almost four times greater than that of men (from 3.1 to 6.9 = 3.8 per 100 000 men). The mortality rate from thyroid cancer was stable between 1975 and 2009 (approximately 0.5 deaths per 100 000). The epidemiology of the increased incidence, however, suggests that it is not an epidemic of disease but rather an epidemic of diagnosis. The problem is particularly acute for women, who have lower autopsy prevalence of thyroid cancer than men but higher cancer detection rates by a 3:1 ratio [6–8].

Thyroid cancer is currently the eighth most common malignancy among women, accounting for 3% of all cancers, compared with 1.7% (and ranking 14th) 20 years ago, with an annual increase of 1.4% since 1990 (see Table 3.2). Although the incidence of thyroid cancer doubled, a nearly five-fold increase in the use of thyroid ultrasound and a nearly seven-fold increase in the use of thyroid FNAC occurred between 2000 and 2012. These findings suggest that the increase in thyroid cancer incidence may be related to increases in the use of thyroid ultrasound (US) and Fine Needle Aspiration Cytology (FNAC) [9, 10, 13]. Despite the rise in incidence, however, the mortality from thyroid carcinoma has remained more or less stable (see Table 3.3) [10].

The primary aim of the preoperative diagnosis of thyroid nodules is to exclude the presence of thyroid malignancy, independent of nodule size. Due to a high prevalence of nodular thyroid disease, it is neither economically feasible nor necessary to submit all thyroid

Cytopathology of the Head and Neck: Ultrasound Guided FNAC, Second Edition. Gabrijela Kocjan.
© 2017 John Wiley & Sons Ltd. Published 2017 by John Wiley & Sons Ltd.
Companion website: www.wiley.com/go/kocjan/clinical_cytopathology_head_neck2e

Table 3.1 The prevalence of thyroid nodules is in direct proportion with the frequency used for Ultrasound examination from Davies L et al., 2014. [5]

Author	Country	Frequency (MHz)	Prevalence (%)
Carroll	USA	10.0	67
Horlocker	USA	10.0	46
Stark	USA	10.0	40
Brander	Finland	7.5	27
Tomimori	Brasil	7.5	17
Woestyn	Belgium	5.5	19

Range: 19–67%

Table 3.2 Thyroid cancer incidence. In the United States, thyroid cancer is currently the eighth most common malignancy among women, accounting for 3% of all cancers, compared with 1.7% (and ranking 14th) 20 years ago, with an annual increase of 1.4% since 1990. (From Davies L et al, 2014) [5]

	Men	Women
USA	4.9	14.9
Europe	5.0	12.9
Italy	5.2	15.5

n. cases/100.000 inhabitants/year

Table 3.3 Trends in Incidence and Mortality of Thyroid Cancer (1973–2002) and Papillary Tumors by Size (1988–2002) in the United States) from *Davies L et al.*, 2014. [5]

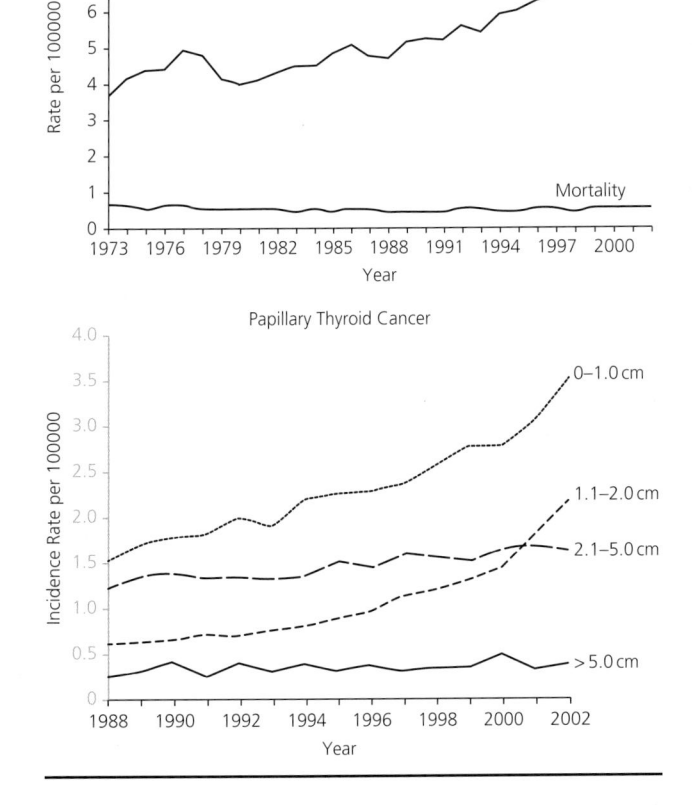

'The most common diagnostic pathway for thyroid nodules takes into account clinical history and physical examination, thyroid function tests, thyroid scintigraphy, neck ultrasonography and FNAC.'

Physical examination assesses the factors suggesting increased risk of malignant potential, such as race, age <20 or >70 years, male sex, persistent dysphonia or dysphagia, firm or hard consistency, fixed nodule, growing nodule, suspicious cervical lymph nodes and increased TSH levels. Clinical history considers at increased risk of thyroid cancer patients who have a history of cancer in one or more first degree relatives, history of cancer syndromes with TC (i.e. FAP, Cowden, etc.), exposure to ionising radiation in childhood or adolescence, environmental factors, prior hemithyroidectomy with discovery of thyroid cancer, MEN2/FMTC-associated RET proto-oncogene mutation, [18]FDG avidity on PET scanning and increased serum calcitonin levels. Of the environmental factors, Hawaii has the highest incidence of thyroid cancer, especially in Chinese men and Pilipino women.

Ideally, a thyroid diagnostic team should consist of an endocrinologist and/or an endocrine surgeon, a dedicated head and neck radiologist, a cytotechnologist who prepares the sample, a cytopathologist who takes the sample under US guidance and interprets it, preferably assessing the adequacy on site and a histopathologist who interprets the surgical specimens.

A good thyroid management is possible only through a multidisciplinary team (MDT) effort (Fig. 3.1).

Cytopathologists are MDT members and FNAC a part of the framework of other clinical, imaging and laboratory investigations. A cytopathologist examining the patient and reporting the FNAC smears should have the results of other investigations available and, if necessary, refer to them in the report. Similarly, if following a microscopic examination, the diagnosis is not apparent and could be elucidated by further investigations, this should be stated in the report. This approach, although requiring a lot of coordination, discipline and mutual understanding, will produce meaningful results and will not alienate the continuing use of FNAC as a key investigation of solitary thyroid lumps.

3.1.1 Ultrasound and FNAC procedure

Apart from the impalpable nodules, the indications for an US guided FNAC are the following: multiple nodules, complex nodules, prior failed FNAC, thyroid bed abnormalities, post thyroidectomy, difficult access and investigation of a recurrent tumour in a residual thyroid lobe. US features that have to be considered are: number of nodules, interval growth, size, internal content of nodules, echogenicity, calcification, margin, shape and vascularity [17]. Suspicious features include: a single nodule, taller than wide shape, solid composition, hypoecogenicity, irregular margins, microcalcifications, intranodular and chaotic vascularisation, suspicious lateral cervical lymph nodes. The risk of malignancy increases as the number of suspicious US features increases [18]. The US reporting system for thyroid nodules stratifying cancer risk for clinical management is shown in Table 3.4 [16].

FNAC of thyroid is deceptively simple, however, it requires skill and practice; most of the difficulties in interpretation arise from a poorly taken sample. Thyroid is a very vascular endocrine organ, much emphasis is on the cellularity and the cell/colloid ratio, the accurate assessment of which depends largely on the collection technique and on cell preparation of the FNAC sample [19]. The excess of

nodules to either surgery or a complete assessment of their structure and function. Instead, it is important to develop and follow a reliable, cost-effective strategy for diagnosis and treatment of thyroid nodules. The most common diagnostic pathway for thyroid nodules takes into account a clinical history and physical examination, thyroid function tests, thyroid scintigraphy, neck US and FNAC [14–16].

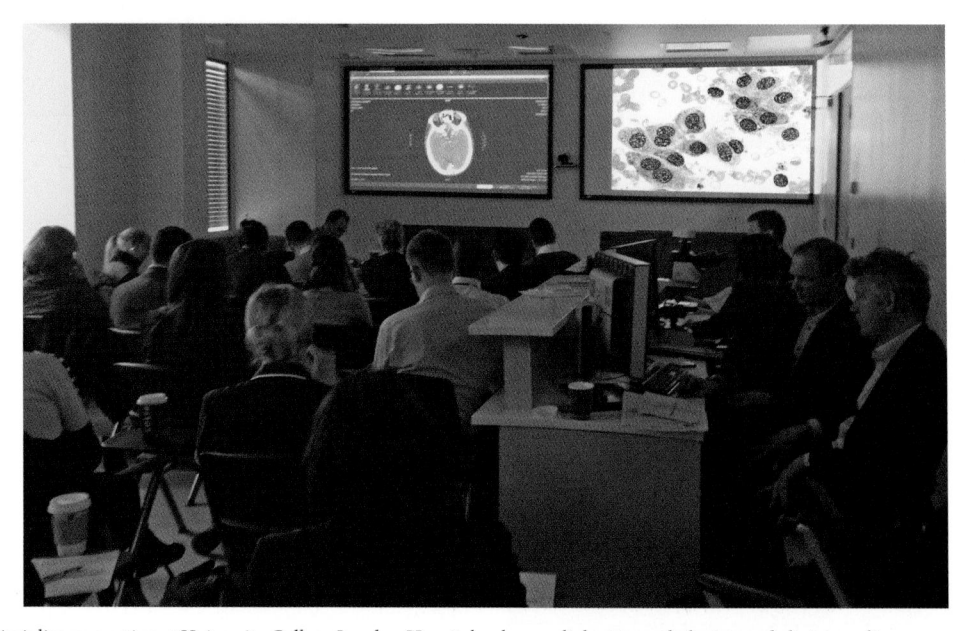

Figure 3.1 Multidisciplinary meeting at University College London Hospitals where radiologists, pathologists and clinicians discuss complex thyroid cases.

Table 3.4 The Society of Radiologists in Ultrasound (SRU) recommendations on which nodules should undergo FNA.

Description of US pattern	US patterns	Malignancy	TIRADS
Anechoic with hyperechoic spots, non-vascularized lesion.	Colloid type 1		
Non-encapsulated, mixed, non-expansile, with hyperechoic spots, vascularized lesion, "grid" aspect (spongiform nodule).	Colloid type 2	0%	TIRADS 2: benign findings
Non-encapsulated, mixed with solid portion, isoechogenic, expansile, vascularized nodule with hyperechoic spots.	Colloid type 3		
Hyper, iso, or hypoechoic, partially encapsulated nodule with peripheral vascularization, in Hashimoto's thyroiditis.	Hashimoto pseudo-nodule	<5%	TIRADS 3: probably benign
Solid or mixed hyper, iso, or hypoechoic nodule, with a thin capsule.	Simple neoplastic pattern	5–10%	TIRADS 4A: undetermined
Hypoechoic lesion with ill-defined borders, without calcifications.	de Quervain pattern		
Hyper, iso, or hypoechoic, hypervascularized, encapsulated nodule with a thick capsule, containing calcifications (coarse or microcalcifications).	Suspicious neoplastic pattern		
Hypoechoic, non-encapsulated nodule, with irregular shape and margins, penetrating. vessels, with or without calcifications	Malignant pattern A	10–80%	TIRADS 4B: suspicious
Iso or hypoechoic, non-encapsulated nodule with multiple peripheral microcalcifications and hypervascularization.	Malignant pattern B	>80%	TIRADS 5: consistent with malignancy
Non-encapsulated, isoechoic mixed hypervascularized nodule with or without calcifications, without hyperechoic spots.	Malignant pattern C		
	Cancer, confirmed by previous biopsy	100%	TIRADS 6: malignant

Note: Horvath E, Majlis S, Rossi R, et al. An ultrasonogram reporting system for thyroid nodules stratifying cancer risk for clinical management. *J Clin Endocrinol Metab* 2009; **94**(5):1748–51. [16]

blood, so often produced by the inexperienced aspirators, can result in the thyroid epithelium being trapped in the strands of fibrin giving a false impression of focal hypercellularity. In this case it is also difficult to study the cell detail due to cell crowding, poor fixation and/or poor penetration of stain. Such suboptimal samples often give rise to 'non-diagnostic', 'indeterminate', 'atypical' or 'suspicious' cytology reports, and are unhelpful in the context of optimal clinical management. The rapid on site assessment (ROSE) of the FNAC sample by the cytotechnologist or a cytopathologist can reduce the number of suboptimal samples. Olson et al. showed that the accuracy of cytotechnologists is comparable with that of cytopathologists in assessing adequacy of thyroid FNAC sample using ROSE [20].

FNAC of palpable thyroid lumps can be performed without the US guidance with a patient in a supine position, neck extended over the support cushion (Fig. 3.2). The procedure is explained to the

patient with a request not to swallow or speak during the insertion of the needle. The thyroid is palpated whilst the patient is asked to swallow. An enlarged nodule, usually situated between the trachea and the anterior edge of the sternocleidomastoid muscle, is fixed between the fingers of the non-dominant hand. After cleaning the skin, the patient is reminded not to swallow or speak. A 23-G, 25-G or lesser calibre needle, preferably without the attached syringe, is passed vertically into the nodule ('capillary technique'). This *non-aspiration* technique produces specimens of better quality and reduces inadequate results and should be preferable to aspiration using the syringe for the cytological evaluation of thyroid nodules [21]. Direction of the needle remains vertical, tangential to the trachea throughout the procedure. Once in the nodule, several fast passes, pushing and withdrawing the needle from the lesion, are made, lasting a few seconds (Fig. 3.3). In view of intranodular

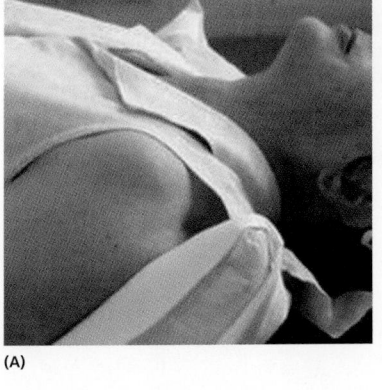
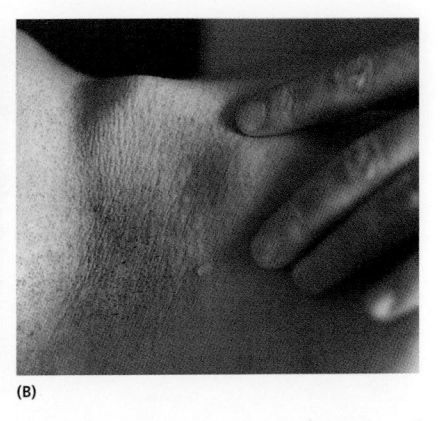

(A)   (B)

Figure 3.2 FNAC thyroid. (A) Procedure is performed with a patient in a supine position with the extended neck. (B) Thyroid is palpated whilst the patient is asked to swallow. Enlarged nodule is fixed between the fingers of the non-dominant hand. Thyroid enlargements are usually situated in the groove between the trachea and the anterior edge of the sternocleidomastoid muscle.

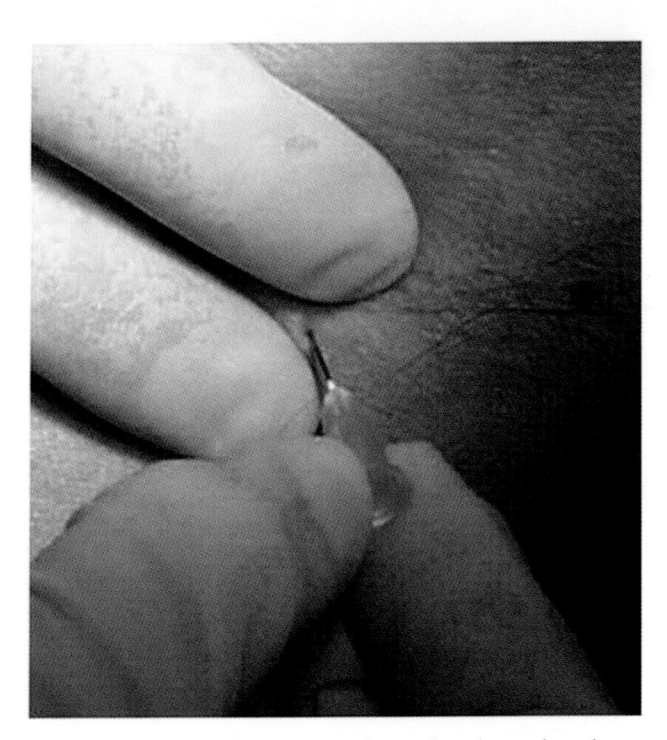

Figure 3.3 FNAC thyroid. A 23 G or smaller needle with or without the attached syringe is passed vertically into the nodule. Direction of the needle remains vertical, tangential to the trachea throughout the procedure. Once in the nodule, several fast passes, pushing and withdrawing the needle from the lesion, are made.

heterogeneity, some authors advise sampling of at least four distinct regions in order to accurately assesses thyroid nodules while minimising non-diagnostic results [22]. After withdrawing the needle, patient is placed in a comfortable position and allowed to swallow and speak. Occasionally, the procedure is repeated except when cysts are drained. If anticipating a cystic lesion, a 20-ml syringe and Cameco syringe holder are used (Fig. 1.5 and Fig. 3.4). Otherwise, capillary action of the needle is usually sufficient to obtain ample diagnostic material. Material is either spread on the glass slides or expelled into a container, or both (Fig. 3.5). Alcohol fixation and air-drying are both used in interpretation of thyroid aspirates so that the method of fixation will vary according to the local preference. The material for ancillary techniques is usually placed in the liquid transport medium.

Rapid on-site assessment (ROSE) is generally associated with an improvement in adequacy, but the impact of ROSE depends heavily on the initial adequacy rate. Sites with lower initial adequacy rates can benefit the most from the implementation of ROSE [23].

3.1.2 FNAC reporting categories

A diverse style of cytology reporting in the past decades, including the use of multiplicity of category names, descriptive reporting (no categories) or by using surgical pathology terminology, made it difficult to compare the results and outcomes of thyroid FNAC. This has brought about a need for a standardised reporting, with a set of defined diagnostic categories, each of which would have clinical relevance and patient management implications including an estimate of the risk of malignancy associated with each reporting category. At the National Cancer Institute (NCI) Thyroid FNAC State of the Science Conference in Bethesda, MD, USA, in 2007, a so-called 'Bethesda' classification for reporting of thyroid samples was established [24, 25]. At the same time, other classifications, such as the UK Royal College of Pathologists (UKRCPath) and Italian *SIAPEC/IAP* classifications have also emerged in a revised edition [26, 27]. In 2009, European cytology societies have agreed to report thyroid FNAC by using a classification system, either adopting a Bethesda classification or use a local/national 'translation' of the Bethesda system (see Table 3.5) [28, 29]. The subsequent use of such diagnostic categories proved to be reproducible and clinically relevant [30, 31].

In particular, the associated risk of malignancy, listed for each category proves useful in patient counselling and planning further management (Table 3.6).

Wu et al. found that by using TBSRTC, based on histological follow-up, the risk of *neoplasm* (including benign and malignant neoplasm) was as follows: benign 14%, AUS 44%, follicular neoplasm 67%, suspicious for malignancy 77%, and malignant 100% and the risk of *malignancy* was: benign 3%, AUS 6%, follicular neoplasm 22%, suspicious for malignancy 56% and malignant 100% [32]. Similarly, Theoharis et al. found that by using the TBSRTC classification, they were able to predict benign versus malignant thyroid nodules [33].

3.1.3 Diagnostic accuracy

3.1.3.1 Ultrasound

It has been reported that certain sonographic features of a thyroid nodule are associated with an increased likelihood of malignancy, although no single predictor has been found to have a high positive predictive value for cancer. Hence, guidelines with various

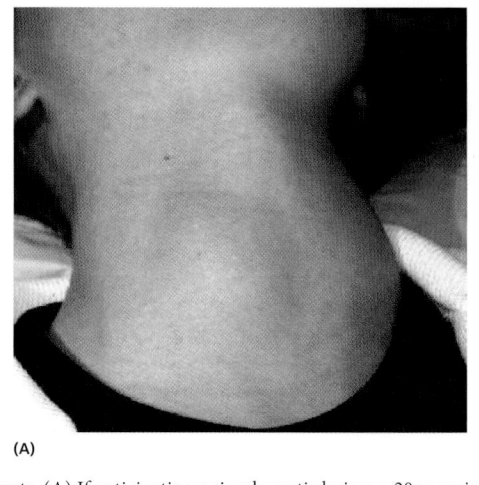
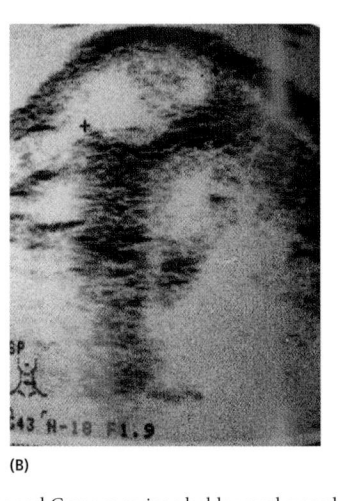

(A)   (B)

Figure 3.4 FNAC thyroid cysts. (A) If anticipating a simple cystic lesion, a 20 m syringe and Cameco syringe holder can be used. Cystic fluid is drained as much as possible without changing the direction of the needle. Repeat aspirates are not advised since they usually produce bleeding into the cystic space and refilling of the cyst. (B) Complex cystic lesions may be aspirated under ultrasound guidance. Ultrasound appearances in this case of a 29-year-old woman show a growth within the cystic space. FNAc showed papillary carcinoma (see Fig. 3.24).

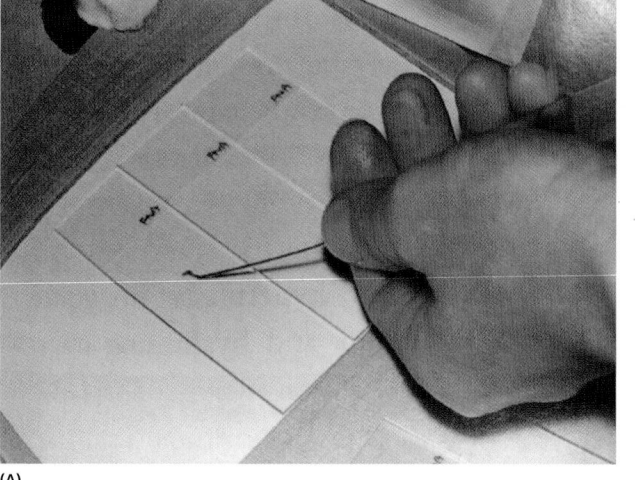
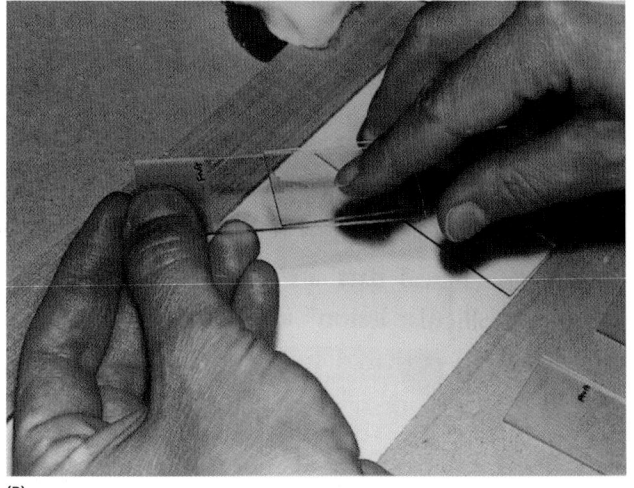

(A)   (B)

Figure 3.5 FNAC thyroid. Material is (A) expelled on the centre of glass slide and (B) spread with the help of another slide positioned flat against the test slide, sliding over it in parallel, avoiding edges that push cells to one side and account for ridge like effects.

Table 3.5 Comparison of TBSRTC (Bethesda) and UK RCPath/BTA thyroid FNAC reporting classifications.

Description	RCPath/BTA (UK)	TBSRTC (Bethesda)
Non-diagnostic for cytological diagnosis	Thy1 Cystic lesion (Thy1c)	I. Cyst fluid only
Non-neoplastic/ benign	Thy2 Thy2c Colloid cyst	II.
Neoplasm possible/Atypia of undetermined significance	Thy3a	III. or follicular lesion of undetermined significance
Neoplasm possible/suggesting follicular neoplasm	Thy3f	IV. Follicular neoplasm or suspicious for a follicular neoplasm or Hürthle cell (oncocytic) type
Suspicious of malignancy	Thy4	V.
Malignant	Thy5	VI.

Table 3.6 Risk of malignancy and clinical management for each category of TBSRTC.

Diagnostic Category	Risk of Malignancy (%)	Usual Management
I. Nondiagnostic or unsatisfactory	1–4	Repeat FNA with ultrasound guidance
II. Benign	0–3	Clinical follow-up
III. Atypia of undetermined significance or follicular lesion of undetermined significance	5–15	Repeat FNA
IV. Follicular neoplasm or suspicious for a follicular neoplasm	15–30	Surgical lobectomy
V. Suspicious for malignancy	60–75	Near-total thyroidectomy or surgical lobectomy
VI. Malignant	97–99	Near-total thyroidectomy

Abbreviations: FNA, fine-needle aspiration; TBSRTC, The Bethesda System for Reporting Thyroid Cytopathology.
Modified from Cibas ES et al. The Bethesda System for Reporting Thyroid Cytopathology *Am J Clin Pathol* 2009; **132**: 658–65.

combinations of ultrasound features that are both sensitive and specific for predicting the presence of cancer have been defined in several studies [14, 34–38].

Imaging Reporting and Data System (TIRADS) was first proposed by Horvath, and stratifies the risk of malignancy of thyroid nodules based on ten ultrasound characteristics. The TIRADS improved patient management and cost-effectiveness, avoiding unnecessary FNAC (Table 3.4) [39]. However, this system was considered to be too complex for implementation in clinical practice and has since modified by several other authors. They scored TIRADS as 4A (one suspicious feature), 4B (two suspicious features), 4C (three or four suspicious features) and 5 (five suspicious features) and demonstrated the fitted probability and risk of malignancy increased as the number of suspicious US features increased. The advantages of this scoring system are its simplicity and ease in implementation in clinical practice. A recent study by the same group proposed a thyroid cancer risk prediction model using features of thyroid nodules found on US and was validated based on multicentre retrospective data [40] By using TIRADS scoring system in our institution, Chng et al. showed that the risk of malignancy increased with advancing TIRADS score: TIRADS 4A (14.3%), TIRADS 4B (23.1%), TIRADS 4C (87.5%) and TIRADS 5 (100%) [41]. Maia et al. showed that thyroid imaging reporting system can be combined with the malignancy risk stratification in nodules with indeterminate cytology [42].

> No single ultrasound criterion is reliable in differentiating all benign from malignant thyroid nodules, but combined US features aid in predicting the benign or malignant nature of a given nodule.

When compared with palpation-only-guided FNAC, the US guided FNAC provides additional information in 60% of those patients in whom conventional FNAC with palpation failed to obtain material. Sensitivity (96%), specificity (91%), accuracy (94%), positive (96%) and negative predictive values (91%) of US-guided FNAC for malignancy are not significantly different from those (88, 90, 88, 95 and 75%, respectively) of palpation-guided FNAC for those nodules where an adequate FNAC is obtained [43]. US is valuable for identifying many malignant or potentially malignant thyroid nodules. No single ultrasound criterion is reliable in differentiating all benign from malignant thyroid nodules, but many US features aid in predicting the benign or malignant nature of a given nodule [44].

3.1.3.2 FNAC

Using the approach suggested by Sebo et al., the false-negative and false-positive rates of 'negative (benign)' and 'positive (malignant)' thyroid FNAC should be no more than 1%; and the prevalence of an 'indeterminate' aspirate – the area in FNAC attracting the most attention for improvement with novel biomarkers – should be 10% or less [45].

Thus, physicians should be capable of managing at least 90% of patients undergoing FNAC in a confident manner without further testing beyond the routine, future re-examination of the patient's nodule to re-assess for any change in its nature or its impact on the patient's quality of life. The other 10% can then be considered for molecular testing in a manner tailored to those individuals truly in need of a more sophisticated – and expensive – approach to the characterisation of their thyroid nodules.

The rates of sensitivity and specificity of FNAC for the diagnosis of thyroid malignancy differ amongst various reported series. The values differ depending on whether only clearly positive and negative results are considered or whether 'positives' include 'suspicious for malignancy'; whether *adenomas* are considered neoplasms in the same category as *carcinomas* and whether only histologically proven cases are taken into calculation without regard for benign cases on clinical follow-up, the latter being the majority of FNAC [46]. When considering *malignant, suspicious for malignancy*, and *indeterminate* cytology readings as 'positive' and *benign cytology* as 'negative', Yoon et al. found the sensitivity of thyroid FNAC was 96.7%, specificity 85.9%, positive predictive value 76.6%, negative predictive value 98.2% and accuracy 89.4% [47]. Our own results, using the UKRCPath diagnostic categories showed the specificity and PPV of the Thy3f, Thy4 and Thy5 (equivalent to the TBSRTC IV, V and VI) were 50, 50 and 100% and 28, 64 and 100%, respectively. The PPV of Thy3f (TBSRTC IV) for diagnosis of 'neoplasms' (benign and malignant) was 63% [31].

When calculating diagnostic accuracy, most commonly, four cytological diagnostic categories are used. Rates for these categories, based on data pooled from recent series, were as follows: benign, 69%; suspicious, 10%; malignant, 4% and nondiagnostic, 17%. Analysis of data suggests a false-negative rate of 1 to 11%, a false-positive rate of 1–8%, a sensitivity of 65–98%, and a specificity of 72–100% [48–61].

There are many reports that diagnostic accuracy of FNAC of thyroid is improved with US guidance, especially for impalpable nodules [62]. When FNAC results were compared with US results, the positive and negative predictive values of the US categories were 59.1 and 97.0%, and those of the cytological results were 93.7 and 98.9% [63].

The US categories were significantly correlated with final diagnosis in the benign (p = 0.014) and suspicious for malignancy (p < 0.001) cytological result groups, but not in the inadequate and indeterminate cytological results groups. The false positive and negative rates of cytological results were 1.9 and 3.2%.

3.1.4 Diagnostic pitfalls

Limitations of FNAC are related to the skill of the aspirator, the expertise of the cytopathologist, and the intrinsic difficulty in distinguishing adenomas from their malignant counterparts [64–66].

The following appearances, often in combination may lead to overdiagnosis: cellularity, little colloid (e.g. in cellular adenoma), pseudopapillary changes due to regression of follicular epithelial cells in a multinodular goitre, cellular atypia of follicular epithelium, thick colloid simulating a psammoma body, but without the characteristic lamellar appearance, papillary hyperplasia in Hashimoto's thyroiditis, cellular atypia of follicular epithelium in Hashimoto's disease, treatment with radioactive iodine, thyroid gland inhibitory or stimulatory drugs, chemotherapy or radiotherapy to the neck.

3.1.5 The role of FNAC thyroid in clinical management

The introduction of FNAC has had a substantial effect on the management of patients with thyroid nodules. The percentage of patients undergoing thyroidectomy has decreased by 25% and the yield of carcinoma in patients who undergo surgery has increased from 15% to at least 30%. FNAC has decreased the cost of care by 25% [48]. As the era of US has matured – just as with the era of serum PSA testing for prostate cancer in men – we have experienced a paradigm shift: Given the incidence of thyroid nodules in the US adult population in comparison with the risk of dying of thyroid malignancy.

The main role of thyroid FNAC is to reduce the need for surgical intervention [45]

In our own institution, University College Hospitals London (UCLH), we compared the rate of thyroid surgery, the rate of pre-operative FNAC and the surgical outcomes in two defined periods: 10 years ago and now. We found that the absolute rate of surgery has stayed more or less the same or has slightly increased. Since the preoperative FNAC diagnosis in patients undergoing surgery has increased dramatically, the surgical outcomes in terms of benign/malignant ratios have reversed in favour of malignancy. FNAC is the most accurate tool for diagnosing malignancy and selecting candidates for surgery [67]. It has decreased costs substantially because it enables selection of patients who need surgery. Introduction of FNAC reduces the cost of thyroid operations by 25% and doubles the yield of carcinoma [68–70].

There is much concern expressed in the literature regarding the lack of predictive power of the thyroid FNAC approach to defining the nature of clinically detected thyroid nodules. This has been exacerbated in the past decade or more by the routine use of US in examining the thyroid as well as the introduction of molecular testing in the realm of thyroid pathology. Some have even gone so far as to suggest replacing the FNAC with molecular signature testing to reduce the degree of uncertainty for a specific cytological diagnosis. Sebo addresses those concerns with a re-emphasis on understanding the basic 'keys' to successful evaluation of a patient with a thyroid nodule by routine FNAC examination [45]. These 'keys' are, firstly, an integrated MDT approach, secondly, an acute focus on the FNAC cytological categories and, thirdly, an understanding of the predictive ability of molecular testing in a given patient when the cytological interpretation creates too much uncertainty. With this practical approach in mind, Sebo suggests that the false-negative and false-positive rates of 'negative (benign)' and 'positive (malignant)' thyroid FNAC should be no more than 1%; and the prevalence of an 'indeterminate' result should be 10% or less. Thus, clinicians should be capable of managing at least 90% of patients undergoing FNAC in a confident manner without further testing beyond the routine, future re-examination of the patient's nodule to re-assess for any change in its nature or its impact on the patient's quality of life. The other 10% can then be considered for molecular testing in a manner tailored to those individuals truly in need of a more sophisticated – and expensive – approach to the characterisation of their thyroid nodules (Table 3.7).

3.1.6 FNAC versus frozen section and core biopsy histology

FNAC is used to assist in planning surgical strategy for differentiated thyroid cancer mainly by determining the likely extent of contralateral lobe resection and nodal dissection required [71]. Frozen section (FS), which was traditionally used as the surgeon's guide, and FNAC both have varying accuracy rates [72–74]. In a series by Kopald et al., carcinoma was diagnosed by FS in 69% cases of true positive carcinomas. FS analysis was incorrect in 5–31% of cases of carcinoma diagnosed on FNAC and confirmed on definitive histology [75, 76]. FS examination is therefore indicated for intraoperative decision-making in patients with a 'suspicious', 'cellular' or 'indeterminate' FNAC diagnosis but is unnecessary when the FNAC diagnosis is either benign or malignant [76–80]. When combining the results of US and FNAC, the malignancy rate of thyroid nodules read as 'suspicious for PTC' on US-FNAC was 87.1% [81].

When a thyroid nodule with 'suspicious for PTC' diagnosis on FNAC has also suspicious malignant US features, FS may be unnecessary due to a very high risk of malignancy (94.9%). In contrast, when a thyroid nodule read as 'suspicious for PTC' on FNAC has no suspicious malignant US features, FS can help surgeons determine the extent of surgery. FNAC is at least as accurate as FS with less morbidity and expense. When papillary carcinoma of the thyroid is definitively diagnosed on FNAC, the surgeon can perform definitive thyroidectomy without frozen section because of the high specificity for cancer [69, 76, 83]. If FS is not diagnostic of malignancy, a thyroid lobectomy/isthmusectomy is recommended because 71% have a benign lesion. This systematic approach to papillary carcinoma of the thyroid will avoid unnecessary FS while maintaining excellent diagnostic specificity.

Core needle biopsy (CNB) can reduce the false negative and inconclusive results of conventional FNAC and should be considered as an additional method in assessing solid thyroid nodules at high risk of malignancy. However, it is still not helpful for the differential diagnosis in 36% of nodules that are suspicious for follicular neoplasm seen on US [84, 87]. The complication rate after US-guided CNB for thyroid lesions is reported as 0.81% [87a].

When comparing both methods, some authors found US-FNAC is a more valuable method for the diagnosis of suspected malignant nodules [88].

Table 3.7 University College London Hospitals Multidisciplinary Team Guidelines for clinical management of thyroid nodules, following a cytological diagnosis.

UCLH ultrasound and cytological assessment of thyroid nodules		
Finding	**Imaging required**	**Management**
Benign MNG	No USS follow-up	No concerns about symptoms Normal TFTs Discharge – re-refer if change in size
Thy 1 (Inadequate) Thy1c (Cystic)	Repeat USS and FNA (3–6 mo)	Non-diagnostic, need repeat FNA and rescan, in particular if haemorrhagic cyst
Thy2 (Benign) Colloid cystic Hashimotos	Consider USS at clinician's discretion	Benign. Repeat biopsy only at the discretion of the clinician such as new symptoms or change in size
Thy 3a (Atypia)	Consider serial USS/further FNA (6 months)	Cases should be discuss in MDT Discuss surgery vs repeat FNA/serial USS
Thy 3f (Follicular-lesion)	No further USS	Cases to be discussed in MDT to support the decision of surgery (hemithyroidectomy)
Thy4 (Suspicious of malignancy)	No further USS	Cases to be discussed in MDT to decide if further investigation is necessary to guide surgery (hemi or total thyroidectomy)
Thy 5 (Malignant)	Consider further USS for assessment of lymph nodes	Cases to be discussed in MDT and refer for surgery or other oncology (lymphoma, sarcoma)

Note: Thyroid MDT group Updated 3rd September 2012 by Dr Teng Teng Chung based on BTA guidelines 2007 [70a]

3.1.7 Ancillary techniques

Immunocytochemistry: A spectrum of markers has been used in to distinguish between benign/reactive and neoplastic thyroid nodules. Immunocytochemical staining of thyroid FNAC specimens for CD44, showed positivity in 88% classic, surgically confirmed, PTC on FNAC with no staining of benign aspirates [89]. The authors conclude that most papillary carcinomas of the thyroid express the cell adhesion molecule CD44. However, Matesa et al. found CD44v6 expression in 33% of Hashimoto thyroiditis and in 18% of nodular goitre [89a].

The monoclonal antibody, HBME-1, has been shown to have significant reactivity in histologicalal sections of follicular-derived thyroid malignancies. Sack et al. concluded that a positive immunostaining for HBME-1 on a thyroid FNAC is supportive evidence that the lesion is a carcinoma, that a negative result for HBME-1 does not preclude the diagnosis of thyroid carcinoma [90]. Ohta et al. reported the sensitivity and specificity of HBME-1 for follicular varioant of papillary carcinoma (FVPTC) as 92 and 89%, respectively, while those of CD15 were 23 and 100%, respectively and conclude that HBME-1 is a sensitive marker of papillary carcinoma, including both usual type and FVPTC, in cytological specimens [91]. On the other hand, Das et al., whilst finding CD44 and galectin 3 helpful in diagnosing PTC, found HMBE1 unhelpful [91a].

Other ICC markers, such as CD19, TROP, CD56 have also been used with variable success in an attempt to triage patients with inconclusive FNAC results for surgery [91b]. ICC panels help in reducing the number of thyroidectomies and providing a more adequate clinical and/or surgical selection [92].

Molecular testing has been proposed as a useful adjunct to cytology establishing the risk stratification in indeterminate cases. A series of molecular markers have been used in an attempt to refine cytological diagnosis. The best known molecular alterations in thyroid cancer include BRAF and RAS point mutations, RET/PTC and PAX8/PPAR γ rearrangements [93]. These non-overlapping genetic alterations are found in more than 70% of papillary and follicular thyroid carcinomas and can be detected in surgically resected samples as well as FNAC samples from thyroid nodules, particularly in those with indeterminate findings (AUS/FLUS, FN/SFN). The analysis may also help in the management of thyroid nodules with benign cytology, two or more suspicious US features and positive BRAF(V600E) mutation. In these cases, thyroidectomy should be considered [94].

Adeniran et al. showed that the sensitivity and specificity of BRAF mutation in detecting PTC in FNAC specimens with indeterminate diagnosis was 59.3 and 100%, respectively, while the positive and negative predictive values were 100 and 65.6%, respectively, thus supporting the use of BRAF mutation analysis to predict the risk of malignancy in patients with indeterminate thyroid FNAC [95]. On the other hand, Colanta et al. report that BRAF mutation analysis did not provide a significant increase in the accuracy of thyroid FNAC diagnosed as suspicious or atypical [96]. The BRAF V600E mutation has been associated with aggressive disease, therefore, in addition to the diagnostic use, BRAF V600E mutation can also be used for tumour prognosis [93, 96]. The BRAFV600E mutation has been correlated with older age, classical variant of PTC and advanced stages in patients >45 years [97]. It is significantly more common in conventional papillary thyroid carcinoma (58% versus 31% in FVPC) [98]. Smith and colleagues alert to the importance of the technical excellence in BRAF detection and report increased detection of BRAF V600E in FNAC specimens

using allele-specific/blocking probe PCR, which has an analytical sensitivity of 0.01% [99].

Jordan et al. explore the potential use of high-resolution magic angle spinning proton magnetic resonance spectroscopy as an ancillary diagnostic technique for PTC in thyroid FNAC [100]. The method has already been shown to be effective in the classification of various other non-thyroid cancers.

Recent advances in the understanding of the molecular pathogenesis of thyroid cancer and in next generation sequencing (NGS) technologies have exponentially increased the number of genetic alterations that can be interrogated in a single nodule aspirate. Nikiforov and colleagues recently reported a high sensitivity (90%) and specificity (93%) for the ThyroSeq v2 NGS panel in nodules with FN/SFN cytology at a single institution [100a]. Le Mercier et al. also evaluated the added value of NGS and found that 71% of the mutation-positive FNAC samples had a malignant diagnosis after surgery [101]. Although NGS is a promising technique for the molecular testing of thyroid FNAC specimens, thyroid-specific cancer gene panels are not commercially available. Conversely, the Ion AmpliSeq Cancer Hotspot Panel v2 (CHPv2), which includes the genes most frequently mutated in thyroid neoplasms, is commercially available and may represent an alternative to thyroid-specific panels[101a]. Alexander and colleagues reported a sensitivity of 90% and a specificity of 52% for the Afirma gene expression classifier (AGEC) in thyroid nodules with AUS/FLUS or FN/SFN cytology. This is a microarray-based test combining seven distinct classifiers and interrogating the expression levels of 167 genes. It can detect benign nodules with a high NPV of 94%. With a specificity of 52%, the AGEC would indeed reduce by 52% the rate of avoidable surgeries, from 76% of all nodules evaluated without molecular testing (24% cancer prevalence observed) to 37% after AGEC testing (101b). Several studies have reported the potential diagnostic utility of miRNAs in preoperative thyroid nodules FNAC [101c].

In conclusion, it can be expected that, given the high PPV and NPV of the molecular preoperative testing in patients with atypical/suspicious (AUS/FLUS or FN/SFN) FNAC, a diagnostic algorithm combining molecular information and FNAC will enable that patients with positive (malignant) molecular preoperative tests results may be sent to surgery while patients with negative (benign) molecular results may benefit from a more conservative management, ie, active follow up without surgery [101c]. It is estimated that this approach could potentially result in a 6.7-fold reduction in the number of unnecessary diagnostic surgeries, independently of variations in cancer prevalence [101c].

3.1.8 Complications of FNAC

A single case is reported in the literature of a slow-growing papillary carcinoma of the thyroid that caused clinically apparent implantation along the tract of a FNAC. This appears to be the first report of a cutaneous needle tract metastasis from a papillary thyroid carcinoma. It represents a highly unusual complication of an FNAC of an indolent, slow-growing tumour [103].

Histological changes, such as infarction, following FNAC thyroid can be varied and should always be kept in mind in order to avoid misdiagnoses [104, 105]. Potential problems in such cases are: (1) post-FNAC infarction may obscure the nature of a cytologically diagnosed neoplasm, making histological confirmation difficult, and (2) FNAC of an infarcted nodule may have difficulties in obtaining diagnostic material, potentially resulting in a

false-negative diagnosis. Review of the literature on thyroid infarction shows it to be a rare event, with most reported cases occurring after FNAC of a neoplasm. The finding of necrosis and fibrosis in a surgical specimen may suggest the presence of a neoplasm.

3.2 Non-neoplastic and inflammatory conditions

3.2.1 Colloid goitre (non-toxic goitre, adenomatous hyperplasia, multinodular goitre)

Multinodular non-toxic goitre (MNG) used to be the commonest form of thyroid gland enlargement; it was an endemic abnormality in areas with iodine deficiency, which is now extremely uncommon due to the addition of iodine to table salt (Fig. 3.6). Sporadic forms are encountered in clinical practice by primary care doctors, endocrinologists and head and neck surgeons. Epidemiological data suggest that in the non-endemic areas (e.g. USA), the incidence of such goitres is approximately 0.1–1.5% per year, translating into 250 000 new nodules annually. Nodular goitre is more common in women than in men, with advancing age, and after exposure to external irradiation. These goitres may be asymptomatic, with normal TSH levels (non-toxic), or may be associated with systemic thyrotoxic symptoms (toxic multinodular goitre or Plummer's disease).

Diagnostic evaluation of patients with MNG consists of clinical evaluation, biochemical testing, imaging and FNAC. The serum TSH level is a sensitive and reliable index of thyroid function. FNAC results are pivotal to assess cancer risk in patient management for prominent palpable and suspicious nodules. Chest radiography, high-resolution US and computed tomography help to delineate the size and extent of goitre in evaluating compression symptoms. Indications for treatment in patients with MNG include hyperthyroidism; local compression symptoms attributed to the goitre, cosmesis and concern about malignancy based on FNAC results. Management of toxic MNG by surgery is well established. Radioiodine is also effective therapy for many of these patients. The management policy, for patients who have small, non-toxic MNG that are clinically asymptomatic, who are biochemically euthyroid according to serum TSH levels, and who have prominent palpable or suspicious nodules, benign by FNAC, is yearly evaluation with

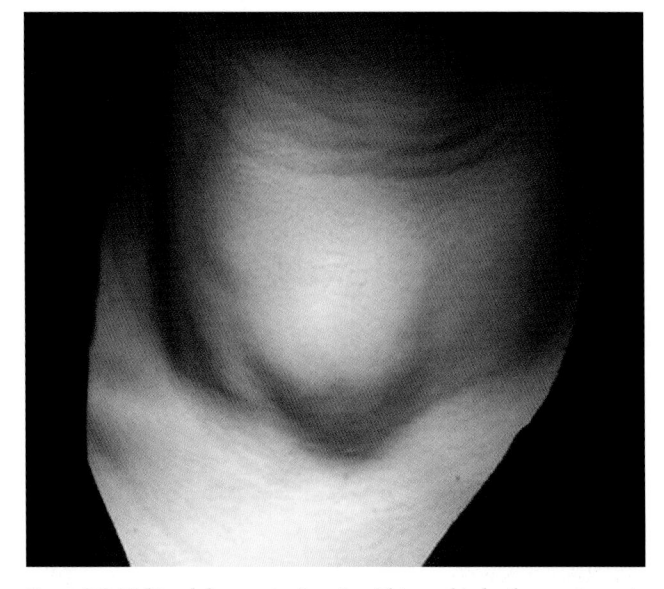

Figure 3.6 Multinodular non-toxic goitre. This used to be the commonest form of thyroid gland enlargement.

serum TSH determinations and thyroid ultrasound. For large non-toxic MNG with local compression symptoms, the preferred treatment is surgery [106]. Routine performance of repeated FNAC in the follow-up of females with MNG, without any clinical changes, is of limited usefulness [107].

Histologically, MNG is composed of variably sized, partly encapsulated nodules composed of follicles, which also vary in size. There are usually extensive regressive changes (oedema, infarction, haemorrhage, fibrosis, calcification and occasional bone formation) The follicular epithelium is often oncocytic and sometimes shows clear cell metaplasia. The gland may show diffuse nodularity, focal nodularity or solitary hyperplastic nodules.

The distinction between an adenoma and a solitary, hyperplastic, adenomatous nodule is arbitrary. The term adenoma is usually used to describe solitary lesions with a microscopically complete capsule; the thyroid gland parenchyma in an adenoma differs in that in the surrounding thyroid gland, the follicles are compressed by the extensive growth of the adenoma. Also in adenoma, extensive regressive changes may be seen. It is not certain if all solitary nodules are true adenomata (neoplasms) or if some of them represent hyperplastic (physiological) lesions.

[See BOX 3.1. Summary of ultrasound features: Colloid Nodule on www.wiley.com/go/kocjan/clinical_cytopathology_head_neck2e]

The cytological features of multinodular goitre are variable [108]. FNAC from adenomatous areas are cellular with little colloid (a low 'cell/colloid ratio'); aspirates from a MNG contain abundant thin colloid (pale blue on MGG staining) with sparse follicular epithelium (Fig. 3.7). Thyroid epithelium is uniform, arranged in loose aggregates or flat sheets lying within the colloid. Individual cells have oval or round pyknotic nuclei, inconspicuous nucleoli and poorly defined cytoplasm. They are regular in size and monotonous in appearance. They may be difficult to differentiate from lymphocytes. Minor variations in size of the nuclei are common. Microfollicles may be present, usually enveloped in a hyaline stroma. Occasionally, oncocytic change may be noted: sharply circumscribed cell borders, abundant finely granular grey/blue cytoplasm, anisonucleosis and occasionally prominent nucleoli (Fig. 3.8). In heavily bloodstained aspirates, the concentration of cells along the strands of fibrin may give an impression of hypercellularity. However, a lack of consistency of this finding throughout the sample is important. Macrophages are often seen even in a predominantly colloid goitre. Fragments of hyaline stroma may be seen in generously sampled aspirates. Calcium oxalate crystals showing birefringence may be seen. Although they can be seen in all, they are more commonly seen in MNG than in adenomas or carcinomas [109]. Psammoma bodies may be seen (Fig. 3.9). Psammoma bodies are not pathognomonic of papillary carcinoma, and their presence, in the absence of other cytological criteria for malignancy, should not necessarily lead to diagnosis of carcinoma [110]. However, the presence of psammoma bodies in an FNAC smear cytologically consistent with a colloid goitre should raise the possibility of coexistent papillary hyperplasia or neoplasia. Because of the strong statistical association of psammoma bodies with malignant thyroid neoplasms, histological confirmation is mandatory in such cases [111]. Occasionally, multicentric papillary hyperplasia presents with cytological features suggestive of thyroid papillary carcinoma. While the cytological criteria for papillary thyroid carcinoma are well defined, occasional diagnostic difficulties can arise. Cytologically, the presence of focal papillary aggregates, the

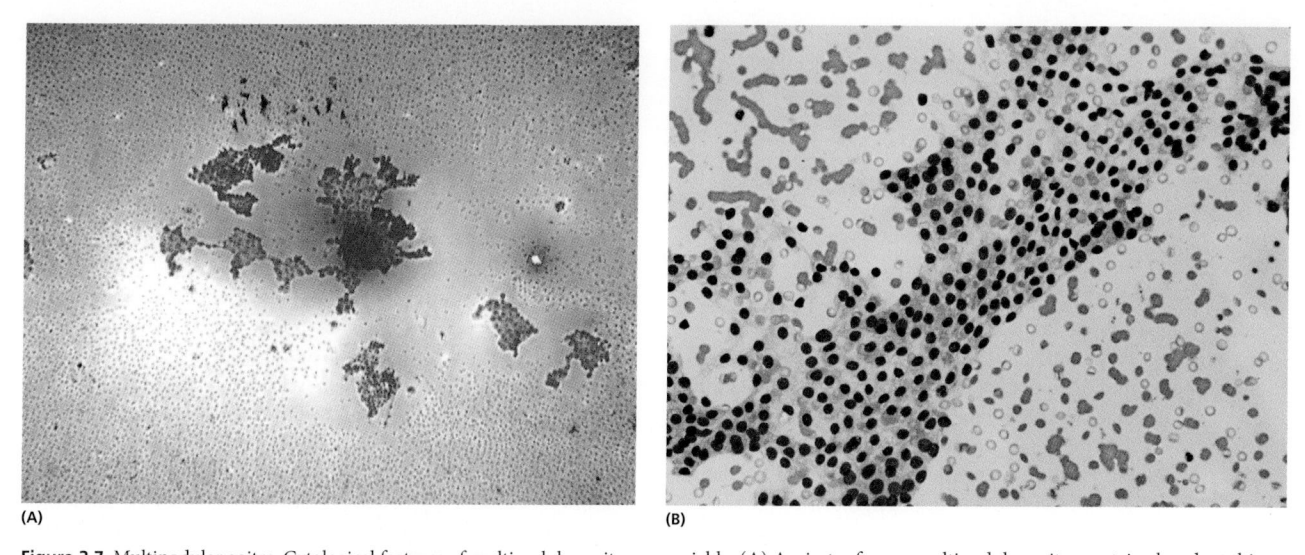

(A)

(B)

Figure 3.7 Multinodular goitre. Cytological features of multinodular goitre are variable. (A) Aspirates from a multinodular goitre contain abundant thin colloid (pale blue or pink on MGG staining) with sparse follicular epithelium. Cells are uniform, arranged in loose aggregates or flat sheets lying within the colloid. (B) Individual cells have oval or round pyknotic nuclei, inconspicuous nucleoli and poorly defined cytoplasm. They are regular in size and monotonous in appearance.

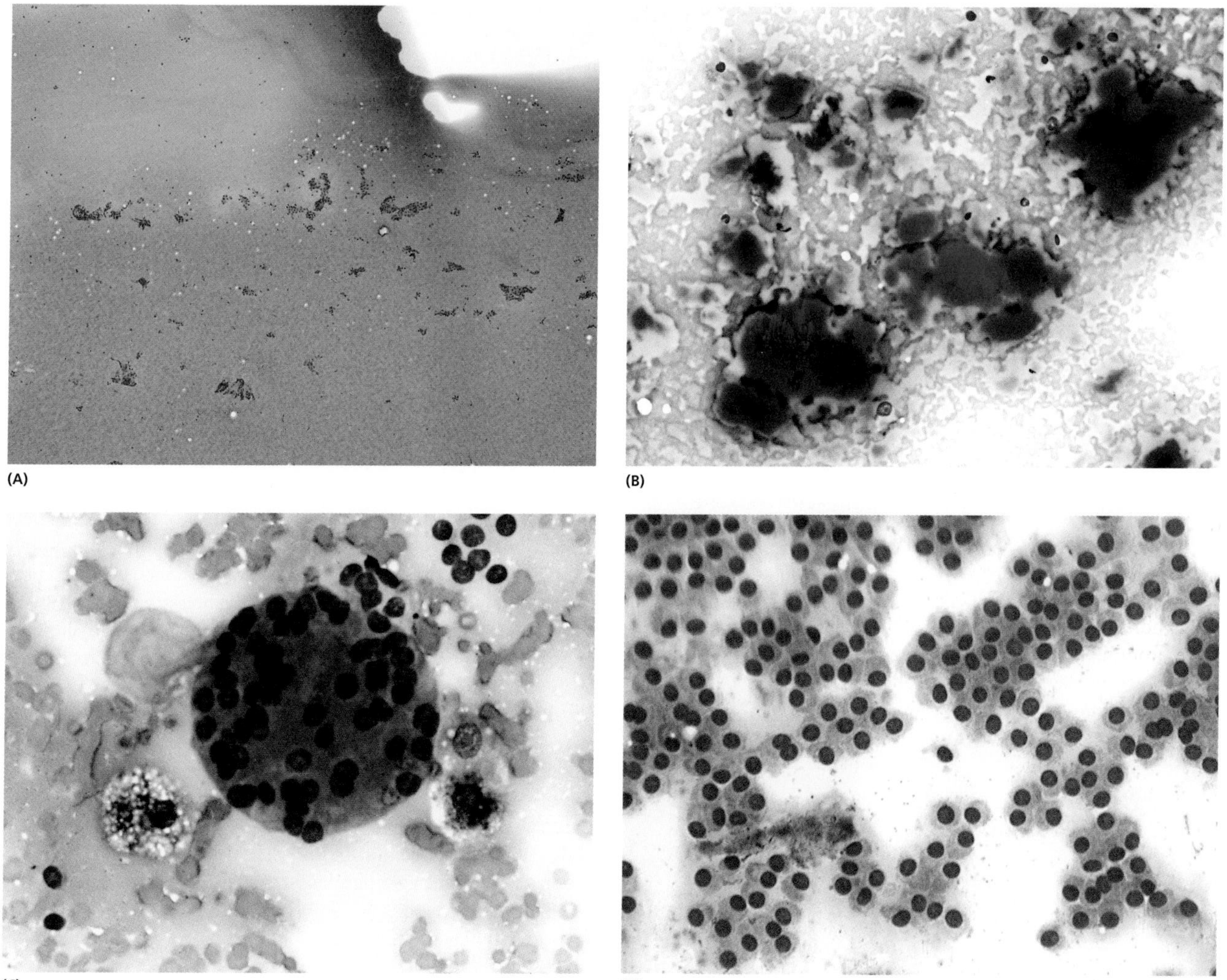

(A)

(B)

(C)

(D)

Figure 3.8 Multinodular goitre. (A) Thin and (B) thick colloid may be seen. Minor variations in size of the nuclei are common. (C) Microfollicles may be present. (D) Occasionally, there is oncocytic change: sharply circumscribed cell borders, abundant finely granular grey/blue cytoplasm, anysonucleosis and occasionally prominent nucleoli.

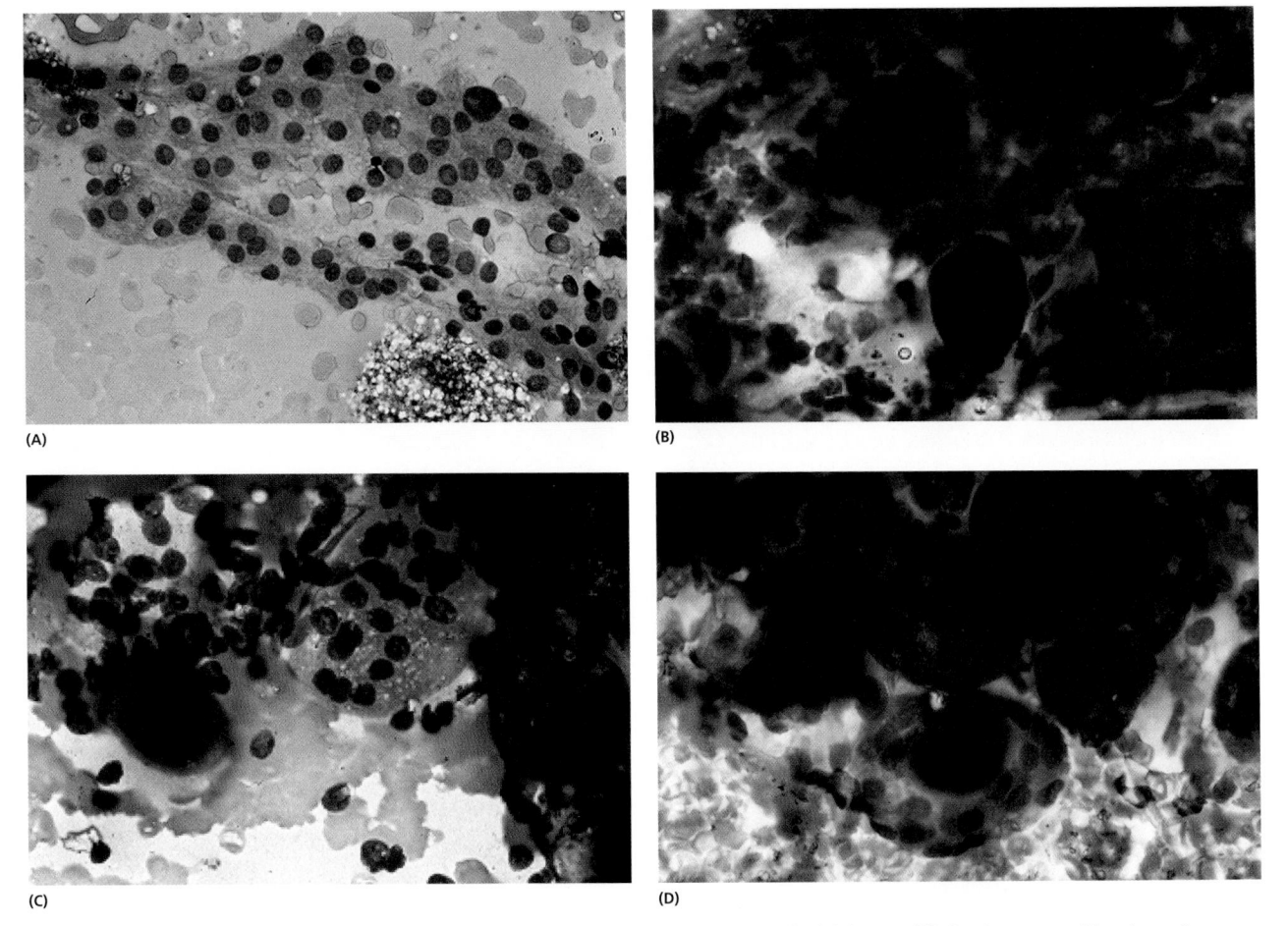

Figure 3.9 Multinodular goitre. (A) Aspirates from adenomatous areas are cellular with thin colloid. (B) Microfollicles showing overklapping and crowding. Some thick colloid attached to the cell groups. (C) Inspissated colloid mimicking psammoma bodies may be seen within the epithelial clusters. (D) High power view shows psammoma bodies. Apart from papillary carcinoma, psammoma bodies may be present in colloid goitre. Their presence, in the absence of other cytological criteria for malignancy, should not necessarily lead to diagnosis of carcinoma. However, the presence of psammoma bodies in an FNAC smear cytologically consistent with a colloid goitre should raise the possibility of coexistent papillary hyperplasia or neoplasia. Because of the strong statistical association of psammoma bodies with malignant thyroid neoplasms, histological confirmation is mandatory in such cases.

presence of a psammoma body within a background of copious colloid and scattered follicular cells may lead to diagnostic errors [112]. Thyroid epithelium may show degenerative changes; foamy cytoplasm containing granules makes epithelium indistinguishable from macrophages (Fig. 3.10). Sometimes follicular epithelium may be spindle shaped, particularly in the wall of the cystic goitre and have prominent nucleoli resembling repair epithelium (Fig. 3.11). Large bare nuclei with structureless chromatin may be seen in hypothyroidism. Antithyroid drug treatment, Hashimoto's disease, chemotherapy and radiotherapy can all produce marked degenerative changes that may be source of diagnostic errors (Fig. 3.12).

According to the current thyroid reporting classifications (see Section 3.1.2) a minimum of six aggregates, each comprising at least 10 epithelial cells, has to be identified in order for the sample to be considered as diagnostic or adequate for a reliable assessment. In these cases, a repeat FNAC is usually recommended. Jo et al. report the overall risk of malignancy as 4% following a single non-diagnostic FNAC and 6.3% after repeated non-diagnostic FNACs concluding that there is no modification of malignancy risk when repeated FNACs are non-diagnostic [113]. Clinical management for a non-diagnostic FNAC should remain repeat aspiration along with clinical and sonographic correlation. Since BRAF(V600E)

mutation analysis is a highly sensitive diagnostic tool in the diagnosis of papillary thyroid carcinomas, this analysis may help in the management of thyroid nodules with benign cytology but positive BRAF(V600E) mutation. In these cases, thyroidectomy should be considered in nodules which have two or more suspicious US features and are considered discordant on image-cytology correlation [114].

3.2.2 Cysts

In MNG with cyst formation, macrophages, colloid and often blood are seen. Macrophages may be multinucleated and contain haemosiderin. Epithelial cells with degenerative changes may be seen, anisonucleosis and anisocytosis may be present although the nucleo cytoplasmic (N/C) ratio remains normal (Figs 3.13 and 3.14). Cystic thyroid lesions often contain blood and/or colloid only with very few or no epithelial cells in which case they are considered as suboptimal for assessment. According to the current classifications, such FNAC samples have to be repeated to avoid a false negative finding, particularly that of a papillary carcinoma which can be cystic and very sparsely cellular. The issue of adequacy criteria in the case of cystic thyroid

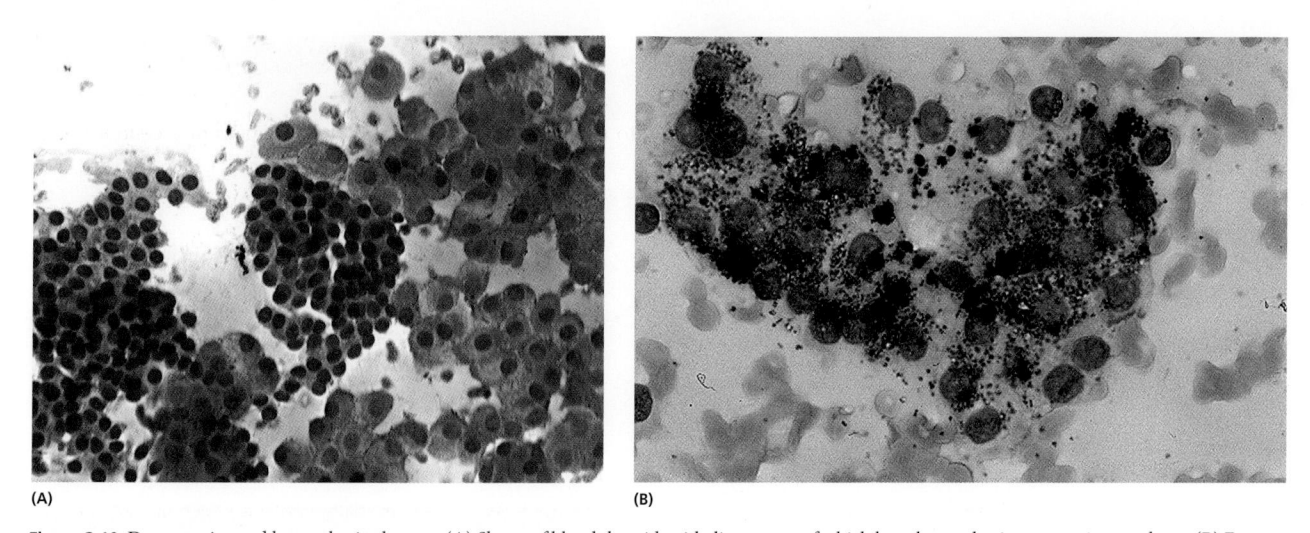

(A)　　　　　　　　　　　　　　　　　　　　　(B)

Figure 3.10 Degenerative and hyperplastic changes. (A) Sheets of bland thyroid epithelium some of which have hyperplastic, oncocytic cytoplasm. (B) Foamy cytoplasm containing granules makes epithelium indistinguishable from macrophages (MGG ×600, oil immersion).

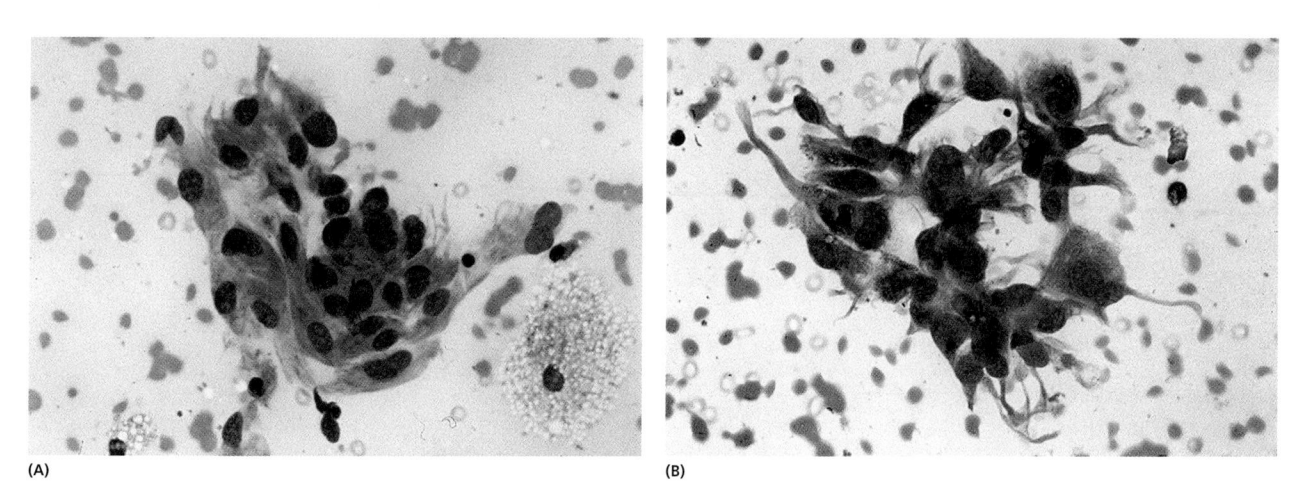

(A)　　　　　　　　　　　　　　　　　　　　　(B)

Figure 3.11 Regenerative changes. (A) Spindle shaped follicular epithelium and macrophages (MGG ×600, oil immersion). (B) Spindle epithelial cells from the wall of the cystic goitre have prominent nucleoli resembling repair epithelium and may be misleading into diagnosis of a mesenchymal lesion (MGG × 600, oil).

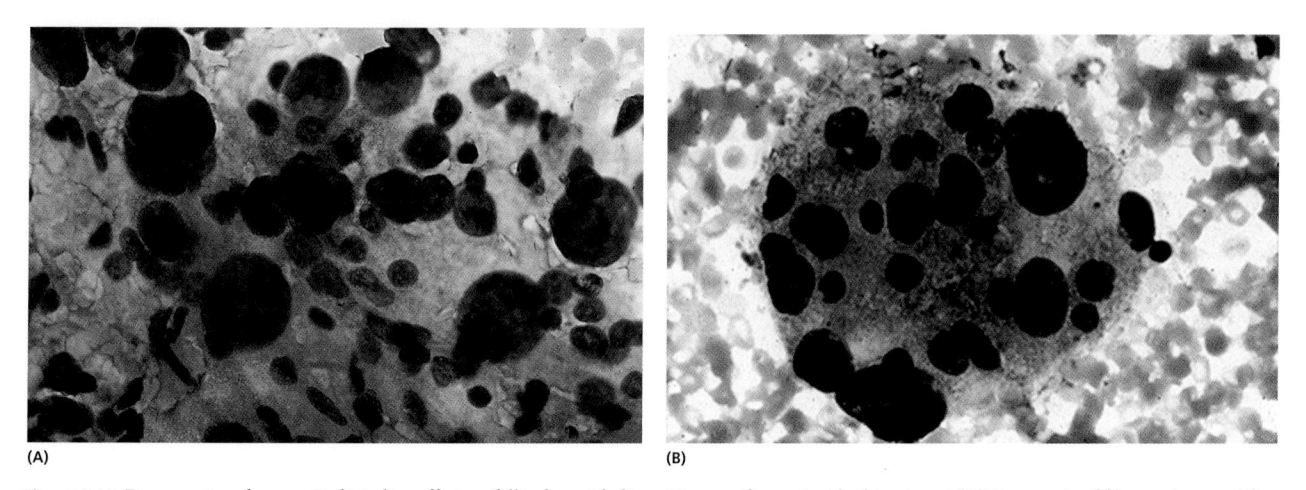

(A)　　　　　　　　　　　　　　　　　　　　　(B)

Figure 3.12 Degenerative changes. Radioiodine effect on follicular epithelium 30 years after patient had treatment (A) Fragments of fibrous stroma with large bare nuclei (MGG ×400). (B) Bare nuclei with structureless chromatin but prominent anisonucleosis and alarming pleomorphism (MGG ×1000, oil immersion).

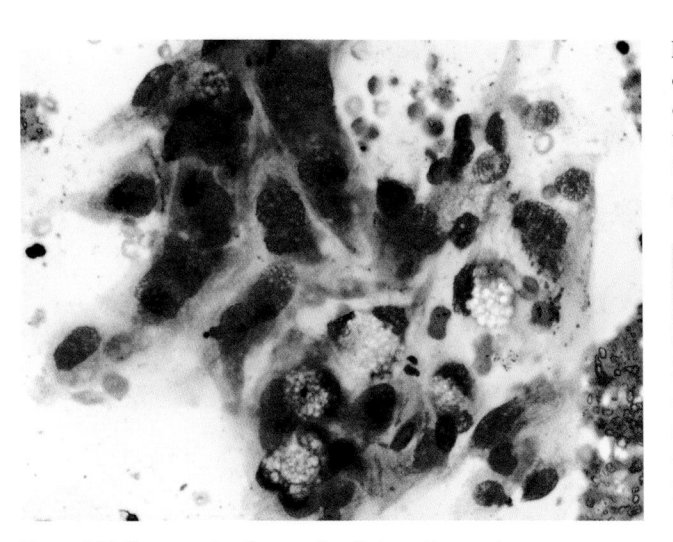

Figure 3.13 Degenerative changes. Cyst lining cells may show apparent pleomorphism due to multinucleation and degenerate changes such as cytoplasmic vacuolation.

lesions is controversial. In some instances, given the appropriate clinical and radiological context, the presence of abundant colloid, even in the absence of thyroid epithelium, is considered to be an adequate finding for the diagnosis of a colloid nodule (see 3.1.2 and 3.4.1.11). This is particularly common in areas of endemic goitre.

3.2.3 Hyperactive goitre (toxic goitre, thyrotoxicosis, primary hyperthyroidism, Graves' disease)

FNAC smears from a hyperactive goitre usually show an increased quantity of (Fig. 3.15) thyroid epithelium, which is arranged in flat sheets but also in microfollicles or acini. Obvious anisonucleosis is seen. Marginal vacuoles (fire flare cells) and fine red granulation are present in the cytoplasm (Fig. 3.16). Apart from the hyperactive (thyrotoxic goitre) in which marginal vacuoles are seen in 100% of cases, they are also seen in 42.6% of hyperplastic nodules, 5.2% of colloid goitre and 13.3% of neoplasms. Marginal vacuoles are limited to neoplasms with a follicular component; that includes 15% of follicular

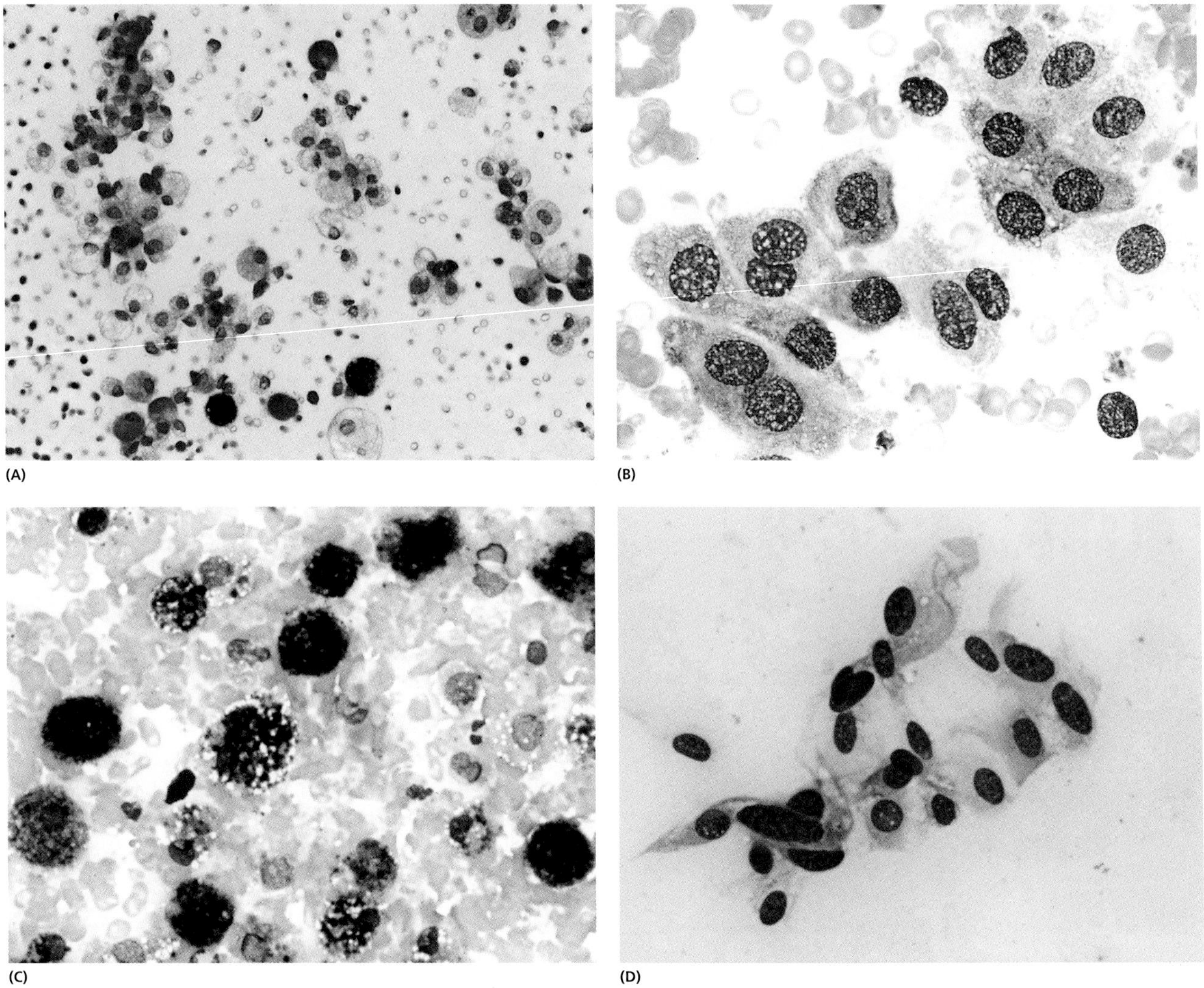

(A)

(B)

(C)

(D)

Figure 3.14 Thyroid cyst. In multinodular goitre with cyst formation, macrophages are often seen. (A) Low power view typical of a benign thyroid cyst. Sparse follicular epithelium and macrophages (MGG ×200). (B) Epithelium shows degenerative changes. Macrophages are filled with haemosiderin (MGG ×400). (C) Foamy macrophages and colloid (MGG ×600, oil immersion). (D) Spindle cells, overlapping and cytoplasmic vacuolation may be seen in the cells of a cyst wall and are not to be confused with other spindle cell pathology in the thyroid. (MGG ×600)

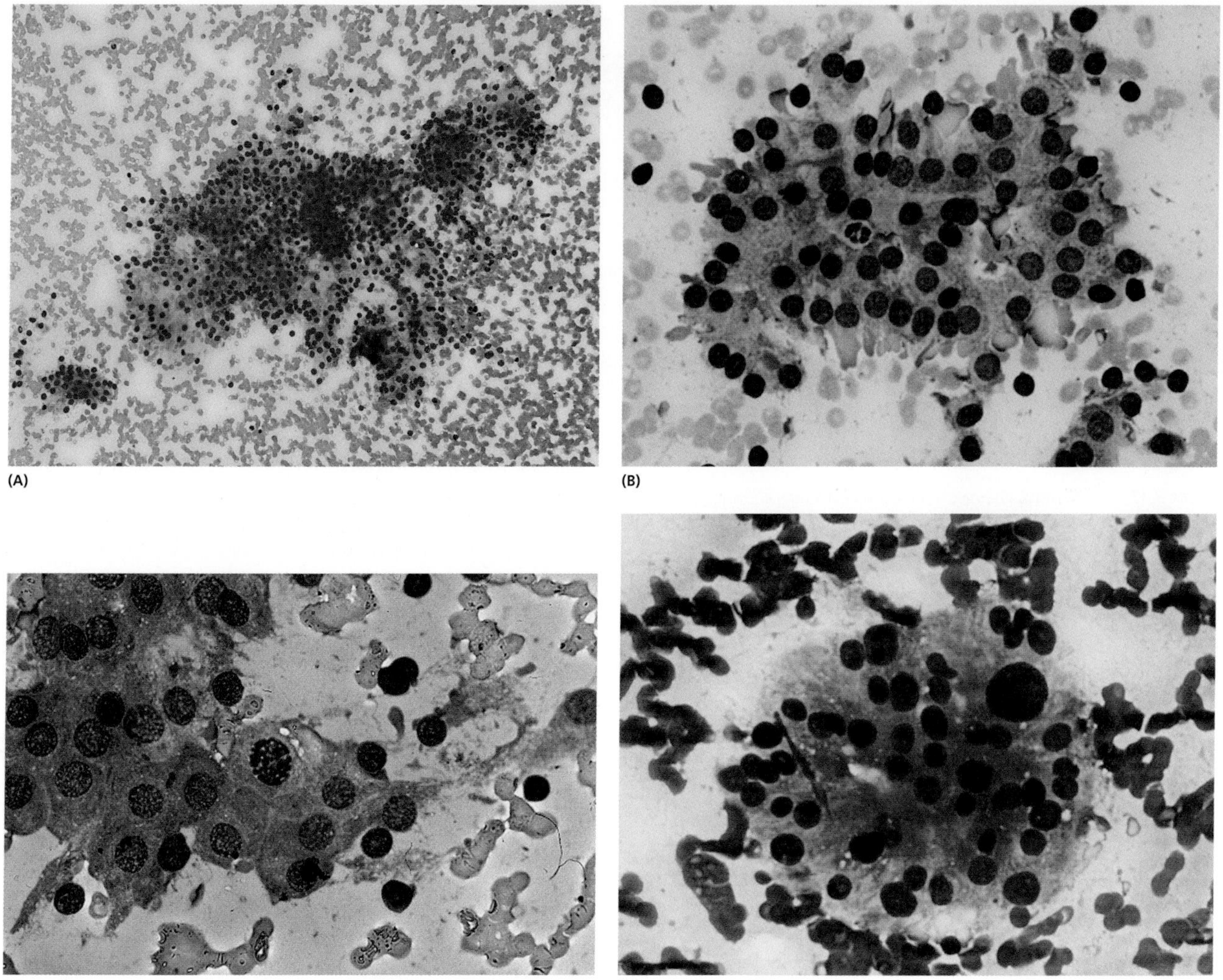

Figure 3.15 Hyperactive, toxic goitre. (A) FNAC smears from hyperactive goitre may show little colloid. Follicular epithelium may be hypercellular, arranged in microfollicles or acini. (B, C, D) Marginal vacuoles (fire flare cells) and fine red granulation are present in the cytoplasm (MGG ×600, ×1000, oil immersion).

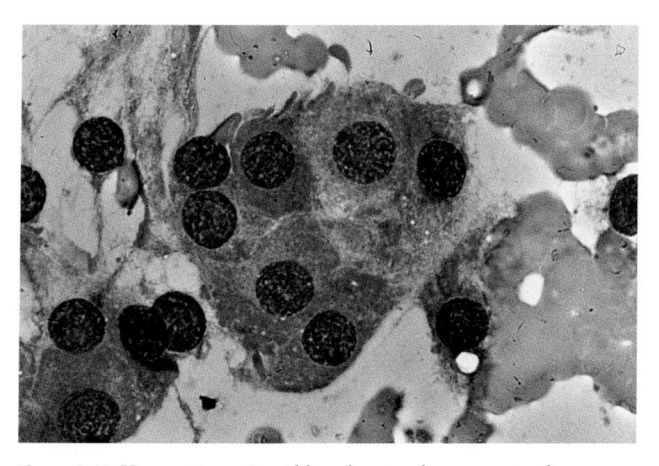

Figure 3.16 Hyperactive goitre. Although not pathognomonic of hyperactive nodules, fire-flare appearance of the cytoplasm of the follicular cells and a good cellularity of the smears are the features most frequently observed. Appearances of a well outlined cytoplasm of oncocytic type with scalloped edges may be misleading (see Fig. 3.24) (MGG ×600).

neoplasms and 50% of follicular variant of papillary carcinoma. A multiparametre study of FNAC from toxic goitre showed that a 'fire-flare' appearance of the follicular cells and a good cellularity of the smears were the features most frequently observed in these cases [115]. Oncocytic change was present in 47% of the cases, and small numbers of lymphocytes were seen in smears from 41% of the cases. Epithelioid cell granulomata and multinucleated giant cells were observed in less than one-fourth of the cases. About half of the cases showed some degree of pleomorphism of the thyroid epithelial cells. Occasionally, cases showing focal cytological or architectural changes out of keeping with the rest of the sample, have to be reported as 'atypical' (BTS RTC III, UKRCPath Thy 3a) (see Section 3.1.2. and Table 3.5) and FNAC repeated at a later date (Fig. 3.17).

[See BOX 3.2. Summary of ultrasound features: Thyrotoxicosis Graves' disease on www.wiley.com/go/kocjan/clinical_cytopathology_head_neck2e]

Hyperthyroidism is sometimes associated with thyroid malignancy. Gul et al. set to evaluate the role of preoperative US guided

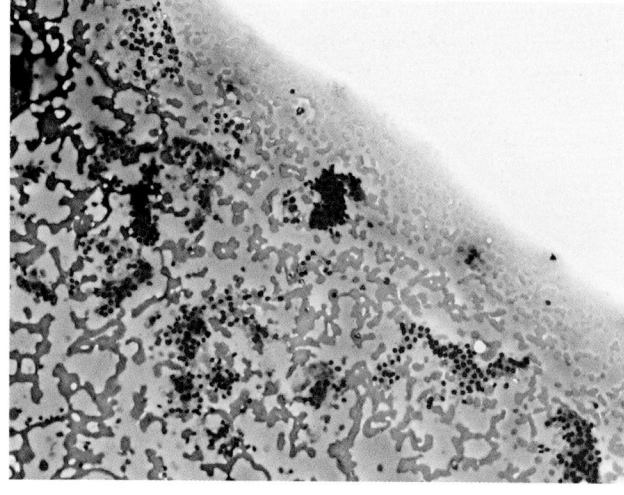

Figure 3.17 Adenomatous goitre versus follicular adenoma. FNAC of the thyroid is limited in differentiating hyperplastic nodular goitres from true follicular neoplasms. This is the edge of an aspirate from an adenomatous/hyperplastic colloid goitre. Although the aspirate is cellular, note plenty of thin colloid in the background.

thyroid FNAC in diagnosis of thyroid carcinoma in patients with hyperthyroidism and found that the malignancy rates were 16% in toxic MNG, 6.4% in autonomous functioning thyroid nodule and 12.6% in Graves' disease [116].

3.2.4 Thyroiditis

3.2.4.1 Acute

Acute thyroiditis is rarely seen. The cause is bacteria, fungi or parasites. Differential diagnosis includes anaplastic carcinoma, which can be associated with a background with numerous granulocytes. Granulocytes may also be seen in subacute thyroiditis.

3.2.4.2 Subacute (granulomatous thyroiditis, De Quervain's thyroiditis)

Subacute thyroiditis presents usually in young females, frequently after viral respiratory infection. There is painful asymmetrical thyroid gland enlargement. Clinically, there is a raised ESR, occasionally fever and mild hypothyroidism. Patients complain of pain in the thyroid typically irradiating into the ear. The illness lasts several weeks to several months and usually ends in complete recovery. Histologically there is destruction of follicular epithelium with a granulomatous reaction to colloid. There is variably dense lymphocytic infiltrate and variable fibrosis. The cause is unknown and is assumed to be viral.

Granulomatous thyroiditis has a variably cellular appearance with multinucleated giant cells, sometimes of Langhans' type with fragments of colloid, epithelioid cells, macrophages, lymphocytes, fibroblasts and frequently small epithelial cells with degenerative changes (Fig. 3.18). Hürthle cells may be seen. Stromal cells with large pleomorphic nuclei may be present.

Apart from subacute thyroiditis, multinucleate giant cells may be seen in papillary carcinoma and Hashimoto's thyroiditis, thyroid granulomas, adenomatous goitre and Hürthle-cell adenoma [117]. Anaplastic carcinoma of the thyroid may also cause painful swelling of the gland with inflammatory cells, spindle cells and osteoclast like giant cells.

3.2.4.3 Lymphocytic (Hashimoto)

Lymphocytic thyroiditis occurs most often in females above the age of 40 and causes a symmetrical diffuse thyroid gland enlargement (Fig. 3.19). Initially there is often mild hyperthyroidism; eventually the patient is clinically hypothyroid. Histologically, there is intralobular fibrosis, a dense lymphoplasmacytic infiltrate with lymphoid follicle formation, extension of the infiltrate around atrophic follicles and extensive oncocytic metaplasia of the follicular epithelium. The epithelium often shows nuclear enlargement, nuclear overlap and occasionally clearing of the nuclear structure to produce appearances similar to that of papillary carcinoma. Squamous cell metaplasia may be seen. The cause is autoimmune; high levels of different antibodies, including antibodies to thyroglobulin, are found in serum.

See BOX 3.3. Summary of ultrasound features: Hashimoto's thyroiditis (autoimmune or chronic lymphocytic)on www.wiley. com/go/kocjan/clinical_cytopathology_head_neck2e]

Hashimoto's thyroiditis is the commonest thyroiditis encountered by the cytopathologists and, given its variable cytological appearances, one of the most frequent causes of thyroid FNAC consultations. In classical cases, FNAC samples are cellular with an abundance of lymphocytes and lymphoid follicle centre cells, centrocytes, centroblasts and plasma cells (Fig. 3.20). Oncocytic epithelial cells are seen. They may have prominent anisonucleosis and anisocytosis with prominent nucleoli. Multinucleated giant cell histiocytes may also be seen [118]. FNAC is highly sensitive in diagnosing Hashimoto's thyroiditis, with a diagnostic accuracy rate of 92% [119]. However, more often than this classical presentation, FNAC samples have a predominance of epithelium and a relative scarcity of lymphoid cells, which need to be examined with care.

The potential pitfalls in diagnosis relate to both, the lymphoid and the epithelial component [120]. Epithelial atypia may be interpreted as malignancy, particularly if associated with multinucleated giant cells as in papillary carcinoma (Fig. 3.21). On the other hand, pleomorphic oncocytic cells may be present in aspirates from oncocytic cell neoplasms and underdiagnosed as Hashimoto's thyroiditis, especially when they are associated with a few lymphocytes [121].

Differential diagnosis of thyroid entities containing *oncocytic* cells is vast. These cells have been identified in benign oncocytic lesions, such as senescent thyroids, exposure to radiation, nodular goitre, Graves' disease and thyroiditis. Oncocytic cells are also components of oncocytic neoplasms including oncocytic papillary thyroid carcinoma (PTC), tall cell PTC, Warthin-like PTC, Hürthle cell adenoma and Hürthle cell carcinoma. Oncocytic cells in one-third of Hashimoto's thyroiditis cases can show atypical nuclear features with focal regions demonstrating optically clear nuclei, prominent cytoplasmic invaginations, intranuclear cytoplasmic inclusions, and occasional grooves, mimicking papillary thyroid carcinoma [122–124].

Sheets of oncocytic cells with a single small nucleolus is indicative of Hashimoto's thyroiditis, while papillary arrangements of oncocytic cells without nucleoli suggest the presence of PTC [125].

PTC and anaplastic carcinomas may have lymphocytic infiltrates. Non-Hodgkin lymphoma of the thyroid arises against a background of lymphocytic thyroiditis (see Fig. 3.32, Section 3.4.1.1). False positive diagnoses may arise on the basis of epithelial atypia or suspicion of a lymphoma. False negative results may be due to lymphocytic infiltrates in tumours, particularly papillary carcinoma with a thyroiditis component.

Differential diagnosis of Hashimoto's thyroiditis includes subacute thyroiditis, oncocytic hyperplasia, oncocytic tumours, follicular tumours, PTC and malignant lymphoma.

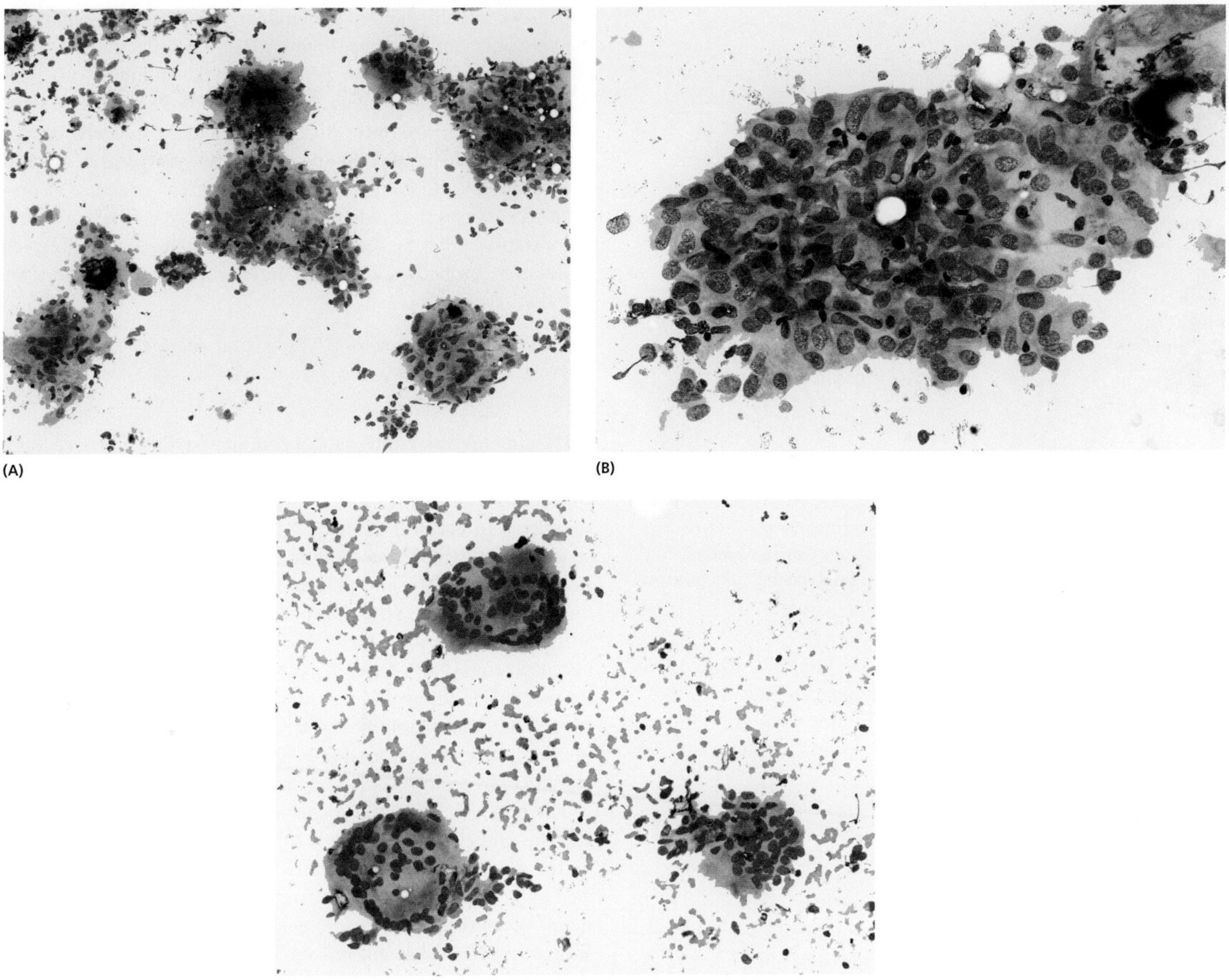

(A)

(B)

(C)

Figure 3.18 Granulomatous thyroiditis. (A) Low power view shows variably cellular appearance with multinucleated giant cells with fragments of colloid, epithelioid cells and macrophages (MGG ×100). (B) Epithelioid cells forming granulomas often replace any thyroid epithelium in aspirates (MGG ×600, oil immersion). (C) Multinucleate giant cells may be of Langhans type (MGG ×600, oil immersion).

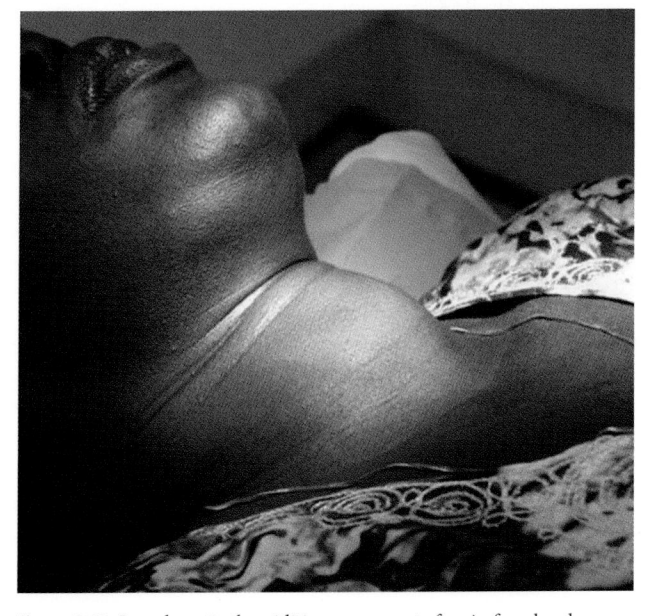

Figure 3.19 Lymphocytic thyroiditis occurs most often in females above the age of 40 and causes a symmetrical diffuse thyroid gland enlargement.

3.2.4.4 Riedel's

Riedel's thyroiditis (RT) is a rare form of chronic thyroiditis, characterised by a fibro-inflammatory process that partially destroys the thyroid and often involves surrounding tissues (vessels, muscles, oesophagus, trachea upper mediastinum), sometimes causing severe compression and dislocation of trachea and oesophagus. It is relatively frequent in women aged 45–50 years or over. The clinical presentation can be hypothyroidism associated with a solitary firm to hard cold nodule replacing the entire right lobe of thyroid gland. The aetiology of RT is unknown but speculation is that it lies between a primary fibrotic and an autoimmune process [126]. Today, we know that the combination of Riedel's disease and fibrosing Hashimoto's thyroiditis is rare and coincidental, as both represent two distinct clinicopathological entities (Figs. 3.20D and 3.22D) [127, 128].

There are reports of association of RT with subacute thyroiditis. Antithyroid antibodies have been detected in over 50% of the patients with RT. Since the 1960s, RT has been considered to be part of multifocal systemic fibrosclerosis (MSF). MSF is a multisystem disease, which often mimics malignancy. Sclerosing cholangitis, retroperitonealfibrosis, RT, fibrotic pseudotumour of the orbit and fibrosis of the salivary glands have all been reported to be part of the spectrum of

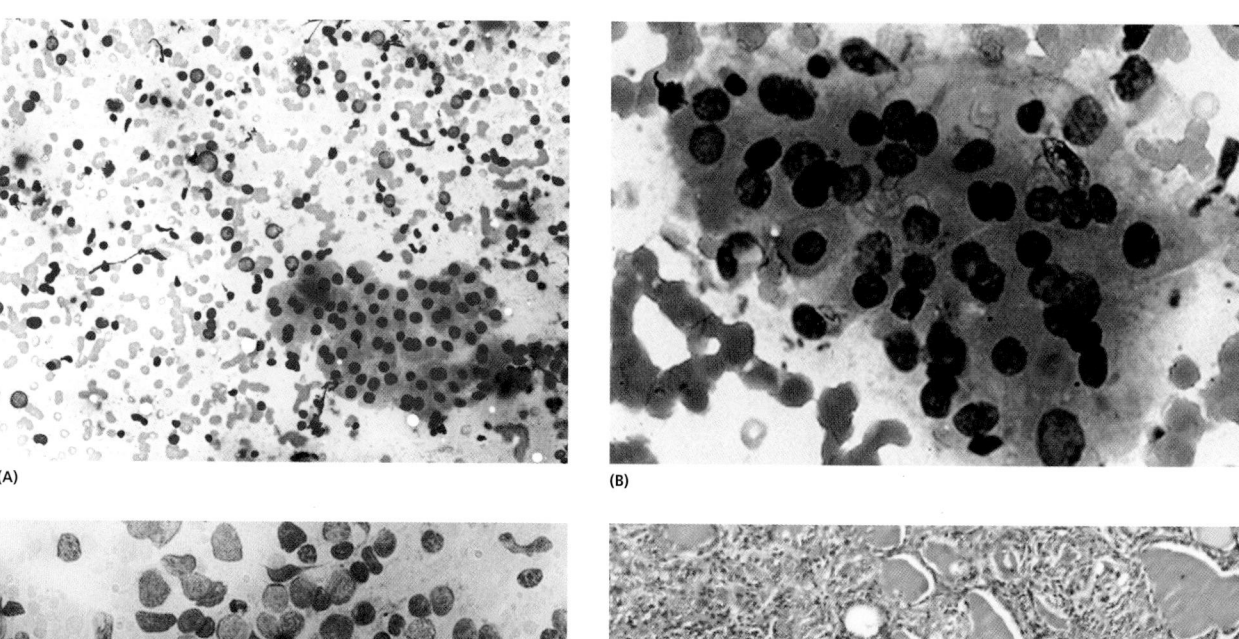

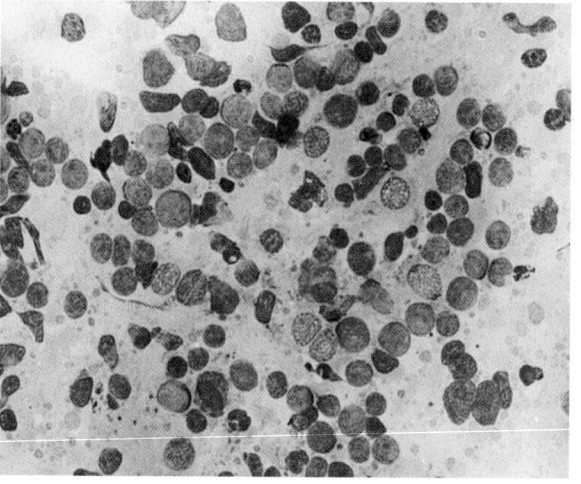
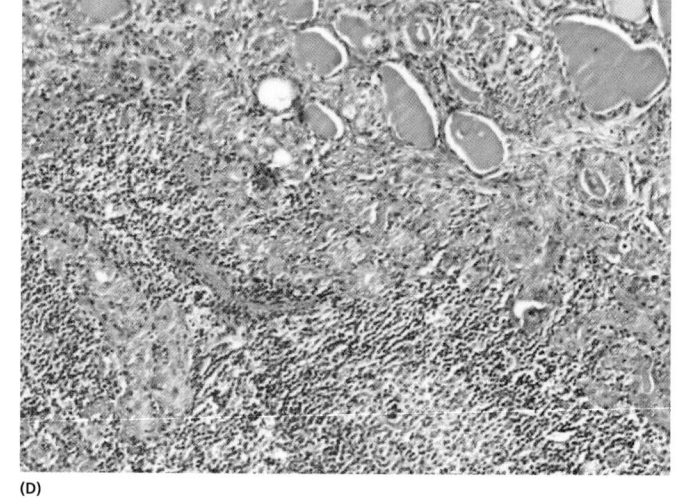

Figure 3.20 Lymphocytic thyroiditis. (A) Smears are cellular with lymphocytes and lymphoid follicle centre cells, centrocytes, centroblasts, plasma cells and oncocytic epithelial cells (MGG ×400). (B) Oncocytic epithelial cells (×600, oil immersion). (C) Lymphoid cells including folllicle centre cells (MGG ×400). (D) Histology of the fibrosing variant of Hashimotos thyroiditis.

this condition [129]. More recently, Nield et al. [130] have referred to this condition as the hyper IgG disease, characterised histologically by a lymphoplasmacytic inflammation with IgG4-positive cells and exuberant fibrosis, which leaves dense fibrosis on resolution. A typical example of a hyper IgG disease is idiopathic retroperitoneal fibrosis.

[See BOX 3.4. Summary of ultrasound features: Reidel's Thyroiditis on www.wiley.com/go/kocjan/clinical_cytopathology_head_neck2e]

Cytological features of Riedel's thyroiditis show moderate cellularity with fragments of fibrous tissue with bland spindle-shaped cells, dispersed singly and in small clusters (Fig. 3.22) [131]. The spindle cells vary from bland-appearing fibroblasts with a uniform pale nucleus to more active-appearing myofibroblast-like cells with more abundant basophilic cytoplasm. These show no mitoses and lack any increase in the nuclear-to cytoplasmic ratio. Scattered inflammatory cells consisting of a mixed population of lymphocytes, plasma cells, neutrophils, and rare eosinophils may be seen. The background of the smears displays no necrosis or malignant diathesis. Neither germinal centre cells nor Hürthle cells are identified to support the diagnosis of a fibrosing variant of Hashimoto's thyroiditis. Similarly, multinucleated giant cells and clusters of epithelioid cells are not seen. FNAC of Riedel's thyroiditis may be mistakenly diagnosed as anaplastic thyroid carcinoma [131].

3.3 Indeterminate cytological findings: follicular lesions

FNAC is the primary testing modality for identifying malignancy in patients with a thyroid nodule. A majority of thyroid FNAC specimens, generally in the range of 60–70%, are classified as 'benign', and approximately 20–30% in total fall into the three categories of 'suspicious for a follicular neoplasm' (SFN), 'suspicious for malignancy' and 'malignant' [132, 133].

3.3.1 Atypia of uncertain significance (AUS)/ Follicular lesion of uncertain significance (FLUS) (TBSRTC III, UK Thy 3a)

The Bethesda 2007 Thyroid Cytology Classification (TBSRTC) defines *follicular lesion of undetermined significance* (AUS/FLUS) as a heterogeneous category of cases that are not convincingly benign nor sufficiently atypical for a diagnosis of *follicular neoplasm or suspicious for malignancy* [134–136].

By definition, AUS/FLUS includes a variety of abnormal architectural, cellular or nuclear features and, as such, implementation of this category among cytopathologists, at least initially, is expected to be variable. In many instances, a predisposing

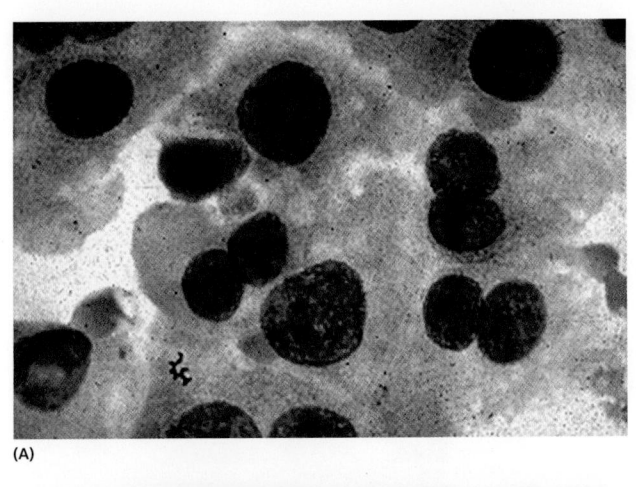

(A)

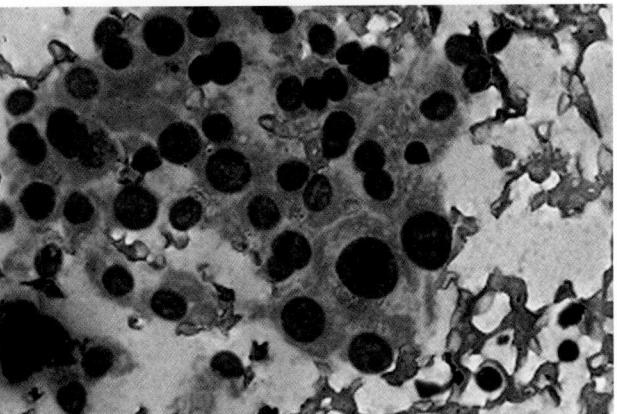

(B)

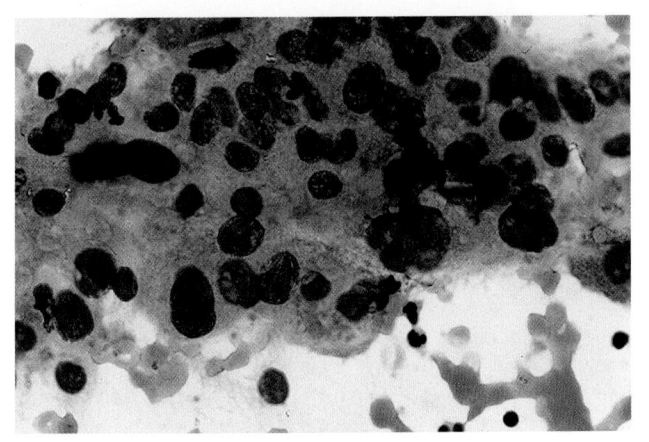

(C)

Figure 3.21 Lymphocytic thyroiditis. (A,B,C) Oncocytic epithelial atypia that occurs in longstanding lymphocytic thyroiditis may be interpreted as malignancy, particularly if associated with multinucleated giant cells as in papillary carcinoma (MGG ×1000).

condition for an AUS/FLUS is a suboptimal sample and a repeat FNAC often resolves the dilemma. At the time of its implementation, the authors of the TBSRTC recommended that the AUS/FLUS category should not exceed 7% of thyroid FNAC diagnoses. Although the associated risk of malignancy for this category was anticipated to be in the range of 5–15%, intermediate between that of the benign and suspicious categories (see Table 3.6), recent series that reported experiences with the TBSRTC categories showed that the AUS/FLUS category exhibited a marked

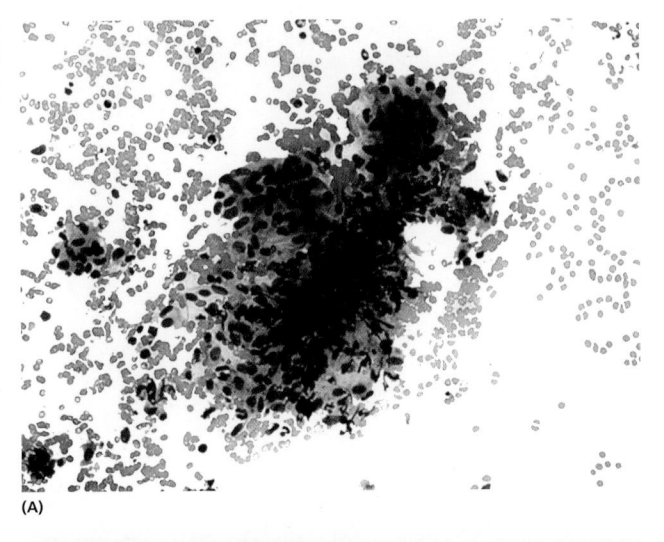

(A)

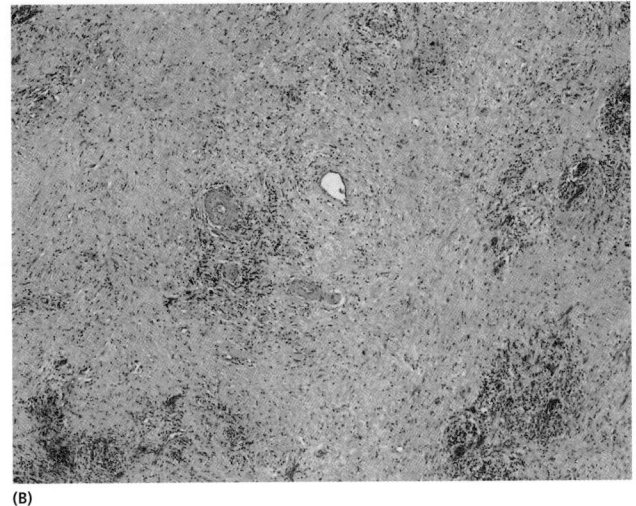

(B)

Figure 3.22 Riedel's thyroiditis. Usually a paucicellular sample, composed of spindle cells in poorly organised aggregates and as single bare nuclei. It is frequently confused with an anaplastic carcinoma or a soft tissue lesion. (B) Histology of Riedel's thyroiditis. Compare with image 3.20d.

variability in incidence (0.7–18%) and malignant outcome (2–48%) in resection specimens. Review of the literature revealed institutional differences in technical aspects, interpretation and application of criteria, analysis of outcome data and clinicopathologic interactions [137].

Whilst TBSRTC indicated that the initial follow-up of thyroid FNAC diagnosed as AUS/FLUS should be a repeat FNAC (Tables 3.6 and 3.7), UK RCPath recommends that indeterminate cases should be reviewed at the multidisciplinary meetings (MDM). Our own experience of using AUS/FLUS (Thy3a) category showed a poor interobserver agreement [138] and a relatively high positive predictive value (PPV), that is, risk of malignancy of 40%. This figure is unusually high partly because of the small number of cases within this category that underwent surgery [29, 131, 139–145].

Our experience is supported by that of others who found that malignancy rates in nodules with AUS/FLUS (Thy 3a) cytology are higher than previously estimated, with 26.6–37.8% of AUS/FLUS nodules harbouring cancer. These data imply that Bethesda Category III nodules in some practice settings may have a higher risk of malignancy than traditionally believed, and that guidelines recommending repeat FNAC or observation merit reconsideration [146–148].

Morphologically, the majority of indeterminate cases fall into one of the two most common scenarios: (1) low cellularity with predominant microfollicular architecture and absence of colloid and (2) nuclear features not characteristic of benign lesions (nuclear atypia) [134].

Architectural atypia in AUS/FLUS (Thy 3a) is shown as an abnormal arrangement of follicular cells with each other, this can raise concern for a neoplasm under several different circumstances without being sufficiently convincing to warrant the interpretation of *'suspicious for follicular neoplasm'* (SFN). A subset of microfollicles is normal in a benign thyroid FNAC specimen; many benign thyroid nodules demonstrate a mixture of macrofollicles and microfollicles, but usually with a predominantly macrofollicular cytoarchitectural pattern. However, a subset of thyroid FNAC specimens are paucicellular and contain only a few well-formed microfollicles, trabeculae or crowded groups (Fig. 3.23A). Some of these cases may not even meet minimal adequacy criteria of TBSRTC (see Table 3.6) (at least 6 groups of follicular cells with 10 cells per group), yet to interpret the aspirate as 'non-diagnostic' would ignore the architectural atypia that is present. Another pattern of concerning architectural atypia occurs when only a subset of smears (such as a single slide from 1 pass) exhibits a predominance of microfollicles whereas other smears from the same case demonstrate a benign macrofollicular pattern. Still another instance of architectural atypia is subtle but persistent crowding of follicular cells throughout a paucicellular aspirate.

Nuclear atypia in AUS/FLUS (Thy 3a) can present in several patterns raising the spectre of PTC but are quantitatively and/or qualitatively insufficient for an interpretation of 'suspicious for malignancy'. These include a hypocellular aspirate (sometimes in the setting of extensive cystic degeneration) with only rare follicular cells exhibiting nuclear atypia suggestive of PTC (Fig. 3.23B). Alternatively, similar rare cells may be present in a cellular background that has an otherwise benign appearance, obscuring the significance of the rare atypical cells. In some instances, more diffuse but mild nuclear changes can be appreciated, with nuclear enlargement, crowding and pallor, but without other supporting features (e.g. intranuclear pseudoinclusions, grooves and nuclear

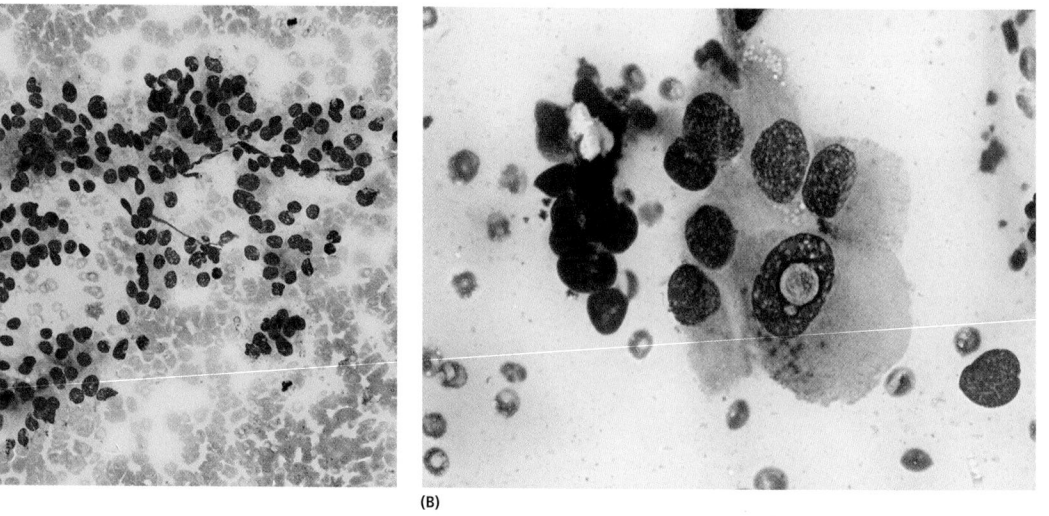

(A)

(B)

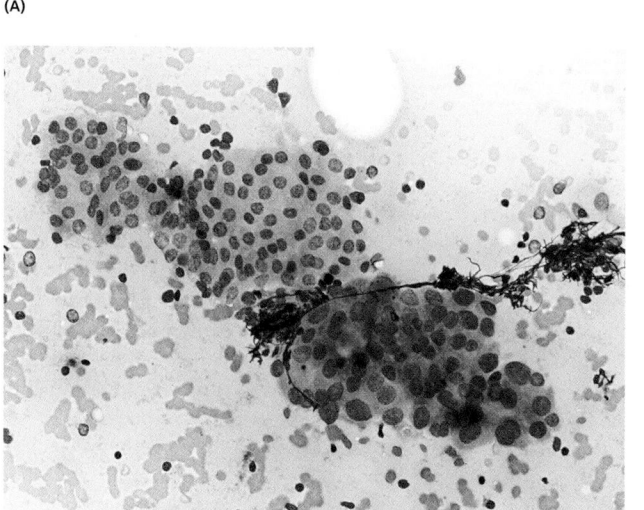

(C)

(D)

Figure 3.23 Atypical architectural and nuclear features in AUS/FLUS (UK Thy 3a) (A) An abnormal arrangement of follicular cells with each other, so-called 'architectural atypia', can raise concern for a neoplasm under several different circumstances without being sufficiently convincing to warrant the interpretation of a follicular neoplasm. (B) A hypocellular aspirate (sometimes in the setting of extensive cystic degeneration) with only rare follicular cells exhibiting nuclear atypia suggestive of papillary carcinoma, (C) More diffuse but mild nuclear changes can be appreciated, with nuclear enlargement, crowding, and pallor, but without other supporting features (e.g., intranuclear pseudoinclusions, grooves, and nuclear contour irregularities) of PTC. (D) nuclear atypia due to radioiodine treatment.

contour irregularities) of PTC (Fig. 3.23C). Focal and/or mild changes that suggest PTC are occasionally encountered in settings known to mimic the cytologic atypia of PTC, therefore raising doubt about the significance of the findings. Such confounding situations include patients with chronic lymphocytic thyroiditis (Hashimoto thyroiditis [HT]) and those with a history of external beam radiation, radioiodine therapy or thyroid suppressive agents, most notably for Graves' disease (Fig. 3.23D).

Some paucicellular thyroid aspirates are comprised of a virtually exclusive population of *oncocytes* (grouped or isolated) while lacking lymphocytes or significant numbers of benign, non-oncocytic follicular cells. The paucicellularity mitigates against the interpretation of 'SFN, oncocytic (Hürthle) cell type' (SFNHCT), but the exclusive or virtually exclusive population of Hürthle cells precludes an interpretation of 'benign' (Fig. 3.24). Aspirates with this pattern are better placed in the AUS/FLUS (Thy3a) category, and patients may benefit from a repeat FNAC performed within 3–6 months (see Table 3.7).

The differential diagnosis of thyroid entities containing oncocytic cells, as mentioned earlier, includes benign oncocytic lesions, such as senescent thyroids, exposure to radiation, nodular goitre, Graves' disease and thyroiditis. Oncocytic cells are also components of oncocytic neoplasms including oncocytic PTC, tall cell PTC, Warthin-like PTC, oncocytic (Hürthle) cell adenoma and oncocytic (Hürthle) cell carcinoma.

Atypia secondary to preparation artefact is not sufficient to warrant the interpretation of AUS/FLUS. Nevertheless, some thyroid FNAC specimens contain atypical cells that are hard to observe and assess confidently because of obscuring blood, clotting artefact, or poor fixation or staining (Fig. 3.25). Excessive blood and microclots can obscure the architectural pattern of follicular cells, in some instances making the groups appear falsely crowded or microfollicular. When improperly fixed or stained slides are used, cells may appear larger than usual, especially at the periphery of the smear. Nuclei can appear enlarged and the chromatin can resemble the 'salt-and-pepper' pattern observed in medullary thyroid carcinoma. True atypical cells (with grooves and nuclear enlargement) can be admixed with such artefacts and lead to a false-positive interpretation. Similarly, if the stain is very pale, the chromatin pattern can raise the possibility of PTC.

Atypical cyst-lining cells are a potential pitfall encountered with cystic thyroid nodules [149]. Benign cyst-lining cells exhibit a range of appearances from elongated, reactive-appearing cells to markedly enlarged cells with nuclear features that mimic PTC. Benign cyst-lining cells are typically polygonal or fusiform, with abundant dense cytoplasm; well-defined cellular borders; occasionally enlarged, grooved nuclei; and small, distinct nucleoli (Fig. 3.26). In the context of a cystic aspirate with admixed macrofollicles and colloid, the benign cyst-lining cells are easily recognised as benign. However, in isolation, it can be difficult to exclude PTC. In the latter instance, the aspirate is better classified as AUS/FLUS to reflect the uncertainty regarding the findings.

Ultrasound findings play a complementary role in the diagnosis of thyroid nodules with AUS/FLUS. In case of highly suspicious US findings such as 'TDW and marked hypoechogenicity', could be very helpful in the diagnosis of malignancy. Malignancy was associated with taller-than-wide shape, ill-defined margin and marked hypoechogenicity [150].

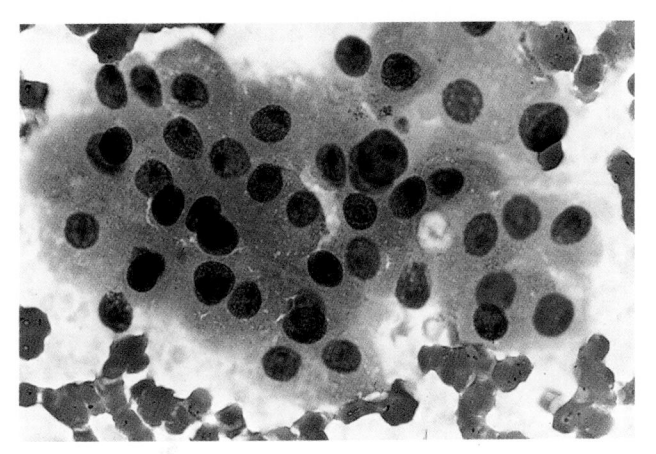

Figure 3.24 Oncocytic change as part of the AUS/FLUS category (UK Thy 3a) Some paucicellular thyroid aspirates are comprised of a virtually exclusive population of oncocytes (grouped or isolated) while lacking lymphocytes or significant numbers of benign, nononcocytic follicular cells.

3.3.2 'Follicular lesions' (TBSTRC IV: Follicular neoplasm or suspicious for a follicular neoplasm) (UK: Thy 3f)

FNAC of the thyroid has a limited role in differentiating hyperplastic nodular goitres from true follicular neoplasms (Fig. 3.17) and, to date, no role in separating follicular adenomas from follicular carcinomas. Similarly, cytological differential diagnosis of a hyperplastic colloid nodule and a follicular variant of papillary carcinoma (FVPC) is difficult using the common morphological features. FVPC can sometimes be differentiated from a colloid nodule based on nuclear changes, which include a larger size, higher N/C ratio, and presence of pseudoinclusions and nuclear grooves. In the instances where it is not possible to distinguish between these entities, namely a hyperplastic goitre, follicular adenoma, follicular carcinoma and a FVPC, an indeterminate cytology report of a *'suggestive of follicular neoplasm'* or *'follicular lesion'* is issued (BTSRTC IV, UKRCPath Thy 3f). Current thyroid reporting classifications (see Section 3.1.2. Table 3.5) recommend that these cases be discussed at the multidisciplinary team meetings (MDM) with a view to surgery, usually a hemithyroidectomy, to exclude a neoplasm (see Table 3.7). Ancillary techniques may be applied to try and refine the

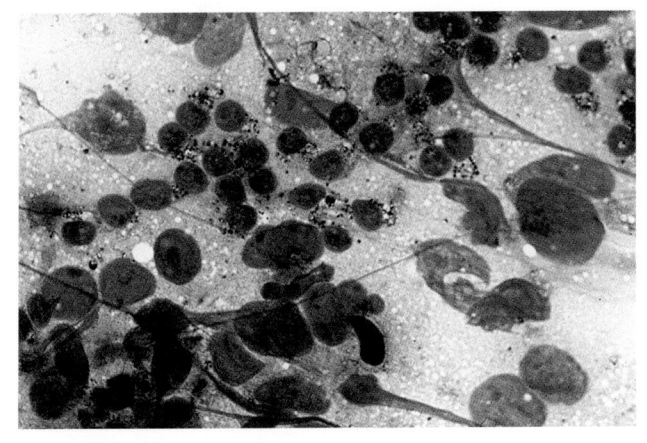

Figure 3.25 Preparation artefact as AUS/FLUS (UK Thy 3a). Some thyroid FNA specimens contain atypical cells that are hard to observe and assess confidently because of obscuring blood, clotting artifact, or poor fixation or staining.

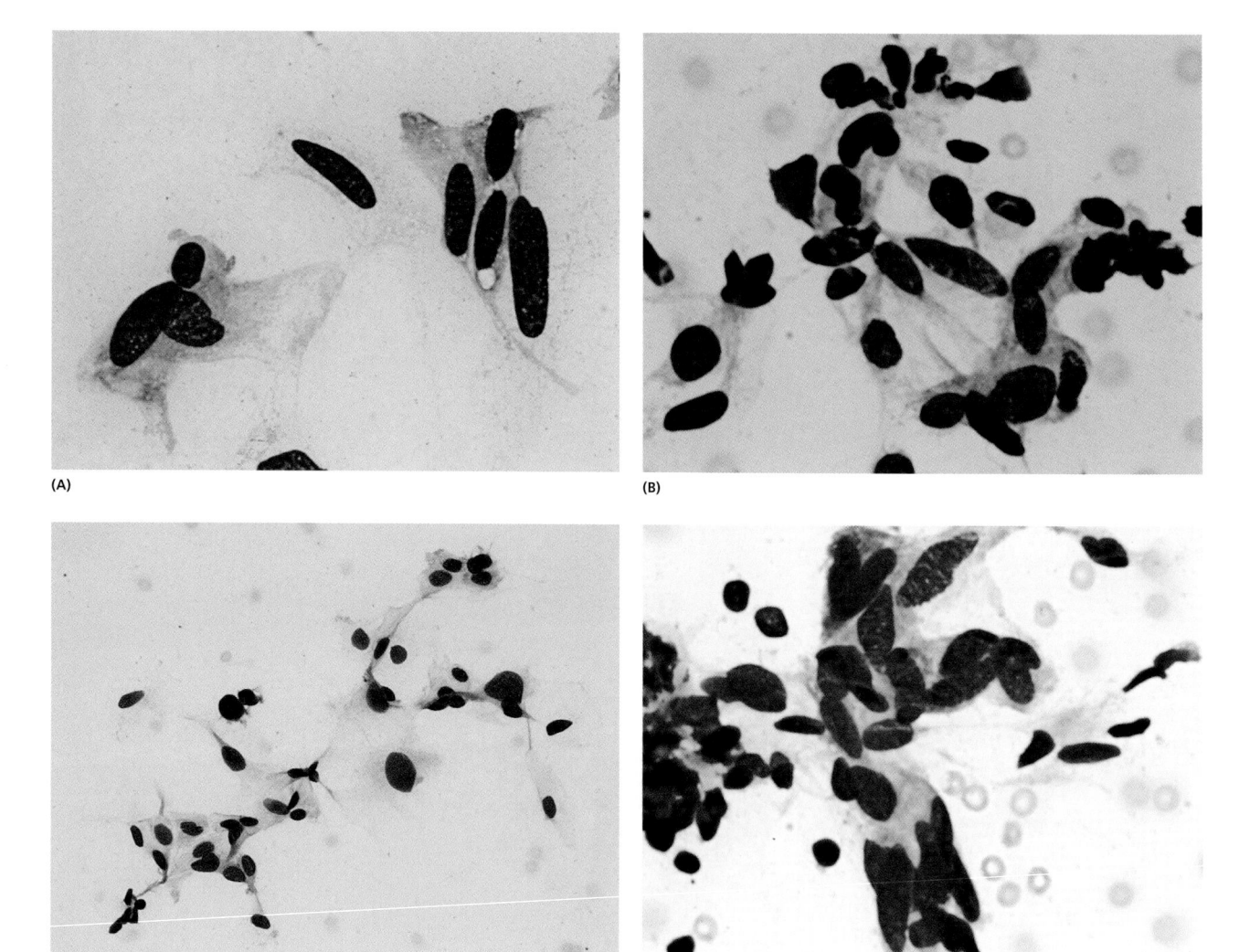

Figure 3.26 Atypical cyst lining cells as AUS/FLUS (UK Thy3 a) (A) Plump, spindle cell nuclei, in isolation, may be misleading. (B) Hyperchromasia, irregular hromatin pattern and overlapping are in this case all due to a technical artefact but may be difficult to ignore. (C) Out of the blue, anisonucleosis may not be explained. (D) Plump hyperchromatic nuclei may mimick a stromal lesion.

diagnosis in 'follicular lesions'. By using HBME-1 immunocyto-chemistry in FNAC led to reduction of the incidence of false-nega-tive diagnoses of FVPTC. Although CD15 is apparently inferior in terms of sensitivity for FVPTC, its excellent specificity will support the definitive diagnosis of thyroid malignancies, including FVPTC, after screening with HBME-1 [91]. While 'follicular lesion' FNAC had a 28% risk of malignancy, the risk increased up to 71% for mutation positive follicular lesions, and decreased to 18% for muta-tion negative follicular lesions thus helping a presurgical diagnosis [151] (see Section 3.1.7). Whilst accepting the shortcomings of cytomorphology in the indeterminate category of 'follicular lesions', audits of laboratory performance have shown a high interobserver reproducibility for its interpretation [138] and a comparable range of positive predictive value ('risk of malignancy'), which helps in counselling the patients in whom a diagnosis of 'follicular lesion' is made [31].

3.3.2.1 Follicular adenoma

Follicular adenoma is a solitary encapsulated lesion composed of a proliferation of follicular epithelium. Patients usually have normal thyroid gland function and present with a palpable lesion, which by immunoscintigraphy is usually 'cold' (non-hormonally active).

[See BOX 3.5. Summary of ultrasound features: Follicular lesion on www.wiley.com/go/kocjan/clinical_cytopathology_head_neck2e]

Histologically, the lesion is usually round, encapsulated and has an expansive growth pattern with compression of the surrounding thyroid gland tissue. The growth pattern may vary with macrofolli-cles (colloid adenoma), microfollicles (foetal adenoma), trabeculae and solid areas (embryonal adenoma). The cell type may vary bet-ween oncocytic/Hürthle cell, clear cell and signet ring cell. These microscopic variations have no clinical significance. The distinction between follicular adenoma and follicular carcinoma may be diffi-cult even on histology due to pseudoinfiltrative growth in the cap-sule and the often extremely close relationship between the follicular epithelium and thin walled blood vessels. Pseudopapillary hyper-plastic structures, cellular atypia and nuclear pleomorphism (espe-cially in Hürthle cell tumours) may also cause diagnostic difficulty [152]. A rare variant, hyalinising trabecular adenoma, a tumour with

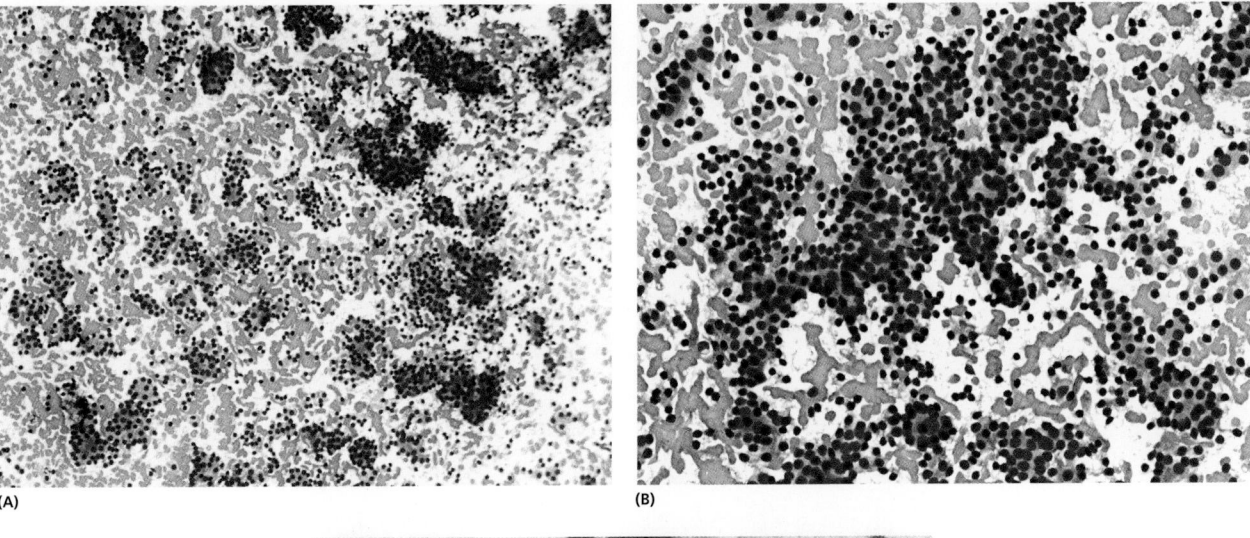

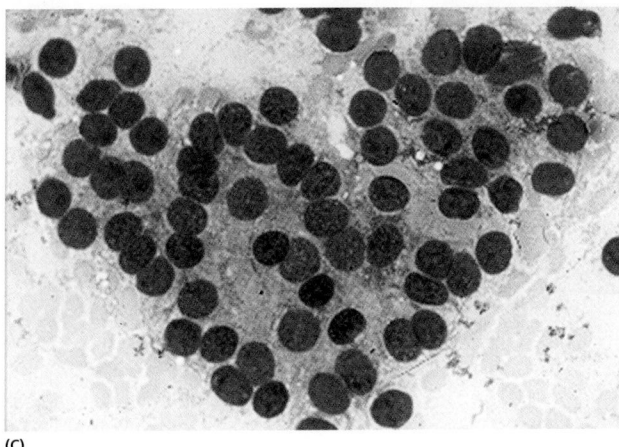

Figure 3.27 Follicular neoplasm cannot be excluded (TBSRTC IV, 'Follicular lesion' UKThy3f). (A, B) In microfollicular adenoma, the aspirate is cellular, with cells arranged in follicular structures. These are arranged in the form of rings or rosettes with cytoplasm centrally and without obvious cytoplasmic borders. There is little or no colloid present (MGG ×600, oil immersion). When present, colloid is seen in particles within the microfollicles (MGG ×600, oil immesrsion). (C) Follicular adenomas usually show little pleomorphism and nucleoli are small.

a large cell type, may be confused microscopically with a medullary or papillary carcinoma. The term atypical adenoma is used for encapsulated lesions with cytological atypia, mitoses and necrosis. Follow-up studies have shown that these lesions are benign.

Cytological features of follicular adenoma are indistinguishable from follicular carcinoma, a hyperplastic thyroid nodule or a FVPC, hence it is categorised as *'follicular neoplasm'*, *'suspicious for follicular neoplasm'* or *'follicular lesion'* (see Table 3.5) (Fig. 3.27A). In microfollicular adenoma, the aspirate is cellular, with cells arranged in follicular structures in the form of rings or rosettes with cytoplasm centrally and without obvious cytoplasmic borders. There is little or no colloid present. When present, it is seen in particles within the microfollicles. Pleomorphism, although usually absent, can be pronounced in follicular adenoma whilst the anisonucleosis is common (Fig. 3.28). Follicular lesions with even subtle nuclear atypia have been shown to have a high positive predictive value for malignancy and therefore should be distinguished from other follicular lesions because these cases require more aggressive surgical management [151a]. Nucleoli are usually small. In macrofollicular adenoma, there is usually abundant colloid and the appearance may be similar to that of MNG.

3.3.2.2 Oncocytic (Hürthle) cell tumours

The differential diagnosis of thyroid entities containing oncocytic cells includes benign oncocytic lesions, such as senescent thyroids, exposure to radiation, nodular goitre, Graves', disease and thyroiditis. Oncocytic cells are also components of oncocytic neoplasms including oncocytic PTC, tall cell PTC, Warthin-like PTC, oncocytic cell adenoma, and oncocytic (Hürthle) cell carcinoma. FNACs from oncocytic adenomas are predominantly composed of large monomorphic cells with oval nuclei, prominent nucleoli, and abundant, well-defined, granular cytoplasm, presenting singly, in follicular arrangement, and in monolayered sheets of variable sizes. Nuclear pleomorphism is noted (Fig. 3.29). Occasional small syncytial tumour cell clusters and a few naked tumour cell nuclei are observed [153]. Although oncocytic (Hurthle) cell adenoma and oncocytic cell carcinoma cannot be reliably distinguished on FNAC alone, some authors claim that the presence of small tumour cells with ill-defined cytoplasm and prominent nucleoli in syncytial clusters and abundant naked tumour cell nuclei in the FNAC of a thyroid nodule should alert the observer about the strong possibility of a oncocytic cell carcinoma [154]. However, other authors trying to find out whether the presence or absence of certain

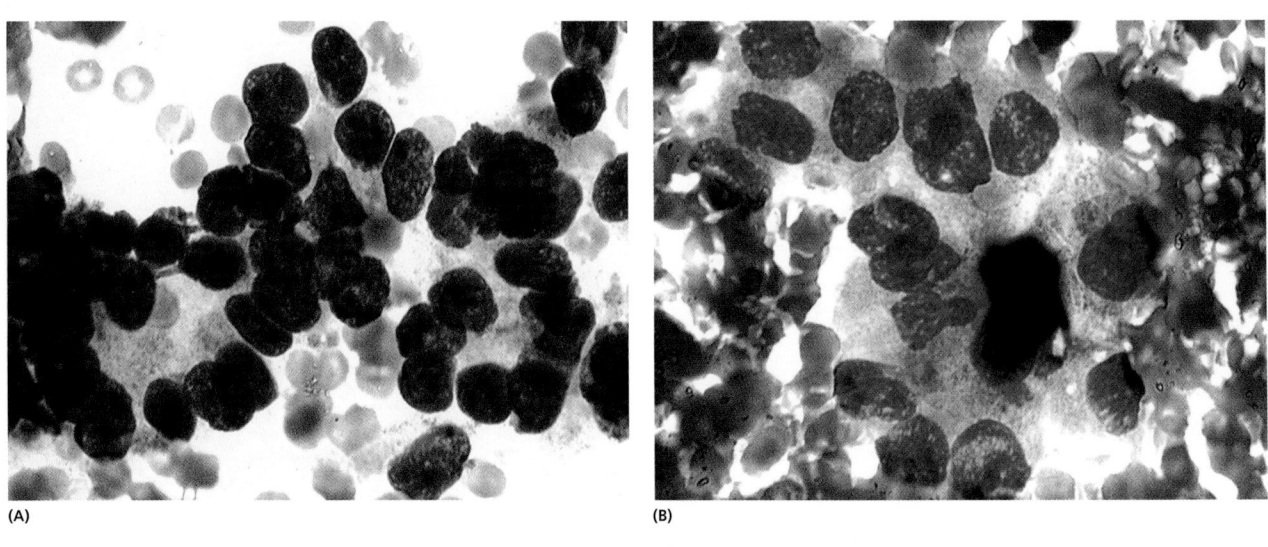

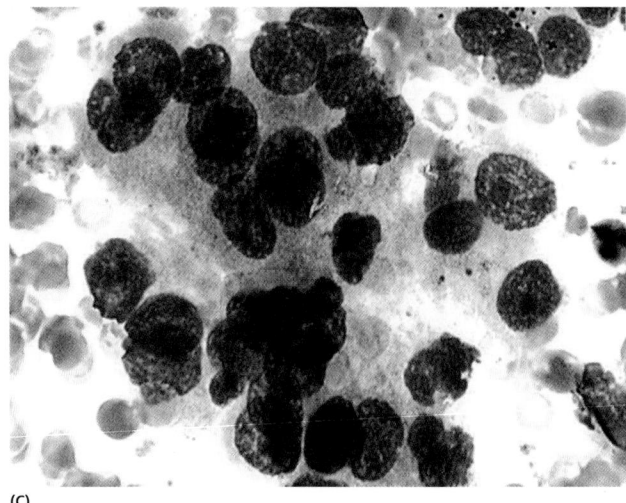

Figure 3.28 Follicular neoplasm cannot be excluded (TBSRTC IV, 'Follicular lesion' UKThy3f). Cytological atypia in follicular adenoma may be misinterpreted as carcinoma. (A) Occasionally, cellularity and pleomorphism may be tempting to diagnose follicular proliferation as a follicular carcinoma. (B) high power view of individual follicles with dense colloid in the centre. (C) The lesion was a follicular adenoma. Follicular lesions with even subtle nuclear atypia have been shown to have a high positive predictive value for malignancy and therefore should be distinguished from other follicular lesions.

cytological features, such as microfollicular arrangement, discohesive single cells, small cell dysplasia, large cell dysplasia, transgressing blood vessels and colloid, can exclude oncocytic (Hürthle cell) carcinoma in thyroid FNAC to minimise unnecessary surgery, conclude that none of the cytological features, including abundant colloid, can exclude oncocytic carcinoma. Oncocytic carcinoma can only be excluded by thorough histological examination of thyroidectomy specimens. A molecular marker is needed to triage oncocytic lesions in thyroid FNAC [155].

In the classification of 'follicular lesions' of the thyroid by FNAC, adherence to strict cytological criteria helps identify those patients who will benefit most from surgery [155]. When assessing the 'risk of malignancy', that is, PPV of 'follicular lesions', using the TBSRTC classification, cat IV ('Follicular neoplasm or suspicious for a follicular neoplasm or Hürthle cell (oncocytic) type'), this was found to be in the region of 15–30% (see Table 3.6) [156]. Molecular testing is becoming of increasing importance in the triage of patients that require surgery (See 3.1.7.)

3.3.2.3 Hyalinising trabecular adenoma

Hyalinising trabecular adenoma (HTA) is a benign thyroid tumour, almost exclusively occurring in females [157]. The morphological features of this entity overlap with both papillary and medullary carcinomas to varying extents. This, in turn, creates a situation of serious diagnostic pitfall particularly for a false positive diagnosis of papillary carcinoma in FNAC. False consideration of medullary carcinoma is also possible by the unwary especially if staining for Congo red and/or immunostaining for calcitonin is not resorted to.

HTAs contain cells with mild nuclear atypia, nuclear grooves and nuclear pseudoinclusions but lack psammoma bodies, high cellularity and papillary structures. Collections of an amorphous colloid-like material are noted surrounded by follicular cells. This purplish red stromal deposits corresponding to accumulations of basement membrane material helps to prevent cytological over-diagnosis of malignancy in this rare benign tumour [158, 159] (Fig. 3.30) Inflammatory cells in the background may suggest the possibility of a thyroiditis [160]. Immunohistochemistry using

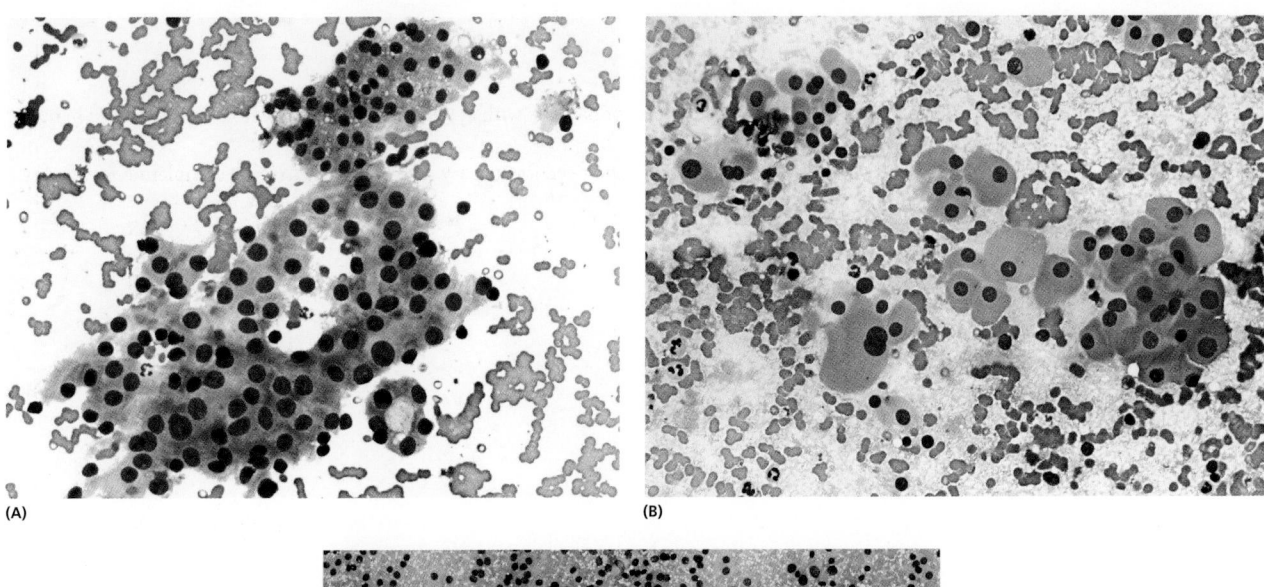

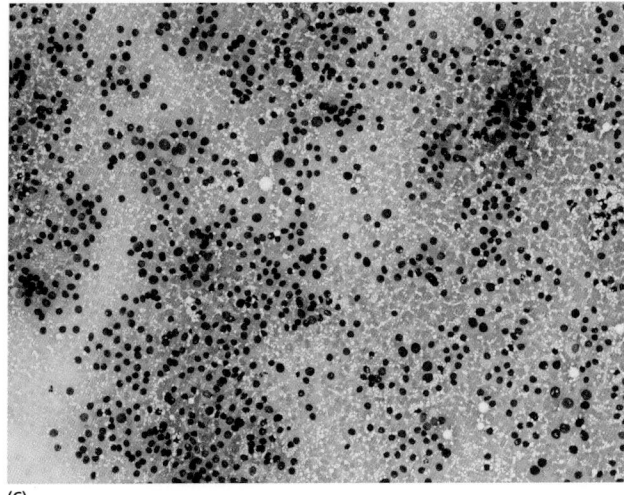

Figure 3.29 Oncocytic (Hürthle) cell tumours. (A) FNACs from Hürthle cell adenomas are predominantly composed of large monomorphic Hürthle cells with oval nuclei, prominent nucleoli, and abundant, well-defined, granular cytoplasm present singly, in acinar arrangement, and in monolayered sheets of variable sizes. (B) Anisonucleosis and prominent nucleoli may be misleading into diagnosis of malignancy. (C) The presence of small tumour cells with ill-defined cytoplasm and prominent nucleoli in syncytial clusters and abundant naked tumour cell nuclei should alert the observer about the strong possibility of a oncocytic cell carcinoma.

anti-calcitonin and anti-thyroglobulin antibodies is helpful in distinguishing these tumours from medullary carcinoma. The low Ki-67 (nuclear) index and absence of p53 immunostaining are consistent with the benign behaviour of this tumour [161]. Tumour cells of HTA reveal an intense cytoplasmic immunopositivity for MIB1. In contrast, cytoplasmic immunostaining for MIB1 was negative in all other thyroid tumours and non-neoplastic lesions. Positive cytoplasmic immunostaining for MIB1 is a characteristic finding of HTA and is useful in differentiating it from other thyroid tumours [162]. All of the HTA cases in a series by Goellner et al. had been initially interpreted as either suspicious or positive for malignancy. On retrospective review, many of the cytological features did mimic those of other lesions, particularly papillary carcinoma. The smears were hypercellular, nuclei were often slightly enlarged with pale chromatin, intranuclear holes and longitudinal grooving of the nuclear membrane. On the other hand, some cytological features were more suggestive of medullary carcinoma – poor cohesion of cells with elongated and spindle cell forms

and hyaline acellular areas. Authors suggest awareness of the histological and cytological features of HTA which may enable the cytopathologist to avoid a false positive diagnosis of papillary carcinoma or medullary carcinoma, although they consider unrealistic to expect a definitive diagnosis of HTA on FNAC [159, 163–169].

3.4 Malignant tumours

Approximately 95% of malignant thyroid gland tumours arise from the follicular epithelium and the remainder from C-cells. The commonest carcinomas are papillary, follicular, anaplastic and medullary.

3.4.1 Papillary carcinoma

Papillary carcinoma (PTC) is the commonest type of thyroid carcinoma. It is commoner in females than in males, presents in all age groups. Histologically, papillary carcinoma is characterised

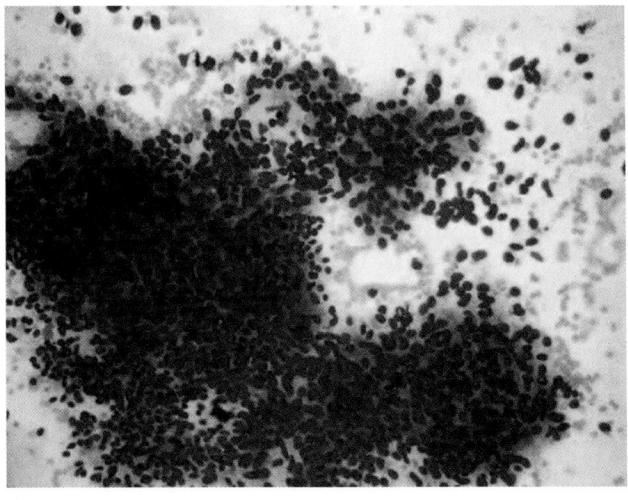

Figure 3.30 Hyalinising trabecular adenoma. Cells with mild nuclear atypia, nuclear grooves and nuclear pseudoinclusions but lacking psammoma bodies, high cellularity and papillary structures. Collections of an amorphous colloid-like material are noted surrounded by follicular cells. This purplish red stromal deposits corresponding to accumulations of basement membrane material helps to prevent cytological overdiagnosis of malignancy.

by characteristic cytological features and papillary structures. Papillae are complex with a variable amount of stroma and lined by a single layer of epithelium. Occasionally, the entire tumour may be follicular without papillary structures. The biological behaviour of both, classical and follicular type is similar. Apart from the classical and follicular variants, other histological types of PTC include papillary microcarcinoma, tall cell, oncocytic, columar cell, diffuse sclerosing, solid, clear cell, cribriform morular, macrofollicular, PTC with prominent hobnail features, PTC with fasciitis-like stroma, combined papillary and medullary carcinoma, PTC with de-differentiation to anaplastic carcinoma and papillary Hürthle cell carcinoma with lymphoplasmacytic stroma (Warthin-like variant).

PTC may become cystic, particularly in lymph node metastases. Psammoma bodies in the stroma are characteristic but may be seen in other conditions. PTC tends to spread via the lymphatics. Distant metastases are infrequent. Prognosis is good (20-year survival is 90%). Unfavourable prognostic features are old age at presentation, extension of the tumour outside the thyroid gland and the presence of poorly differentiated areas. The relevance of different tumour types on the prognosis is not entirely clear. To date, a loco-regional spread of disease has a greater prognostic importance than the histological type of papillary carcinoma [170].

[See BOX 3.6a. Summary of ultrasound features: Papillary carcinoma on www.wiley.com/go/kocjan/clinical_cytopathology_head_neck2e]

When PTC is definitively diagnosed on FNAC, the positive predictive value of the diagnosis is 97–99% (Table 3.6), the surgeon can perform definitive thyroidectomy without frozen section. If the FNAC is *suspicious for papillary carcinoma* of the thyroid (TBSRTC V, UKRCPath Thy4; see Table 3.5), the risk of malignancy is 60–75%. Patients with these conditions should be discussed at the MDM (Fig. 3.1) and undergo a partial thyroidectomy to establish the nature of the lesion. The US is very useful in planning the extent of surgery in patients with a FNAC reading of 'suspicious for PTC'.

The probability of malignancy is much lower in thyroid nodules with benign US findings even if the FNAC is read as 'suspicious for PTC'. However, as thyroid malignancy occurs in approximately 26% of patients with cytology readings 'suspicious for PTC' and benign-appearing US, the US reading alone is not sufficient to determine the need for surgery. The US and FNAC are complementary to each other and should be useful when providing informed consent before thyroid surgery [171].

This multidisciplinary approach to papillary carcinoma of the thyroid will maintain excellent diagnostic specificity [82, 172, 173]. *Cytological features* of classical PTC are characteristic enough to enable accurate tumour typing [174] (Fig. 3.31). FNAC smears are cellular, often displaying papillary architecture in either flat or three-dimensional aggregates. Follicular cells with dense cytoplasm, well-defined cell margins and presence of papillary clusters are the most consistent features observed. Intranuclear cytoplasmic inclusions, though characteristic, are found in 66.6% of cases [175]. Psammoma bodies may be seen but are not pathognomonic for papillary carcinoma (see Section 3.3.2: HTA) [108]. Isolated psammoma bodies are an unreliable predictor of PTC in the absence of cytological features [110, 176]. Nuclear grooves are also a useful criterion in the diagnosis (Fig. 3.31C). Eighty-eight percent of PTC have nuclear grooves in *greater than or equal to 20% tumour cells*, whereas none of the other thyroid diseases exceed this level [177–179]. Nuclear grooves are better seen in H&E and PAP stained smears. However, in MGG-stained smears the number of cells with nuclear grooves is also significantly higher as compared to other thyroid disorders (MNG, follicular adenoma, Hürthle cell adenoma, pure thyroiditis, thyroiditis with nodular hyperplasia [180]). Therefore, nuclear grooving, when seen in abundance, can be considered a reliable criterion for the diagnosis of PTC. The presence of occasional grooves, however, should be regarded as a non-specific finding [181. Grooved nuclei are somewhat difficult to recognise in the aspiration smears, particularly in air dried smears, although lobulated nuclei are identified easily. The latter are also a significant feature in the diagnosis of PTC. Ultrastructurally, grooved nuclei show a deep linear indentation of the nuclear membranes. Lobulated nuclei are characterised by multiple indentations that divided the nucleus into several lobules [182]. Well defined cytoplasmic borders with scalloping of the cytoplasm is often seen (Fig. 3.31D). Cystic change may be present (Fig. 3.31E) [183]. Multinucleate giant cells are frequently present in a classic papillary carcinoma and FVPC. They are usually absent from follicular adenomas (Fig. 3.31F) [184].

3.4.1.1 Follicular variant

Follicular variant of papillary thyroid carcinoma (FVPC) presents significant diagnostic difficulty in FNAC [185]. Diagnoses by FNAC vary considerably and usually are categorised as 'follicular lesions' [186] (Fig. 3.32) or 'suspicious' of papillary carcinoma (TBSRTC V) (UK Thy 4) (Table 3.5). The smears reveal thick colloid balls in the background, multilayered microfollicles (rosettes), absence of calcification and papillary clusters [187]. Nuclei are twice the size of red blood cells, have smooth contours, are hyperchromatic, and vary in shape but not much in size. Nuclear overlapping is common. Some nuclei have one small and almost pointed end, thereby resembling arrowheads. Although present, intranuclear inclusions, multinucleated histiocytes, and psammoma bodies are uncommon [188, 189]. Marginal vacuoles may be seen in 50% of FVPC [190]. Cases of other 'follicular lesions', notably a follicular adenoma, follicular carcinoma and a hyperplastic goitre, share many of these features, but lack inclusions and abundant nuclear

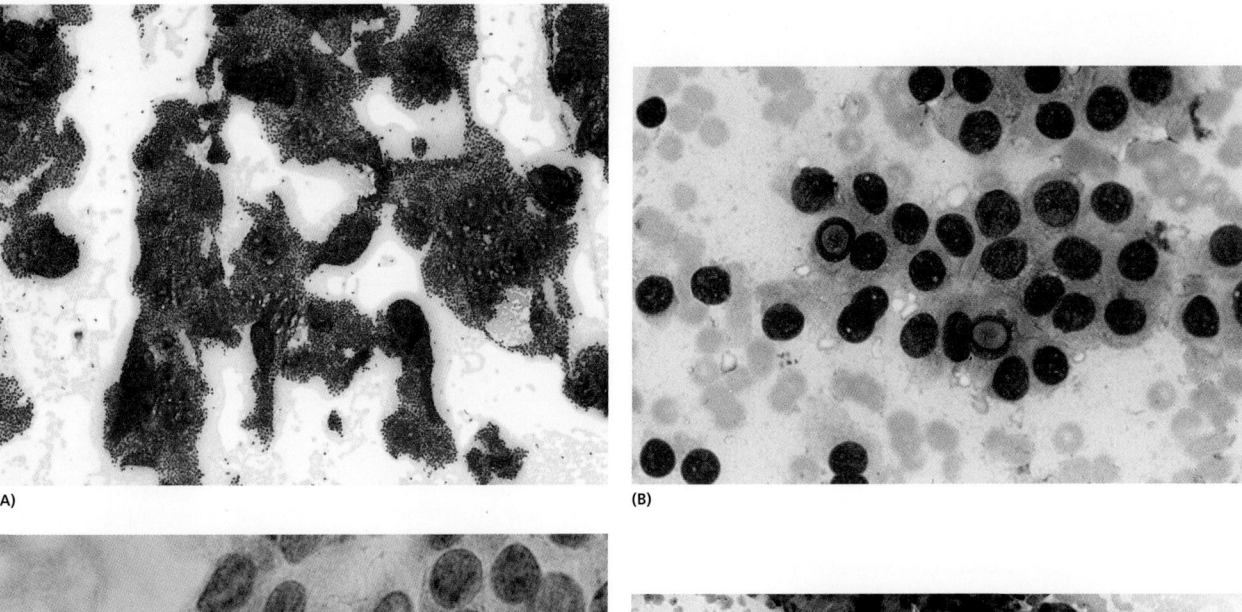

(A)

(B)

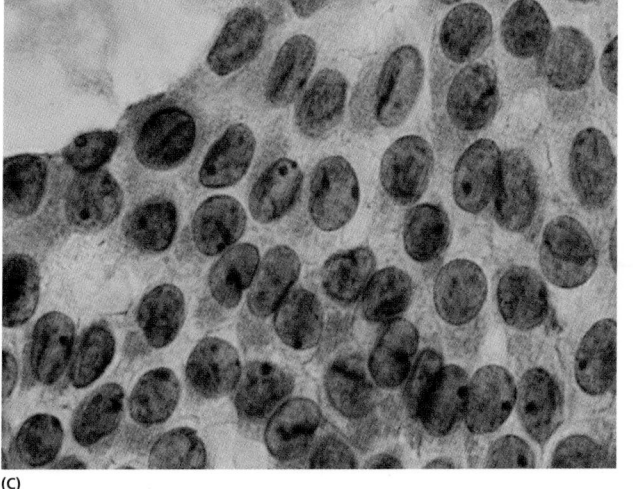

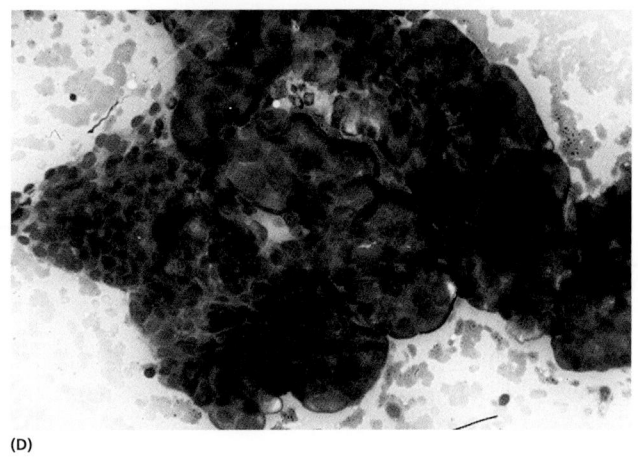

(C)

(D)

Figure 3.31 Papillary carcinoma. (A) FNAC smears are cellular. Follicular cells with dense cytoplasm, well defined cell margins, and presence of papillary clusters are the most consistent features observed. (B) Intranuclear cytoplasmic inclusions, though characteristic, are found in 66.6% of cases. (C) Nuclear grooves are also a useful criterion in the diagnosis of papillary thyroid carcinoma. Eighty-eight percent of papillary carcinomas have nuclear grooves in > or = 20% tumour cells. They are better appreciated on PAP stained smears and H&E. (D) Well-defined cytoplasmic borders with scalloping of the cytoplasm is often seen.

grooves [191]. A careful microscopic search for nuclear grooves should be attempted in aspirates yielding a diagnosis of *'follicular lesion'* (TBSRTC IV, UKRCPAth Thy3f) that could otherwise be indistinguishable from FVPC [192]. FVPC usually presents with a higher number of follicular and tubular formations, marginal vacuoles and a lower number of cases with nuclear grooves [193]. Given the variable presence of characteristic nuclear features, in order to avoid a false negative report, suspicion of a FVPC should be conveyed in the cytopathology report, which may prompt a MDM discussion and a surgical intervention such as hemithyroidectomy [194] (see Fig. 3.1 and Table 3.7).

Ohta et al. found that HBME-1 is a sensitive marker of papillary carcinoma, including both usual type and FVPC, in cytological specimens. In recent studies, molecular techniques including MicroRNA (miRNA) are being used to determine whether miRNA expression profiles may help distinguish between non invasive follicular proliferations versus follicular adenomas and infiltrative FVPC. If helpful, these tests could be applied to presurgical FNAC,

especially for lesions classified as indeterminate thyroid nodules [91, 192a]. For molecular testing please see section 3.1.7.

Macrofollicular variant of PTC is defined as a combination of numerous macrofollicles occupying 50% of the tumour and foci of the conventional follicular variant of papillary carcinoma [195, 196].

3.4.1.2 Tall cell variant

Tall cell variant of PTC (TCV-PTC) represents 8.5% of all papillary carcinomas. 'Tall cells' are defined as cells with abundant eosinophilic, elongated cytoplasm; the height of these cells is twice their width or more, and they have to constitute >30% of the tumour cell population (Fig. 3.33). They show round or oval tall columnar cells with basal nuclei with finely granular or stippled chromatin pattern (ground glass), pseudonuclear inclusions, small or inconspicuous nucleoli, nuclear grooves and abundant oxyphilic cytoplasm, which can be vacuolated and have indistinct borders. Mitoses are seen. The identification of both, tall cells and mitotic figures in the same smears is highly indicative of TCV-PTC [197–204].

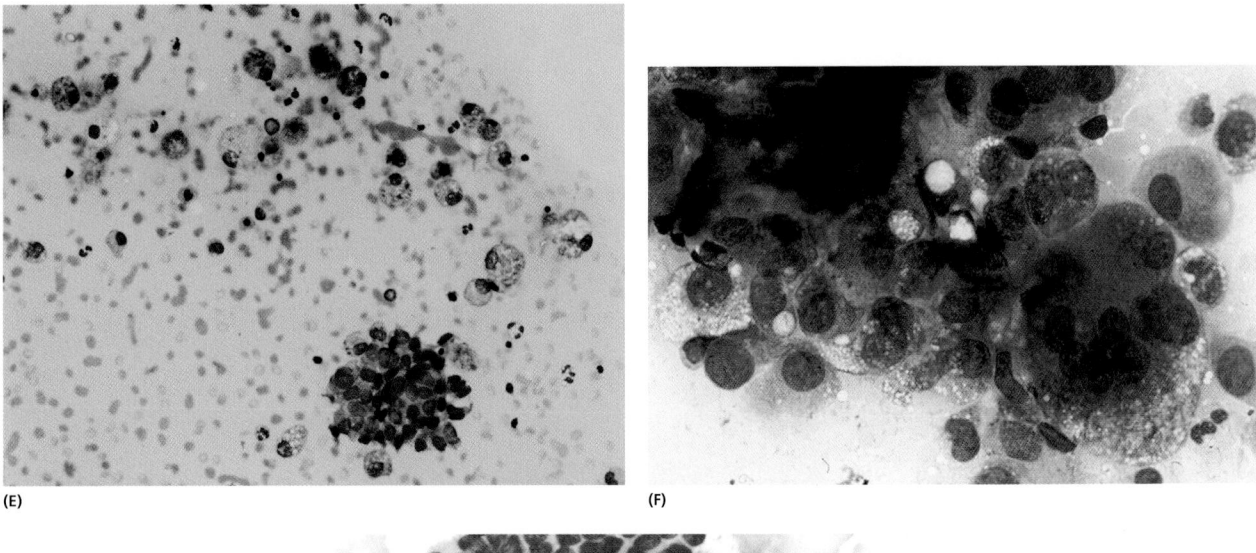

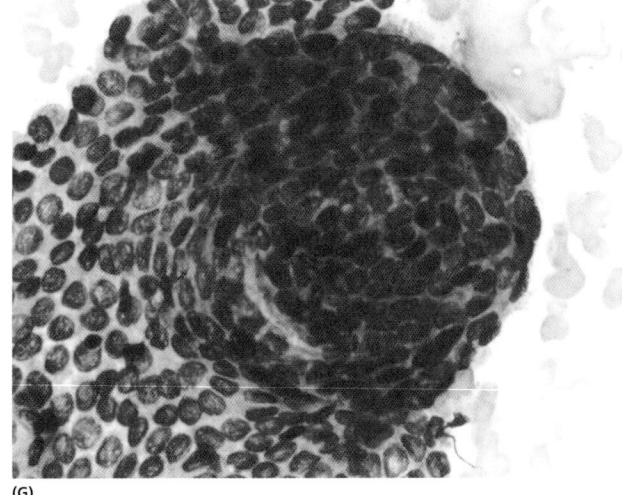

Figure 3.31 (*Continued*) (E) Cystic change may be present. (F) Multinucleate giant cells are frequently present in papillary carcinoma and follicular variant of papillary carcinoma. (G) Cell whorls with well defined edges and psammoma bodies may be seen.

3.4.1.3 Columnar cell variant

The columnar (CCV-PC) and tall cell variants (TCV-PC) of PTC are uncommon and have generally been regarded as more aggressive forms in comparison to the more common classic papillary and follicular subtypes, although this is controversial. FNAC sampling is composed of monolayered sheets, papillary clusters and microfollicles of tall, columnar cells with oval nuclei and uniform, finely granular chromatin (Fig. 3.33). These cells are arranged in a pseudostratified manner around well-defined fibrovascular cores. There are no intranuclear inclusions or well-defined nuclear grooves in the cells of the aspirate. There is also absence of colloid despite the presence of well-formed follicles. Some cells may have supranucleur and subnuclear cytoplasmic vacuoles. Some tumours may resemble endometrial or colonic adenocarcinomas [205, 206]. Nuclear pseudostratification, resembling that seen in respiratory epithelial cells, is present in some of the cell clusters [203]. Occasional cells may show squamous or oncocytic cell metaplasia.

TCV-PC can be distinguished from CCV-PC by the oxyphilia of the tumour cells and the absence of nuclear pseudostratification. The differential diagnosis of CCV includes medullary carcinoma of thyroid and metastatic adenocarcinoma (colorectal and endometrial adenocarcinomas) [203]. As with many PTCs, columnar cell variant tumours that are completely encapsulated are less likely to metastasize.

3.4.1.4 Oncocytic variant

Oncocytic variant of papillary carcinoma (OVPTC) oncocytic (Hürthle) cells of the thyroid can be identified within a wide spectrum of entities encompassing multinodular goitre, inflammatory and autoimmune conditions, benign tumours and malignant tumours, such as the, tall cell variant of PTC, Warthin-like variant of PTC and Hürthle cell carcinoma [207]. OVPTC requires the presence of large crowded cells with ground-glass ('Orphan Annie' eye) nuclei, nuclear grooves and nuclear pseudoinclusions in addition to abundant eosinophilic granular cytoplasm within >50% of the neoplastic cells. Smears show scattered papillary groups and monolayered sheets (Fig. 3.34) [208]. Psammoma bodies and colloid are not identified. Histologically, the tumours consist predominantly of oxyphilic cells arranged in papillary pattern and with nuclear features of the classical papillary carcinoma. OVPTC can be diagnosed in FNAC smears composed predominantly of large oxyphilic cells but showing features associated with classical

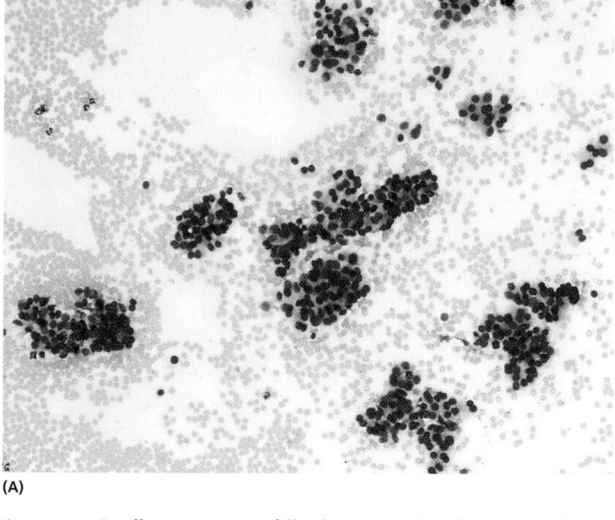

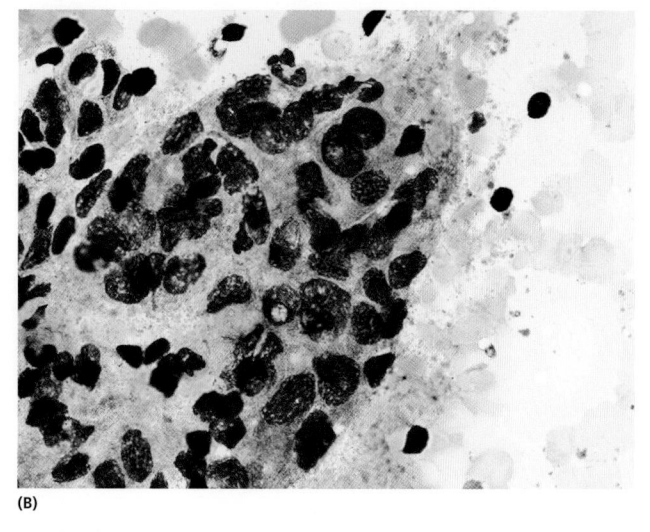

(A)   (B)

Figure 3.32 Papillary carcinoma, follicular variant. (A) The smears of FVPTC reveal multilayered microfollicles (rosettes). (B) Numerous nuclear grooves and inclusions in the follicular cells, very rare giant cells with absence of calcification and papillary clusters.

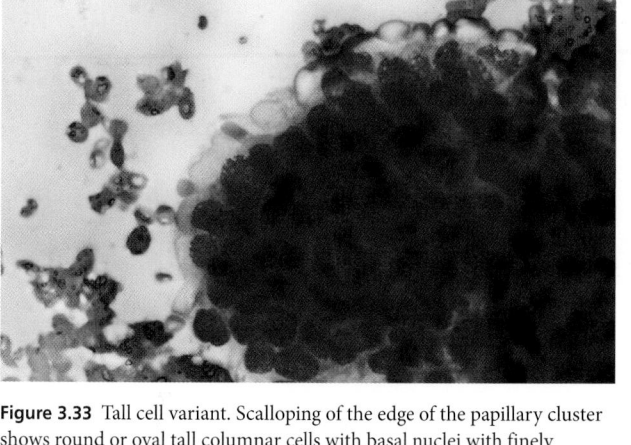

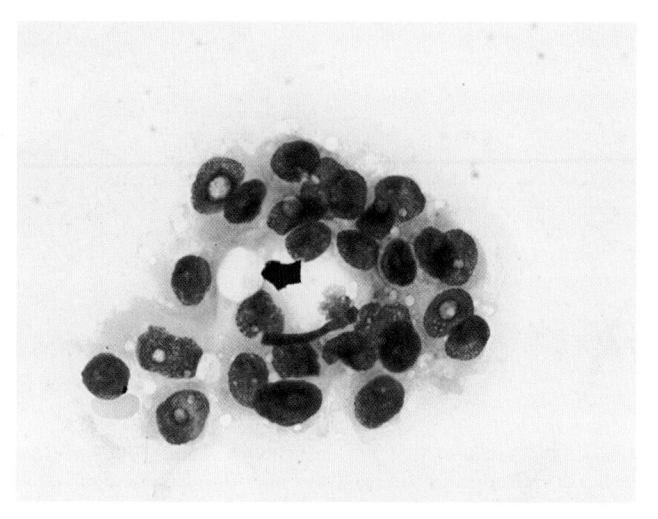

Figure 3.33 Tall cell variant. Scalloping of the edge of the papillary cluster shows round or oval tall columnar cells with basal nuclei with finely granular or stippled chromatin pattern (ground glass), pseudonuclear inclusions, small or inconspicuous nucleoli, nuclear grooves and abundant oxyphilic cytoplasm which can be vacuolated and have indistinct borders.

Figure 3.34 Papillary carcinoma, oxyphilic variant. The large, neoplastic cells have abundant, granular cytoplasm and eccentrically placed nuclei. Intra and extracellular eosinophilic granular material is present. Nuclear grooves and intranuclear inclusions are variably present. Nucleoli are not prominent.

papillary carcinoma and can be cytologically distinguished from follicular oxyphilic (Hürthle cell) tumours and the classical papillary carcinoma [208]. When differentiating OVPTC from Hashimoto's thyroiditis, it has been suggested that sheets of oncocytic cells with a single small nucleolus is indicative of Hashimoto's thyroiditis, while papillary arrangements of oncocytic cells without nucleoli suggest the presence of PTC [125].

3.4.1.5 Papillary Hürthle cell carcinoma with lymphoplasmacytic stroma

Papillary Hürthle cell carcinoma with lymphoplasmacytic stroma (Warthin-like variant) is a newly recognised variant of PTC. FNAC findings yield cellular smears, mostly in large and small papillary clusters of Hürthle cells, with nuclear grooves and rare nuclear inclusions in a lymphoplasmacytic background. Isolated oncocytic cells and multinucleated giant cells are also seen. The presence of

papillary clusters with nuclear features of papillary carcinoma and oxyphilic cytoplasm in a lymphoplasmacytic background should raise the diagnosis of Warthin-like tumour of the thyroid [209, 210]. This variant is often associated with Hashimoto's thyroiditis and has a similar prognosis compared to conventional PTC [211].

3.4.1.6 Cribriform-morular variant

A diagnosis of cribriform-morular variant of papillary carcinoma of the thyroid could be established on FNAC, prompting exclusion of familial adenomatous polyposis and distinguishing it from other, more aggressive variants of thyroid carcinoma, such as columnar cell carcinoma [212]. Histology shows a circumscribed neoplasm composed of tubular, papillary, cribriform and solid areas. The pseudostratified columnar tumour cells show occasional nuclear grooves and rare nuclear inclusions (Fig. 3.35). Immunohistochemistry

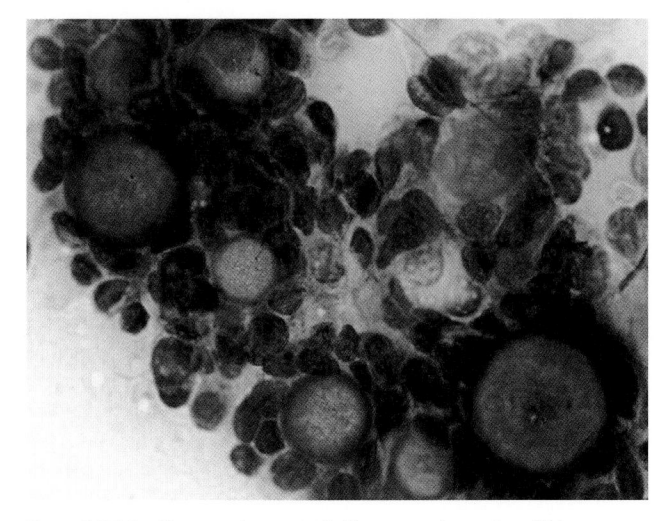

Figure 3.35 Papillary carcinoma, cribriform morular variant. This rare tumour appears similar to adenoid cystic carcinoma: follicle-like structures with hyaline globules in the centre nuclear grooves and intranuclear cytoplasmic inclusions.

shows positive staining with antibodies to cytokeratin AE1/AE3, oestrogen and progesterone receptor proteins. Focal immunoreactivity is also noted with antibodies to thyroglobulin (in the epithelium, hyaline globules are negative) epithelial membrane antigen, 34betaE12 and cytokeratin CK7 [213]. On FNAC, smears show high cellularity, papillary arrangement with fibrovascular cores as well as morula-like groupings with magenta hyaline globules [214].

3.4.1.7 Diffuse sclerosing variant

This is a rare tumour with aggressive behaviour that requires aggressive treatment. It affects young people [215]. Despite characteristic clinical and histological features that easily permit diagnosis, pre-operative FNAC diagnosis is often challenging and thus delays diagnosis. It is characterised by diffuse involvement of one or both thyroid lobes showing histologically prominent sclerosis, an intense lymphocytic infiltrate, numerous psammoma bodies and squamous metaplasia together with the characteristic cytoarchitectural pattern of classical papillary carcinoma. A diagnosis of DSPC on FNAC should be considered when a combination of clinico-cytological features consisting of numerous psammoma bodies, lymphocytes, squamous metaplasia and absence of stringy colloid are noted with otherwise typical cytoarchitectural features of papillary carcinoma obtained from diffusely nodular, firm thyroid enlargement [216, 217]. Ultrasonograpy may show a heterogeneous enlargement of both thyroid lobes suspicious for a lymphoproliferative syndrome. Flow cytometry may show a suspect B-lymphocyte population. FNAC may show an overwhelming presence of slightly atypical monomorphic small lymphocytes. Ultrasound features may also be difficult to interpret

[See BOX 3.6b. Summary of ultrasound features: Papillary carcinoma on www.wiley.com/go/kocjan/clinical_cytopathology_head_neck2e]

3.4.1.8 Papillary carcinoma with a nodular fasciitis like stroma

The presence of a prominent nodular fasciitis-like stromal component may result in low-power microscopic appearances resembling

fibroadenoma, phyllodes tumour, or fibrocystic disease of the breast. The carcinomatous component grows in the form of anastomosing narrow tubules, clustered glands, solid sheets with or without squamous differentiation and/or papillae, and exhibits the typical nuclear features of papillary thyroid carcinoma. The abundant stroma may have a nodular fasciitis-like quality and be composed of short fascicles of spindle cells separated by varying amounts of mucoid matrix, collagen and extravasated red blood cells; this is interpreted as an exuberant mesenchymal reaction to the carcinoma. The importance of recognising this variant of PTC is that, when one encounters a fibroproliferative lesion of the thyroid, a diligent search should be made for PTC. This variant also must be distinguished from the vastly more aggressive PTC with anaplastic transformation and the so-called carcinosarcomas [218–221]. Epithelium of PTC may occasionally assume a spindle shape [222].

When correlating cytological features and the different histological variants of PTC, Leung et al. noted that single cells, monolayers and papillary fragments were present in all the variants. The presence of follicles was not restricted to FVPC. Nuclear grooves and cytoplasmic pseudoinclusions were present in most of the cases; with nuclear grooves the most common finding in all the variants (92.3–100%). Psammoma bodies were an infrequent finding (0–25%) and were absent from the FVPC. Colloid was present in all the variants and was a frequent finding in the FVPC (84.6%). The findings suggest that the exact histological variant of PTC cannot be predicted from the appearance of the FNAC [223].

3.4.1.9 Immunohistochemical markers

Immunohistochemical markers such as TTF-1 and thyroglobulin are very helpful in confirming the thyroid origin of PTC, especially when the tumour is present outside of the thyroid gland. TTF-1 is also expressed in lung carcinomas and small cell carcinomas in many sites, so it is most useful when combined with thyroglobulin. Because of difficulties in distinguishing some FVPC from adenomas and adenomatoid nodules, markers such as HBME-1 and CITED-1 have been used with increasing frequency [224]. Lloyd et al. consider HBME-1 and CITED 1 as very useful in such settings, but as with most markers, they have to be used with the appropriate histological and cytological findings. Other markers such as cytokeratin 19, Galectin 3, CD56, PAX 8 and thyroid peroxidase have not been as useful in these differential diagnosis because of lower sensitivity and specificity [225, 226].

3.4.1.10 Molecular markers

Molecular markers in papillary thyroid carcinoma, such as the BRAF mutation (V600E) has proven to be relatively restricted to PTC and anaplastic thyroid carcinomas, and is very useful in the differential diagnosis of difficult thyroid tumours. Unfortunately, the FVPC, often difficult to diagnose of FNAC, has a BRAF mutation in only 5–20% of the time while conventional PTC shows a BRAF mutation more often (35–70%) (39–42) Recently, uncommon BRAF mutations were not detected in a clasical variant but only in FVPC [226a]. Apart from diagnostic use, BRAF mutations have been reported to be predictive of tumour behaviour and response to radioactive iodine (79, 80), but more studies are needed in this area.

RET/PTC rearrangement is found mainly in PTC with a highly variable frequency (5–80%) in different geographic regions and in different studies [227] FVPC has a higher frequency of RAS mutations than other PTC. However, RAS mutations are also present in follicular carcinomas and adenomas [227].

HMGA2 and insulin-like growth factor II mRNA binding protein 3 (IMP3) are highly expressed during foetal development and then tissue levels are very low to absent in adult tissues. Recent studies have shown that in many malignant neoplasms HMGA2 and IMP3 have increased levels of expression [228, 229]. These studies have shown that normal thyroid tissues and follicular adenomas express low levels of HMGA2 and IMP3 mRNA compared to PTC and follicular carcinomas. The measurements of the levels of expression by quantitative RT–PCR helps to separate benign from low grade malignant thyroid neoplasms in most cases [228, 229] These observations have been examined in thyroid tissues and molecular assays including MicroRNA are being developed to distinguish follicular adenomas from PTC and follicular carcinomas in cytological specimens as well as in tissues using formalin fixed paraffin embedded tissues [230, 291a] (See also 3.1.7).

3.4.1.11 Differential diagnosis
Differential diagnosis of PTC includes the following: Papillary proliferation in MNG and Hashimoto's thyroiditis where other features of papillary carcinoma are absent, adenomatoid nodules with focal papillary hyperplasia where the presence of focal papillary aggregates, the presence of a psammoma bodies within a background of copious colloid and scattered follicular cells, all may lead to diagnostic confusion [112]. PTC may be cystic causing diagnostic problems, mainly due to poor cellularity and the bland appearance of the cells in a fluid (Fig. 3.36) (see Section 3.2.2). In the FVPC nuclear vacuoles may suggest the appropriate diagnosis. If the appearance is predominantly of single tumour cells, the appearances can mimic a medullary carcinoma. A thymoma with a dominant epithelial component has to be considered in the differential diagnosis [231].

Mahajan et al.'s analysis of the reasons for overcall of suspicious cases includes findings of pseudopapillae, syncytial sheets, nuclear grooves and pinpoint nucleoli in chronic lymphocytic thyroiditis and Hürthle cell neoplasms, and intranuclear inclusions in parathyroid adenoma, hyalinising trabecular adenoma and mesenchymal repair [232].

The primary reasons for undercall of PTC as suspicious includes: cystic aspirates with minor features of PTC such as histiocytoid cells, bubble gum colloid, syncytial sheets and cellular swirls. Cases

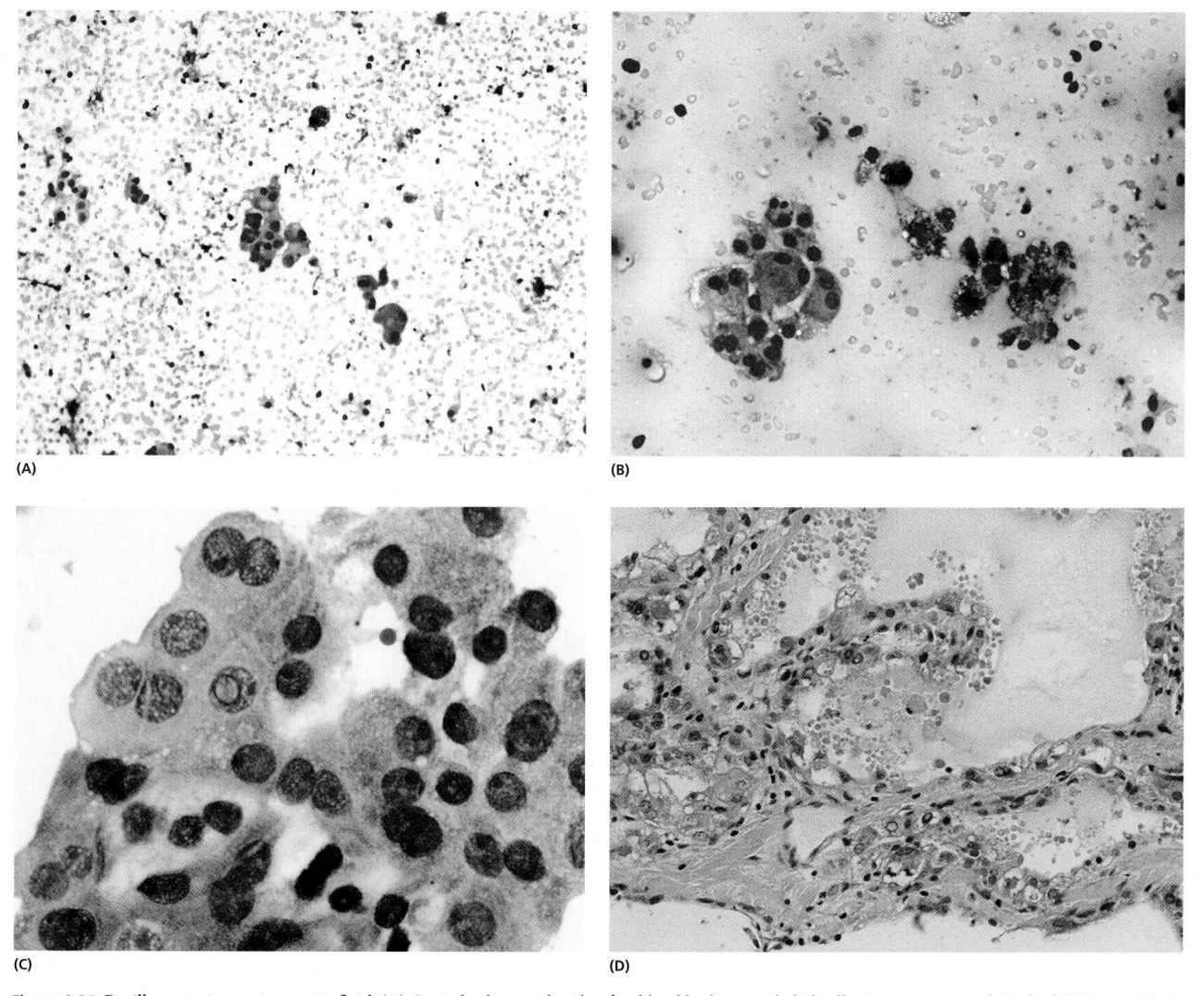

(A)　　　　(B)
(C)　　　　(D)

Figure 3.36 Papillary carcinoma in a cystic fluid. (A) Cystic background with a few bland looking epithelial cells, in aggregates and single. (B) Haemosiderin laden macrophages, epithelium mimicking macrophages and thin colloid in the background. (C) A single intranuclear inclusion was spotted on the review of the case which was initially reported as a benign cystic goitre. (D) Thyroid resection specimen shows features of papillary carcinoma.

with cytoplasm similar to Hürthle cells were also noted to cause difficulty in accurate classification. These examples reiterate that no single cytological feature should be used independently in the cytological diagnosis of thyroid lesions. Tumour cellularity and papillary tissue fragments should not be equated with neoplasia per se; all cytomorphological features should be evaluated [233].

> No single cytological feature should be used independently in the cytological diagnosis of thyroid lesions.

3.4.2 Follicular carcinoma

Follicular carcinoma is an infrequent thyroid gland tumour and represents 15% of all thyroid gland carcinomas. It presents as a solitary swelling in the gland, is never seen as an occult tumour and the mean age of presentation is 50 years.

Histologically, it is a minimally invasive carcinoma, which is macroscopically encapsulated and microscopically has a follicular, trabecular, cribriform and/or solid growth pattern. The cytological features of PTC are not seen. The morphological appearance may vary between monomorphic and pleomorphic. Currently, it is not possible to differentiate morphologically from benign follicular proliferations such as follicular adenoma and adenomatous hyperplastic nodule. Criteria for diagnosis of malignancy are histological: capsular and/or vascular invasion. Nuclear atypia, mitoses and necrosis are not features of malignancy in follicular tumours and can be present in follicular adenomas as well as in carcinomas (Fig. 3.38).

The prognosis of follicular carcinoma with minimal invasion is good (10-year survival 85%). In contrast to PTC, follicular carcinoma metastasises haematogenously with a preference for lung and bone. Metastases are often better differentiated than the primary tumour; may be detected and treated by radioactive iodine.

Oncocytic or *Hürthle cell variant* of follicular carcinoma has a less favourable prognosis. It has more aggressive behaviour and compromised survival compared with other differentiated thyroid cancers [234]. The diagnosis of malignancy in Hürthle cell tumours has the same general diagnostic criteria as for ordinary follicular carcinoma (capsular and/or vascular invasion). *Clear cell variant* is designated by some as a separate entity and by others as a variant of Hürthle cell type.

Cytological features of a well differentiated follicular carcinoma are the same as a microfollicular adenoma: cellular, follicular groups, follicles that are irregular in form with nuclear overlap, occasionally single cells and little or no colloid (Figs 3.37 and 3.38). If colloid is present, it is present in particles. In these cases, the diagnosis of *'follicular lesion'* (TBSRTC IV, UKRCPath Thy3f, see Table 3.5) is appropriate. In follicular carcinoma, haemorrhage, necrosis and calcifications may be seen. If the cells have the appearance of clear cells than it is more likely that the tumour is a carcinoma than and adenoma. Clear cell carcinoma is fat negative in contrast with metastases of renal cell carcinoma with which it may be confused. Oncocytic (Hürthle cell) adenoma cannot be reliably differentiated from oncocytic carcinoma and oncocytic variant of PTC. The cells may show anisocytosis, anisonucleosis and large nucleoli whether they originate from Hashimoto's thyroiditis, oncocytic adenoma or carcinoma. Pure oncocytic proliferations are indication for surgery (Fig. 3.39).

Insular variant of follicular carcinoma (ITC), now recognised as a distinct thyroid neoplasm, accounts for 4–7% of thyroid malignancies, is twice as common in males with a mean age of 55.7 years. It presents as a rapidly growing, large mass, cold on radioiodine scintigraphy with associated nodal and distant metastasis in 30%. Many cases have radioiodine refractory metastases, resulting in death. Cytologically (Fig. 3.40), the lesions show many follicular epithelial cells arranged predominantly in rosettes with tissue fragments of empty microfollicles, clusters of cells with scant cytoplasm and crowded nuclei. There are sheets and clusters of atypical cells with enlarged, pleomorphic nuclei and very scanty colloid. Nuclear overlapping is constant. When present, the cytoplasm is poorly outlined [235–238].

3.4.3 Medullary carcinoma

Medullary carcinoma (MC) represents 4–5% of all thyroid carcinomas and arises from C-cells. The mean age at presentation is 50 years. In 10–20% of cases this type of carcinoma is familial when it can present at a younger age. The tumour is often multicentric

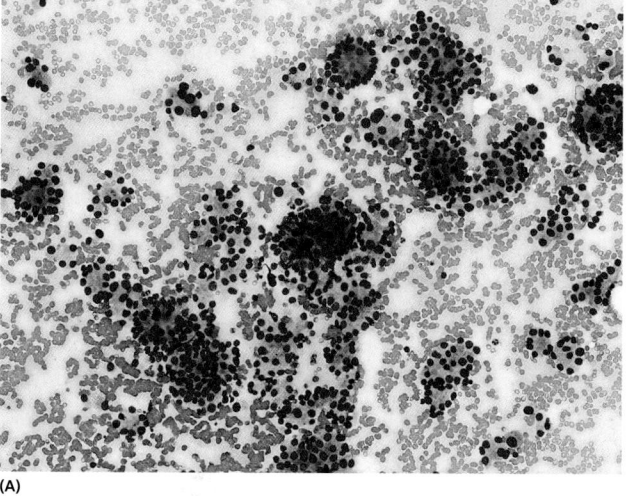

(A)

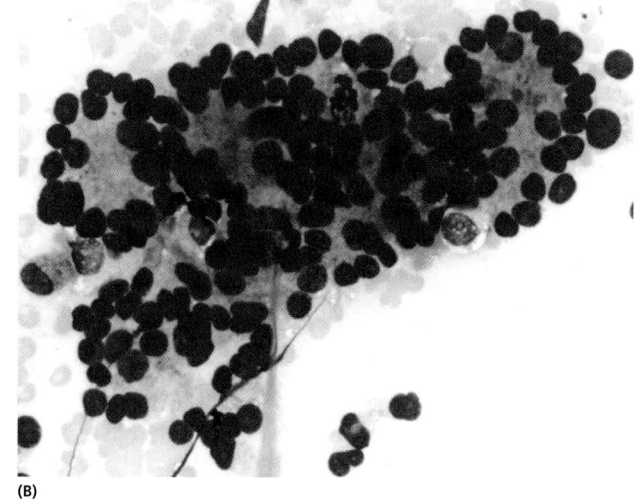

(B)

Figure 3.37 Follicular carcinoma. (A) Well differentiated follicular carcinoma has the same appearance as a microfollicular adenoma: cellular, confluent follicular groups with very little or no colloid in the background. (B) Follicles are irregular in form with nuclear overlap and occasional single cells.

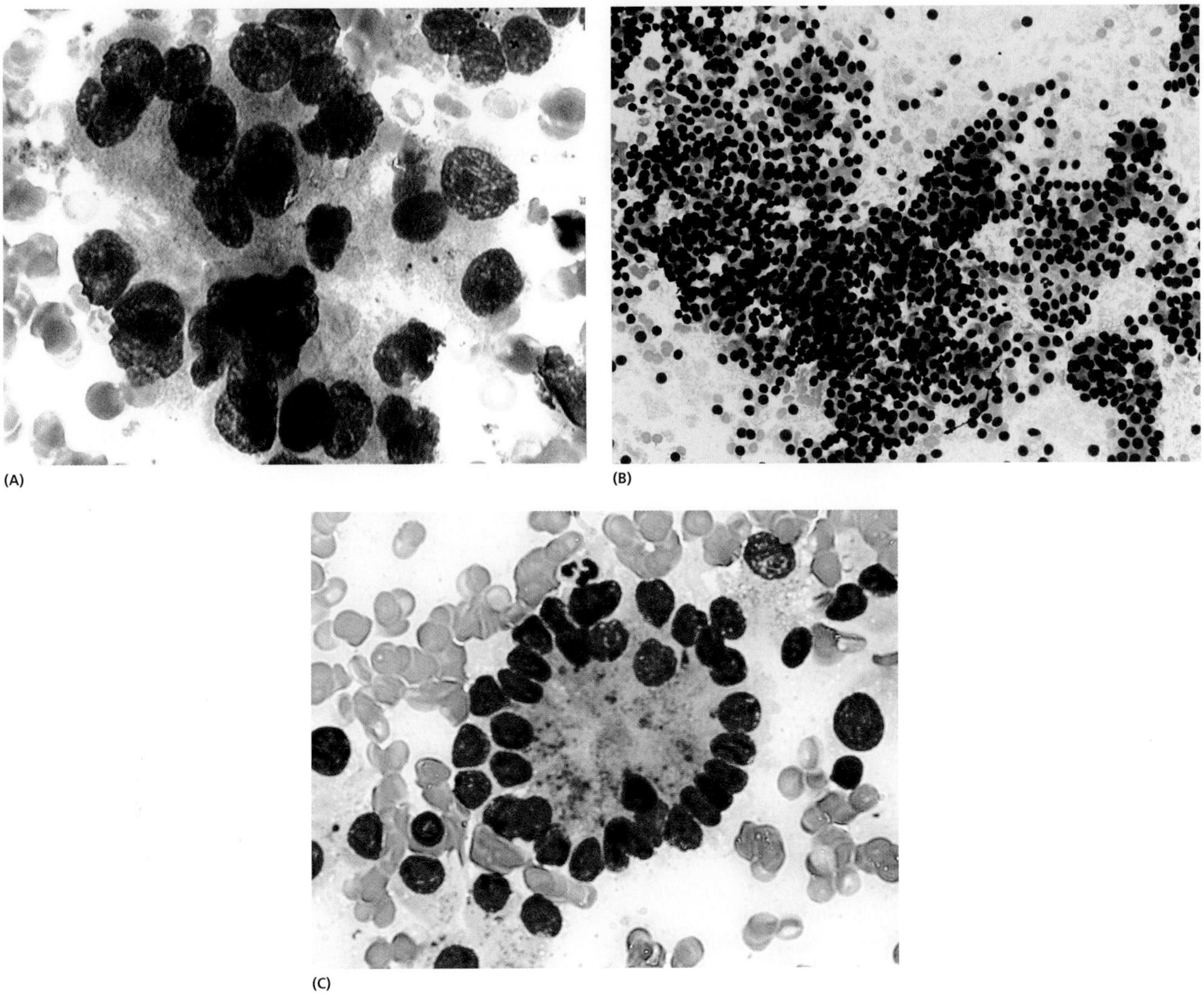

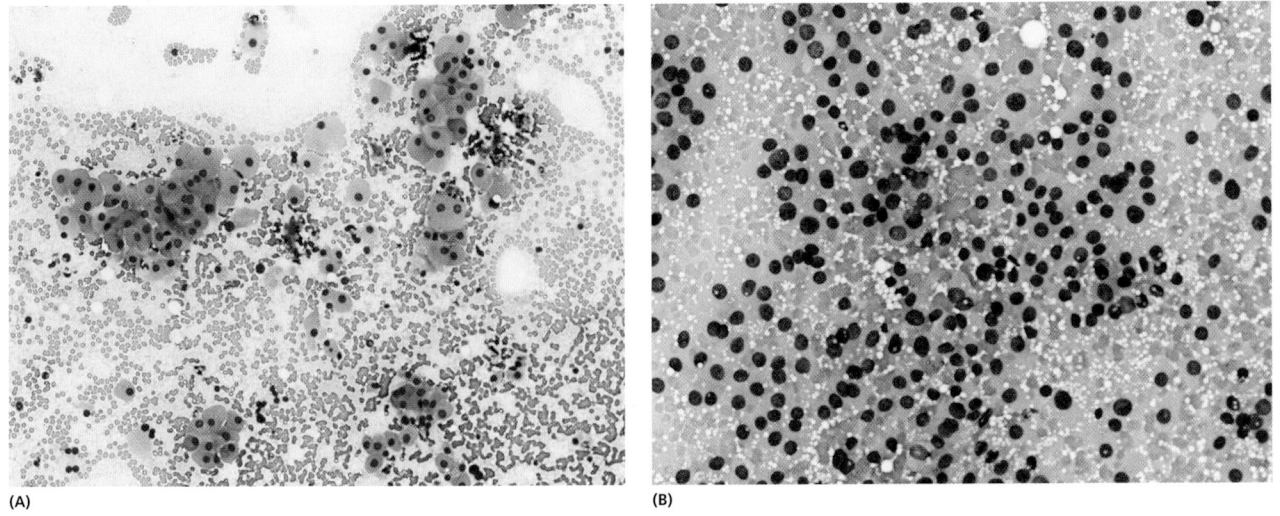

Figure 3.38 Follicular lesion. (A) Follicular adenoma may show anisonucleosis, crowding and overlapping. (B) Follicular hyperplasia may show architectural arrangement and cellularity reminiscent of follicular neoplasms. (C) Follicular carcinoma has microfollicules indistinguishable from follicular adenoma.

Figure 3.39 Oncocytic proliferations. (A) Oncocytic adenoma shows an aggregate of oncocytic cells in the background of blood. (B) Oncocytic carcinoma shows dispersed oncocytic cells.

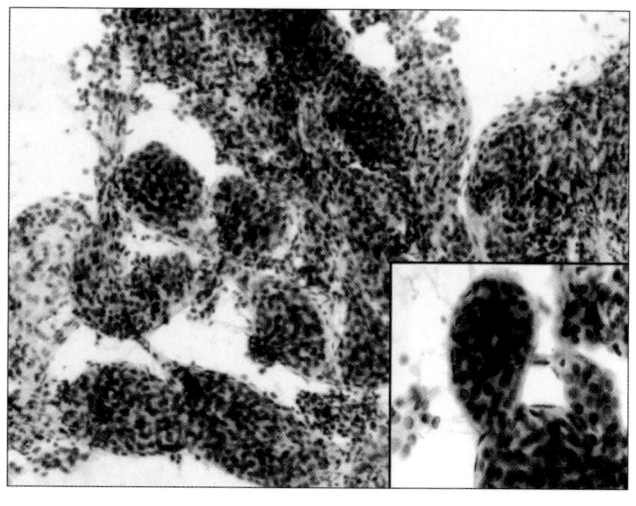

Figure 3.40 Insular carcinoma. Follicular epithelial cells ('tumor cellularity') arranged predominantly in rosettes with tissue fragments of empty microfollicles, clusters of cells with scant cytoplasm and crowded nuclei and sheets and clusters of atypical cells with enlarged, pleomorphic nuclei and with very scanty colloid.

and associated with tumours in other endocrine organs as part of the Multiple Endocrine Neoplasia (MEN) syndrome. Histologically, the commonest type of MC has a monomorphic, small epithelial (plasmacytoid/carcinoid-like) or spindle-cell type and a solid or trabecular growth pattern with hyaline stroma containing amyloid present between the epithelial islands. Variations in growth pattern (papillary, glandular), in cell type (giant cell, small cell) and histochemical variants (mucin producing, melanin containing without amyloid) contribute to the diagnostic difficulty. All these variants are classified as MC on the basis of positive staining for calcitonin. The 10-year survival of medullary carcinoma is 50%. Among patients without initial distant metastatic involvement and with complete resection of the tumour, 20-year survival free of distant metastatic lesions is 81%. Overall 10- and 20-year survival rates are 63 and 44%, respectively [239].

A preoperative diagnosis of medullary carcinoma of the thyroid is essential. It allows for the investigation of associated MEN/pheochromocytoma, and a definitive surgery without the need for frozen section or hemithyroidectomy.

[See BOX 3.7. Summary of ultrasound features: Medullary carcinoma on www.wiley.com/go/kocjan/clinical_cytopathology_head_neck2e]

Criteria for cytodiagnosis are well known but variable patterns of presentation may cause diagnostic difficulty. Although correct diagnosis is made by FNAC in the majority of instances, other tumours may show cytological findings similar to MC. Electron microscopy of FNAC material was found to be useful. Immunocytochemistry may be misleading for rarely performed tests [240, 241].

MC can be easily recognised as malignant on FNAC. Preparations usually contain single cells but may have cell aggregates. The cells may be small and round, elongated or pleomorphic, depending on the type of MC (Fig. 3.41). Nuclei are oval and eccentric. There are prominent nucleoli. Triangular shaped cells are characteristic. The cytoplasm may have fine red granulation, which may also be seen in follicular carcinoma and metastases of breast carcinoma. Occasional

cells are binucleate or multinucleate with pleomorphic nuclei. Nuclear vacuoles may be seen. Intracellular and extracellular amyloid may be seen. In MGG stained preparations it is blue/violet and is Congo Red positive [242–246].

Immunocytochemically, tumour cells react with keratin, calcitonin and chromogranin. Thyroglobulin is usually negative. Grimelius staining is positive.

C-cell hyperplasia can mimic MC biochemically. The possible role of FNAC to distinguish between the two is in patients with elevated serum calcitonin and absence of a discrete thyroid nodule. The finding of clusters of calcitonin-positive cells intermixed with normal follicular cells by FNAC may provide a means of making a pre-surgical diagnosis of C-cell hyperplasia [247].

3.4.4 Anaplastic carcinoma

Anaplastic carcinoma (ATC) of the thyroid is one of the most aggressive tumour types in humans [248]. Histologically it is composed of pleomorphic large cells, often partly spindle celled (pseudosarcomatous) and/or giant cells (often with numerous osteoclast type giant cells). It presents in an older age group (usually over 60 years) as a rapidly progressive, indurated, asymmetrical swelling, which may arise in a longstanding goitre or be associated with a variety of more well-differentiated thyroid carcinomas [219, 249, 250]. It may cause dyspnoea due to tracheal compression. Nearly all patients die shortly after the diagnosis is made due to local tumour extension. Noninvasive ATC is a rare, surgically resectable variant with only four reported cases [251].

FNAC smears from ATC are usually cellular with abundant cell dissociation, easily recognised as malignant (Fig. 3.42). In the largest series of ATC, Us Krasovec et al. described three different cell patterns: (1) pleomorphic cell (2) round cell and (3) spindle cell pattern [252, 253]. ATC with rhabdoid features has been described [254]. Due to the simple technique and high diagnostic accuracy, FNAC is the method of choice in patients with ATC. There are often large nucleoli, abundant mitoses, necrosis and occasionally numerous neutrophils. Leukophagocytosis may be seen in tumour cells, osteoclast type giant cells and rarely squamous type differentiation. In difficult cases of ATC, differential diagnoses may be sarcoma or non-Hodgkin lymphoma. Immunocytochemistry is essential in these cases. Tumour cells are immunoreactive for keratins AE1/AE3, CAM5.2 and CK19; PAX-8 and p63, but negative for S-100, HMB-45, calcitonin, TTF-1, thyroglobulin, CD56, HBME-1, glypican-3, PAX-5, myogenin, CD31 and INI-1. However, ATC may be cytokeratin negative and vimentin positive.

Differential diagnosis of ATC also includes active fibroblasts and histiocytes in granulomatous inflammation, regressive changes in follicular epithelial cells, particularly after I-131 treatment, MC, metastases of a poorly differentiated carcinoma, for example squamous cell carcinoma and purulent thyroiditis.

The main reasons for inadequate or non-representative FNAC sampling are: (1) tumour regressive changes (necrosis, haemorrhage, leukocytic infiltration), (2) extensive tumour fibrosis and (3) distinct differentiated and anaplastic patterns in the same tumour [252].

3.4.5 Thyroid lymphoma

Thyroid lymphomas are rare and almost always arise in the background of chronic lymphocytic thyroiditis (Hashimoto's thyroiditis) (Fig. 3.43) [255–258]. They occur predominantly in elderly females. Most patients have a short history of an enlarging thyroid or a neck mass causing tracheal compression [259].

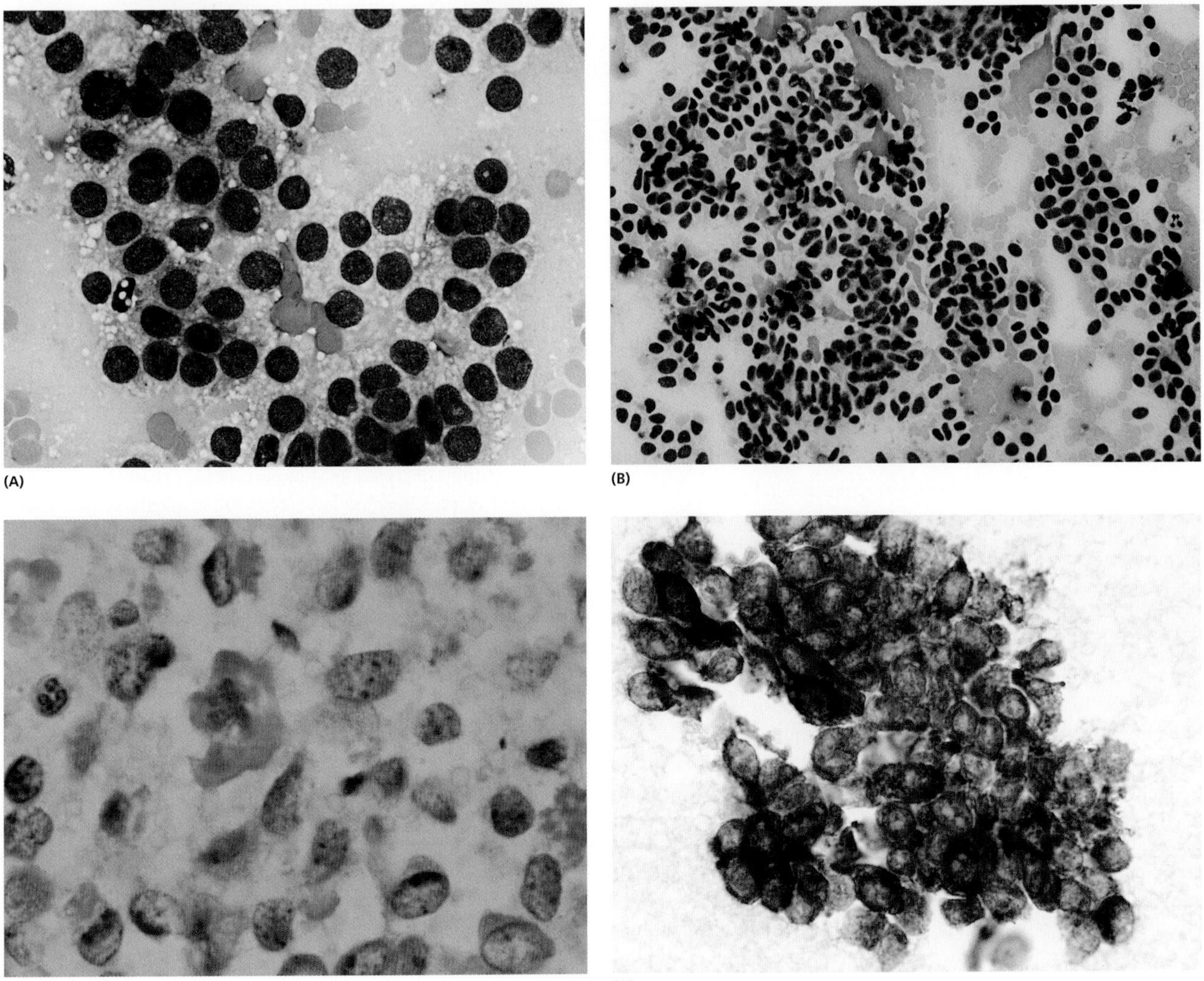

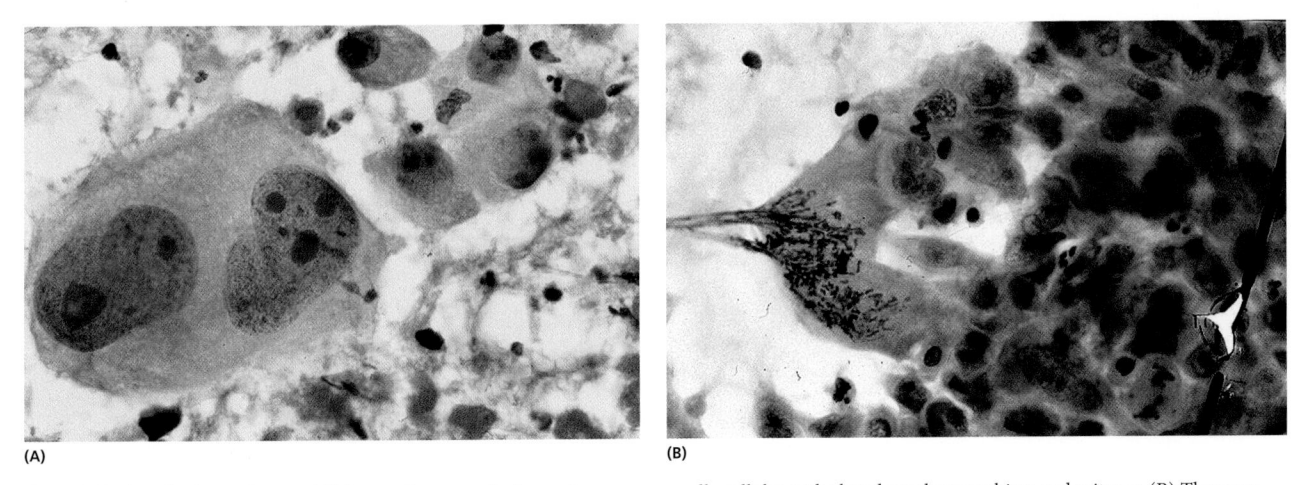

Figure 3.41 Medullary carcinoma. (A) Cellular aspirates usually contain single cells but may have cell aggregates (MGG ×400). (B) The cells may be small and round, elongated or pleomorphic, depending on the type of medullary carcinoma. (C) Congo Red staining of amyloid in medullary carcinoma). (D) Tumour cells are positive for calcitonin (anticalcitonin).

Figure 3.42 Anaplastic carcinoma. (A) Smears from anaplastic carcinoma are usually cellular with abundant pleomorphism and mitoses. (B) There are often large nucleoli, necrosis and occasionally numerous neutrophils.

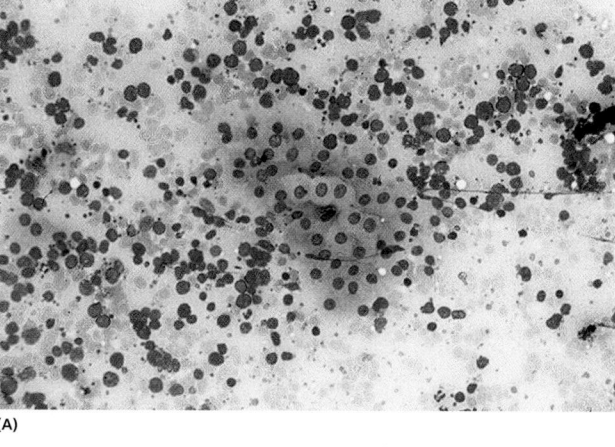

(A)

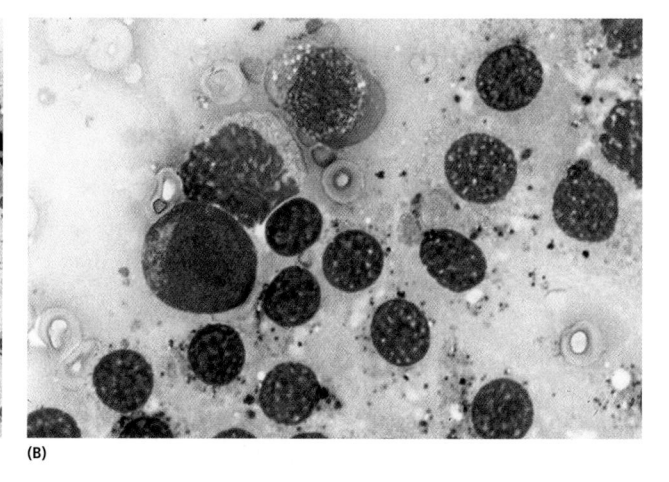

(B)

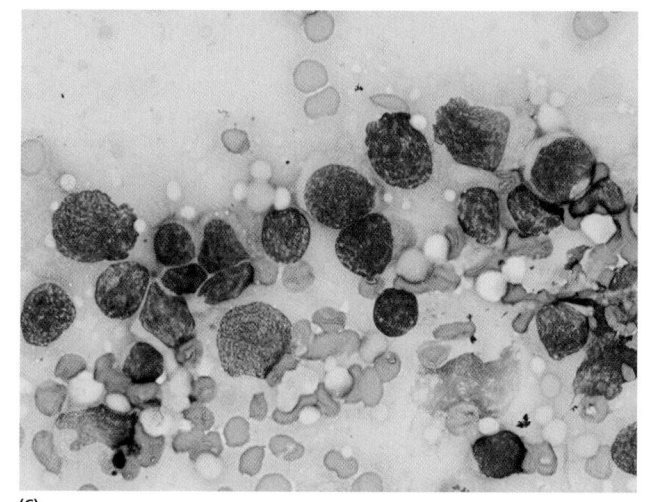

(C)

Figure 3.43 Thyroid lymphoma. (A) Thyroid cells in close proximity with immature lymphoid cells. (B) Lymphoid blasts and thyroid epithelium. (C) Differential diagnosis includes Hashimoto's thyroiditis and post transplant lymphopriliferative disorder.

[See BOX 3.8. Summary of ultrasound features: Thyroid lymphoma on www.wiley.com/go/kocjan/clinical_cytopathology_head_neck2e]

The conventional approach to treatment is a combination of radiation therapy with multi-agent chemotherapy, while there is no significant role for extirpative surgery in the management of thyroid lymphoma [260]. The prognosis of localised tumours (stage IE, Ann Arbor classification) is excellent. Extrathyroidal involvement (stage IIE-IVE) reduces the 5-year survival rate to about 70%, provided that current therapy regimens are respected [255]. Thyroid lymphoma usually represents a neoplasm of *mucosa-associated lymphoid tissue (MALT)* [261]. This can sometimes be associated with amyloid deposition [262].

Diffuse large cell lymphoma is an aggressive disease and usually is not a significant diagnostic challenge from the pathological point of view. 'Small cell' lymphomas, however, can sometimes be difficult to distinguish from chronic lymphocytic thyroiditis. In the past, most thyroid lymphomas were considered to be of follicle centre cell origin. Today, most of the lymphomas in the extranodal sites are thought to originate from the marginal zone of the lymphoid follicles. The distinction between the different types of lymphomas has significant impact on the patient's prognosis, treatment and follow-up [263–265]. It is imperative that clinicians

(endocrinologists and surgeons) and pathologists are aware of these types of lymphomas in order for the most appropriate diagnostic procedures to be selected, specific staging principles to be applied and appropriate disease-specific treatment to be implemented (see Chapter 4, Section 4.4) [266–270].

In addition to morphological evaluation performed on direct smears, core biopsy, immunophenotyping, flow cytometry and molecular studies may assist the diagnosis. These additional studies make a clear distinction between lymphoma and Hashimoto's thyroiditis, which may present a similar cytological picture [271–273] (see Chapter 4).

Diagnostic pitfalls include ATC of the small-cell type, lymphocytic thyroiditis and a posttransplant lymphoproliferative syndrome (PTLS) [274, 275].

3.4.6 Metastatic tumours

Metastases may simulate primary malignant tumours of the thyroid, causing problems in the diagnosis and management of patients with a history of carcinoma. In the 7-year period, 1.5% of thyroid FNAC contained metastatic tumour [276]. The primary sites of origin are most commonly breast, kidney, colon and stomach as well as lymphoma (Fig. 3.44). The cytological features in the FNAC

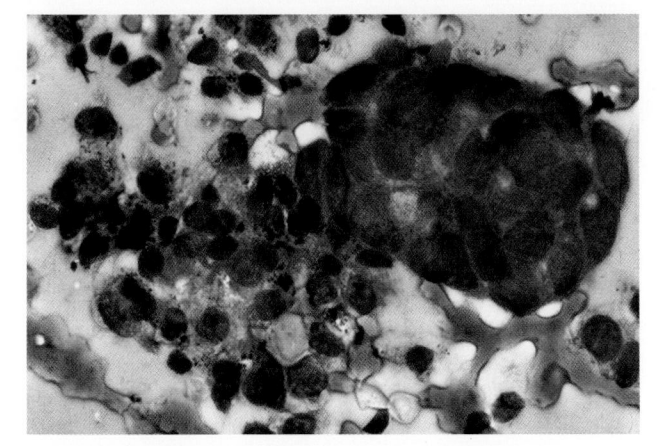

Figure 3.44 Metastatic carcinoma. A cluster of breast carcinoma cells is seen close to the benign thyroid epithelium. Clinical history and immunocytochemistry are helpful.

material are characteristic of the primary tumours. It is of critical importance that primary thyroid neoplasms occurring in patients known to have primary tumours elsewhere be distinguished from disseminated tumours involving the thyroid. FNAC is of considerable value in this differential diagnosis. Needle aspirates of the thyroid are also of value in leading to the diagnosis of unsuspected non-thyroidal primary cancer [277, 278].

[See BOX 3.9. Summary of ultrasound features: Thyroid metastases on www.wiley.com/go/kocjan/clinical_cytopathology_head_neck2e]

This chapter also has online only material. Ultrasound Summary boxes, which have been cited throughout the chapter text as 'Summary of ultrasound features', are available on www.wiley.com/go/kocjan/clinical_cytopathology_head_neck2e for the following diseases:

Box 3.1 Summary of ultrasound features: Colloid Nodule
Box 3.2 Summary of ultrasound features: Thyrotoxicosis Graves' disease
Box 3.3 Summary of ultrasound features: Hashimoto's thyroiditis (autoimmune or chronic lymphocytic)
Box 3.4 Summary of ultrasound features: Reidel's Thyroiditis
Box 3.5 Summary of ultrasound features: Follicular lesion
Box 3.6 Summary of ultrasound features: Papillary carcinoma **a and b**
Box 3.7 Summary of ultrasound features: Medullary carcinoma
Box 3.8 Summary of ultrasound features: Thyroid lymphoma
Box 3.9 Summary of ultrasound features: Thyroid metastases

References

1. Gharib H. Fine-needle aspiration biopsy of thyroid nodules: advantages, limitations, and effect. *Mayo Clin Proc* 1994; **69**(1): 44–9.
2. Ezzat S, Sarti DA, Cain DR, Braunstein GD. Thyroid incidentalomas. Prevalence by palpation and ultrasonography. *Arch Intern Med*. 1994 Aug 22; **154**(16): 1838–40.
3. Mortensen JD, Woolner LB, Bennett WA. Gross and microscopic findings in clinically normal thyroid glands. *J Clin Endocrinol Metab*. 1955 Oct; **15**(10): 1270–80.
4. Tan GH, Gharib H. Thyroid incidentalomas: management approaches to nonpalpable nodules discovered incidentally on thyroid imaging. *Ann Intern Med*. 1997 Feb 1; **126**(3): 226–31.
5. Davies L, Welch HG. Current thyroid cancer trends in the United States. *JAMA Otolaryngol Head Neck Surg*. 2014 Apr; **140**(4): 317–22.
6. Enewold LR, Zhou J, Devesa SS, et al. Thyroid cancer incidence among active duty U.S. military personnel, 1990–2004. *Cancer Epidemiol Biomarkers Prev*. 2011 Nov; **20**(11): 2369–76.
7. Altekruse SF, Kosary CL, Krapcho M, et al. SEER Cancer Statistics Review, 1975–2007. Bethesda, MD: National Cancer Institute [cited 2010 Nov 15]. Available from: http://seer.cancer.gov/csr/1975_2007/.
8. American Cancer Society. *Cancer facts and figures 2011*. Atlanta, GA: American Cancer Society, 2011.
9. Zevallos JP, Hartman CM, Kramer JR et al. Increased thyroid cancer... *Cancer* 2014; Nov 6. doi: 10.1002/cncr.29122.
10. Davies L, Welch HG. Increasing incidence of thyroid cancer in the United States, 1973–2002. *JAMA*. 2006 May 10; **295**(18): 2164–7.
11. Mitchell J, Milas M, Barbosa G et al. Avoidable reoperations for thyroid and parathyroid surgery: effect of hospital volume. *Surgery*. 2008 Dec; **144**(6): 899–906.
12. Leenhardt L, Grosclaude P, Chérié-Challine L. Thyroid Cancer Committee. Increased incidence of thyroid carcinoma in france: a true epidemic or thyroid nodule management effects? Report from the French Thyroid Cancer Committee. *Thyroid*. 2004 Dec; **14**(12): 1056–60.
13. Boyle P, Ferlay J. Cancer incidence and mortality in Europe, 2004. *Ann Oncol*. 2005 Mar; **16**(3): 481–8.
14. Perros P, Boelaert K, Colley S, et al. Guidelines for the management of thyroid cancer. *Clin Endocrinol (Oxf)* 2014; **81**(Suppl 1): 1–122.
15. Gharib H, Papini E, Paschke R, et al. Nodules AAETFoT. American Association of Clinical Endocrinologists, Associazione Medici Endocrinologi, and European Thyroid Association: Medical guidelines for clinical practice for the diagnosis and management of thyroid nodules: executive summary of recommendations. *Endocr Pract* 2010; **16**: 468–475.
16. Cooper DS, Doherty GM, Haugen BR et al. American Thyroid Association Guidelines Taskforce on Thyroid, N., Differentiated Thyroid. Revised American Thyroid Association management guidelines for patients with thyroid nodules and differentiated thyroid cancer. *Thyroid* 2009; **19**: 1167–214.
17. Kwak JY. Indications for fine needle aspiration in thyroid nodules. *Endocrinol Metab (Seoul)*. 2013 Jun; **28**(2): 81–5.
18. Russ G, Leboulleux S, Leenhardt L, Hegedüs L. Thyroid incidentalomas: epidemiology, risk stratification with ultrasound and workup. *Eur Thyroid J*. 2014; **3**(3): 154–63.
19. Pitman MB, Abele J, Ali SZ et al. Techniques for thyroid FNAC: a synopsis of the National Cancer Institute Thyroid FNAC State of the Science Conference. *Diagn Cytopathol* 2008; **36**: 407–24.
20. Olson MT, Tatsas AD, Ali SZ. Cytotechnologist-attended on-site adequacy evaluation of thyroid fine-needle aspiration: comparison with cytopathologists and correlation with the final interpretation. *Ref Am J Clin Pathol*. 2012 Jul; **138**(1): 90–5.
21. Romitelli F, Di Stasio E, Santoro C et al. A comparative study of fine needle aspiration and fine needle non-aspiration biopsy on suspected thyroid nodules. *Endocr Pathol*. 2009; **20**(2): 108–13.
22. Musgrave YM, Davey DD, Weeks JA et al. Assessment of fine-needle aspiration sampling technique in thyroid nodules. *Diagn Cytopathol*. 1998 Jan; **18**(1): 76–80.
23. Witt BL, Schmidt RL. Rapid onsite evaluation improves the adequacy of fine-needle aspiration for thyroid lesions: a systematic review and meta-analysis. *Thyroid*. 2013 Apr; **23**(4): 428–35.
24. Cibas ES, Alexander EK, Benson CB, et al: Indications for thyroid FNAC and pre-FNAC requirements: a synopsis of the National Cancer Institute Thyroid FNAC State of the Science Conference. *Diagn Cytopathol* 2008; **36**: 390–9.
25. Baloch ZW, LiVolsi VA, Asa SL, et al: Diagnostic terminology and morphologic criteria for cytologic diagnosis of thyroid lesions: a synopsis of the National Cancer Institute Thyroid Fine-Needle Aspiration State of the Science Conference. *Diagn Cytopathol* 2008; **36**: 425–37.
26. *Royal College of Pathologists: Guidelines for reporting of thyroid cytology specimens*. Jan 2016 http://ukeps.com/docs/thyroidfna.pdf
27. Nardi F, Basolo F, Crescenzi A et al. Italian consensus for the classification and reporting of thyroid cytology. *J Endocrinol Invest*. 2014 Jun; **37**(6): 593–9.
28. Kocjan G, Cochand-Priollet B et al. Diagnostic terminology for reporting thyroid fine needle aspiration. European Federation of Cytology Societies working group. Lisbon 2009. *Cytopathology* 2010; **21**: 86–92.
29. Cochand-Priollet B, Schmitt F, Toetsch M, Vielh P, European Federation of Cytology Societies' Scientific Committee: The Bethesda terminology for reporting thyroid cytopathology: from theory to practice in Europe. *Acta Cytol* 2011; **55**: 507–11.
30. Kocjan G, Ashish Ch. The interobserver reproducibility of using the UKRCPath thyroid fine needle aspiration classification system. *Am J Clin Pathol* 2011; **135**(6): 852–9.

31. Lobo C, McQueen A, Beale T, Kocjan G. The UK Royal College of Pathologists thyroid fine-needle aspiration diagnostic classification is a robust tool for clinical management of abnormal thyroid nodules. *Acta Cytol* 2011; **55**: 499–506.

32. Wu HH, Rose C, Elsheikh TM. The Bethesda system for reporting thyroid cytopathology: An experience of 1382 cases in a community practice setting with the implication for risk of neoplasm and risk of malignancy. *Diagn Cytopathol*. 2012 May; **40**(5): 399–403.

33. Theoharis CG, Schofield KM, Hammers L et al. The Bethesda thyroid fine-needle aspiration classification system: year 1 at an academic institution. *Thyroid*. 2009 Nov; **19**(11): 1215–23.

34. Gharib H, Papini E, Paschke R et al. Nodules AAETFoT. American Association of Clinical Endocrinologists, Associazione Medici Endocrinologi, and European Thyroid Association: Medical guidelines for clinical practice for the diagnosis and management of thyroid nodules: executive summary of recommendations. *Endocr Pract* 2010; **16**: 468–75.

35. Hambly NM, Gonen M, Gerst SR et al. Implementation of evidence-based guidelines for thyroid nodule biopsy: a model for establishment of practice standards. *AJR Am J Roentgenol* 2011; **196**: 655–60.

36. Kim EK, Park CS, Chung WY et al. New sonographic criteria for recommending fine-needle aspiration biopsy of nonpalpable solid nodules of the thyroid. *AJR Am J Roentgenol* 2002; **178**: 687–91.

37. Park JY, Lee HJ, Jang HW et al. A proposal for a thyroid imaging reporting and data system for ultrasound features of thyroid carcinoma. *Thyroid* 2009; **19**: 1257–64.

38. Russ G, Bigorgne C, Royer B, et al. The Thyroid Imaging Reporting and Data System (TIRADS) for ultrasound of the thyroid. *J Radiol* 2011; **92**: 701–13.

39. Horvath E, Majlis S, Rossi R et al. An ultrasonogram reporting system for thyroid nodules stratifying cancer risk for clinical management. *J Clin Endocrinol Metab* 2009; **94**: 1748–51.

40. Kwak JY, Jung I, Baek JH et al. Image reporting and characterization system for ultrasound features of thyroid nodules: multicentric Korean retrospective study. *Korean J Radiol* 2013; **14**: 110–17.

41. Chng CL, Kurzawinski TR, Beale T. Value of sonographic features in predicting malignancy in thyroid nodules diagnosed as follicular neoplasm on cytology. *Clin Endocrinol (Oxf)*. 2015; **83**(5): 711–6.

42. Maia FF, Matos PS, Pavin EJ, Zantut-Wittmann DE. Thyroid imaging reporting and data system score combined with Bethesda system for malignancy risk stratification in thyroid nodules with indeterminate results on cytology. *Clin Endocrinol (Oxf)* 2015 Mar; **82**(3): 439–44.

43. Takashima S, Fukuda H, Kobayashi T. Thyroid nodules: clinical effect of ultrasound-guided fine-needle aspiration biopsy. *J Clin Ultrasound* 1994; **22**(9): 535–42.

44. Yunus M, Ahmed Z. Significance of ultrasound features in predicting malignant solid thyroid nodules: need for fine-needle aspiration. *J Pak Med Assoc*. 2010 Oct; **60**(10): 848–53.

45. Sebo TJ. What are the keys to successful thyroid FNAC interpretation? *Clin Endocrinol (Oxf)*. 2012 Jul; **77**(1): 13–7. doi: 10.1111/j.1365–2265.2012.04404.x.

46. Cap J, Ryska A, Rehorkova P et al. Sensitivity and specificity of the fine needle aspiration biopsy of the thyroid: clinical point of view. *Clin Endocrinol (Oxf)* 1999; **51**(4): 509–15.

47. Yoon JH, Kwak JY, Moon HJ et al. The diagnostic accuracy of ultrasound-guided fine-needle aspiration biopsy and the sonographic differences between benign and malignant thyroid nodules 3 cm or larger. *Thyroid*. 2011 Sep; **21**(9): 993–1000.

48. Gharib H, Goellner JR. Fine-needle aspiration biopsy of the thyroid: an appraisal. *Ann Intern Med* 1993; **118**(4): 282–9.

49. Altavilla G, Pascale M, Nenci I. Fine needle aspiration cytology of thyroid gland diseases. *Acta Cytol* 1990; **34**(2): 251–6.

50. Hawkins F, Bellido D, Bernal C, et al. Fine needle aspiration biopsy in the diagnosis of thyroid cancer and thyroid disease. *Cancer* 1987; **59**(6): 1206–9.

51. Hussain ST, Beeby I, Missan A, Buxton-Thomas MS. Use of fine needle aspiration cytology in the management of the solitary cold thyroid nodule. *Nucl Med Commun* 1993; **14**(4): 335–8.

52. Merchant WJ, Thomas SM, Coppen MJ, Prentice MG. The role of thyroid fine needle aspiration (FNAC) cytology in a District General Hospital setting. *Cytopathology* 1995; **6**(6): 409–18.

53. Franc B, Allory Y, Hejblum G. Cytopuncture in tumors of the thyroid. *Rev Prat* 1996; **46**(19): 2315–20.

54. Dwarakanathan AA, Ryan WG, Staren ED, Martirano M, Economou SG. Fine-needle aspiration biopsy of the thyroid. Diagnostic accuracy when performing a moderate number of such procedures. *Arch Intern Med* 1989; **149**(9): 2007–9.

55. Anderson JB, Webb AJ. Fine-needle aspiration biopsy and the diagnosis of thyroid cancer. *Br J Surg* 1987; **74**(4): 292–6.

56. Buitrago Ramirez F, Saenz de Santamaria Morales J, Moreno Casado J. Cytological diagnosis of thyroid nodules by fine needle aspiration. A study of 385 cases from primary care. *Aten Primaria* 1989; **6**(10): 714–8.

57. Guimaraes EM, Morais DM, Da Silva SJ, Cremonini NC. The impact of fine needle aspiration biopsy: diagnostic accuracy study. *Rev Assoc Med Bras* 1996; **42**(1): 2–6.

58. Moisson-Meer A, Franc B, Duprey J et al. Reliability of needle biopsy of solitary thyroid nodules in view of surgical indications. *Rev Med Interne* 1996; **17**(9): 732–7.

59. Klemi PJ, Joensuu H, Nylamo E. Fine needle aspiration biopsy in the diagnosis of thyroid nodules. *Acta Cytol* 1991; **35**(4): 434–8.

60. Perez JA, Pisano R, Kinast C et al. Needle aspiration cytology in euthyroid uninodular goiter. *Rev Med Chil* 1991; **119**(2): 158–63.

61. Akerman M, Tennvall J, Biorklund A et al. Sensitivity and specificity of fine needle aspiration cytology in the diagnosis of tumors of the thyroid gland. *Acta Cytol* 1985; **29**(5): 850–5.

62. Nam-Goong IS, Kim HY, Gong G et al. Ultrasonography-guided fine-needle aspiration of thyroid incidentaloma: correlation with pathological findings. *Clin Endocrinol (Oxf)*. 2004 Jan; **60**(1): 21–8.

63. Lee MJ, Hong SW, Chung WY et al. Cytological results of ultrasound-guided fine-needle aspiration cytology for thyroid nodules: emphasis on correlation with sonographic findings. *Yonsei Med J*. 2011 Sep; **52**(5): 838–44.

64. Layfield LJ, Reichman A, Bottles K, Giuliano A. Clinical determinants for the management of thyroid nodules by fine-needle aspiration cytology. *Arch Otolaryngol Head Neck Surg* 1992; **118**(7): 717–21.

65. Baloch ZW, Sack MJ, Yu GH et al. Fine-needle aspiration of thyroid: an institutional experience. *Thyroid* 1998; **8**(7): 565–9.

66. Cusick EL, MacIntosh CA, Krukowski ZH, Williams VM, Ewen SW, Matheson NA. Management of isolated thyroid swellings: a prospective six year study of fine needle aspiration cytology in diagnosis. *BMJ* 1990; **301**(6747): 318–21.

67. Popoveniuc G, Jonklaas J. Thyroid nodules. *Med Clin North Am*. 2012 Mar; **96**(2): 329–49.

68. Gharib H, Goellner JR, Johnson DA. Fine-needle aspiration cytology of the thyroid. A 12-year experience with 11,000 biopsies. *Clin Lab Med* 1993; **13**(3): 699–709.

69. Harach HR. Usefulness of fine needle aspiration of the thyroid in an endemic goiter region. *Acta Cytol* 1989; **33**(1): 31–5.

70. Gagneten CB, Roccatagliata G, Lowenstein A et al. The role of fine needle aspiration biopsy cytology in the evaluation of the clinically solitary thyroid nodule. *Acta Cytol* 1987; **31**(5): 595–8.

70a. http://www.british-thyroid-association.org/news/Docs/Thyroid_cancer_guidelines_2007.pdf

71. Chadwick DR, Harrison BJ. The role of fine-needle aspiration cytology and frozen section histology in management of differentiated thyroid cancer: the UK experience. *Langenbecks Arch Surg* 1998; **383**(2): 164–6.

72. Bugis SP, Young JE, Archibald SD, Chen VS. Diagnostic accuracy of fine-needle aspiration biopsy versus frozen section in solitary thyroid nodules. *Am J Surg* 1986; **152**(4): 411–6.

73. Schmid KW, Ladurner D, Zechmann W, Feichtinger H. Clinicopathologic management of tumors of the thyroid gland in an endemic goiter area. Combined use of preoperative fine needle aspiration biopsy and intraoperative frozen section. *Acta Cytol* 1989; **33**(1): 27–30.

74. Mulcahy MM, Cohen JI, Anderson PE et al. Relative accuracy of fine-needle aspiration and frozen section in the diagnosis of well-differentiated thyroid cancer. *Laryngoscope* 1998; **108**(4 Pt 1): 494–6.

75. Kopald KH, Layfield LJ, Mohrmann R et al. Clarifying the role of fine-needle aspiration cytologic evaluation and frozen section examination in the operative management of thyroid cancer. *Arch Surg* 1989; **124**(10): 1201–4; discussion 1204–5.

76. McHenry CR, Rosen IB, Walfish PG, Bedard Y. Influence of fine-needle aspiration biopsy and frozen section examination on the management of thyroid cancer. *Am J Surg* 1993; **166**(4): 353–6.

77. Hamming JF, Vriens MR, Goslings BM et al. Role of fine-needle aspiration biopsy and frozen section examination in determining the extent of thyroidectomy. *World J Surg* 1998; **22**(6): 575–9; discussion 579–80.

78. Aguilar-Diosdado M, Contreras A, Gavilan I et al. Thyroid nodules. Role of fine needle aspiration and intraoperative frozen section examination. *Acta Cytol* 1997; **41**(3): 677–82.

79. Boyd LA, Earnhardt RC, Dunn JT, Frierson HF, Hanks JB. Preoperative evaluation and predictive value of fine-needle aspiration and frozen section of thyroid nodules. *J Am Coll Surg* 1998; **187**(5): 494–502.

80. Morosini PP, Mancini V, Filipponi S, et al. Comparison between the diagnostic accuracy in diagnosis of thyroid nodules with fine needle biopsy an intraoperative histological evaluation of frozen tissue. *Minerva Endocrinol* 1997; **22**(1): 1–5.

81. Moon HJ, Kwak JY, Kim EK, et al. The combined role of ultrasound and frozen section in surgical management of thyroid nodules read as suspicious for papillary thyroid carcinoma on fine needle aspiration biopsy: a retrospective study. *World J Surg* 2009 May; **33**(5): 950–7.

82. Chen H, Zeiger MA, Clark DP et al. Papillary carcinoma of the thyroid: can operative management be based solely on fine-needle aspiration? *J Am Coll Surg* 1997; **184**(6): 605–10.

83. Davoudi MM, Yeh KA, Wei JP. Utility of fine-needle aspiration cytology and frozen-section examination in the operative management of thyroid nodules. *Am Surg* 1997; **63**(12): 1084–9; discussion 1089–90.

84. Trimboli P, Nasrollah N, Guidobaldi L et al. The use of core needle biopsy as first-line in diagnosis of thyroid nodules reduces false negative and inconclusive data reported by fine-needle aspiration. *World J Surg Oncol.* 2014 Mar 24; **12**: 61.

85. Hahn SY, Shin JH, Han BK et al. Ultrasonography-guided core needle biopsy for the thyroid nodule: does the procedure hold any benefit for the diagnosis when fine-needle aspiration cytology analysis shows inconclusive results? *Br J Radiol.* 2013 May; **86**(1025): 20130007.

86. Ha EJ, Baek JH, Lee JH et al. Sonographically suspicious thyroid nodules with initially benign cytologic results: the role of a core needle biopsy. *Thyroid.* 2013 Jun; **23**(6): 703–8.

87. Choi YJ, Baek JH, Ha EJ et al. Differences in risk of malignancy and management recommendations in subcategories of thyroid nodules with atypia of undetermined significance or follicular lesion of undetermined significance: the role of ultrasound-guided core-needle biopsy. *Thyroid.* 2014 Mar; **24**(3): 494–501.

87a. Ha EJ, Baek JH, Lee JH, Kim JK, Choi YJ, Sung TY, Kim TY. Complications following US-guided core-needle biopsy for thyroid lesions: a retrospective study of 6,169 consecutive patients with 6,687 thyroid nodules. *Eur Radiol.* 2016 Jun **16**. [Epub ahead of print]

88. Zhang S, Niu L. Evaluation of the efficacy and the limitation of ultrasound-guided core-needle biopsy, core-needle aspiration and fine-needle aspiration in micro-nodules of thyroid. *Zhonghua Er Bi Yan Hou Tou Jing Wai Ke Za Zhi.* 2014 Nov; **49**(11): 893–6.

89. Ross JS, del Rosario AD, Sanderson B, Bui HX. Selective expression of CD44 cell-adhesion molecule in thyroid papillary carcinoma fine-needle aspirates. *Diagn Cytopathol* 1996; **14**(4): 287–91.

89a. Matesa N, Samija I, Kusić Z. Galectin-3 and CD44v6 positivity by RT-PCR method in fine needle aspirates of benign thyroid lesions. *Cytopathology.* 2007 Apr; **18**(2): 112–6.

90. Sack MJ, Astengo-Osuna C, Lin BT et al. HBME-1 immunostaining in thyroid fine-needle aspirations: a useful marker in the diagnosis of carcinoma. *Mod Pathol* 1997; **10**(7): 668–74.

91. Ohta M, Ookoshi T, Naiki H, Imamura Y. HBME-1 and CD15 immunocytochemistry in the follicular variant of thyroid papillary carcinoma. *Pathol Int.* 2015 Jan 19: [Epub ahead of print] PubMed PMID: 25597783.

91a. Das DK, Al-Waheeb SK, George SS, Haji BI, Mallik MK. Contribution of immunocytochemical stainings for galectin-3, CD44, and HBME1 to fine-needle aspiration cytology diagnosis of papillary thyroid carcinoma. *Diagn Cytopathol.* 2014 Jun; **42**(6): 498–505.

91b. Bizzarro T, Martini M, Marrocco C, D'Amato D, Traini E, Lombardi CP, Pontecorvi A, Fadda G, Larocca LM, Rossi ED. The Role of CD56 in Thyroid Fine Needle Aspiration Cytology: A Pilot Study Performed on Liquid Based Cytology. 2015 Jul 17; **10**(7).

92. Rossi ED, Bizzarro T, Martini M, Straccia P, Lombardi CP, Pontecorvi A, Larocca LM, Fadda G. The role of fine-needle aspiration in the thyroid nodules of elderly patients. *Oncotarget* 2016; **15**; 7(11): 11850–9.

93. Nikiforov YE. Molecular diagnostics of thyroid tumors. *Arch Pathol Lab Med.* 2011 May; **135**(5): 569–77.

94. Kim SY, Kim EK, Kwak JY et al. What to do with thyroid nodules showing benign cytology and BRAF(V600E) mutation? A study based on clinical and radiologic features using a highly sensitive analytic method. *Surgery.* 2015 Feb; **157**(2): 354–61.

95. Adeniran AJ, Hui P, Chhieng DC et al. BRAF mutation testing of thyroid fine-needle aspiration specimens enhances predictability of malignancy in thyroid follicular lesions of undetermined significance. *Acta Cytologica* 2011; **55**: 570–5.

96. Colanta A, Lin O, Tafe L et al. BRAF mutation analysis of fine-needle aspiration biopsies of papillary thyroid carcinoma: impact on diagnosis and prognosis. *Acta Cytologica* 2011; **55**: 563–69.

97. Pelizzo MR, Boschin IM, Barollo S et al. BRAF analysis by fine needle aspiration biopsy of thyroid nodules improves preoperative identification of papillary thyroid carcinoma and represents a prognostic factor: a mono-institutional experience. *Clin Chem Lab Med.* 2011 Feb; **49**(2): 325–9.

98. Smith RA, Salajegheh A, Weinstein S et al. Correlation between BRAF mutation and the clinicopathological parameters in papillary thyroid carcinoma with particular reference to follicular variant. *Hum Pathol.* 2011 Apr; **42**(4): 500–6. Epub 2010 Dec 16.

99. Smith GD, Zhou L, Rowe LR et al. Allele-specific PCR with competitive probe blocking for sensitive and specific detection of BRAF V600E in thyroid fine-needle aspiration specimens. *Acta Cytologica* 2011; **55**: 576–83.

100. Jordan KW, Adkins CB, Cheng LL, Faquin WC. Application of magnetic-resonance-spectroscopy- based metabolomics to the fine-needle aspiration diagnosis of papillary thyroid carcinoma. *Acta Cytologica* 2011; **55**: 584–9.

100a. Nikiforov YE, Carty SE, Chiosea SI, et al. Highly accurate diagnosis of cancer in thyroid nodules with follicular neoplasm/suspicious for a follicular neoplasm cytology by ThyroSeq v2 next-generation sequencing assay. *Cancer.* 2014; **120**: 3627–3634.

101. Le Mercier M, D'Haene N, De Nève N et al. Next-generation sequencing improves the diagnosis of thyroid FNA specimens within determinate cytology. *Histopathology.* 2015 Jan; **66**(2): 215–24.

101a. Bellevicine C, Sgariglia R, Malapelle U, Vigliar E, Nacchio M, Ciancia G, Eszlinger M, Paschke R, Troncone G. Young investigator challenge: Can the Ion AmpliSeq Cancer Hotspot Panel v2 be used for next-generation sequencing of thyroid FNA samples? *Cancer.* 2016 Sep 26. doi: 10.1002/cncy.21780.

101b. Alexander EK, Kennedy GC, Baloch ZW, et al. Preoperative diagnosis of benign thyroid nodules with indeterminate cytology. *N Engl J Med.* 2012; **367**: 705–715.

101c. Labourier E, Shifrin A, Busseniers AE, et al. Molecular Testing for miRNA, mRNA, and DNA on Fine-Needle Aspiration Improves the Preoperative Diagnosis of Thyroid Nodules With Indeterminate Cytology. *The Journal of Clinical Endocrinology and Metabolism.* 2015; **100**(7): 2743–2750.

101d. Nikiforov YE, Carty SE, Chiosea SI, et al. Highly accurate diagnosis of cancer in thyroid nodules with follicular neoplasm/suspicious for a follicular neoplasm cytology by ThyroSeq v2 next-generation sequencing assay. *Cancer.* 2014; **120**: 3627–3634.

102. Hodak SP, Rosenthal DS. American Thyroid Association Clinical Affairs Committee. Information for clinicians: commercially available molecular diagnosis testing in the evaluation of thyroid nodule fine-needle aspiration specimens. *Thyroid.* 2013 Feb; **23**(2): 131–4.

103. Hales MS, Hsu FS. Needle tract implantation of papillary carcinoma of the thyroid following aspiration biopsy. *Acta Cytol* 1990; **34**(6): 801–4.

104. Lopez JI, Pereda E, Rodil MA, Fernandez-Larrinoa A. Histologicalal changes mimicking papillary carcinoma following fine needle aspiration of the thyroid gland. *Arch Anat Cytol Pathol* 1996; **44**(2–3): 98–100.

105. Layfield LJ, Lones MA. Necrosis in thyroid nodules after fine needle aspiration biopsy. Report of two cases. *Acta Cytol* 1991; **35**(4): 427–30 [the above report in].

106. Hurley DL, Gharib H. Evaluation and management of multinodular goiter. *Otolaryngol Clin North Am* 1996; **29**(4): 527–40.

107. Lucas A, Llatjos M, Salinas I et al. Fine-needle aspiration cytology of benign nodular thyroid disease. Value of re-aspiration. *Eur J Endocrinol* 1995; **132**(6): 677–80.

108. Franklyn JA, Daykin J, Young J et al. Fine needle aspiration cytology in diffuse or multinodular goitre compared with solitary thyroid nodules. *BMJ* 1993; **307**(6898): 240.

109. Katoh R, Kawaoi A, Muramatsu A et al. Birefringent (calcium oxalate) crystals in thyroid diseases. A clinicopathological study with possible implications for differential diagnosis. *Am J Surg Pathol.* 1993 Jul; **17**(7): 698–705.

110. Cooper DS, Tiamson E, Ladenson PW. Psammoma bodies in fine needle aspiration biopsies of benign thyroid nodules. *Thyroidology* 1988(**1**): 55–9.

111. Riazmontazer N, Bedayat G. Psammoma bodies in fine needle aspirates from thyroids containing nontoxic hyperplastic nodular goiters. *Acta Cytol* 1991; **35**(5): 563–6.

112. Fiorella RM, Isley W, Miller LK, Kragel PJ. Multinodular goiter of the thyroid mimicking malignancy: diagnostic pitfalls in fine-needle aspiration biopsy. *Diagn Cytopathol* 1993; **9**(3): 351–5; discussion 355–7.

113. Jo VY, Vanderlaan PA, Marqusee E, Krane JF. Repeatedly nondiagnostic thyroid fine-needle aspirations do not modify malignancy risk. *Acta Cytol.* 2011; **55**(6): 539–43. Epub 2011 Dec 9.

114. Kim SY, Kim EK, Kwak JY, Moon HJ, Yoon JH. What to do with thyroid nodules showing benign cytology and BRAF(V600E) mutation? A study based on clinical and radiologic features using a highly sensitive analytic method. *Surgery.* 2015 Feb; **157**(2): 354–61.

115. Jayaram G, Singh B, Marwaha RK. Grave's disease. Appearance in cytologic smears from fine needle aspirates of the thyroid gland. *Acta Cytol* 1989; **33**(1): 36–40.

116. Gul K, Di Ri Koc A, Ki Yak G et al. Thyroid carcinoma risk in patients with hyperthyroidism and role of preoperative cytology in diagnosis. *Minerva Endocrinol.* 2009 Dec; **34**(4): 281–8.

117. Shabb NS, Tawil A, Gergeos F et al. Multinucleated giant cells in fine-needle aspiration of thyroid nodules: their diagnostic significance. *Diagn Cytopathol* 1999; **21**(5): 307–12.

118. Luca IC, Zamfir C. Fine-needle biopsy cytology in autoimmune thyroiditis [In Process Citation]. *Rev Med Chir Soc Med Nat Iasi* 1998; **102**(3–4): 150–1.

119. Nguyen GK, Ginsberg J, Crockford PM, Villanueva RR. Hashimoto's thyroiditis: cytodiagnostic accuracy and pitfalls. *Diagn Cytopathol* 1997; **16**(6): 531–6.

120. Kumarasinghe MP, De Silva S. Pitfalls in cytological diagnosis of autoimmune thyroiditis. *Pathology* 1999; **31**(1): 1–7.

121. MacDonald L, Yazdi HM. Fine needle aspiration biopsy of Hashimoto's thyroiditis. Sources of diagnostic error. *Acta Cytol* 1999; **43**(3): 400–6.

122. DeMay RM. The art and science of cytopatholgy, volume II. In: DeMay RM, editor. *Thyroid*. Chicago: American Society for Clinical Pathology Press. 1996. p 703–78.

123. Berho M, Suster S. Clear nuclear changes in Hashimoto's thyroiditis. A clinico-pathologic study of 12 cases. *Ann Clin Lab Sci* 1995; **25**: 513–21.

124. Weber D, Brinard J, Chen L. Atypical epithelial cells, cannot exclude papillary carcinoma, in fine needle aspiration of the thyroid. *Acta Cytol* 2008; **52**: 320–4.

125. Koseoglu RD, Onuk Filiz N. The oncocytic variant of papillary thyroid carcinoma. *Turk J Med Sci* 2006; **36**: 387–92.

126. Belsing ZRU, Bendtzen K. Case report. Riedel's thyroiditis: an autoimmune or primary fibrotic disease? *J Intern Med* 1994; **235**: 271–4.

127. Baloch ZW, Saberi M, Livolsi VA. Simultaneous involvement of thyroid by Riedel's [correction of Reidel's] disease and fibrosing Hashimoto's thyroiditis: a case report. *Thyroid* 1998; **8**: 337–41.

128. Best TB, Munro RE, Burwell S, Volpe R. Riedel's thyroiditis associated with Hashimoto's thyroiditis, hypoparathyroidism, and retroperitoneal fibrosis. *J Endocrinol Invest* 1991; **14**: 767–72.

129. De Boer WA. Riedel's thyroiditis, retroperitoneal fibrosis, and sclerosing cholangitis: diseases with one pathogenesis? *Gut* 1993; **34**: 714.

130. Neild GH, Rodriguez-Justo M, Wall C, Connolly JO. Hyper-IgG4 disease: report and characterisation of a new disease. *BMC Med* 2006; **4**: 23.

131. Kocjan G, Ramsay A, Young M et al. Spindle cell lesion of thyroid: a potential pitfall in FNAC diagnosis. *Cytopathology*. 2010 Apr; **21**(2): 123–6.

132. Gharib H, Goellner JR. Fine-needle aspiration biopsy of the thyroid: an appraisal. *Ann Intern Med*. 1993; **118**: 282–9.

133. Cibas ES, Ali SZ; NCI Thyroid FNAC State of the Science Conference. The Bethesda System for Reporting Thyroid Cytopathology. *Am J Clin Pathol*. 2009; **132**: 658–65.

134. Horne MJ, Chhieng DC, Theoharis C et al. Thyroid follicular lesion of undetermined significance: Evaluation of the risk of malignancy using the two-tier sub-classification. *Diagn Cytopathol*. 2012 May; **40**(5): 410–5.

135. Krane JF, Nayar R, Renshaw AA. Atypical cells of undetermined significance. In: Ali SZ, Cibas ES, editors. *The Bethesda System for Reporting Thyroid Cytopathology: Definitions, criteria and explanatory notes*. New York: Springer, 2010: 37–49.

136. Ali SZ, Cibas ES, eds. *The Bethesda System for Reporting Thyroid Cytopathology: Definitions, criteria and explanatory notes*. New York: Springer, 2010.

137. Ohori N, Schoedel KE. Variability in the atypia of undetermined significance/follicular lesion of undetermined significance diagnosis in the Bethesda System for Reporting Thyroid Cytopathology: Sources and recommendations. *Acta Cytologica* 2011; **55**(6): 492–8.

138. Kocjan G, Chandra A, Cross PA et al. The interobserver reproducibility of thyroid fine-needle aspiration using the UK Royal College of Pathologists' classification system. *Am J Clin Pathol*. 2011 Jun; **135**(6): 852–9.

139. Horne MJ1, Chhieng DC, Theoharis C et al. Thyroid follicular lesion of undetermined significance: Evaluation of the risk of malignancy using the two-tier sub-classification. *Diagn Cytopathol*. 2012 May; **40**(5): 410–5.

140. Van der Laan PA, Marqusee E, Krane JF. Clinical outcome for atypia of undetermined significance in thyroid fine-needle aspirations: should repeated FNAC be the preferred initial approach? *Am J Clin Pathol*. 2011; **135**: 770–5.

141. Faquin WC, Baloch ZW. Fine-needle aspiration of follicular patterned lesions of the thyroid: diagnosis, management, and follow-up according to National Cancer Institute (NCI) recommendations. *Diagn Cytopathol*. 2010; **38**: 731–9.

142. Renshaw AA. Should 'atypical follicular cells' in thyroid fine-needle aspirates be subclassified? *Cancer (Cancer Cytopathol)*. 2010; **118**: 186–9.

143. Dincer N, Balci S, Yazgan A et al. Follow-up of atypia and follicular lesions of undetermined significance in thyroid fine needle aspiration cytology. *Cytopathology*. 2013 Dec; **24**(6): 385–90.

144. Jo VY, Stelow EB, Dustin SM, Hanley KZ. Malignancy risk for fine-needle aspiration of thyroid lesions according to the Bethesda System for Reporting Thyroid Cytopathology. *Am J Clin Pathol*. 2010; **134**: 450–6.

145. Ohori NP, Nikiforova MN, Schoedel KE et al. Contribution of molecular testing to thyroid fine-needle aspiration cytology of 'follicular lesion of undetermined significance/atypia of undetermined significance.' *Cancer (Cancer Cytopathol)*. 2010; **118**: 17–23.

146. Ho AS, Sarti EE, Jain KS et al. Malignancy rate in thyroid nodules classified as Bethesda category III (AUS/FLUS). *Thyroid*. 2014; **24**(5): 832–9.

147. Layfield LJ, Morton MJ, Cramer HM, Hirschowitz S. Implications of the proposed thyroid fine-needle aspiration category of 'follicular lesion of undetermined significance': a five-year multi-institutional analysis. *Diagn Cytopathol*. 2009; **37**: 710–4.

148. Rabaglia JL, Kabbani W, Wallace L et al. Effect of the Bethesda system for reporting thyroid cytopathology on thyroidectomy rates and malignancy risk in cytologically indeterminate lesions. *Surgery*. 2010; **148**: 1267–72; discussion 1272–3.

149. Faquin WC, Cibas ES, Renshaw AA. 'Atypical' cells in fine-needle aspiration biopsy specimens of benign thyroid cysts. *Cancer (Cancer Cytopathol)*. 2005; **105**: 71–9.

150. Yoo WS, Choi HS, Cho SW et al. The role of ultrasound findings in the management of thyroid nodules with atypia or follicular lesions of undetermined significance. *Clin Endocrinol (Oxf)*. 2014; **80**(5): 735–42.

151. Eszlinger M, Piana S, Moll A et al. Molecular testing of thyroid fine needle aspirations (FNA) improves cpre-surgical diagnosis and supports the histological identification of minimally invasive follicular thyroid carcinomas. *Thyroid*. 2015; **25**(4): 401–9.

151a. Ustun B, Chhieng D, Van Dyke A, Carling T, Holt E, Udelsman R, Adeniran AJ. Risk stratification in follicular neoplasm: a cytological assessment using the modified Bethesda classification. *Cancer Cytopathol*. 2014 Jul; **122**(7): 536–45.

152. Blumenfeld W, Nair R, Mir R. Diagnostic significance of papillary structures and intranuclear inclusions in Hurthle-cell neoplasms of the thyroid. *Diagn Cytopathol*. 1999 Apr; **20**(4): 185–9.

153. Nguyen GK, Husain M, Akin MR. Cytodiagnosis of benign and malignant Hurthle cell lesions of the thyroid by fine-needle aspiration biopsy. *Diagn Cytopathol* 1999; **20**(5): 261–5.

154. Yang GC, Schreiner AM, Sun W. Can abundant colloid exclude oncocytic (Hürthle cell) carcinoma in thyroid fine needle aspiration? Cytohistological correlation of 127 oncocytic (Hürthle cell) lesions. *Cytopathology*. 2013; **24**(3): 185–93.

155. Busseniers AE, Oertel YC. 'Cellular adenomatoid nodules' of the thyroid: review of 219 fine-needle aspirates. *Diagn Cytopathol* 1993; **9**(5): 581–9.

156. Tuttle RM, Lemar H, Burch HB. Clinical features associated with an increased risk of thyroid malignancy in patients with follicular neoplasia by fine-needle aspiration. *Thyroid*. 1998; **8**(5): 377–83.

157. Karak AK, Sahoo M, Bhatnagar D. Hyalinizing trabecular adenoma – a case report with FNAC histological, MIB-1 proliferative index and immunohistochemical findings. *Indian J Pathol Microbiol* 1998; **41**(4): 479–84.

158. Bondeson L, Bondeson AG. Clue helping to distinguish hyalinizing trabecular adenoma from carcinoma of the thyroid in fine-needle aspirates. *Diagn Cytopathol* 1994; **10**(1): 25–9.

159. Boccato P, Mannara GM, La Rosa F et al. Hyalinizing trabecular adenoma of the thyroid diagnosed by fine-needle aspiration biopsy [clinical conference]. *Ann Otol Rhinol Laryngol* 2000 Feb; **109**(2): 235–8.

160. Strong CJ, Garcia BM. Fine needle aspiration cytologic characteristics of hyalinizing trabecular adenoma of the thyroid. *Acta Cytol* 1990; **34**(3): 359–62.

161. Kaleem Z, Davila RM. Hyalinizing trabecular adenoma of the thyroid. A report of two cases with cytologic, histological and immunohistochemical findings. *Acta Cytol* 1997; **41**(3): 883–8.

162. Hirokawa M, Shimizu M, Manabe T et al. Hyalinizing trabecular adenoma of the thyroid: its unusual cytoplasmic immunopositivity for MIB1. *Pathol Int* 1995; **45**(5): 399–401.

163. Goellner JR, Carney JA. Cytologic features of fine-needle aspirates of hyalinizing trabecular adenoma of the thyroid. *Am J Clin Pathol* 1989; **91**(2): 115–9.

164. Cerasoli S, Tabarri B, Farabegoli P et al. Hyalinizing trabecular adenoma of the thyroid. Report of two cases, with cytologic, immunohistochemical and ultra-structural studies. *Tumori* 1992; **78**(4): 274–9.

165. Fornes P, Lesourd A, Dupuis G et al. Hyalinizing trabecular adenoma of the thyroid gland. Histological and immunohistochemical study. Report of 2 cases. *Arch Anat Cytol Pathol* 1990; **38**(5–6): 203–7.

166. Schmid KW, Mesewinkel F, Bocker W. Hyalinizing trabecular adenoma of the thyroid—morphology and differential diagnosis. *Acta Med Austriaca* 1996; **23**(1–2): 65–8.

167. Akin MR, Nguyen GK. Fine-needle aspiration biopsy cytology of hyalinizing trabecular adenomas of the thyroid. *Diagn Cytopathol* 1999; **20**(2): 90–4.

168. Vassko V, Garcia S, Henry JF, De Micco C. Expression of proliferating cell nuclear antigen in follicular thyroid tumors: correlation with clinicopathological findings. *Oncol Rep* 1999; **6**(2): 359–64.

169. Huss LJ, Mendelsohn G. Medullary carcinoma of the thyroid gland: an encapsulated variant resembling the hyalinizing trabecular (paraganglioma-like) adenoma of thyroid. *Mod Pathol* 1990; **3**(5): 581–5.

170. Cameselle-Teijeiro J, Febles-Perez C, Sobrinho-Simoes M. Cytologic features of fine needle aspirates of papillary and mucoepidermoid carcinoma of the thyroid with anaplastic transformation. A case report. *Acta Cytol* 1997; **41**(4 Suppl): 1356–60.

171. Kwak JY, Kim EK, Kim MJ et al. The role of ultrasound in thyroid nodules with a cytology reading of 'suspicious for papillary thyroid carcinoma'. *Thyroid*. 2008 May; **18**(5): 517–22.

172. Layfield LJ, Mohrmann RL, Kopald KH, Giuliano AE. Use of aspiration cytology and frozen section examination for management of benign and malignant thyroid nodules. *Cancer* 1991; **68**(1): 130–4.

173. Harach HR, Saravia Day E, Zusman SB. Occult papillary microcarcinoma of the thyroid – a potential pitfall of fine needle aspiration cytology? [see comments]. *J Clin Pathol* 1991; **44**(3): 205–7.

174. Kini SR, Miller JM, Hamburger JI, Smith MJ. Cytopathology of papillary carcinoma of the thyroid by fine needle aspiration. *Acta Cytol* 1980; **24**(6): 511–21.

175. Kaur A, Jayaram G. Thyroid tumors: cytomorphology of papillary carcinoma. *Diagn Cytopathol* 1991; **7**(5): 462–8.

176. Ellison E, Lapuerta P, Martin SE. Psammoma bodies in fine-needle aspirates of the thyroid: predictive value for papillary carcinoma. *Cancer* 1998; **84**(3): 169–75.

177. Francis IM, Das DK, Sheikh ZA, Sharma PN, Gupta SK. Role of nuclear grooves in the diagnosis of papillary thyroid carcinoma. A quantitative assessment on fine needle aspiration smears. *Acta Cytol* 1995; **39**(3): 409–15.

178. Shurbaji MS, Gupta PK, Frost JK. Nuclear grooves: a useful criterion in the cytopathologic diagnosis of papillary thyroid carcinoma. *Diagn Cytopathol* 1988; **4**(2): 91–4.

179. Rupp M, Ehya H. Nuclear grooves in the aspiration cytology of papillary carcinoma of the thyroid. *Acta Cytol* 1989; **33**(1): 21–6.

180. Chhieng DC, Ross JS, McKenna BJ. CD44 immunostaining of thyroid fine-needle aspirates differentiates thyroid papillary carcinoma from other lesions with nuclear grooves and inclusions. *Cancer* 1997; **81**(3): 157–62.

181. Akhtar M, Ali MA, Huq M, Bakry M. Fine-needle aspiration biopsy of papillary thyroid carcinoma: cytologic, histological, and ultrastructural correlations. *Diagn Cytopathol* 1991; **7**(4): 373–9.

182. Ruiz-Velasco R, Waisman J, Van Herle AJ. Cystic papillary carcinoma of the thyroid gland. Diagnosis by needle aspiration with transmission electron microscopy. *Acta Cytol* 1978; **22**(1): 38–42.

183. Tabbara SO, Acoury N, Sidawy MK. Multinucleated giant cells in thyroid neoplasms. A cytologic, histological and immunohistochemical study. *Acta Cytol* 1996; **40**(6): 1184–8.

184. Martinez-Parra D, Campos Fernandez J, Hierro-Guilmain CC et al. Follicular variant of papillary carcinoma of the thyroid: to what extent is fine-needle aspiration reliable? *Diagn Cytopathol* 1996; **15**(1): 12–6.

185. Zacks JF, de las Morenas A, Beazley RM, O'Brrien MJ. Fine-needle aspiration cytology diagnosis of colloid nodule versus follicular variant of papillary carcinoma of the thyroid. *Diagn Cytopathol* 1998; **18**(2): 87–90.

186. Kumar PV, Talei AR, Malekhusseini SA et al. Follicular variant of papillary carcinoma of the thyroid. A cytologic study of 15 cases. *Acta Cytol* 1999; **43**(2): 139–42.

187. Gallagher J, Oertel YC, Oertel JE. Follicular variant of papillary carcinoma of the thyroid: fine-needle aspirates with histological correlation. *Diagn Cytopathol* 1997; **16**(3): 207–13.

188. Hugh JC, Duggan MA, Chang-Poon V. The fine-needle aspiration appearance of the follicular variant of thyroid papillary carcinoma: a report of three cases. *Diagn Cytopathol* 1988; **4**(3): 196–201.

189. Das DK, Jain S, Tripathi RP et al. Marginal vacuoles in thyroid aspirates. *Acta Cytol* 1998; **42**(5): 1121–8.

190. Goodell WM, Saboorian MH, Ashfaq R. Fine-needle aspiration diagnosis of the follicular variant of papillary carcinoma. *Cancer* 1998; **84**(6): 349–54.

191. Harach HR, Zusman SB. Cytologic findings in the follicular variant of papillary carcinoma of the thyroid. *Acta Cytol* 1992; **36**(2): 142–6.

192. Das DK, Khanna CM, Tripathi RP et al. Solitary nodular goiter. Review of cytomorphologic features in 441 cases. *Acta Cytol* 1999; **43**(4): 563–74.

192a. Borrelli N, Denaro M, Ugolini C, Poma AM, Miccoli M, Vitti P, Miccoli P, Basolo F. miRNA expression profiling of 'noninvasive follicular thyroid neoplasms with papillary-like nuclear features' compared with adenomas and infiltrative follicular variants of papillary thyroid carcinomas. *Mod Pathol.* 2016 Sep 2. doi: 10.1038/modpathol.2016.157. [Epub ahead of print]

193. Baloch ZW, Gupta PK, Yu GH et al. Follicular variant of papillary carcinoma. Cytologic and histological correlation. *Am J Clin Pathol* 1999; **111**(2): 216–22.

194. Hirokawa M, Shimizu M, Terayama K et al. Macrofollicular variant of papillary thyroid carcinoma. Report of a case with fine needle aspiration biopsy findings. *Acta Cytol* 1998; **42**(6): 1441–3.

195. Mesonero CE, Jugle JE, Wilbur DC, Nayar R. Fine-needle aspiration of the macrofollicular and microfollicular subtypes of the follicular variant of papillary carcinoma of the thyroid. *Cancer* 1998; **84**(4): 235–44.

196. Cameselle-Teijeiro J, Febles-Perez C, Cameselle-Teijeiro JF et al. Cytologic clues for distinguishing the tall cell variant of thyroid papillary carcinoma. A case report. *Acta Cytol* 1997; **41**(4 Suppl): 1310–6 [the above report in].

197. Hui PK, Chan JK, Cheung PS, Gwi E. Columnar cell carcinoma of the thyroid. Fine needle aspiration findings in a case. *Acta Cytol* 1990; **34**(3): 355–8.

198. Gamboa-Dominguez A, Candanedo-Gonzalez F, Uribe-Uribe NO, Angeles-Angeles A. Tall cell variant of papillary thyroid carcinoma. A cytohistological correlation. *Acta Cytol* 1997; **41**(3): 672–6.

199. Perez F, Llobet M, Garijo G et al. Fine-needle aspiration cytology of columnar-cell carcinoma of the thyroid: report of two cases with cytohistological correlation. *Diagn Cytopathol* 1998; **18**(5): 352–6.

200. Harach HR, Zusman SB. Cytopathology of the tall cell variant of thyroid papillary carcinoma. *Acta Cytol* 1992; **36**(6): 895–9.

201. Kaw YT. Fine needle aspiration cytology of the tall cell variant of papillary carcinoma of the thyroid [letter]. *Acta Cytol* 1994; **38**(2): 282.

202. Pilotti S, Collini P, Sampietro G et al. Thyroid papillary carcinoma of columnar cell type: a clinicopathologic study of 16 cases [letter; comment]. *Cancer* 1998; **83**(11): 2421–3.

203. Putti TC, Bhuiya TA, Wasserman PG. Fine needle aspiration cytology of mixed tall and columnar cell papillary carcinoma of the thyroid. A case report. *Acta Cytol* 1998; **42**(2): 387–90.

204. Dina R, Capitano A, Damiani S. A morphometric analysis of cytological features of tall cell variant and classical papillary carcinoma of the thyroid [In Process Citation]. *Cytopathology* 2000 Apr; **11**(2): 124–8.

205. Jayaram G. Cytology of columnar-cell variant of papillary carcinoma [In Process Citation]. *Diagn Cytopathol* 2000 ; **22**(4): 227–9.

206. Ylagan LR, Dehner LP, Huettner PC, Lu D. Columnar cell variant of papillary thyroid carcinoma. Report of a case with cytologic findings. *Acta Cytol.* 2004; **48**(1): 73–7.

207. Montone KT, Baloch ZW, LiVolsi VA. The thyroid Hürthle (oncocytic) cell and its associated pathologic conditions: a surgical pathology and cytopathology review. *Arch Pathol Lab Med* 2008; **132**: 1241–50.

208. Doria MI, Jr., Attal H, Wang HH et al. Fine needle aspiration cytology of the oxyphil variant of papillary carcinoma of the thyroid. A report of three cases. *Acta Cytol* 1996; **40**(5): 1007–11.

209. Vasei M, Kumar PV, Malekhoseini SA, Kadivar M. Papillary Hurthle cell carcinoma (Warthin-like tumor) of the thyroid. Report of a case with fine needle aspiration findings. *Acta Cytol* 1998; **42**(6): 1437–40.

210. Chen KT. Fine-needle aspiration cytology of papillary Hurthle-cell tumors of thyroid: a report of three cases. *Diagn Cytopathol* 1991; **7**(1): 53–6.

211. Lee J, Hasteh F. Oncocytic variant of papillary thyroid carcinoma associated with Hashimoto's thyroiditis: a case report and review of the literature. *Diagn Cytopathol.* 2009 Aug; **37**(8): 600–6.

212. Chuah KL, Hwang JS, Ng SB et al. Cytologic features of cribriform-morular variant of papillary carcinoma of the thyroid: a case report. *Acta Cytol.* 2005; **49**(1): 75–80.

213. Ng SB, Sittampalam K, Goh YH, Eu KW. Cribriform-morular variant of papillary carcinoma: the sporadic counterpart of familial adenomatous polyposis-associated thyroid carcinoma. A case report with clinical and molecular genetic correlation. *Pathology.* 2003; **35**(1): 42–6.

214. Mandal S, Jain S. Adenoid cystic pattern in follicular variant of papillary thyroid carcinoma: a report of four cases. *Cytopathology.* 2010; **21**(2): 93–6.

215. Koo, JS, Hong S, Park CS. Diffuse sclerosing variant is a major subtype of papillary thyroid carcinoma in the young. *Thyroid.* 2009; **19**(11): 1225–31.

216. Caruso G, Tabarri B, Lucchi I, Tison V. Fine needle aspiration cytology in a case of diffuse sclerosing carcinoma of the thyroid. *Acta Cytol* 1990; **34**(3): 352–4.

217. Kumarasinghe MP. Cytomorphologic features of diffuse sclerosing variant of papillary carcinoma of the thyroid. A report of two cases in children. *Acta Cytol* 1998; **42**(4): 983–6.

218. Chan JK, Carcangiu ML, Rosai J. Papillary carcinoma of thyroid with exuberant nodular fasciitis-like stroma. Report of three cases. *Am J Clin Pathol* 1991; **95**(3): 309–14.

219. Vinette DS, MacDonald LL, Yazdi HM. Papillary carcinoma of the thyroid with anaplastic transformation: diagnostic pitfalls in fine-needle aspiration biopsy. *Diagn Cytopathol* 1991; **7**(1): 75–8.

220. Us-Krasovec M, Golouh R. Papillary thyroid carcinoma with exuberant nodular fasciitis-like stroma in a fine needle aspirate. A case report. *Acta Cytol* 1999; **43**(6): 1101–4.

221. Yang YJ, LiVolsi VA, Khurana KK. Papillary thyroid carcinoma with nodular fasciitis-like stroma. Pitfalls in fine-needle aspiration cytology. *Arch Pathol Lab Med* 1999; **123**(9): 838–41.

222. Woyke S, al-Jassar AK, al-Jarallah MA, Temmim L. Papillary carcinoma of the thyroid with numerous spindle-shaped tumor cells in fine needle aspiration smears. A case report. *Acta Cytol* 1994; **38**(2): 226–30.

223. Leung CS, Hartwick RW, Bedard YC. Correlation of cytologic and histological features in variants of papillary carcinoma of the thyroid. *Acta Cytol* 1993; **37**(5): 645–50.

224. Scognamiglio T, Hyjek E, Kao J, Chen YT. Diagnostic usefulness of HBME1, galectin-3, CK19, and CITED1 and evaluation of their expression in encapsulated lesions with questionable features of papillary thyroid carcinoma. *Am J Clin Pathol.* 2006; **126**: 700–8.

225. Khan A, Nose V. Recent developments in the molecular biology of the parathyroid. In: Lloyd RV, ed. *Endocrine pathology: differential diagnosis and molecular advances*, 2nd edn. New York: Springer, 2010; p. 181–236.

226. DeLellis RA, Lloyd RV, Heitz PU, Eng C, eds. Pathology and genetics of tumours of endocrine organs. In: Kleihues P, Sobrin LH, series editors. *World Health Organization. Classification of tumours.* Lyon: IARC Press, 2004.

226a. Rossi ED, Martini M, Bizzarro T, Capodimonti S, Cenci T, Lombardi CP, Pontecorvi A, Fadda G, Larocca LM. Uncommon BRAF mutations in the follicular variant of thyroid papillary carcinoma: New insights. *Cancer Cytopathol.* 2015 Oct; **123**(10): 593–602.

227. Nikiforova MN, Nikiforov YE. Molecular genetics of thyroid cancer: implications for diagnosis treatment and prognosis. *Expert Rev Mol Diagn.* 2008; **8**: 83–95.

228. Lappinga PJ, Kip NS, Jin L et al. HMGA2 gene expression analysis performed on cytologic smears to distinguish benign from malignant thyroid nodules. *Cancer Cytopathol.* 2010; **118**: 287–97.

229. Jin L, Seys AR, Zhang S et al. Diagnostic utility of IMP3 expression in thyroid neoplasms: a quantitative RT-PCR study. *Diagn Mol Pathol.* 2010; **19**: 63–9.

230. Cancer Genome Atlas Research Network. Integrated genomic characterization of papillary thyroid carcinoma. *Cell.* 2014 Oct 23; **159**(3): 676–90.

231. Oertel YC. Thymoma mimicking thyroid papillary carcinoma: another pitfall in fine-needle aspiration. *Diagn Cytopathol* 1997; **17**(1): 61–3.

232. Mahajan A, Lin X, Nayar R. Thyroid Bethesda reporting category, 'suspicious for papillary thyroid carcinoma', pitfalls and clues to optimize the use of this category. *Cytopathology.* 2013 Apr; **24**(2): 85–91; doi: 10.1111/j.1365–2303. 2012.00966.x.

233. Faser CR, Marley EF, Oertel YC. Papillary tissue fragments as a diagnostic pitfall in fine-needle aspirations of thyroid nodules. *Diagn Cytopathol* 1997; **16**(5): 454–9.

234. Goffredo P, Roman SA, Sosa JA. Hurthle cell carcinoma: a population-level analysis of 3311 patients. *Cancer.* 2013 Feb 1; **119**(3): 504–11.

235. Oertel YC, Miyahara-Felipe L. Cytological features of insular carcinoma. *Diagn Cytopathol.* 2006 Aug; **34**(8): 572–5.

236. Sironi M, Collini P, Cantaboni A. Fine needle aspiration cytology of insular thyroid carcinoma. A report of four cases. *Acta Cytol* 1992; **36**(3): 435–9.

237. Guiter GE, Auger M, Ali SZ et al. Cytopathology of insular carcinoma of the thyroid. *Cancer* 1999; **87**(4): 196–202.

238. Kuhel WI, Kutler DI, Santos-Buch CA. Poorly differentiated insular thyroid carcinoma. A case report with identification of intact insulae with fine needle aspiration biopsy. *Acta Cytol* 1998; **42**(4): 991–7.

239. Gharib H, McConahey WM, Tiegs RD et al. Medullary thyroid carcinoma: clinicopathologic features and long-term follow-up of 65 patients treated during 1946 through 1970. *Mayo Clin Proc* 1992; **67**(10): 934–40.

240. Forrest CH, Frost FA, de Boer WB et al. Medullary carcinoma of the thyroid: accuracy of diagnosis of fine-needle aspiration cytology. *Cancer* 1998; **84**(5): 295–302.

241. Kini SR, Miller JM, Hamburger JI, Smith MJ. Cytopathologic features of medullary carcinoma of the thyroid. *Arch Pathol Lab Med* 1984; **108**(2): 156–9.

242. Bauman A, Strawbridge HT, Bauman WA. The clinical value of fine needle aspiration biopsy in a patient with medullary thyroid carcinoma and pseudofollicular carcinoma. *N Y State J Med* 1989; **89**(9): 527–9.

243. Zeppa P, Vetrani A, Marino M et al. Fine needle aspiration cytology of medullary thyroid carcinoma: a review of 18 cases. *Cytopathology* 1990; **1**(1): 35–44.

244. Collins BT, Cramer HM, Tabatowski K et al. Fine needle aspiration of medullary carcinoma of the thyroid. Cytomorphology, immunocytochemistry and electron microscopy. *Acta Cytol* 1995; **39**(5): 920–30.

245. Gomez-Fernandez C, Kraemer HJ, Ganjei P. Metastatic medullary thyroid carcinoma in liver diagnosis by aspiration cytology. *Diagn Cytopathol* 1994; **11**(3): 277–80.

246. Kaur A, Jayaram G. Thyroid tumors: cytomorphology of medullary, clinically anaplastic, and miscellaneous thyroid neoplasms [see comments]. *Diagn Cytopathol* 1990; **6**(6): 383–9.

247. Aulicino MR, Szporn AH, Dembitzer R et al. Cytologic findings in the differential diagnosis of C-cell hyperplasia and medullary carcinoma by fine needle aspiration. A case report. *Acta Cytol* 1998; **42**(4): 963–7.

248. O'Neill JP, Shaha AR. Anaplastic thyroid cancer. *Oral Oncol.* 2013 Jul; **49**(7): 702–6.

249. Brooke PK, Hameed M, Zakowski MF. Fine-needle aspiration of anaplastic thyroid carcinoma with varied cytologic and histological patterns: a case report. *Diagn Cytopathol* 1994; **11**(1): 60–3.

250. Bauman ME, Tao LC. Cytopathology of papillary carcinoma of the thyroid with anaplastic transformation. A case report. *Acta Cytol* 1995; **39**(3): 525–9.

251. Dibelius G, Mehra S, Clain JB et al. Noninvasive anaplastic thyroid carcinoma: report of a case and literature review. *Thyroid.* 2014; **24**(8): 1319–24.

252. Us-Krasovec M, Golouh R, Auersperg M et al. Anaplastic thyroid carcinoma in fine needle aspirates. *Acta Cytol* 1996; **40**(5): 953–8.

253. Schneider V, Frable WJ. Spindle and giant cell carcinoma of the thyroid: cytologic diagnosis by fine needle aspiration. *Acta Cytol* 1980; **24**(3): 184–9.

254. Feng G, Laskin WB, Chou PM, Lin X. Anaplastic thyroid carcinoma with rhabdoid features. *Diagn Cytopathol.* 2015 Jan 22; **43**(5): 416–20.

255. Fehr-Merhof A, Flury R, Ruttimann S. From Hashimoto thyroiditis to B-cell lymphoma of the thyroid gland. *Schweiz Med Wochenschr* 1999; **129**(23): 883–9.

256. Scholefield JH, Quayle AR, Harris SC, Talbot CH. Primary lymphoma of the thyroid, the association with Hashimoto's thyroiditis. *Eur J Surg Oncol* 1992; **18**(2): 89–92.

257. Zeman V. Hashimoto's lymphocytic thyroiditis and simultaneous malignant tumors of the thyroid gland. *Vnitr Lek* 1979; **25**(4): 360–5.

258. Fenton JE, Stack J, Kelly P, TP OD. Lymphoma and Hashimoto's thyroiditis. *J Laryngol Otol* 1995; **109**(8): 781–3.

259. Paraf F, Brousse N. Primary lymphoma of the thyroid: terminology, diagnostic criteria and relationship to Hashimoto's thyroiditis [letter]. *Presse Med.* 1992; **21**(21): 997.

260. Matsuzuka F, Miyauchi A, Katayama S et al. Clinical aspects of primary thyroid lymphoma: diagnosis and treatment based on our experience of 119 cases. *Thyroid.* 1993; **3**(2): 93–9.

261. Anscombe AM, Wright DH. Primary malignant lymphoma of the thyroid–a tumour of mucosa-associated lymphoid tissue: review of seventy-six cases. *Histopathology* 1985; **9**(1): 81–97.

262. Nobuoka Y, Hirokawa M, Kuma S et al. Cytologic findings and differential diagnoses of primary thyroid MALT lymphoma with striking plasma cell differentiation and amyloid deposition. *Diagn Cytopathol.* 2014; **42**(1): 73–7.

263. Das DK, Gupta SK, Francis IM, Ahmed MS. Fine-needle aspiration cytology diagnosis of non-Hodgkin lymphoma of thyroid: a report of four cases. *Diagn Cytopathol* 1993; **9**(6): 639–45.

264. Matsuda M, Sone H, Koyama H, Ishiguro S. Fine-needle aspiration cytology of malignant lymphoma of the thyroid. *Diagn Cytopathol* 1987; **3**(3): 244–9.

265. Jayaram G, Rani S, Raina V et al. B cell lymphoma of the thyroid in Hashimoto's thyroiditis monitored by fine-needle aspiration cytology. *Diagn Cytopathol* 1990; **6**(2): 130–3.

266. Kossev P, Livolsi V. Lymphoid lesions of the thyroid: review in light of the revised European-American lymphoma classification and upcoming World Health Organization classification. *Thyroid* 1999; **9**(12): 1273–80.

267. Garcia Erce JA, Alvarez Alegret R, Damborenea Tajada J, et al. The limitations of fine-needle aspiration puncture in the diagnosis of primary thyroid lymphoma (letter; comment). *Rev Clin Esp* 1999; **199**(10): 693.

268. Zdziarska B, Zuk E, Listewnik M. A case of centroblastic lymphoma of the thyroid gland. *Pol Merkuriusz Lek* 1998; **4**(19): 29–31.

269. Kuma K, Matsuzuka F. Diagnosis and therapy of malignant thyroid lymphoma. *Nippon Naika Gakkai Zasshi* 1997; **86**(7): 1190–5.

270. Herranz MT, Corrales A, Molina MA, et al. Thyroid lymphoma in a 51-year-old woman. *An Med Interna* 1993; **10**(3): 132–4.

271. Detweiler RE, Katz RL, Alapat C et al. Malignant lymphoma of the thyroid: a report of two cases diagnosed by fine-needle aspiration. *Diagn Cytopathol* 1991; **7**(2): 163–71.

272. Takashima S, Tomiyama N, Morimoto S et al. Nonpalpable primary thyroid lymphoma diagnosed by ultrasound-guided fine needle biopsy. *J Clin Ultrasound* 1992; **20**(2): 142–5.

273. Frederiksen JK, Sharma M, Casulo C, Burack WR. Systematic review of the effectiveness of fine-needle aspiration and/or core needle biopsy for subclassifying lymphoma. *Arch Pathol Lab Med.* 2015 Feb; **139**(2): 245–51.

274. Matsuda M, Sone H, Koyama H et al. Needle aspiration cytology of malignant lymphoma of the thyroid. *Gan No Rinsho* 1987; **33**(1): 21–6.

275. Aozasa K, Takakuwa T. Differential diagnosis of Hashimoto's thyroiditis from thyroidal neoplastic diseases. *Nippon Rinsho* 1999; **57**(8): 1894–8.

276. Chacho MS, Greenebaum E, Moussouris HF, Schreiber K, Koss LG. Value of aspiration cytology of the thyroid in metastatic disease. *Acta Cytol* 1987; **31**(6): 705–12.

277. Lasser A, Rothman JG, Calamia VJ. Renal-cell carcinoma metastatic to the thyroid. Aspiration cytology and histological findings. *Acta Cytol* 1985; **29**(5): 856–8.

278. Smith SA, Gharib H, Goellner JR. Fine-needle aspiration. Usefulness for diagnosis and management of metastatic carcinoma to the thyroid. *Arch Intern Med* 1987; **147**(2): 311–2.

CHAPTER 4

Lymph nodes

Chapter contents

4.1   Introduction, 112
    4.1.1   Distribution of lymph node pathology, 112
    4.1.2   Diagnostic accuracy, 113
    4.1.3   Diagnostic pitfalls, 113
    4.1.4   Ancillary techniques, 113
        4.1.4.1   Flow cytometry, 114
        4.1.4.2   Molecular techniques, 116
    4.1.5   Core biopsy or FNAC?, 117
    4.1.6   Elastography or FNAC?, 117
4.2   Non-neoplastic lymphoproliferative conditions, 118
    4.2.1   Follicular hyperplasia, 118
    4.2.2   Sinus histiocytosis with massive lymphadenopathy
        (Rosai Dorfman), 119
    4.2.3   Granulomatous lymphadenitis, 122
        4.2.3.1   Mycobacterial infection, 122
        4.2.3.2   Cat scratch disease, 122
        4.2.3.3   Fungal diseases (mycoses), 125
        4.2.3.4   Toxoplasmosis, 126
        4.2.3.5   Leishmaniasis, 127
    4.2.4   Chronic lymphadenitis, 128
        4.2.4.1   Kikuchi's lymphadenitis, 128
        4.2.4.2   Infectious mononucleosis, 128
        4.2.4.3   Acquired immunodeficiency
                syndrome (AIDS), 130
    4.2.5   Drug reactions, 131
    4.2.6   Miscellaneous lymphadenopathies, 131
        4.2.6.1   Castleman's disease, 131
        4.2.6.2   Langerhans cell histiocytosis, 132
        4.2.6.3   Post-transplant lymphadenopathy, 135
        4.2.6.4   Kimura's disease, 135
4.3   Hodgkin's lymphoma, 137
    4.3.1   Nodular Lymphocyte Predominant Hodgkin's lymphoma, 139
4.4   Non-Hodgkin's lymphoma, 139
    4.4.1   Introduction, 139
    4.4.2   Obtaining appropriate material, 142
    4.4.3   Classification of Non-Hodgkin's lymphoma, 142
    4.4.4   Precursor lesions, 142
        4.4.4.1   Lymphoblastic leukaemia/
                lymphoma, 142
    4.4.5   B-cell lymphomas, 143
        4.4.5.1   B-cell small lymphocytic lymphoma, 143
        4.4.5.2   Lymphoplasmacytic lymphoma
                (immunocytoma), 144
    4.4.6   Mantle zone lymphoma, 144
    4.4.7   Follicular lymphoma, 147
    4.4.8   Marginal zone lymphoma (MALT type), 148
    4.4.9   Diffuse large B-cell lymphoma, 150
    4.4.10   Primary effusion lymphoma, 151
    4.4.11   Burkitt's lymphoma, 152
    4.4.12   T/NK-cell lymphomas, 154
        4.4.12.1   Peripheral T-cell lymphoma, 154
    4.4.13   Anaplastic large cell lymphoma, 154
4.5   Metastatic carcinoma in lymph nodes, 160
References, 170

4.1 Introduction

The role of imaging and FNAC in the initial diagnosis of primary lymphadenopathies is, *firstly*, to confirm that the lesion is a lymph node, *secondly*, to exclude metastatic disease or specific infection and, *thirdly*, to distinguish between benign and malignant lymphoid proliferations. Used in the proper setting, FNAC will provide a definitive diagnosis in the majority of cases, especially relating to lymphoid versus non-lymphoid pathology, metastatic disease and infection [1]. Whilst primary diagnosis of lymphoma by FNAC is still controversial, it is helpful in triaging the patients that may require biopsy (Fig. 4.1) [2]. Patients with a definitive cytological diagnosis may be spared unnecessary surgery and reviewed through follow up [3] (see Table 4.1).

4.1.1 Distribution of lymph node pathology

In the survey of 1043 FNAC specimens in a 10 year period in our practice, we have observed that patients most frequently presented with a lump of unknown origin, persistent lymphadenopathy, as a follow up of a known clinical condition or staging of a known malignant tumour. Of the specimens adequate for assessment (77%), the most commonly diagnosed categories were: metastatic carcinoma (34%), benign/reactive/inflammatory (31%) and lymphoma or suspicious of lymphoma (11%) [4].

Similarly, in a survey of the role of FNAC in Nigeria, Thomas et al. found that the most common diagnosis was reactive change/non-specific inflammation (33.4%), tuberculosis and metastatic lesions (25.7 and 22.4%, respectively) and lymphoma (16.9%) [5]. The survey from India showed tuberculous lymphadenitis as the most common finding (46.7%), reactive hyperplasia the commonest presentation (45%) in patients less than 20 years of age, malignancy accounted for 13.7% of cervical lymph node enlargement, most of which was due to metastatic squamous cell carcinoma (67.7%) [6]. Following the FNAC, biopsies were performed in the total of 20% of patients with adequate FNAC material. Biopsies were performed in 10% of reactive/inflammatory conditions and in 47% of lymphomas, both categories guided by the appropriate clinical setting and patient's history (Fig. 4.2).

Cytopathology of the Head and Neck: Ultrasound Guided FNAC, Second Edition. Gabrijela Kocjan.
© 2017 John Wiley & Sons Ltd. Published 2017 by John Wiley & Sons Ltd.
Companion website: www.wiley.com/go/kocjan/clinical_cytopathology_head_neck2e

4.1.2 Diagnostic accuracy

With an overall accuracy rate of 96–99% and a typing accuracy rate of 96.5%, FNAC yields a high rate of conclusive cytological diagnoses in the assessment of metastatic malignancies [4, 7–10], a high rate of conclusive diagnoses in the assessment of high grade non-Hodgkin's lymphomas (79–90%) and Hodgkin's disease (with the exception of the Nodular Lymphocytic Predominant variant), but has significant limitations in the assessment of low grade non-Hodgkin's lymphomas [4, 11, 12]. FNAC is also a useful and accurate adjunct for the evaluation of paediatric cervical lymphadenopathy [13]. FNAC should be part of the initial evaluation of paediatric patients with cervical lymphadenopathy before determining the treatment plan.

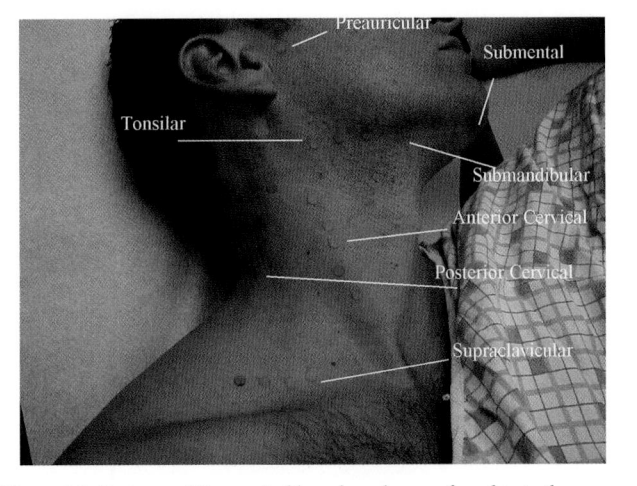

Figure 4.1 Anatomy of the cervical lymph nodes as referred to in the clinical communication.

4.1.3 Diagnostic pitfalls

Diagnostic pitfalls in FNAC of lymph nodes can broadly be listed into seven categories: differentiating low grade B- and T-cell lymphomas from reactive hyperplasia; distinguishing between the small lymphocytic lymphomas (lymphocytic lymphoma, mantle zone lymphoma, marginal zone lymphoma, lymphocyte predominant Hodgkin's disease, progressive transformation of lymph nodes); overlooking lymphoma when metastases are suspected; Hodgkin's disease (lymphocyte depleted) versus anaplastic large cell (Ki-1, CD30 positive) lymphoma; Ki-1 anaplastic large cell lymphoma versus other non-lymphoid tumours; lymphoma versus other malignancies and problems with immunophenotyping [14, 15]. The most commonly encountered diagnostic difficulty is in distinguishing low-grade lymphoma from reactive hyperplasia. This is particularly evident in follicular lymphomas. In the case of low grade non-Hodgkin's lymphomas, morphological and immunocytochemical methods need to be supplemented by flow cytometry, evaluation of proliferative activity by Ki-67 and molecular techniques in order to achieve conclusive diagnoses [14].

4.1.4 Ancillary techniques

Immunocytochemistry. Immunocytochemical studies performed on FNAC material in conjunction with the cytological diagnosis lead to an increase in diagnostic accuracy as well as providing means for sub-classification of neoplastic lymphoid cells. This technique gives results comparable to those obtained by histopathological and immunohistochemical analysis on surgically removed lymph nodes [16]. Apart from phenotypic markers, proliferation markers appear to predict biological behaviour and responses to therapy in NHL. Antibody against Ki-67, a marker for cycling cells, measured by either visual scoring or image analysis,

Table 4.1 Algorithm of management following FNAC of lymph nodes.

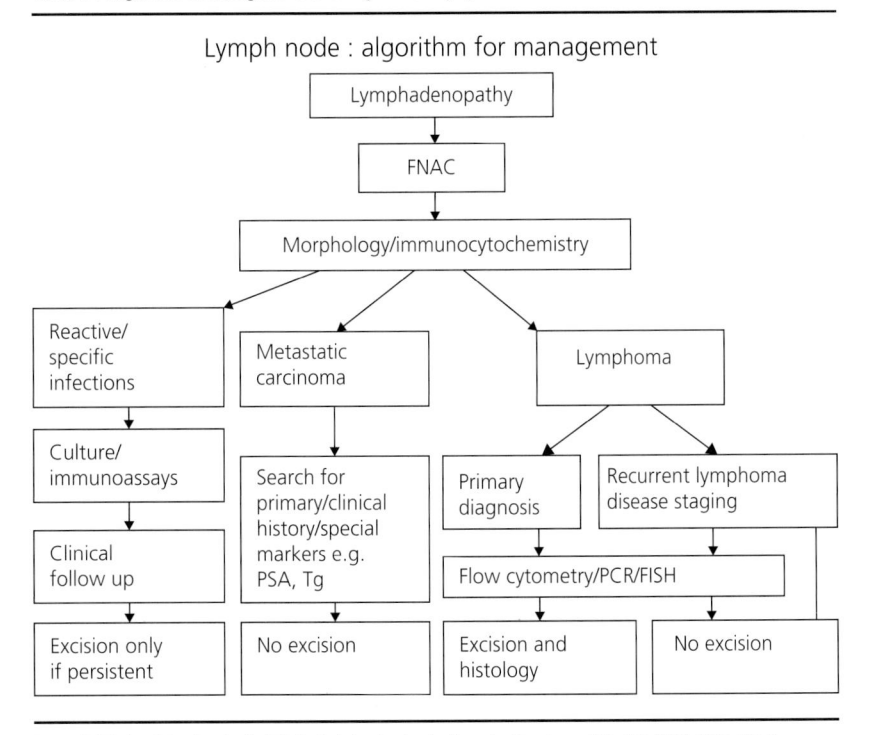

Source: [3a] Kocjan G. Best Practice No 185. Cytological and molecular diagnosis of lymphoma. *J Clin Pathol* 2005; **58**(6): 561–7.

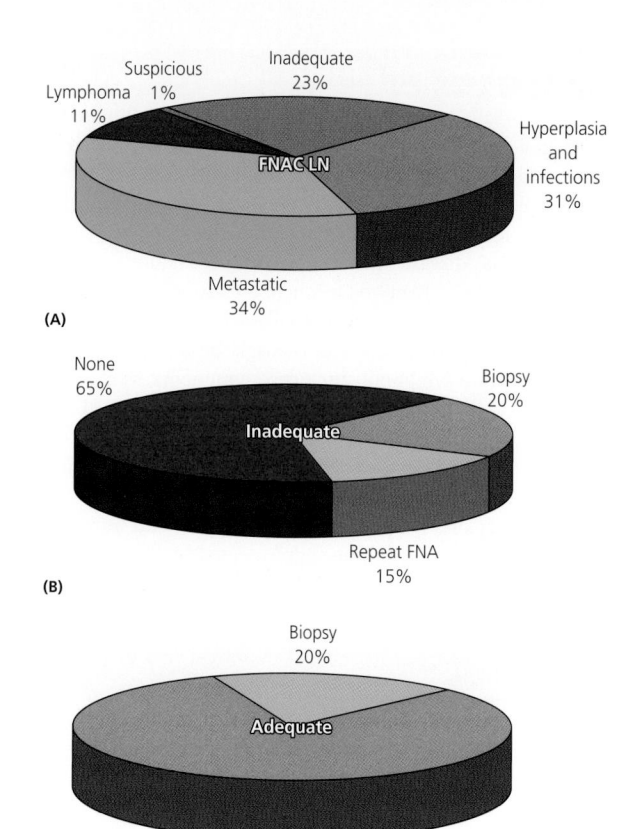

(A)

(B)

(C)

Figure 4.2 (A) Relative proportions of FNAC diagnoses in a survey of 1043 FNAC of lymph nodes in the past 10 years at University College London Hospitals. Metastatic carcinoma and hyperplasias/infections represent the majority of lymph node FNAC diagnoses. (B) Management of inadequate FNAC: Total 234 (23%). Repeat FNAC 15%, biopsy 20% and follow up 65%. (C) Total number of LN biopsies avoided by the use of FNAC (total no = 1043). Biopsy was avoided in 80% of patients with adequate FNAC.

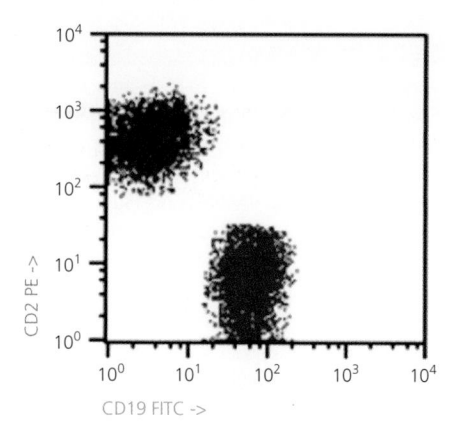

Figure 4.3 Flow cytometry of a lymph node aspirate. B (CD19) and T (CD2) lymphocytes. Modified from Barroca H, Marques C, Candeias J. Fine needle aspiration cytology diagnosis, flow cytometry immunophenotyping and histology in clinically suspected lymphoproliferative disorder: a comparative study. *Acta Cytol.* 2008; **52**(2): 124–32 [27a].

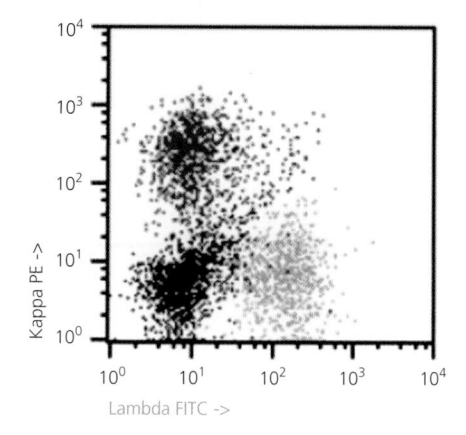

Figure 4.4 Kappa (violet) and lambda (yellow) light chain. The B population is polyclonal, with a normal ratio (red = B-lymphocytes, blue = T-lymphocytes). Modified from Barroca H, Marques C, Candeias J. Fine needle aspiration cytology diagnosis, flow cytometry immunophenotyping and histology in clinically suspected lymphoproliferative disorder: a comparative study. *Acta Cytol.* 2008 Mar-Apr; **52**(2): 124–32 [27a].

correlates positively with increasing grade of lymphoma [17]. The excellent correlation between histological and cytological preparations indicates that FNAC material is suitable for the immunocytochemical assessment of the growth fraction of NHL [11, 18]. Immunophenotyping facilitates patient management in the setting of the recurrence or suspected recurrence of a known lymphoproliferative disorder [19].

4.1.4.1 Flow cytometry

Immunophenotyping can be accomplished via immunocytochemistry or flow cytometry [20, 21]. In the experience of Simsir et al., 85% of the cases were immunophenotyped by both techniques. The advantage of immunocytochemistry is the preservation of cytomorphology, particularly in cases with very few well preserved cells. The advantages of flow cytometry are in the detection of a small population of monoclonal cells in a background of reactive cells (particularly useful in effusion samples in which the predominant cell population is often reactive T lymphocytes), in the increased diagnostic precision through evaluation of objective parameters, and in the use of multiple markers with dual labelling. Flow cytometry enables clonality analysis and immunophenotyping and is therefore a helpful addition in the diagnosis and classification of reactive lymphoid hyperplasia and malignant

lymphoma [22, 23]. Zeppa et al. found the sensitivity, specificity, PPV and NPV of FNAC combined with flow cytometry in differentiating malignant and benign lymphoproliferations to be 73.9, 83.3, 94.4 and 45.5%, respectively [24–26].

Clonality analysis is achieved measuring the immunoglobulin light chain ratio (LCR). Reactive lymphoid hyperplasia is polyclonal by FCM (LCR < 2/1). Most of B-cell non-Hodgkin's lymphoma are monoclonal (LCR > 3/1) [27] (Figs 4.3–4.7). Analysis of CD5, CD10 and CD23 expression by flow cytometry enables subclassification of mantle cell lymphoma, small lymphocytic lymphoma and some lymphomas of follicle centre cell origin [27–29]. When comparing the cytospin analysis and flow cytometry, both appear equally capable of immunotyping aspirated lymphoid samples reliably [22, 29–32]. The successful primary classification of most intra-abdominal non-Hodgkin's lymphomas can be achieved with a combination of cytology and flow cytometry, and this can be the initial approach in patients with deep-seated lesions [33].

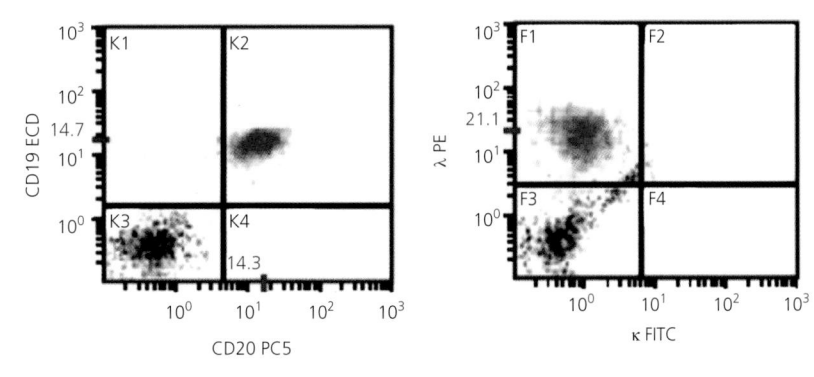

Figure 4.5 Flow cytometric histograms gated on lymphocytes of classic chronic lymphocytic leukemia (CLL). Classic CLL cases show dim CD20 and dim light chain expression. Modified from Ho AK, Hill S, Preobrazhensky SN, Miller ME, Chen Z, Bahler DW. Small B-cell neoplasms with typical mantle cell lymphoma immunophenotypes often include chronic lymphocytic leukemias. *Am J Clin Pathol.* 2009 Jan; **131**(1): 27–32 [27b].

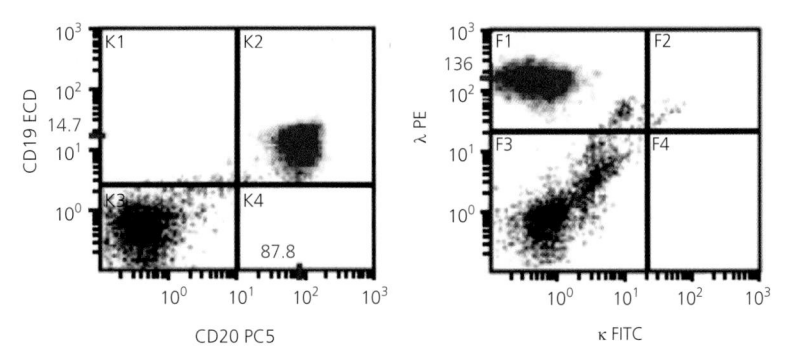

Figure 4.6 Flow cytometric histograms gated on lymphocytes of typical mantle cell lymphoma (MCL) Strong CD20 and light chain expression compared with dim expression of these antigens in CLL (see Fig. 4.5). Modified from Ho AK, Hill S, Preobrazhensky SN, Miller ME, Chen Z, Bahler DW. Small B-cellneoplasms with typical mantle cell lymphoma immunophenotypes often include chronic lymphocytic leukemias. *Am J Clin Pathol.* 2009; **131**(1): 27–32 [27b].

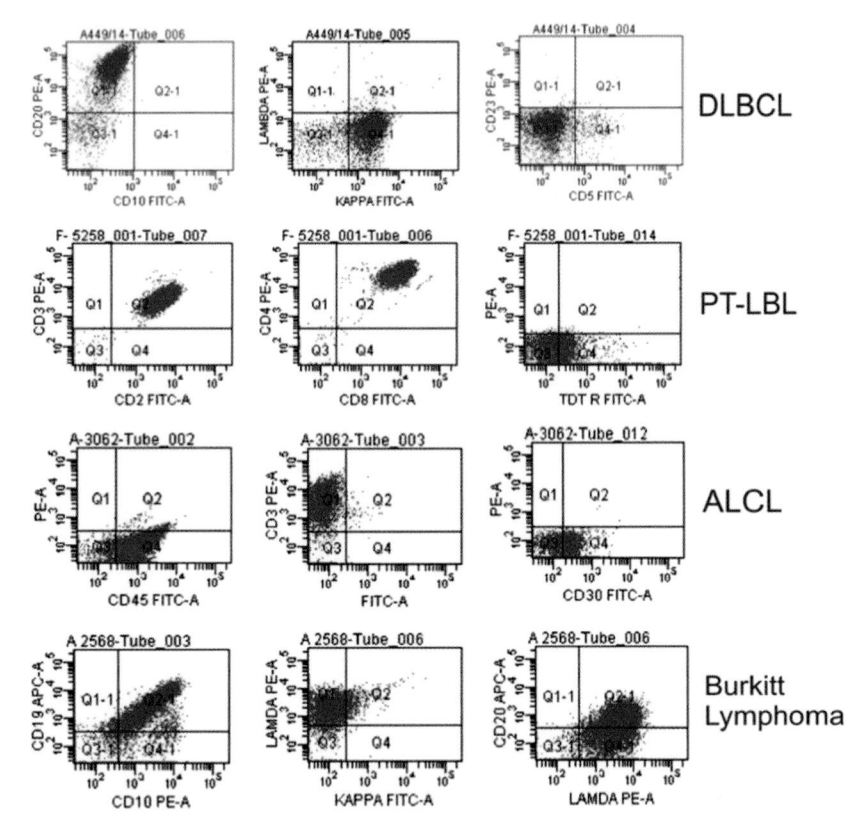

Figure 4.7 Flow cytometry histograms for Diffuse Large B cell lymphoma (DLBL) shows CD20+/kappa+, Precursor T lymphoblastic lymphoma (PT-LBL) shows CD2+/CD3+/CD5+/dual CD4 and 8+/TdT+, Anaplastic Large cell Lymphoma (ALCL) shows CD45+/CD30+ and Burkitt's lymphoma shows CD19+/CD10+/CD20+/lambda+. Image and text Modified from Paul T, Gautam U, Rajwanshi A, Das A, Trehan A, Malhotra P, Srinivasan R. Flow cytometric immunophenotyping and cell block immunocytochemistry in the diagnosis of primary Non-Hodgkin's Lymphoma by fine-needle aspiration: Experience from a tertiary care center. *J Cytol.* 2014 Jul; **31**(3): 123–30 [27c].

4.1.4.2 Molecular techniques

Polymerase chain reaction (PCR) The application of polymerase chain reaction (PCR) to cytological material can be used to identify monoclonal rearrangements of the immunoglobulin heavy chain gene, T-cell receptor and translocations involving the bcl-1 and bcl-2 genes [34, 35]. The detection rate of the t(14;18), the most common translocation in B-cell lymphomas, which results in rearrangement of the immunoglobulin heavy chain and BCL2 genes, has been examined in fresh and archival cytological smears (Fig. 4.8) [36–38]. The results of the technique on FNAC material are highly comparable to those in excision biopsies [39]. The infrequent identification of monoclonal rearrangements and translocations in reactive processes requires cautious application of molecular data [38, 39]. Bogdanic et al showed that FNAC can be used for morphological, molecular and cytogenetic diagnosis of lymphoma with atypical clinical presentation [39a]. Genotyping by antigen-receptor gene rearrangement appears to be redundant in cases with mature B-cell phenotypes that demonstrate monoclonality by immunophenotyping [40].

More recently, human herpesvirus-8 (HHV-8) has been identified by PCR amplification of DNA from FNAC samples isolated from various forms of KS. All of the cases diagnosed as KS and 1 of the lymphoid hyperplasia cases were PCR-positive for HHV-8 DNA, while all other cases of spindle-cell lesions were negative. The

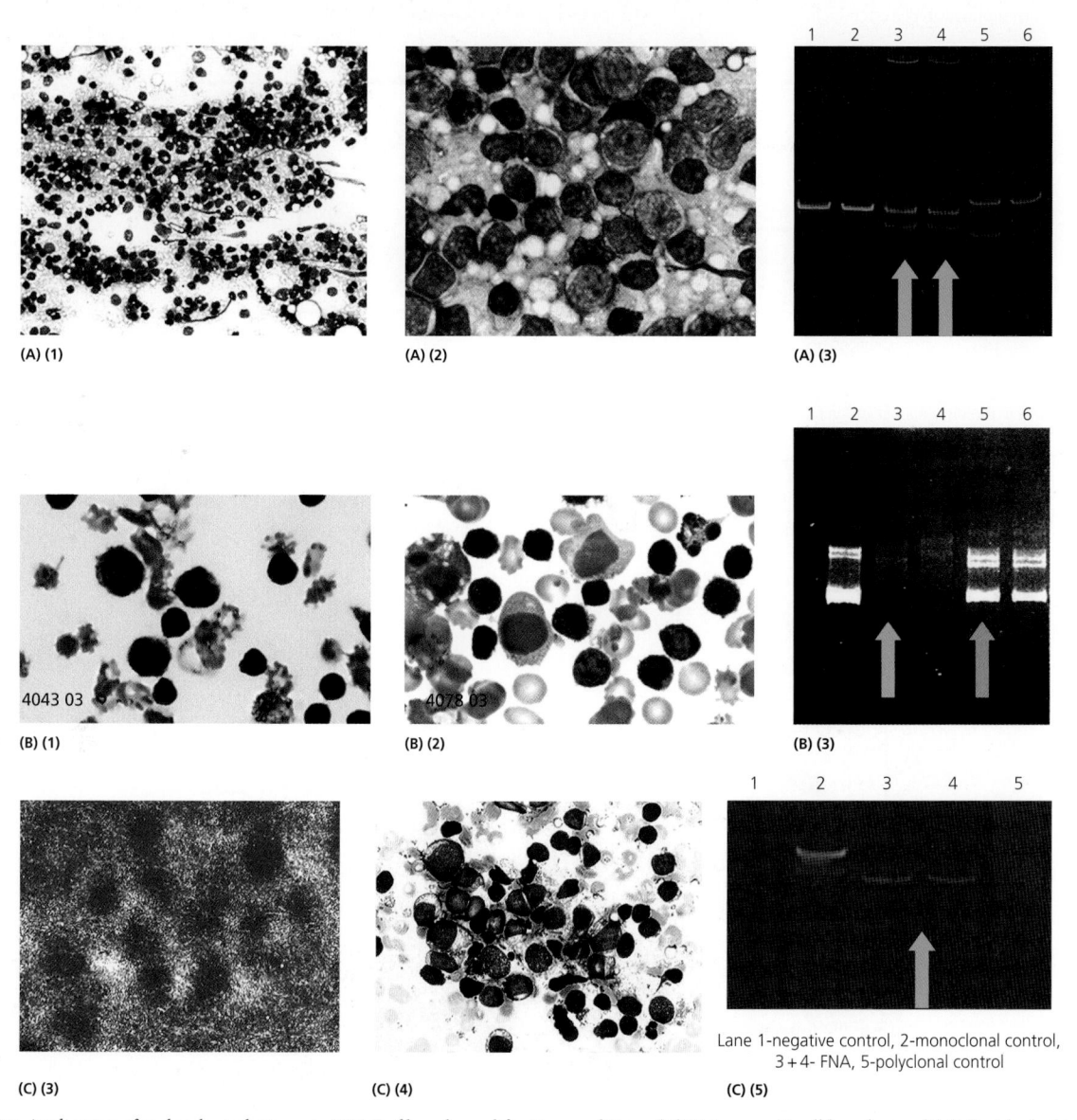

(A) (1)   (A) (2)   (A) (3)

(B) (1)   (B) (2)   (B) (3)

(C) (3)   (C) (4)   Lane 1-negative control, 2-monoclonal control,
3 + 4- FNA, 5-polyclonal control

(C) (5)

Figure 4.8 Application of molecular techniques to FNAC of lymphoproliferative conditions. (A) Cutaneous T-cell lymphoma. (1) Patient had a history of T-cell cutaneous NHL, now presents with a nodule in the buttock and forearm. Low power appearances of the FNA sample show a mixture of lymphoid cells (MGG ×400). (2) High power view shows medium size lymphocytes admixed with follicle centre cells (MGG ×600, oil immersion). (3) PCR amplification of TCR-gamma chain gene shows a biallelic rearrangement (lanes 3 and 4), confirming the presence of neoplastic clone(s).
(B) Follicular lymphoma. Two patients with pleural effusions, both with the previous history of follicular lymphoma. Now there is suspected recurrence. (1) Case one. Small and medium size lymphocytes. (2) Case two. A mixture of small and medium size lymphocytes. (MGG ×600, oil immersion). (3) PCR shows a background smear in Case one (4043 03) (lanes 2 and 3, green arrow) and amplification of IGH in case two (4078/03) (lanes 4 and 5, orange arrow). (C) MALT lymphoma. (3) FNA smear showing dense population of lymphoid cells with prominence of residual follicle centre fragments. (4) High power view shows a monotonous population of centrocyte like cells. (5) PCR of IgH shows monoclonal band confirming the diagnosis.

molecular demonstration of HHV-8 DNA may be a useful adjunct in the diagnosis of KS by FNAC [41].

In situ hybridisation. Southern blot analysis is a useful technique for establishing tumour cell lineage, clonality, and the presence of oncogene rearrangements in fine-needle aspiration specimens of NHL [42]. The assessment of immunoglobulin light chain expression is a useful adjunct to morphology of reactive and malignant lymphoid proliferations [43].

The relative contribution of immunocytochemistry, in situ hybridisation for immunoglobulin light chain mRNA, and polymerase chain reaction for immunoglobulin heavy chain gene rearrangement, towards the final clinicopathological diagnosis is estimated to be: Immunocytochemistry 86%, in situ hybridisation 77%, PCR in 62%. With the help of ancillary techniques, FNAC cytology accurately distinguished reactive lymphoid hyperplasia from malignant lymphoma in 97% of cases [44]. The sensitivity of PCR and FNAC in diagnosis of neoplastic B-cell proliferations was 92 and 78%, respectively [45].

4.1.5 Core biopsy or FNAC?

The World Health Organization system for lymphoma classification relies on histological findings from excisional biopsies [46]. In contrast to expert guidelines, clinicians increasingly rely on FNAC and core needle biopsies (CNB) rather than excisional biopsies to diagnose lymphomas. Like other initially competing methods, FNAC and core needle biopsy (CNB) have achieved not only individual but also combined utility in the diagnosis of mass lesions. Frederiksen et al. reviewed 42 studies published in the literature concerning the use of FNAC/CNB to diagnose and sub-classify lymphoma, focusing on the rate at which these methods result in full sub-classification of lymphomas adequate to guide subsequent management (Table 4.2) [47]. They found the median rate at which FNAC and CNB yielded a subtype-specific diagnosis of lymphoma was 74%. Strictly adhering to expert guidelines, which state that follicular lymphoma cannot be graded by these techniques, decreased the diagnostic yield further to 66%. Thus, 25–35% of FNAC and/or CNB of nodes must be followed by an excisional lymph node biopsy to fully classify lymphoma [48–87].

In the setting of recurrent lymphoma, a specific sub-classification is often not needed to guide therapy. Including less-specific lymphoma diagnoses as actionable increases the median actionable diagnosis rate to 87%. When comparing FNAC and CNB in the Head and Neck, the *sensitivity* of the FNAC-group (85%) compared to the CNB-group (80%), the *negative predictive value* (92 vs 71%) and also the *false negative value* of the FNAC (5 vs 13%) were superior to the results of the CNB-group [88]. However, the *specificity* (87 vs 94%) as well as the *positive predictive value* (64 vs 97%) was lower for FNAC then for CNB. A useful use of both methods is when the pathologist is called upon to assist a radiologist in the minimally invasive retrieval of tissue for diagnosis, FNAC is done initially for adequacy assessment, followed by CNB, only if (based on adequacy assessment) additional tissue is needed. This is an efficient and cost-effective approach that also parallels a recent shift in the literature from the almost exclusive advocation of CNB over FNAC to a renewed recognition of the benefits of FNAC, including the value of FNAC compared to, and combined or in tandem with, CNB [89]. In our own experience, 33.5% of the patients who had an initial FNAC had a subsequent CNB with an overall sensitivity of 85 versus 68%,

Table 4.2 Diagnosis of lymphoma by FNAC and core needle biopsy.

Study	FNAC	CNB	IHC/ICC	FC	FISH	CG/MD
Liemark et al, [48] 1989	X		X			
Sneige et al, [49] 1990	X		X			
Sneige et al, [50] 1991	X		X	X		
Sapia et al, [51] 1995	X			X		
Ben-Yehuda et al, [52] 1996		X	X			
Hughes et al, [53] 1998	X		X	X		
Jeffers et al, [54] 1998	X			X		CG
Young et al, [55] 1998	X			X		
Ravinsky et al, [56] 1999	X			X		
Mayall et al, [57] 2000	X		X	X		
Meda et al, [58] 2000	X			X		
Siebert et al, [59] 2000	X	X	X	X		
Demharter et al, [60] 2001		X	X			
Dong et al, [61] 2001	X			X		
Liu et al, [62] 2001	X			X		
Ribeiro et al, [63] 2001	X		X	X		
Mourad et al, [64] 2003	X			X		
Zeppa et al, [65] 2004	X		X	X	X	
Landgren et al, [66] 2004	X		X			
Hehn et al, [67] 2004	X		X	X		
Gong et al, [68] 2004	X	X	X	X		
Ravinsky et al, [69] 2005	X	X	X	X		
Li et al, [70] 2005		X	X			
Dey et al, [71] 2006	X			X		
Mathiot et al, [72] 2006	X			X		CG
Venkatraman et al, [73] 2006	X		X			MD
De Kerviler et al, [74] 2007		X	X			MD
De Larrinoa et al, [75] 2007		X	X			MD
Lachar et al, [76] 2007		X	X	X		MD
Barroca et al, [27a] 2008	X		X	X		
Loubeyre et al, [77] 2009		X	X	X	X	MD
Pfeiffer et al, [78] 2009		X	X			
Huang et al, [79] 2010		X	X			
Kuveždić et al, [80] 2010	X		X			
Pedote et al, [81] 2010		X	X			
Senjug et al, [82] 2010	X			X		
Yuan and Li, [83] 2010		X	X			
Zeppa et al, [24] 2010	X			X		
Amador-Ortiz et al, [84] 2011	X	X	X	X	X	MD
Burke et al, [85] 2011	X	X				
Metzgeroth et al, [86] 2012	X	X	X	X		
Stacchini et al, [87] 2012	X		X	X		

Abbreviations: CG, cytogenetics; CNB, core needle biopsy; FC, flow cytometry; FISH, fluorescence in situ hybridization; FNAC, fine-needle aspiration cytology; IHC/ICC, immunohistochemistry/immunocytochemistry; MD, molecular diagnostics.
Source: Frederiksen JK et al. *Arch Pathol Lab Med.* 2015; 139: 245–51 [47].

specificity of 91 versus 81%, a PPV of 93 versus 87% and a NPV of 74 versus 59% [4].

The choice of FNAC/CNB or excisional biopsy is guided by numerous considerations, which include reliability (will there be a definitive diagnosis?), accuracy (will the diagnosis be correct?), turnaround time (is a diagnosis needed urgently?), morbidity, cost-effectiveness, and patient compliance. FNAC/CNB yields a definitive diagnosis about 65–75% of the time [47]. Therefore, in about a quarter of cases, FNAC/CNB will fail to yield an actionable diagnosis, in turn further delaying therapy.

4.1.6 Elastography or FNAC?

Elastography is an imaging technique aiming to obtain a 'virtual biopsy' by assessing differences in elasticity between the normal and pathological – usually malignant – tissue. However, Popescu et al. conclude that elastography is not yet ready to replace FNAC in

its indications, but should complement it in various settings, especially for the assessment of lymph nodes, particularly in situations where FNAC is regarded as a contraindication [90].

4.2 Non-neoplastic lymphoproliferative conditions

4.2.1 Follicular hyperplasia

Lymph nodes of the head and neck are often the site of lymph node enlargement. This may be as a response to known local antigenic stimuli, for example tonsillitis, or part of generalised lymphadenopathy due to systemic disease, for example rheumatoid arthritis (Fig. 4.9). In follicular hypeplasia, lymph node follicles increase both in size and in number. Enlarged germinal centres may contain mitoses and tingible body macrophages as a result of high cell turnover.

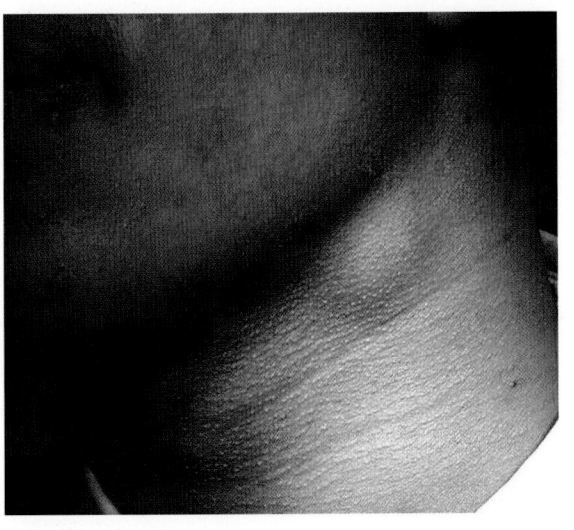

Figure 4.9 Lymph node hyperplasia. 23-year-old patient presented with a history of 1 month's swelling in the left side of the neck. Clinically, it was mobile and soft. Patient was referred to the FNAC clinic for investigation.

[See BOX 4.1. Summary of ultrasound features: Normal (reactive) lymph node on www.wiley.com/go/kocjan/clinical_cytopathology_head_neck2e]

Cytological features. FNAC material from an enlarged lymph node reflects germinal centres ('secondary follicles') that are often present in large numbers and are seen as residual follicle centre fragments (RFCF) (Fig. 4.10A, B). These aggregates are centred around dendritic reticulum cells (follicular dendritic cells) and are composed mainly of centroblasts and centrocytes (Fig. 4.11). Centroblasts are large round cells with a thin rim of evenly spaced basophilic cytoplasm (MGG) and nucleus containing several visible nucleoli. Centrocytes are smaller than centroblasts and contain irregularly shaped nuclei with coarse chromatin and nucleoli and large, ill-defined interlacing cytoplasm that appears to encompass the RFCFs. This is particularly well visible on medium power view at the initial screen. Folliclular dendritic cells have oval nuclei, prominent nucleoli and ill-defined interlacing cytoplasm which appears to encompass RFCFs. These areas stand out as pale blue zones (MGG) in whose network the concentration of follicle centre cells is seen. Their presence can be confirmed with immunocytochemistry (CD21) (Fig. 4.12). The non-lymphoid cells in the lymph node, sinus macrophages and tingible body macrophages are also seen. Hyperplastic germinal centres often contain plasma cells and immunoblasts, sometimes in large numbers (Figs 4.13 and 4.14). In cases of protracted follicular hyperplasia, enlarged germinal centres appear to disintegrate. The expanded node is occupied mainly by small lymphocytes and some larger lymphocytes. This process is known as 'progressive transformation of germinal centres'.

Morphological distinction between reactive lymph node hyperplasia and low-grade non- Hodgkin's lymphoma is the most difficult area in lymph node FNAC. Diagnosis of low grade lymphoma on cytological preparations is based on finding of a monotonous cell population of lymphoid cells as contrasted with the typically polymorphous population seen in reactive proliferations [91, 92]. Potential errors may occur when reactive conditions appear to contain atypical cells or when lymphomas contain admixture of cells. For this reason, excision biopsy is advised in case of an inappropriately persisting lymphadenopathy for which no cause can be found (Table 4.1).

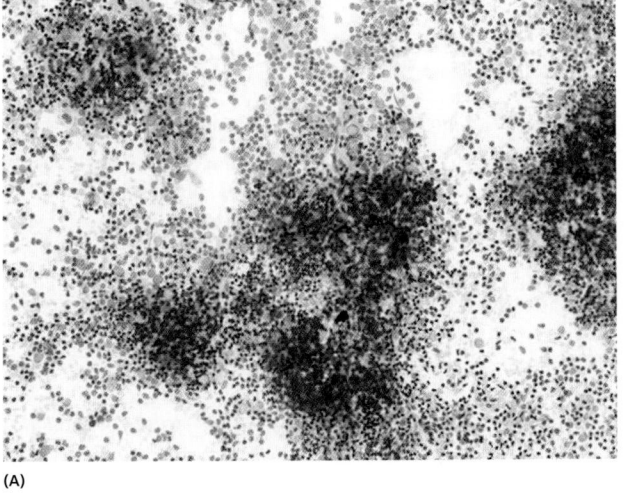

(A)

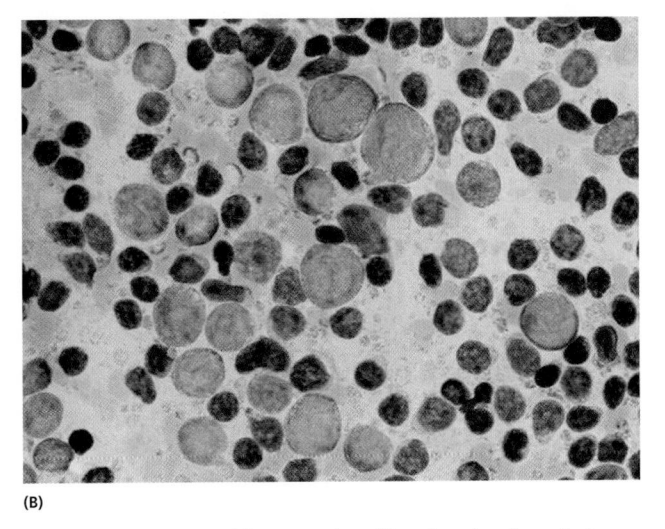

(B)

Figure 4.10 Lymph node hyperplasia. Patient from Fig. 4.9. (A) Low magnification of the FNAC material from an enlarged lymph node reflects the large germinal centres ('secondary follicles'), which are often present in large numbers and are seen as residual follicle centre fragments (RFCF). These aggregates are centred around dendritic reticulum cells (follicular dendritic cells). (B) Higher power reveals residual follicle centre fragment with centrocytes and centroblasts.

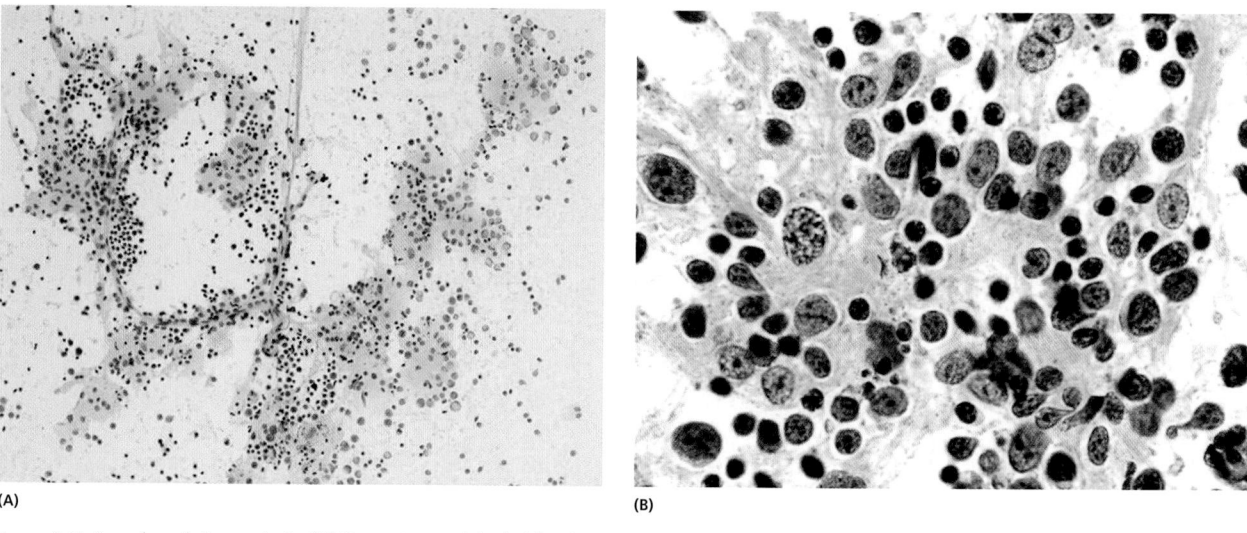

Figure 4.11 Lymph node hyperplasia. (A) Pap staining of alcohol fixed preparations shows residual follicle centre fragment aggregates are centred around dendritic reticulum cells (follicular dendritic cells). (B) RFCF-s are composed mainly of centroblasts and centrocytes. Centroblasts are large round cells with a thin rim of evenly spaced cytoplasm and nucleus containing several visible nucleoli. Centrocytes are smaller than centroblasts and contain irregularly shaped nuclei with coarse chromatin and thin rim of cytoplasm. Follicular dendritic cells have oval nuclei, prominent nucleoli and large, ill-defined interlacing cytoplasm.

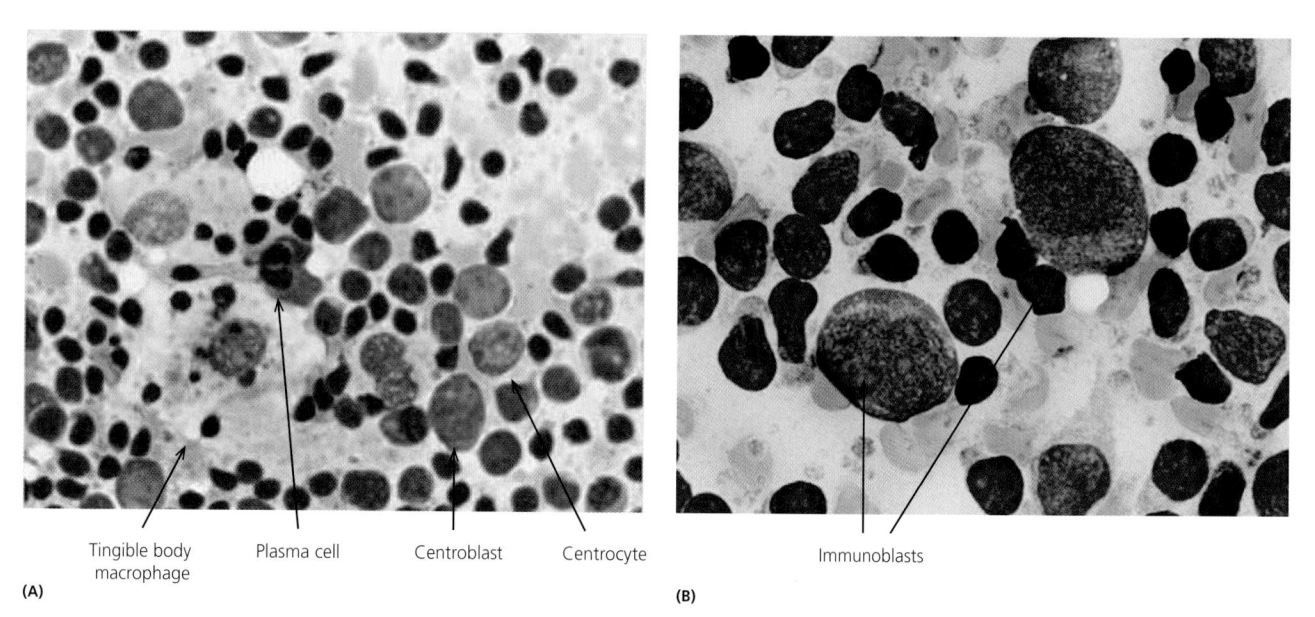

Figure 4.12 Lymph node hyperplasia. (A) Tingible body macrophages, plasma cells, centroblasts and centrocytes form a follicle centre fragment. (B) Immunoblasts are large cells with eccentric nuclei and may have prominent nucleoli.

On the other hand, cytological diagnosis of lymph node hyperplasia, in an appropriate clinical setting, supports conservative management in many cases and reduces the need for biopsy [44].

4.2.2 Sinus histiocytosis with massive lymphadenopathy (Rosai Dorfman)

Sinus histiocytosis with massive lymphadenopathy (SHML) is an uncommon entity of unknown aetiology affecting lymph nodes and extranodal sites (Table 4.3). Originally, it was described as occurring in young males. Since then, over 423 histologically proven cases of SHML have been documented, including many extranodal sites. Sinuses of affected lymph nodes (usually cervical) are filled with very large distinctive macrophages, frequently containing engulfed lymphocytes in their cytoplasm. The condition is self-limiting but lymphadenopathy may persist for a long time. It is more common in black people.

Cytological features of SHML include increased numbers of large, non-cohesive histiocytes associated with a polymorphous, cellular background composed of mixed small mature lymphocytes and plasma cells (Fig. 4.15). The large histiocytes (120–150 μm) have oval nuclei with smooth nuclear contour, one or two small but distinct nucleoli, abundant foamy cytoplasm and well defined cytoplasmic margins. Many histiocytes contain lymphocytes, red cells or plasma cells in their cytoplasm [93]. Lymphophagocytosis (emperipolesis) is a prominent feature [94–98]. Emperipolesis is emphasised by a halo around the lymphocyte and fine vacuoles in the cytoplasm. Identification of an

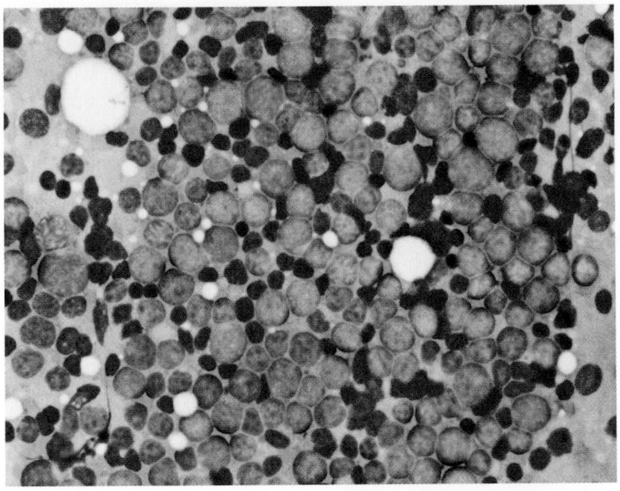

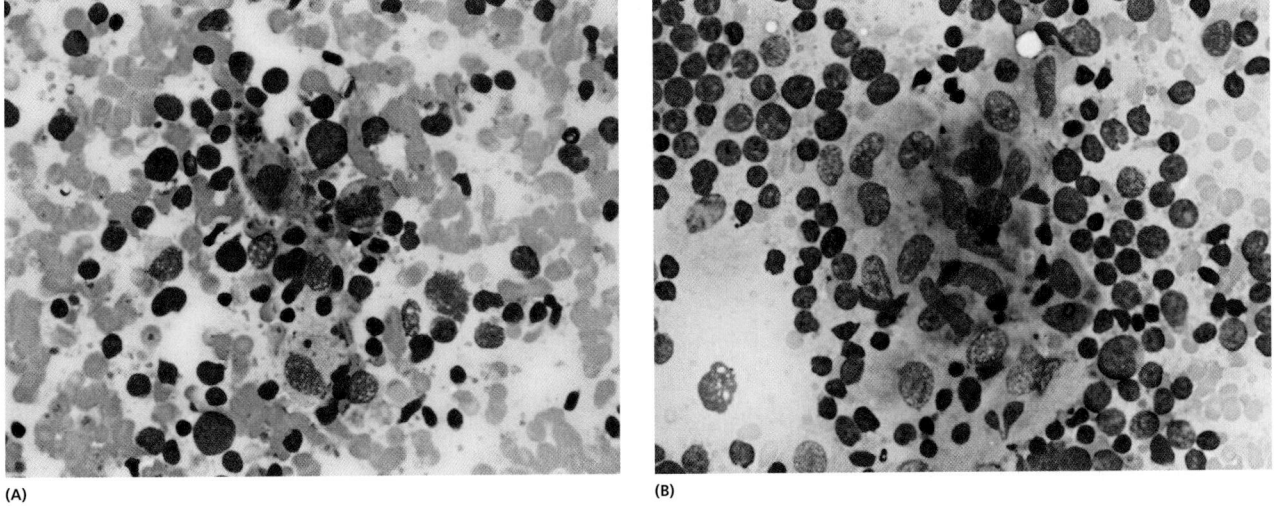

Figure 4.13 Lymph node hyperplasia. (A) Hyperplastic lymph node may look at first glance very monotonous, particularly in cases of interfollicular hyperplasia. (B) Capillary meshwork. (C) Prominent endothelium should not be mistaken for metastatic disease.

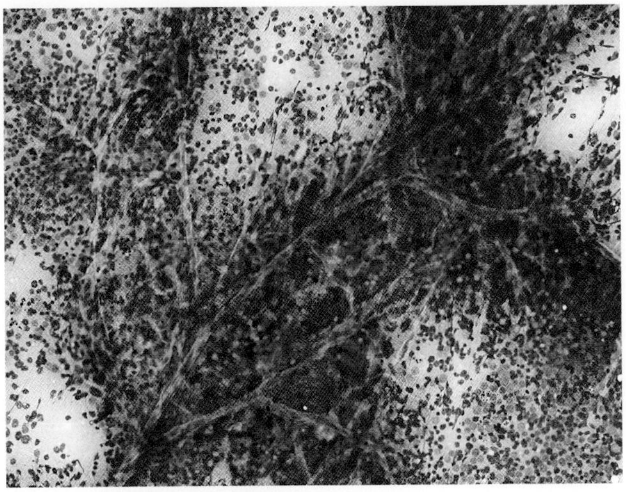

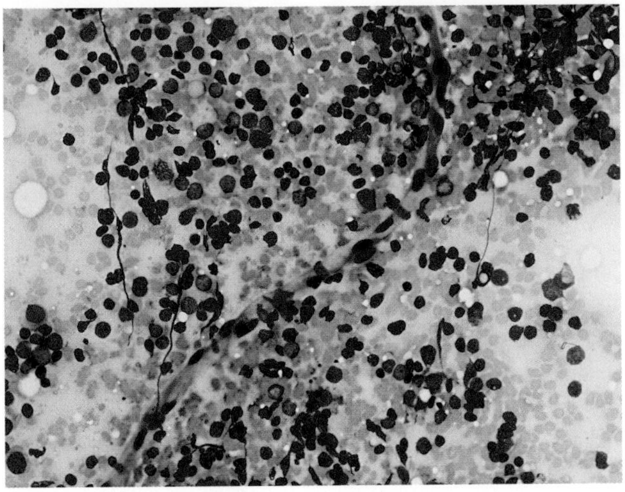

Figure 4.14 Lymph node hyperplasia. (A) Residual follicle centre fragments may show mitotic figures in the follicular dendritic cells. (B) Follicular dendritic cells may be difficult to distinguish from epithelioid cells forming a granuloma. CD21 and CD68, respectively, may be used to distinguish the two.

Table 4.3 Review of main benign, noninfectious causes of lymphadenopathy: clinical features and cytomorphology. (Source: Monaco SE, Khalbuss WE, Pantanowitz L. Benign non-infectious causes of lymphadenopathy. *Diagn Cytopathol*. 2012; 40: 925–38.) [93a]

Diagnosis	Clinical features	Cytomorphology
Histiocytic necrotizing lymphadenitis (Kikuchi-Fujimoto disease and Kikuchi disease)	Frequency in young Asian women Sx: Painless cervical lymphadenopathy, fever, and night sweats	Necrotizing lymphadenopathy with prominent Karyorrhectic debris Absence of neutrophils in the background Two characteristic cell types present: macrophages with crescent-shaped nuclei and plasmacytoid dendritic cells
Kimura disease	Usually male patients with painless lymphadenopathy Mainly in the head and neck region and associated with eosinophilia	Reactive lymphoid hyperplasia with Warth in-Finkeldey-type multinucleated giant cells Background of numerous eosinophils
Sinus histiocytosis with massive lymphadenopathy (SHML and Rosai-Dorfman disease)	Young patients with bilateral, painless, cervical lymphadenopathy	Emperipolesis (histiocytes engulf other viable cells) Background lymphocytes and plasma cells Histocytes stain positive for CD68 and S 100, but are negative for CD 1a
Dermatopathic lymphadenitis (lipomelanosis reticularis of Pautrier)	Lymph node enlargement in response to an exfoliative dermatitis	Numerous melanin-laden macrophages and histocytoid cells with nuclear grooves and positive for $ 100 Proliferative postcapillary venules
Castleman disease (Castleman lymphadenopathy, giant lymph node, or angiofollicular lymph node hyperplasia)	Lymphadenopathy and/or localized extranodal lymphoid tumors Unicentric or multicentric Patients can be very ill with systemic symptoms (fever and hypergammaglobu linemia) Human herpesvirus-8 (HHV-8) association	Similar to RLH Clusters of atypical follicular dendritic cells Traversing capillaries, increased plasma cells, and hyalinized material Fewer tangible body macrophages than in RLH LNA-1 (HHV-8) immunoreactive in HIV-positive patients
Extramedullary hematopoiesis (EMH or myeloid proliferation)	Occurs in patients with hyposplenism, compromised marrow space (e.g., myelofibrosis), chronic anemia states, or after the administration of hematopoietic growth factors	Varying amounts of myeloid precursors, erythroid cells, and/or megakaryocytes Mimics metastases
Lymphadenopathy in autoimmune diseases	Young women with autoimmune-related symptoms and lymphadenopathy Occurs in 26-65% SLE patients and 82% RA patients	Features of reactive lymphoid hyperpolasia In RA plasma cells are seen with eosinophilic, cytoplasmic inclusions (Russell bodies) and polymorphous lymphoid background In SLE there is a necrotic/apoptotic background, with dispersed karyorrhectic nuclear debris (hematoxylin bodies), and an absence of neutrophils

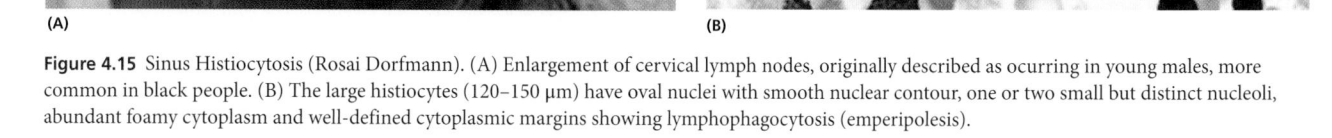

(A)　　　　　　　　　　　　　　　　　　　　　　　(B)

Figure 4.15 Sinus Histiocytosis (Rosai Dorfmann). (A) Enlargement of cervical lymph nodes, originally described as ocurring in young males, more common in black people. (B) The large histiocytes (120–150 μm) have oval nuclei with smooth nuclear contour, one or two small but distinct nucleoli, abundant foamy cytoplasm and well-defined cytoplasmic margins showing lymphophagocytosis (emperipolesis).

empty halo around engulfed lymphocyte is usually better seen on alcohol fixed smears and histologically [99, 100]. Immunophenotypic study of the histiocytes, performed on the FNAC smears and on paraffin-embedded sections shows reactivity for S-100 protein and alpha-1-antichymotrypsin and negativity for lysozyme [101]. Multinucleated histiocytes resembling Touton giant cells may be present. Neutrophils, eosinophils and aggregates of epithelioid cells are absent. A reactive lymphadenopathy may be diagnosed in the majority of cases on FNAC alone although occasionally histiocytes show atypia and may be mistaken for Hodgkin cells [102].

Differential diagnosis includes Langerhans cell histiocytosis, granulomatous disease, large cell lymphoma, malignant histiocytosis, haemophagocytic syndrome, histoplasmosis and dermatopathic lymphadenopathy. Langerhans cell histiocytosis, apart from having

typical Langerhans cells with nuclear folds, contains prominent eosinophilic infiltrate. Granulomatous lymphadenitis due to a variety of infectious agents usually presents as aggregates of cohesive histiocytes/epithelioid cells. These have ill-defined cytoplasm and elongated nuclei. Anaplastic large cell lymphoma and malignant histiocytosis have a more monotonous population of large atypical lymphoid cells. Haemophagocytosis may be seen in malignant histiocytosis and in haemophagocytic syndrome but emperipolesis is typical of sinus histiocytosis with massive lymphadenopathy and is not seen in other conditions. Histoplasmosis is characterised by finding the fungi in the cytoplasm. Dermatopathic lymphadenopathy is histologically characterised by preserved cortical follicles with hyperplastic germinal centres and progressive expansion of interdigitating reticulum cells associated with eosinophils and macrophages containing lipid and melanin pigment.

Cytological features of *dermatopathic lymphadenpathy* are consistent with lymph node hyperplasia. Finding of melanin pigment and appropriate clinical setting may help in reaching the diagnosis. Difficulties arise when a node draining the area of skin involvement with a low grade lymphoma, such as mycosis fungoides, is aspirated. Molecular techniques, in particular detection of the T-cell receptor gene rearrangement, may be helpful in distinguishing a low grade T-cell lymphoma from dermatopathic lymphadenopathy (Fig. 4.8a).

Given the rarity of sinus histiocytosis (Rosai Dorfman) and the clinical suspicion of lymphoma, biopsy of the node is advised. The morphological finding of emperipolesis and immunocytochemical staining for S100 should however be sufficient to allow a confident diagnosis in the follow up of patients with recurrent disease or extranodal progression.

4.2.3 Granulomatous lymphadenitis

4.2.3.1 Mycobacterial infection

Tuberculosis is the most frequent diagnosis in the FNAC of nodes in a developing country and was the most commonly diagnosed infective condition, particularly in those under the age of 20 [5]. The posterior triangle of the neck is the most prevalent site [98]. In developing countries, where there are limited funds and facilities, FNAC has an important role in the investigation of peripheral lymphadenopathy as an alternative to surgical excision biopsy. However, tuberculous lymphadenopathy is not an infrequent finding in the UK, particularly in the inner city immigrant population and in the immunosuppressed (Figs 4.16–4.20). The sensitivity and specificity of lymph node FNAC in the diagnosis of tuberculosis are 78 and 99%, respectively [98, 103].

[See BOX 4.2. Summary of ultrasound features: Tuberculous (TB) lymph node on www.wiley.com/go/kocjan/clinical_cytopathology_head_neck2e]

FNAC of peripheral lymph nodes of patients with TB is an effective diagnostic test. *Cytological features* include aggregates of epithelioid cells, multinuclear giant cells of Langerhans type and necrosis, which can be seen in various ratios ranging from completely necrotic to more granulomatous (Figs 4.17–4.19). The different morphological patterns of tuberculosis, challenges and application of ancillary techniques for cytological diagnosis of tuberculosis are described by Chatterjee [104]. Acid fast bacilli may be detected with Ziehl–Nielsen stain in up to 44% of cases with caseous necrosis [105] (Fig. 4.19B). FNAC material is routinely sent to microbiology

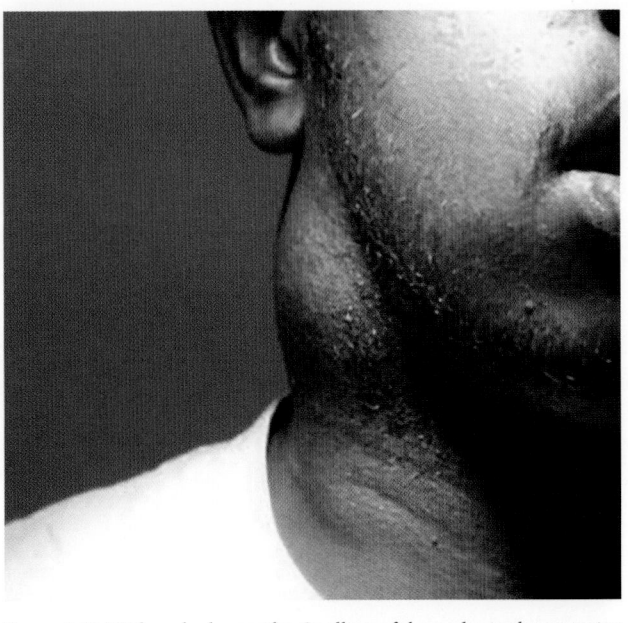

Figure 4.16 TB lymphadenopathy. Swelling of the nodes in the posterior triangle. Patient had night sweats and weight loss. Node was soft and fluctuant.

for confirmation. In the immunosuppressed, the infection with MAI (Mycobacterium Avium Intracellulare) may be detected through presence of numerous macrophages that contain acid fast bacilli in large numbers (Fig. 4.20).

When comparing features of TB infection in Human Immunodeficiency Virus (HIV) positive and HIV negative patients, Lapuerta et al. found that identification of granulomatous inflammation occurs at a similar rate in FNAC specimens from patients with HIV infection (16%) and without HIV infection (21%). Necrosis was the sole reported finding in a significant subset of cases (16%), occurring in patients with and patients without HIV infection. Authors conclude that the granulomatous inflammation and other FNAC findings in peripheral lymph nodes of patients with TB are similar in those with and those without HIV infection [106].

Apart from tuberculosis, *granulomatous lymphadenitis* may be encountered in sarcoidosis (Fig. 4.21) (where it usually does not include necrosis), *cat scratch fever, brucellosis, toxoplasmosis, some fungal infections, leishmaniasis, lepromatous and tuberculoid leprosy, primary syphilis, lymphogranuloma venereum, chronic tularemia and rheumatoid arthritis*. Sarcoidosis is the most common cause of granulomatous lymphadenitis in developed countries. Sarcoid like granulomas may also be provoked by non-infectious causes such as berylliosis and in reaction to other mineral substances including silicones and starch. Malignancies, such as Hodgkin's and, rarely, non-Hodgkin's lymphomas, anaplastic thyroid carcinoma, squamous cell carcinoma, nasopharyngeal carcinoma and others may also show granulomatous reaction (Fig. 4.22) [107].

4.2.3.2 Cat scratch disease

Cat scratch disease (CSD) is usually a benign, self-limited lymphadenitis, characterised by suppurative granulomas, caused by a small Gram-negative bacillus. It affects children and adults, usually in autumn and winter months and is usually associated with a cat scratch or bite 2–4 weeks prior to lymphadenopathy, although it can

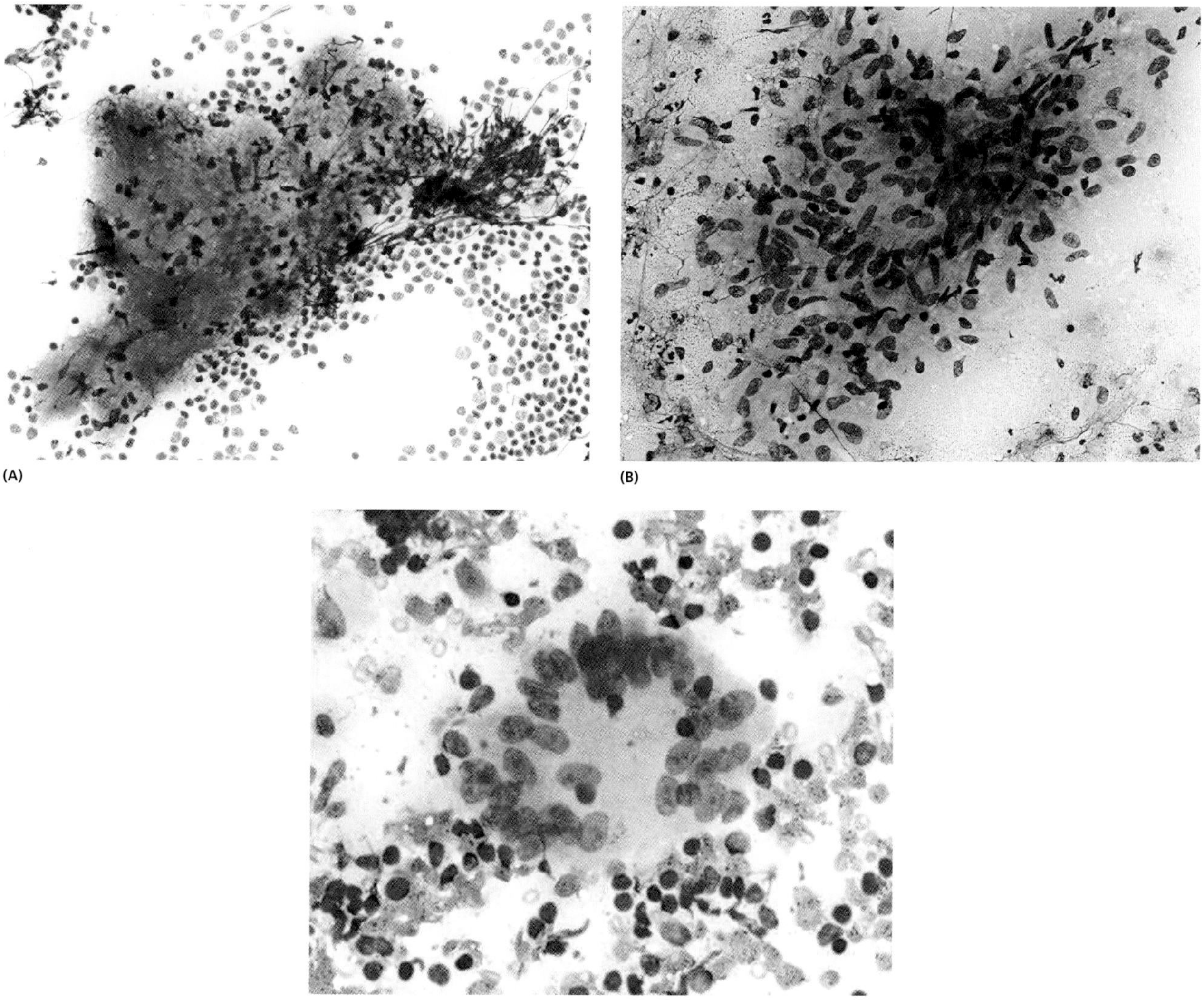

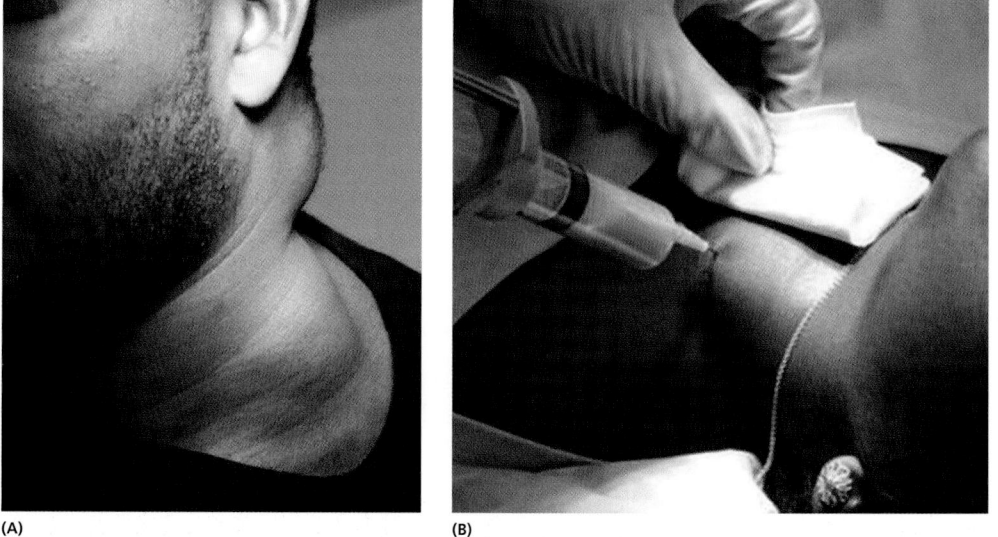

(A)

(B)

(C)

Figure 4.17 Tuberculous lymphadenitis. aggregates of epithelioid cells, multinuclear giant cells of Langhans type and necrosis can be seen in various ratios ranging from completely necrotic to more granulomatous. Acid fast bacilli may be detected with Ziehl–Nielsen stain. (A) Low power view reveals inflammatory, necrotic background (MGG ×200). (B) Aggregates of epithelioid cells and (C) Langhans giant cells.

(A)

(B)

Figure 4.18 Tuberculous lymphadenitis. (A) NA fluctuant neck swelling and (B) FNAC drainage of the necrotic tuberculous lymph node in a different patient. FNAC is performed with a pathologist and an assistant wearing a mask and protective clothing. Slides are not left in the air to dry but are contained in a transport box or handled in a grade 3 safety cabinet. The remaining fluid is sent to microbiology.

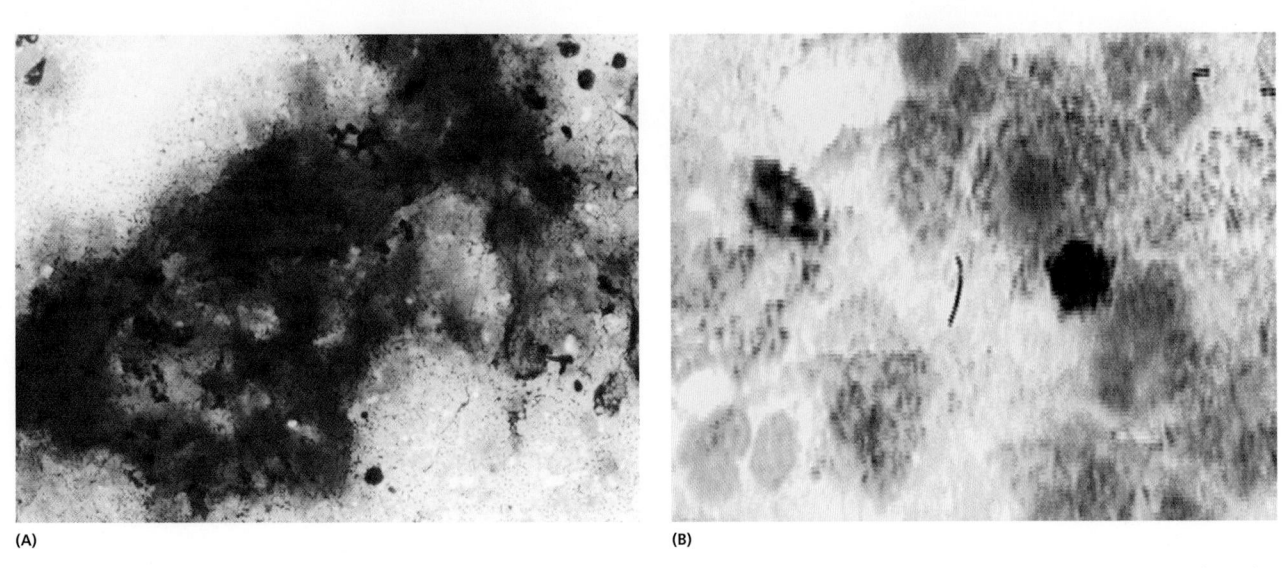

(A)

(B)

Figure 4.19 Tuberculous lymphadenitis. (A) Caseous necrosis produces necrotic background with no viable cells. (B) Ziehl–Nielsen staining confirms the diagnosis by showing an acid fast bacillus.

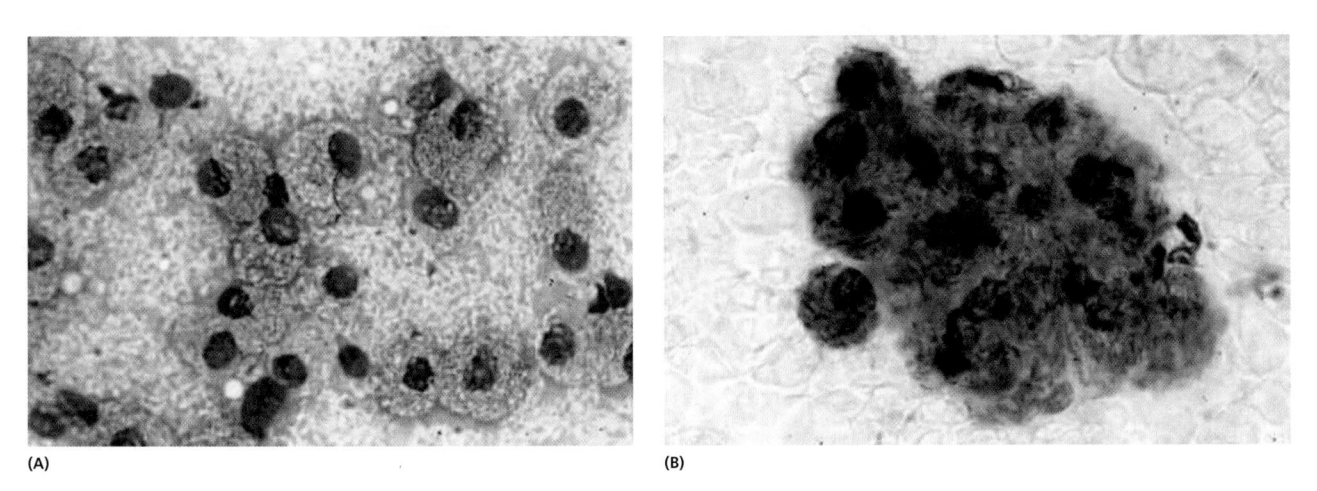

(A)

(B)

Figure 4.20 Mycobacterium avium intracellulare. (A) Lymphoid tissue is replaced by large histiocytes with voluminous finely vacuolated, ill-defined cytoplasm containing numerous bacilli. (B) Ziehl–Nielsen stain shows numerous intracytoplasmic rods.

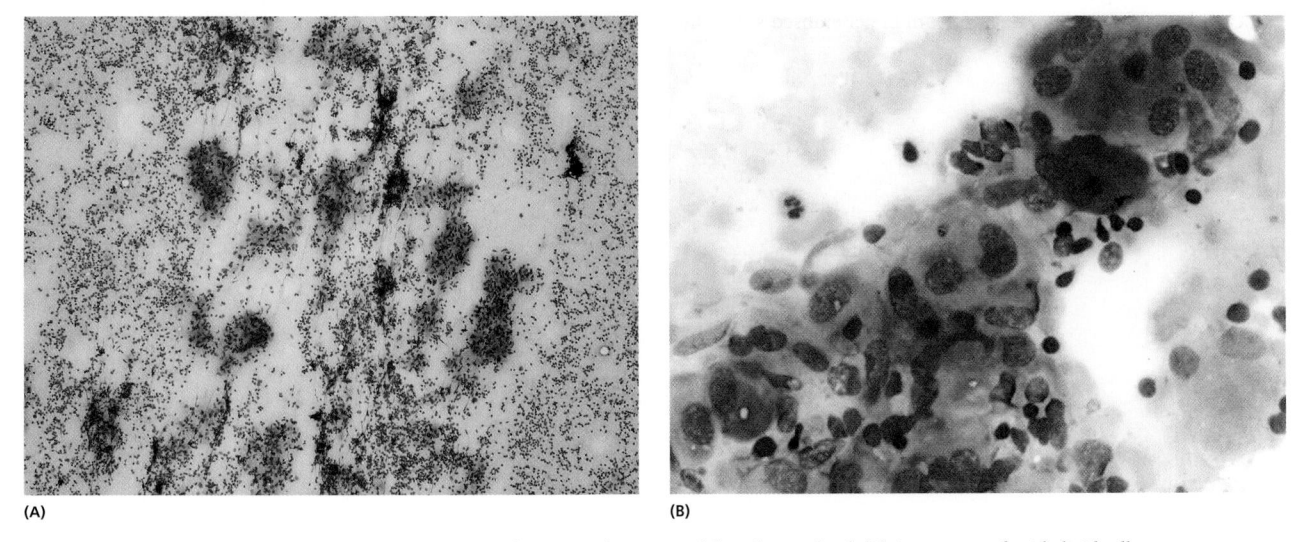

(A)

(B)

Figure 4.21 Sarcoidosis. (A) Numerous non caseating granulomata in the FNAC of the salivary gland. (B) Aggregates of epithelioid cells.

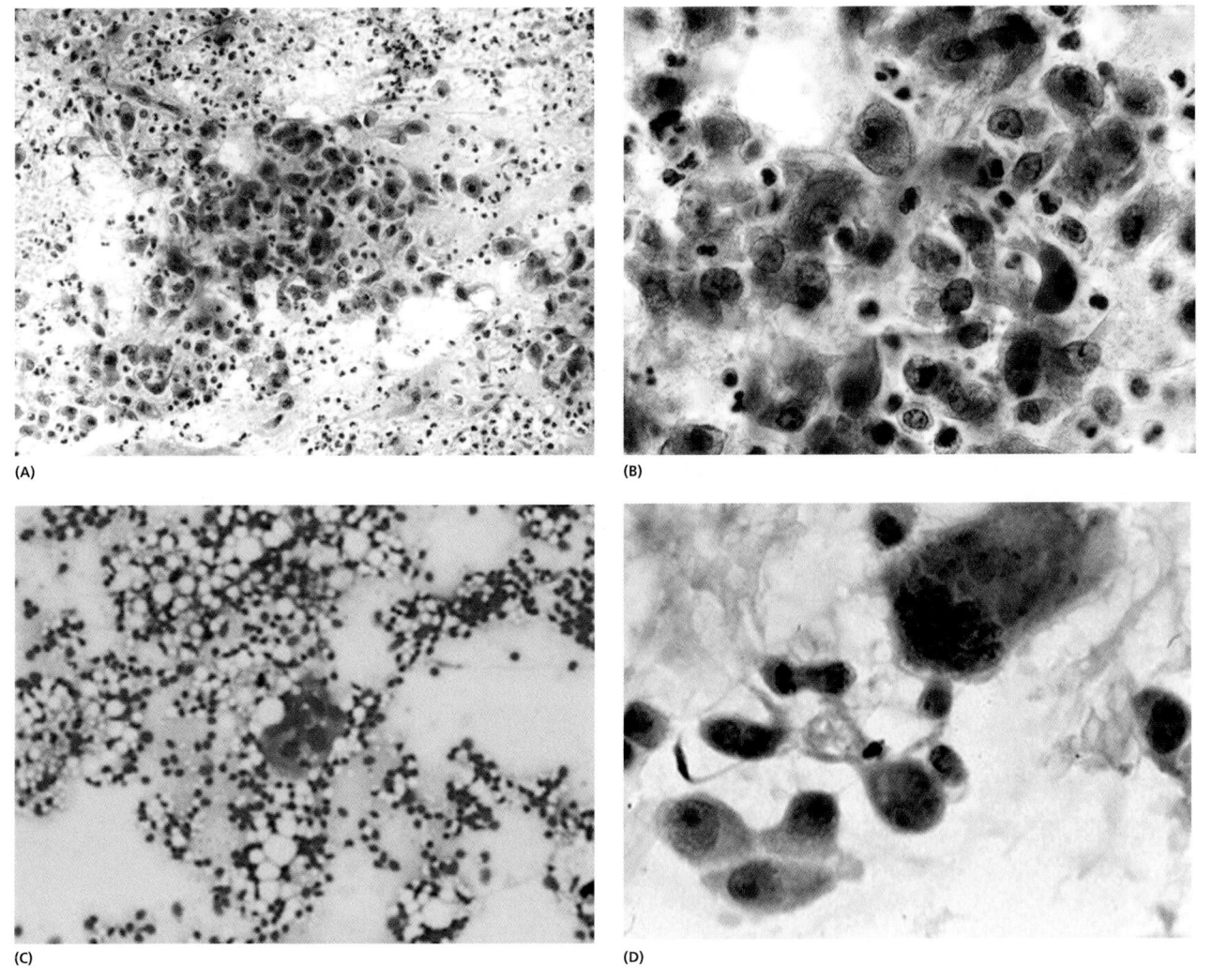

Figure 4.22 Granulomatous reaction. (A) Numerous macrophages, fibroblasts and inflammatory cells in a suture granuloma of the postoperative skin lesion. (B) High power view of this lesion may cause concern unless clinical data are known. (C) Silicone granuloma in the FNAC of the breast contains giant cells and macrophages. (D) Giant cells in anaplastic carcinoma of the thyroid should not be mistaken for lymphocytic or granulomatous thyroiditis.

be acquired through the skin without a visible lesion. It may be associated with fever and wide spectrum of generalised symptoms. Lymphadenopathy is most commonly parotid, cervical or axillary. In children, it may be dramatic and clinically mimic malignancy (Fig. 4.23). Neoplasia is initially suspected clinically in 38% of the cases [108]. Histologically, numerous abscesses or small areas of necrosis surrounded by histiocytic reaction, occasionally granulomas, are found. Diagnosis is confirmed by a positive intradermal skin test.

Cytological features include heterogenous mix of cell types, confluent epithelioid cells admixed with neutrophils against a background of polymorphic inflammatory cells to include lymphocytes, immunoblasts, plasma cells, neutrophils, histiocytes and rare eosinophils (Fig. 4.24). Rare multinucleate giant cells may also be seen. A varying number of medium-sized to large lymphoid cells with an appearance suggestive of monocytoid B lymphocytes are associated with the epithelioid cells [109, 110]. Warthin–Starry silver stain-positive bacteria are detected in 69% of cases and are not limited to those preparations with suppurative granulomas [108, 109]. The most distinctive cytological feature is that of a granuloma,

present in 77% of cases, suppuration is present in 66% and epithelioid histiocytes in 46% and suppurative granulomas in 38% [108]. Neither granulomas nor suppurative inflammation are seen in all cases. The diagnosis is generally one of exclusion since cultures, smears and tissue staining may be negative.

The cytological differential diagnosis includes all lymphadenopathies with suppurative granulomas. These include *LGV, yersinia lymphadenitis, tularemia, brucellosis, listeriosis and meliodosis* [110].

4.2.3.3 Fungal diseases (mycoses)

These are rarely encountered in the UK except in travellers and the immunosuppressed. The most frequently encountered infections are histoplasmosis and cryptococcosis. Histoplasmosis, although primarily affecting lung, may also affect lymph nodes causing necrotising granulomatous lesions that may calcify. Histoplasma capsulatum is readily demonstrated on MGG and PAS stained preparations as intracellular organisms (Fig. 4.25). Cryptococcosis, although a disease of hot climates, is seen in immunosuppressed and may involve lymph nodes. Cryptococcus evokes little cellular

response and is readily recognised on silver staining as oval budding spores (Fig. 4.26).

4.2.3.4 Toxoplasmosis

Toxoplasmosis is a disease caused by protozoan *Toxoplasma gondii*. In humans, disease occurs as congenital and acquired. Congenital form can cause foetal death, hydrocephaly, microcephaly, encephalitis or chorioretinitis. Acquired form usually presents as a mild, usually asymptomatic lymphadenopathy, which occurs sporadically. Toxoplasmic lymphadenopathy is a fairly common (15%) cause of unexplained lymphadenopathy and surgical biopsy is often performed because of a suspicion of

lymphoma. Since the disease is generally self-limited, no treatment is necessary, and FNAC can spare the patient unnecessary hospitalisation and surgery [111]. Disease presents as cervical lymphadenopathy either acutely or of some months' duration, usually in children and young adults [112]. The main reservoir of infection is a domestic cat. Disease can be diagnosed by serological tests but the diagnosis is complicated by the high prevalence of antibodies in the normal population.

Cytological features include polymorphous population of lymphocytes that vary in size, from small mature lymphocytes that predominate, to larger, transformed lymphocytes, plasma cells and immunoblasts (Fig. 4.27). Prominent follicular dendritic cells and germinal centre histiocytes filled with phagocytised karyorrhectic debris are also present. The characteristic finding is that of epithelioid cells are seen in small, loose aggregates. This finding prompts the suggestion of toxoplasmosis. Although not pathognomonic of toxoplasmosis, the finding of small aggregates of epithelioid cells against a background of lymph node hyperplasia, with the absence of giant cells and necrosis, is highly suggestive of toxoplasmosis.

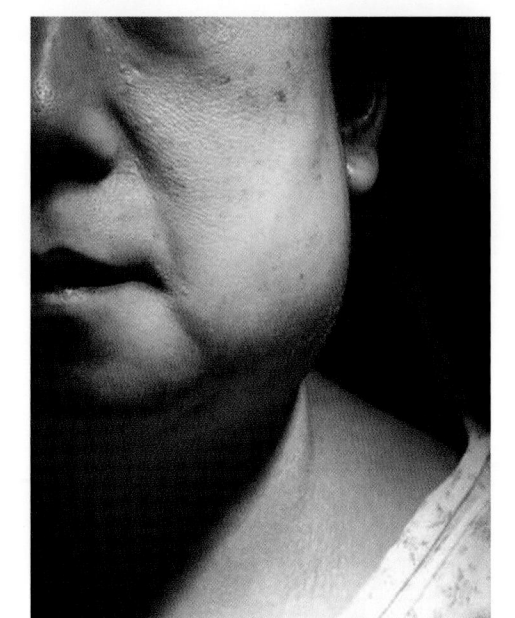

Figure 4.23 Cat scratch disease. Lymphadenopathy is most commonly parotid, cervical or axillary. This patient presented with a 4-week history of hard diffuse swelling at the angle of mandible which was clinically thought to be malignancy.

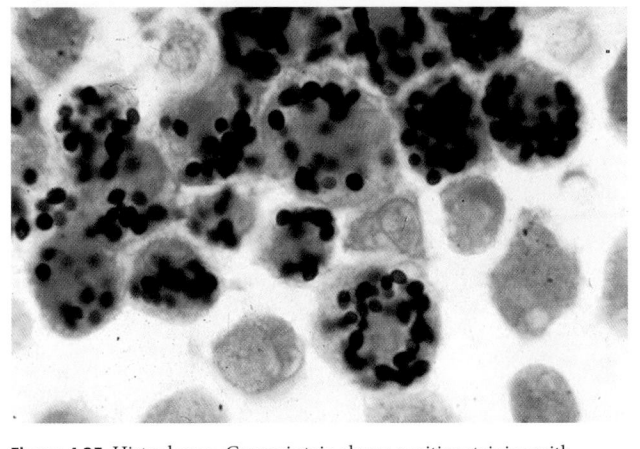

Figure 4.25 Histoplasma. Gomori stain shows positive staining with intracellular organisms. They can be also seen on routine MGG and Diff Quick staining.

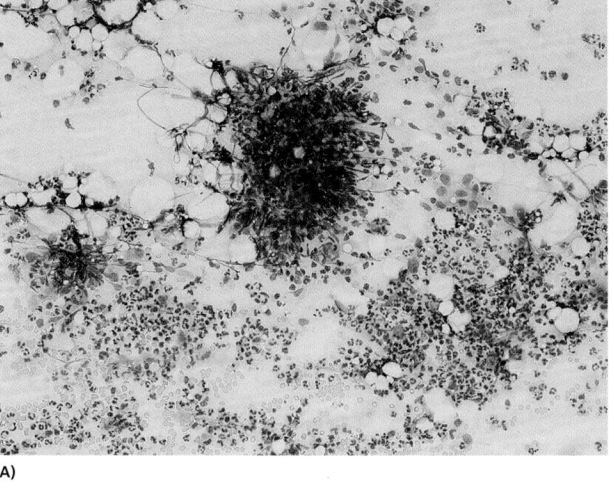

(A)

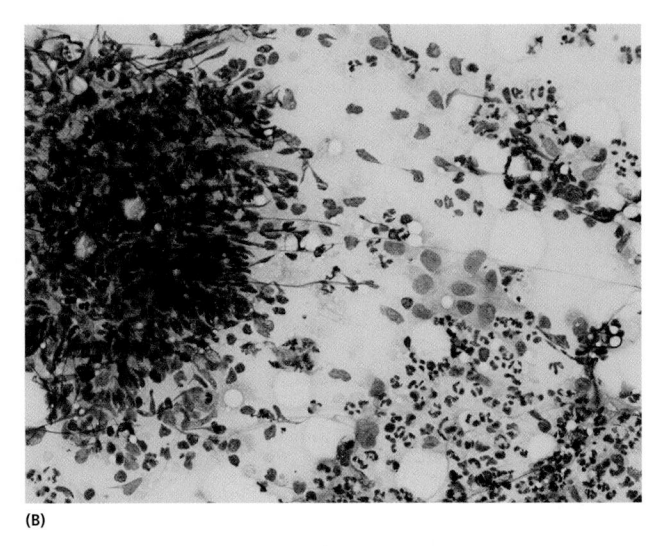

(B)

Figure 4.24 Cat scratch disease. (A) Low power view shows a heterogenous mix of cell types, confluent epithelioid cells admixed with neutrophils against a background of inflammatory cells including polymorphs (MGG ×200). (B) High power view shows lymphocytes, immunoblasts, plasma cells, neutrophils, histiocytes and rare eosinophils. Rare multinucleate giant cells may also be seen (×600, oil immersion).

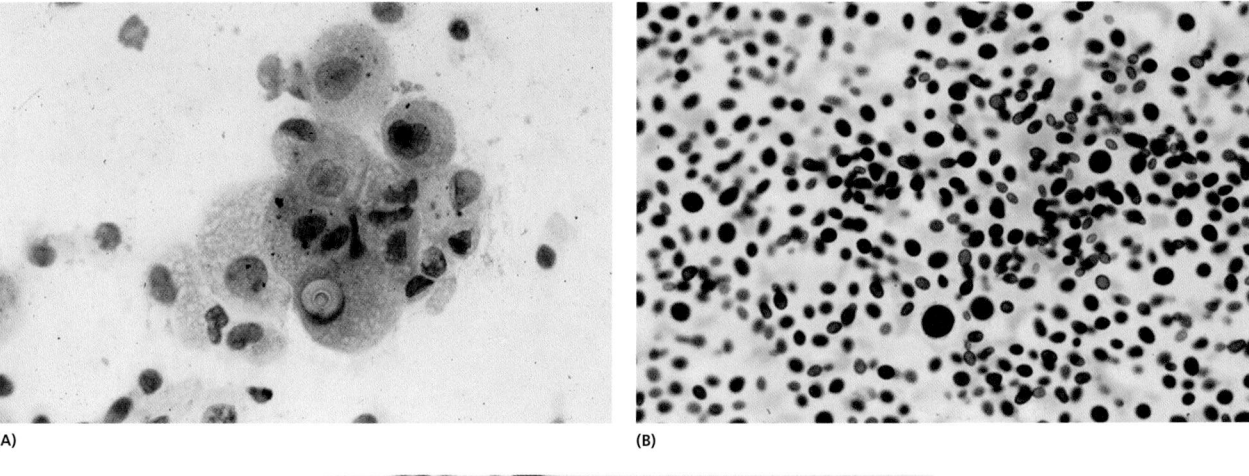

(A)

(B)

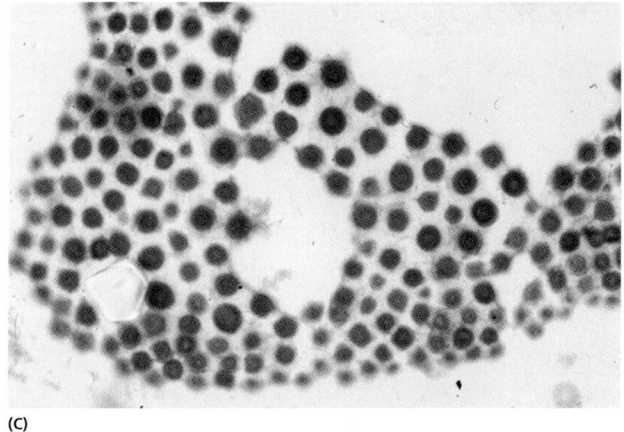

(C)

Figure 4.26 Cryptococcal infection. (A) High power view reveals detail of the refractile, pale bodies in the macrophages (PAP ×1000, oil immersion). (B) Methenamine silver (Grocott) shows numerous oval fungal spores with characteristic budding (MS ×200, ×1000, oil immersion). (C) A mucicarmine stain highlights the mucopolysaccharide capsule of the *Cryptococcus*.

Occasionally, microorganisms can be identified in the cytological preparations. Zaharopoulos et al. described toxoplasma cysts in a Papanicolaou-stained smear and dispersed tachyzoites, and a pseudocyst in MGG preparations [113]. As a fairly rare occurrence, numerous tachyzoites may be seen dispersed free in exudate, and also within cells, forming pseudocysts. Immuno-cytochemistry for the *Toxoplasma gondii* antigen is positive. The tachyzoites seen in MGG preparations, when subjected to fluorescence microscopy, emit autofluorescence, facilitating their identification. Besides the use of immunocytochemistry in the diagnosis of the disease, air-dried preparations stained by the MGG method are valuable for the demonstration of such parasites through careful search, along with the possible use of fluorescence microscopy.

4.2.3.5 Leishmaniasis

Leishmaniasis is a parasitosis caused by protozoa of the genus Leishmania that multiply in the cells of hematopoietic system. Transmission of the parasite occurs through the vector (Phlebotomus). The main reservoirs are humans and dogs. Leishmania has a world-wide distribution with five large known areas of location: Russia and China, South America, India and Pakistan, north and east Africa and countries of the Mediterranean. Clinically, disease presents as cutaneous, muco-cutaneous or visceral (Kala-azar) infection. Patients present with

lymphadenopathy. Histologically, lymph nodes show histiocytic microgranulomas confluent with epithelioid cells, multinucle-ated giant cells and occasionally areas of necrosis. Organism can be cultured on Novy-MCNeal-Nicolle (NNN) medium, which takes approximately 2 weeks to grow, or by the Leishmania skin test, which becomes positive 3 months after the onset of disease. Cytological material can be obtained by either scraping the skin lesions or by FNAC. However, FNAC is recommended as the method of choice of confirming the diagnosis [114].

Cytological features The pathognomonic cytological picture consists of lymphocytes, plasma cells and epithelioid granulomas intermingled with histiocytes. Multinucleated giant cells may be seen. Numerous Leishmania organisms are seen in the cytoplasm of histiocytes and extracellularly [115]. Under oil immersion, these Leishmania–Donovan bodies measure 1.5–3 μm and are small rounded cells with a fine membrane, a relatively large nucleus and a paranucleus (kinetoplast) [116]. Some kinetoplasts are observed within the intracytoplasmic vesicles (phagolysosomes) and some extracellularly. Apart from lymph nodes, organisms can be found in the spleen and bone marrow.

Differential diagnosis includes all granulomatous lymphadenop-athies (tuberculosis, atypical mycobacteria, toxoplasmosis, syphilis, leprosy, LGV, brucellosis and mycotic infections). In the case of skin disease, other skin diseases that contain parasitised macrophages are rhinoscleroma, LGV and histoplasmosis.

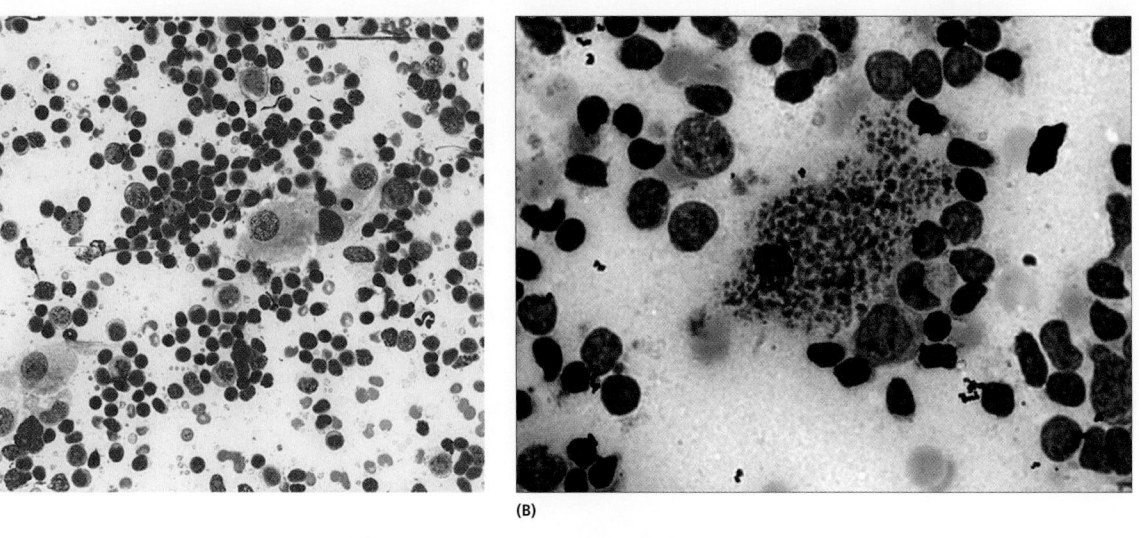

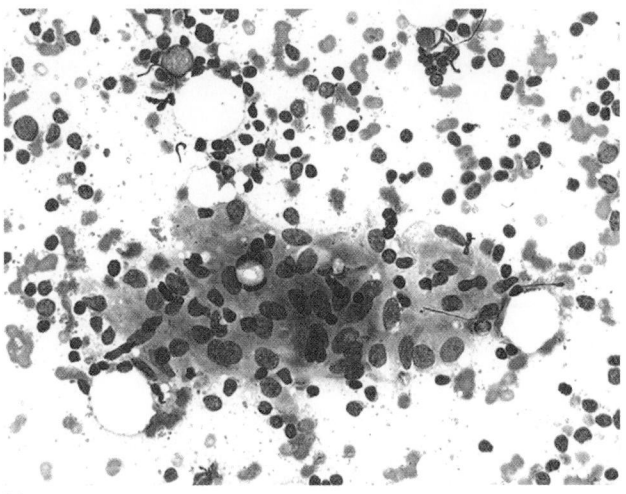

Figure 4.27 Toxoplasmosis. FNAC of a 9-year-old child presenting with large submandibular lymph node without any generalised symptoms. (A) Low power view showing polymorphous population of lymphocytes and prominent follicular dendritic cells. (B) Germinal centre histiocytes filled with phagocytised karyorrhectic debris (MGG ×600, ×100, ×1000, oil immersion). (C) Epithelioid cells are seen in small, loose aggregates. This finding prompts the suggestion of toxoplasmosis (MGG ×600).

4.2.4 Chronic lymphadenitis

4.2.4.1 Kikuchi's lymphadenitis

Kikuchi's lymphadenitis (Table 4.3) is a self-limiting condition typically affecting young women. Patients present with cervical lymphadenopathy affecting one or more lymph nodes, sometimes accompanied by malaise and pyrexia. Sometimes lymphadenopathy may be extensive, clinically mimicking lymphoma. Histologically, there are foci of necrosis in the lymph nodes with numerous nuclear fragments giving an impression of polymorphs although polymorphs are conspicuously absent.

Cytological features: Characteristic FNAC findings are those of karyorrhectic and granular debris and distinctive phagocytic histiocytes. These phagocytic histiocytes have peripherally placed 'crescentic' nuclei and abundant cytoplasm containing phagocytosed karyorrhectic or eosinophilic granular debris, easily distinguishable from tingible-body macrophages, which have centrally placed round nuclei. Also found are plasmacytoid monocytes, medium-sized cells with eccentrically placed round nuclei, condensed chromatin and a moderate amount of amphophilic cytoplasm.

Nonphagocytic histiocytes with twisted nuclei and delicate chromatin and immunoblasts that sometimes show atypical features such as irregular foldings of the nuclei can also be seen (Fig. 4.28) [117, 118], Neutrophils are sparse or absent. FNAC findings of lymph nodes involved by various reactive processes, tuberculosis, and lymphoma for comparison show that although tingible-body macrophages and debris are not uncommon, very few phagocytic histiocytes with crescentic nuclei or plasmacytoid monocytes are observed. The features described here permit diagnosis of Kikuchi's lymphadenitis by FNAC [119]. Because of morphologic similarities between lupus lymphadenitis and Kikuchi's lymphadenitis, however, serologic studies are warranted to exclude systemic lupus erythematosus.

4.2.4.2 Infectious mononucleosis

Infectious mononucleosis (glandular fever) is caused by Epstein–Barr virus that is also associated with Burkitt's lymphoma and nasopharyngeal carcinoma. Disease may be subclinical or manifest itself as generalised lymphadenopathy and flu-like illness. Diagnosis is made by a positive Paul–Bunnel heterophil antibody test or 'monospot' test.

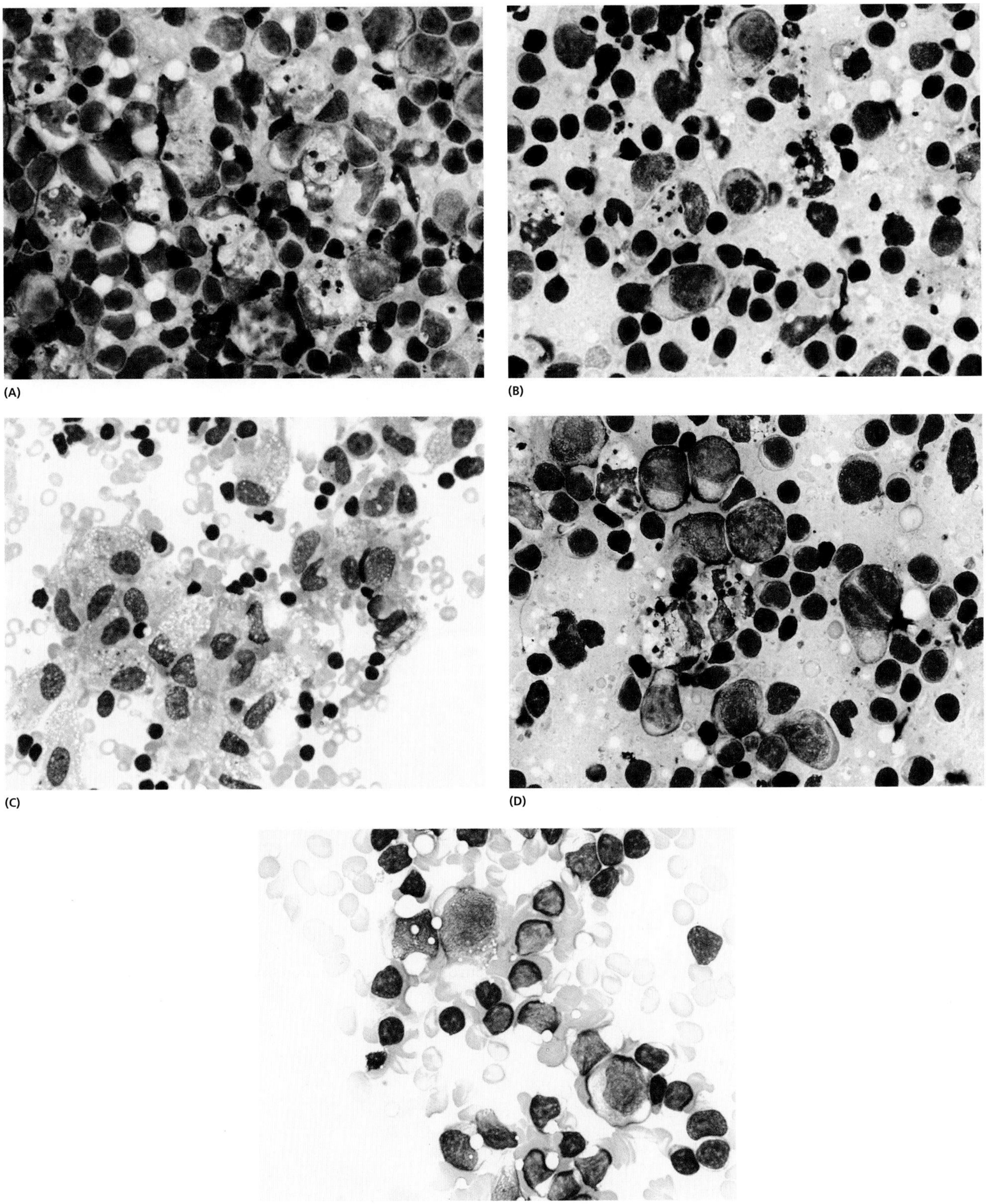

(A)

(B)

(C)

(D)

(E)

Figure 4.28 Kikuchi's lymphadenitis. FNAC lymph node in a 35-year-old patient presenting with clinically alarming cervical lymphadenopathy. (A) Karyorrhectic and granular debris and distinctive phagocytic histiocytes (MGG ×600, oil immersion). (B, C) Phagocytic histiocytes have peripherally placed 'crescentic' nuclei and abundant cytoplasm containing phagocytosed karyorrhectic or eosinophilic granular debris, easily distinguishable from tingible-body macrophages, which have centrally placed round nuclei (MGG ×1000, oil immersion). (D) Plasmacytoid monocytes, medium-sized cells with eccentrically placed round nuclei, condensed chromatin, and a moderate amount of amphophilic cytoplasm (MGG ×1000). (E) Nonphagocytic histiocytes and immunoblasts that sometimes show atypical features such as irregular foldings of the nuclei (×1000, oil immersion).

Histologically, there may be florid blast transformation of lymphocytes with blurring of normal architecture. Occasional large blasts may mimic Reed–Sternberg cells. Patients are referred for FNAC usually for clinically suspected malignant lymphoma, due to often sizeable, sometimes unilateral, cervical lymphadenopathy (Fig. 4.29).

Cytological features: Smears show greater numbers of large immunoblastic lymphocytes than are usually seen in the reactive lymph node. Features may be mistaken for a malignant lymphoma but include a considerable background of polymorphic immunoblasts. Since several reactive and neoplastic processes mimic this pattern, cases should be confirmed by either confirmatory serologic studies and/or resolution of lymphadenopathy (Fig. 4.30). Failing this, an excisional lymph node biopsy should follow [120].

4.2.4.3 Acquired immunodeficiency syndrome (AIDS)

Human Immunodeficiency Virus (HIV) infected patients in the early stages of infection may present with a widespread painless lymphadenopathy accompanied with malaise and listlessness. This is known as Persistent Generalised Lymphadenopathy (PGL) (Fig. 4.31). Immunological function is still preserved although a

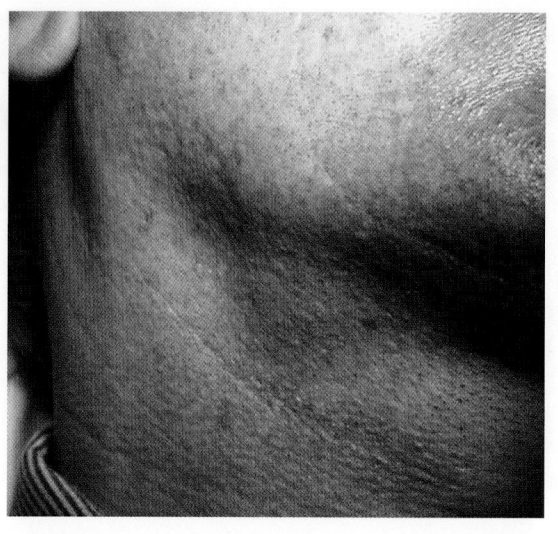

Figure 4.29 Infectious mononucleosis. Patient was referred for FNAC for clinically suspicious, persistent, unilateral, cervical lymphadenopathy.

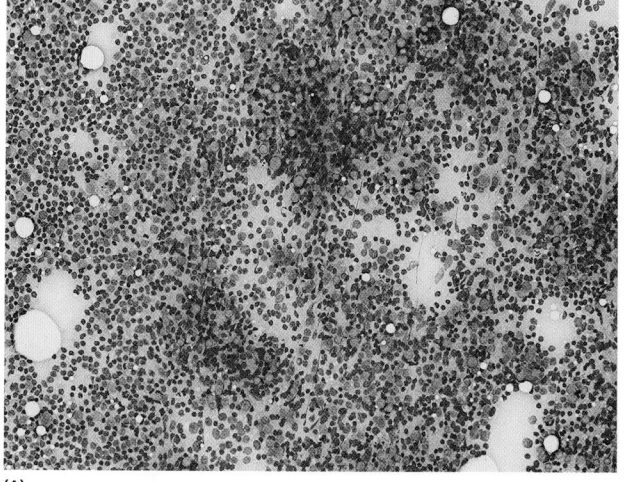

(A)

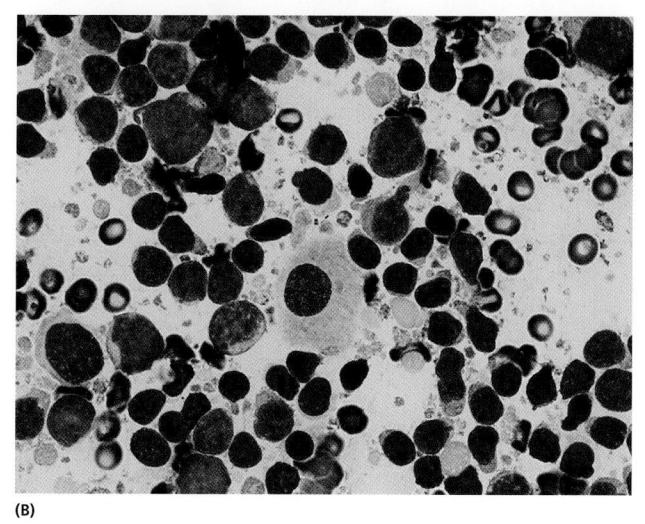

(B)

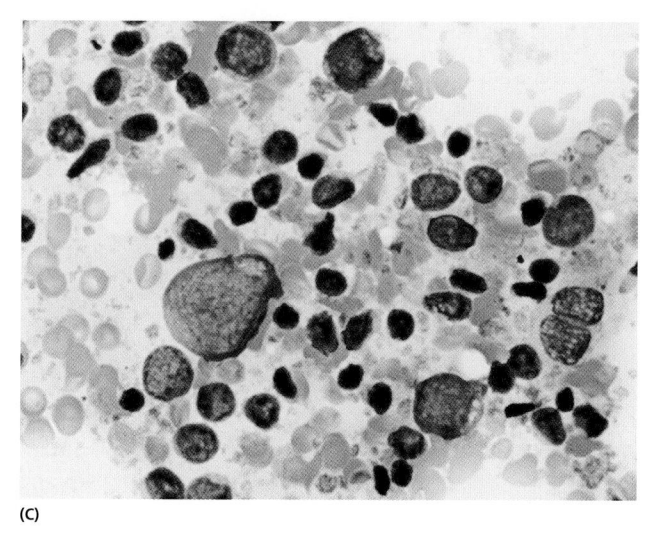

(C)

Figure 4.30 Infectious mononucleosis. (A) Smears show greater numbers of immunoblasts than are usually seen in the reactive lymph node (×600, oil immersion. (B, C) Features may be mistaken for a malignant lymphoma but include a considerable background of polymorphic immunoblasts (×1000, oil immersion). Since several reactive and neoplastic processes mimic this pattern, cases should be confirmed by either confirmatory serologic studies and/or resolution of lymphadenopathy. Otherwise, they should be referred for excision.

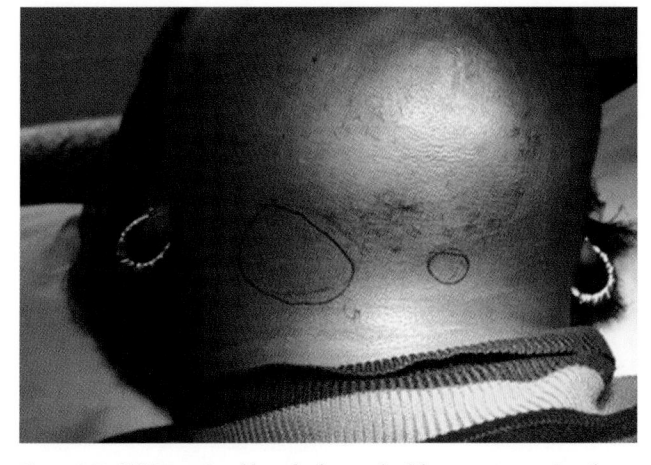

Figure 4.31 HIV associated lymphadenopathy. The commonest site of FNAC in HIV positive patients are cervical lymph nodes. Patients may present at any stage of the disease with enlarged lymph nodes. Clinically, differential diagnosis is either PGL, specific infection, lymphoma or Kaposi's sarcoma. FNAC is useful in distinguishing between these entities and sparing the patient unnecessary biopsy.

progressive reversal of TH/TS ratio may be observed. After a time, lymphadenopathy disappears and is superseded by the phase of immune deficiency where loss of weight, diarrhoea and cerebral impairment are common symptoms. Opportunistic infections are frequent in this phase. The lymph nodes in the terminal stage are small and difficult to find.

Histologically, lymph nodes in PGL show striking follicular hyperplasia with large and irregular germinal centres with poorly developed mantle zones and paracortex relatively depleted of lymphocytes. In the later stages, follicles shrink and disappear with scanty aggregates of B-lymphocytes in place of follicle centres. Proliferation of endothelial venules in the paracortex is noted.

Palpable or radiologically identified masses in patients infected with the HIV are amenable to FNAC to differentiate between the infections and neoplasms [121]. FNAC offers a rapid, simple and cost effective approach for diagnosis. The commonest site of FNAC in HIV positive patients is cervical lymph nodes (54%). Reactive lymphadenopathy (PGL) is the most commonly diagnosed condition, followed by infection and malignancy [122–124]. Part of the FNAC specimen is sent for bacterial culture, fungal culture and acid-fast smear and PCR. Some of the infections detected in FNAC include toxoplasmosis, histoplasmosis, tuberculosis, atypical mycobacterium, cryptococcosis and methicillin-resistant staphylococcal infection. Shapiro et al. found that all patients with either unilateral lymphadenopathy or lymph nodes 3 cm or larger had positive aspirates. Tenderness and recent enlargement are important indicators [125]. A statistically significant difference between patients with lymph nodes smaller than 2 cm and those with nodes larger than 2 cm was found [126]. Cervical node biopsy is not indicated in the HIV or AIDS patient with nontender or nonenlarging nodes [127].

Cytological features of lymphadenopathy associated with HIV infection vary depending on the stage of disease. In the initial stage, PGL may be reflected by a florid proliferation of follicle centre cells with many centroblasts, immunoblasts and tingible body macrophages reflecting the high cell turnover (Fig. 4.32). In the later stages, follicle depletion described in histology is reflected by relatively hypocellular aspirates with only the small lymphocytes and follicular dendritic cells remaining as a residue of follicles.

4.2.5 Drug reactions

Lymphadenopathy is a recognised feature of some drug hypersensitivity reactions, namely penicillin, sulphonamides, certain antimalarials and non-steroidal anti-inflammatory drugs. Generalised symptoms usually prompt the drug to be withdrawn and lymphadenopathy to subside before it had been further investigated. Some anticonvulsant drugs, in particular the hydantoin and carbamazepine may cause lymphadenopathy and gum hypertrophy as side effects (Fig. 4.33) [128]. Histologically and cytologically, the T-cells of the paracortex show blastic transformation similar to infectious mononucleosis. Atypical blasts may also be present. Histological features in the skin are those of a cutaneous pseudolymphoma, including CD30+ cells [128]. Development of malignant lymphoma in some of these nodes has been reported [129].

4.2.6 Miscellaneous lymphadenopathies

4.2.6.1 Castleman's disease

Castleman's disease (Table 4.3) is a rare atypical lymphoproliferative disorder whose morphology, soon after the original presentation of Castleman et al. [129a] has been subdivided in a hyaline vascular and plasma cell histopathological patterns, with intermediate variants. The former occurs much more frequently than the latter and is usually localised to the mediastinum or pulmonary hilum (Fig. 4.34). The plasma cell type involves lymph nodes separately or in aggregates and often displays multicentricity with systemic symptoms including autoimmune phenomena and aggressive course. Infections are the most frequent cause of patient demise in these cases, followed by malignancies such as Kaposi's sarcoma, malignant lymphoma or carcinoma. Histologically, the hallmarks of Castleman's disease are: increase of follicular dendritic reticulum cells, often dysplastic, in the germinal centre and marginal zone, broad marginal zone expansion with prominence of immunophenotypically aberrant B-cells (Ki B3-negative, CD5-positive), possible predominance of paracortical plasma cells often with clusters of clonal λ-light chain restricted plasma cells, increase of paracortical plasmacytoid monocytes. *Hyaline vascular type* shows small hyalinised and hypervascular germinal centres with hypervascular interfollicular stroma and sinus effacement. *Plasma cell type* contains plasma cell aggregates in lymph node paracortex and partially spared sinuses. The two types are frequently concomitant. A key event in the pathogenesis of Castleman's disease has been recently suggested to be an abnormal production of a B-cell growth factor, such as IL-6, leading to lymphoproliferation and plasma cell differentiation and being involved in the oncogenesis of plasmacytoma. In this event, Kaposi's sarcoma associated virus (HHV-8), which has been found in many cases of Castleman's disease, especially in the multicentric form, could play a crucial role both in producing IL-6 and releasing angiogenic factors. A possible differentiation block may lead to the development of a malignant lymphoma, Kaposi's sarcoma or other malignant neoplasias probably as a consequence of the immunodeficiency typical of Castleman's disease.

Cytological features: Castleman's disease of the hyaline vascular subtype is an uncommon lesion; experience with FNAC of this tumour is limited to rare case reports [130]. In the clinical context of orophranygeal and mediastinal mass, hypercellular smears with mature small lymphoid population associated with larger atypical cells, which are consistent with follicular dendritic cells, can be suggestive of Castleman's disease. Confirmation of a polytypic B-cell population by flow cytometry, supported by immunohistochemistry, is very helpful. Biopsy is advised.

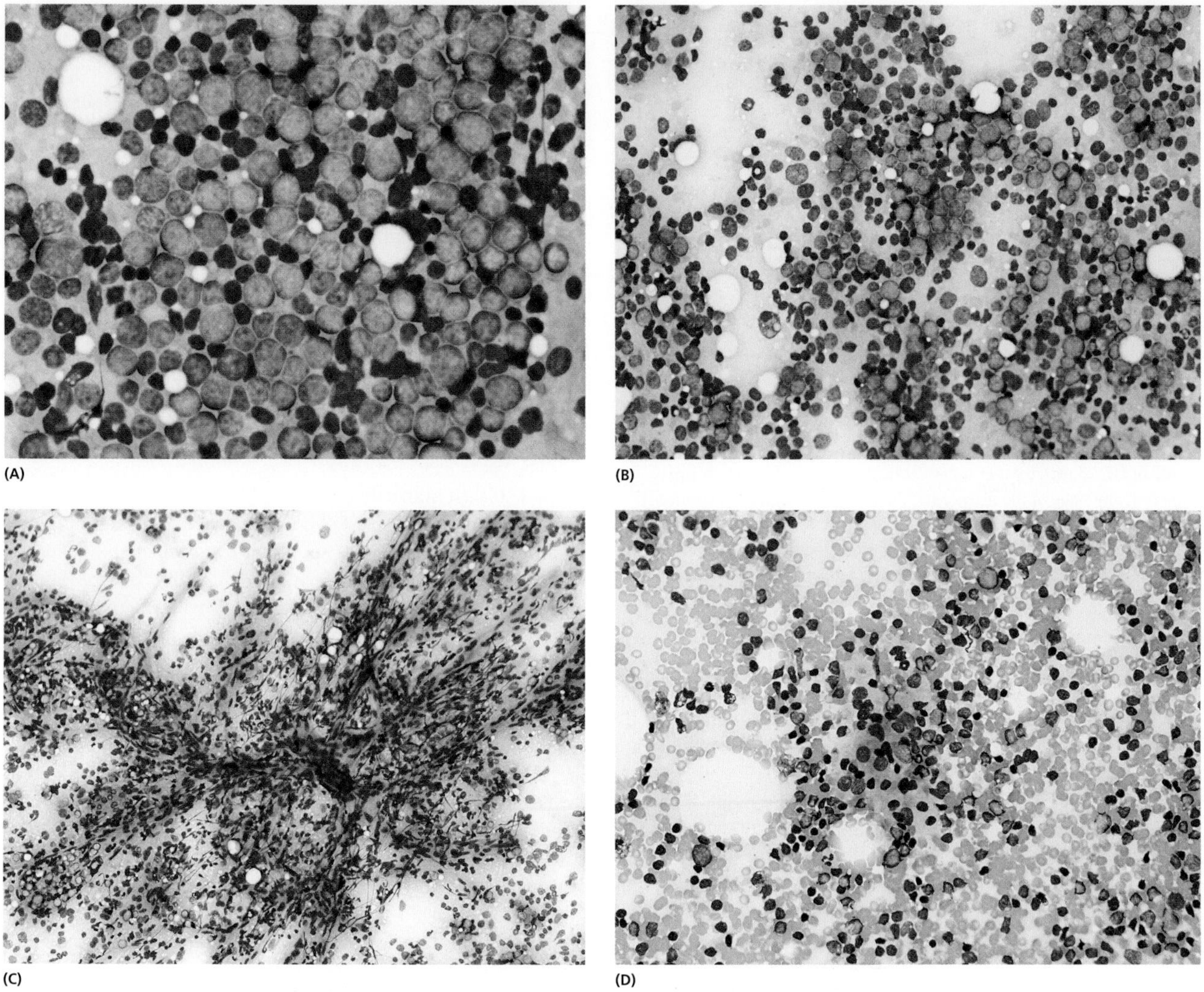

Figure 4.32 HIV associated lymphadenopathy. (A, B, C) In the initial stage, PGL may show a florid proliferation of follicle centre cells with many centroblasts, immunoblasts and tingible body macrophages reflecting the high cell turnover (MGG ×400, ×1000, ×1000, oil immersion). (D) In the later stages, follicle depletion is reflected by relatively hypocellular aspirates with only the small lymphocytes, plasma cells and follicular dendritic cells remaining as a residue of follicles (MGG ×200, ×600, oil immersion).

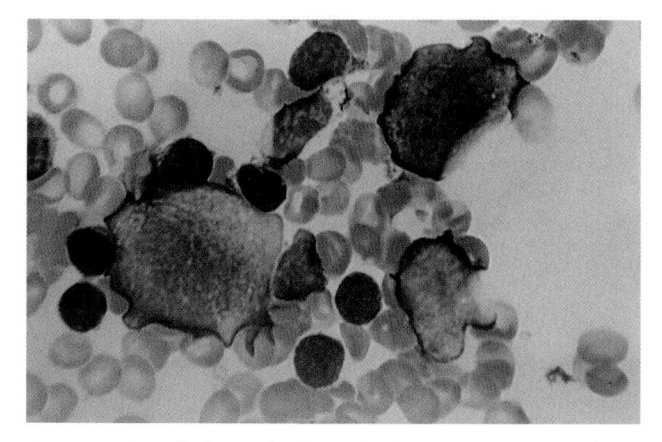

Figure 4.33 Lymphadenopathy due to the drug reaction. T-cells of the paracortex show blastic transformation similar to infectious mononucleosis.

4.2.6.2 Langerhans cell histiocytosis

Langerhans cell histiocytosis is a non-neoplastic condition of unknown aetiology. It is regarded as a reactive disorder reacting to an unknown inciting agent(s). Clinically, it includes a triad of related disorders, *Letterer-Siwe*, *Hand Schüller-Christian* and *Eosinophilic granuloma*, with variable organ involvement of infiltration and characteristic proliferation of Langerhans cells, a special kind of histiocyte of dendritic type. Cytological material may be obtained from different sites including lymph nodes and bone marrow but also more unusual sites including thyroid [131, 132], effusions [133] and solitary bone lesions (Fig. 4.35) [134–138]. Lymph node involvement in Langerhans cell histiocytosis can be seen as a component of the systemic form, or it may be the initial and sometimes exclusive manifestation of the disease [139].

Cytological features of Langerhans cell histiocytosis diagnosed by FNAC include numerous Langerhans cells admixed with eosinophils, neutrophils, lymphocytes, macrophages and multinucleated giant cells. Characteristic Langerhans cells have abundant pale non-phagocytic cytoplasm and somewhat irregular, folded or

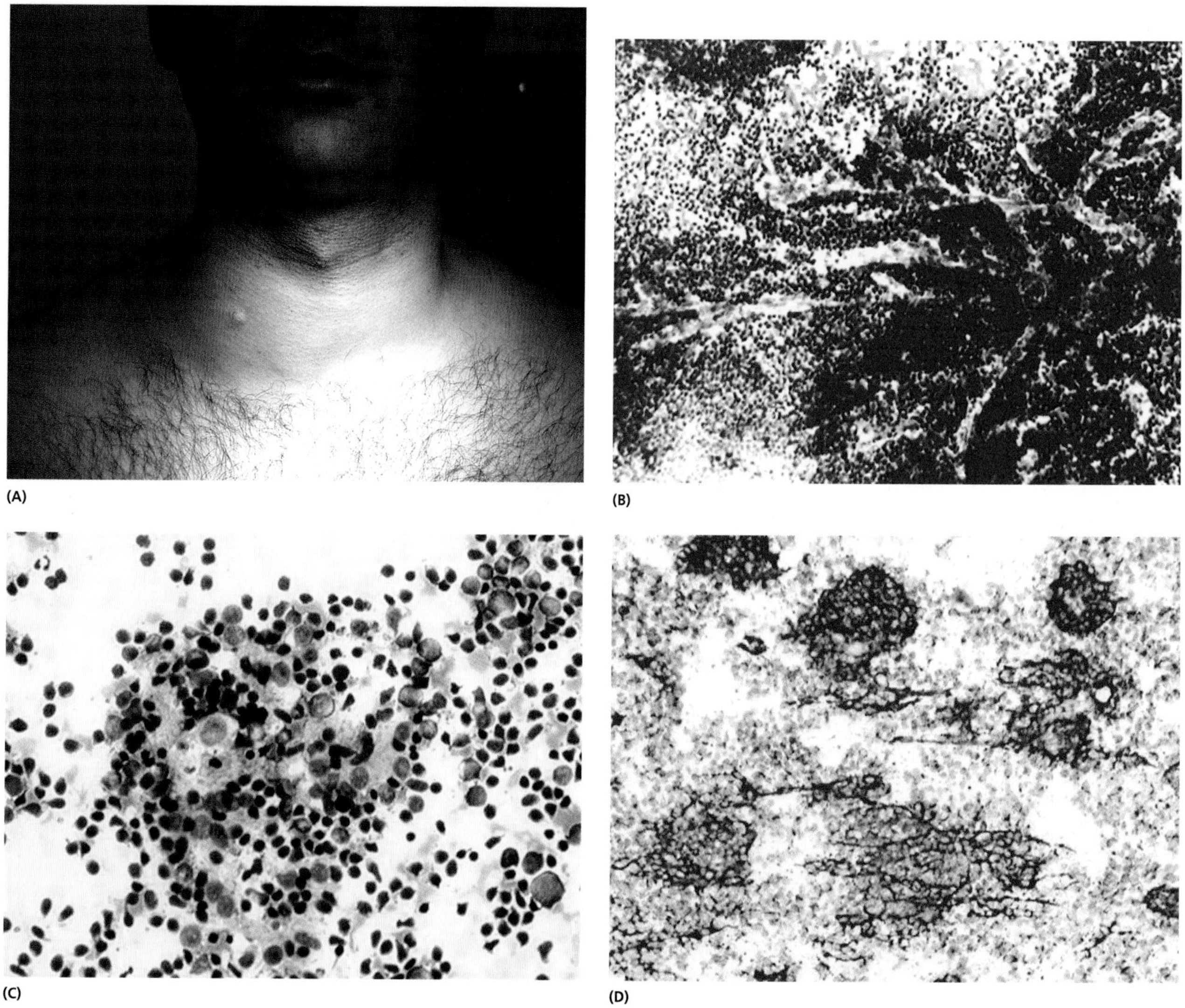

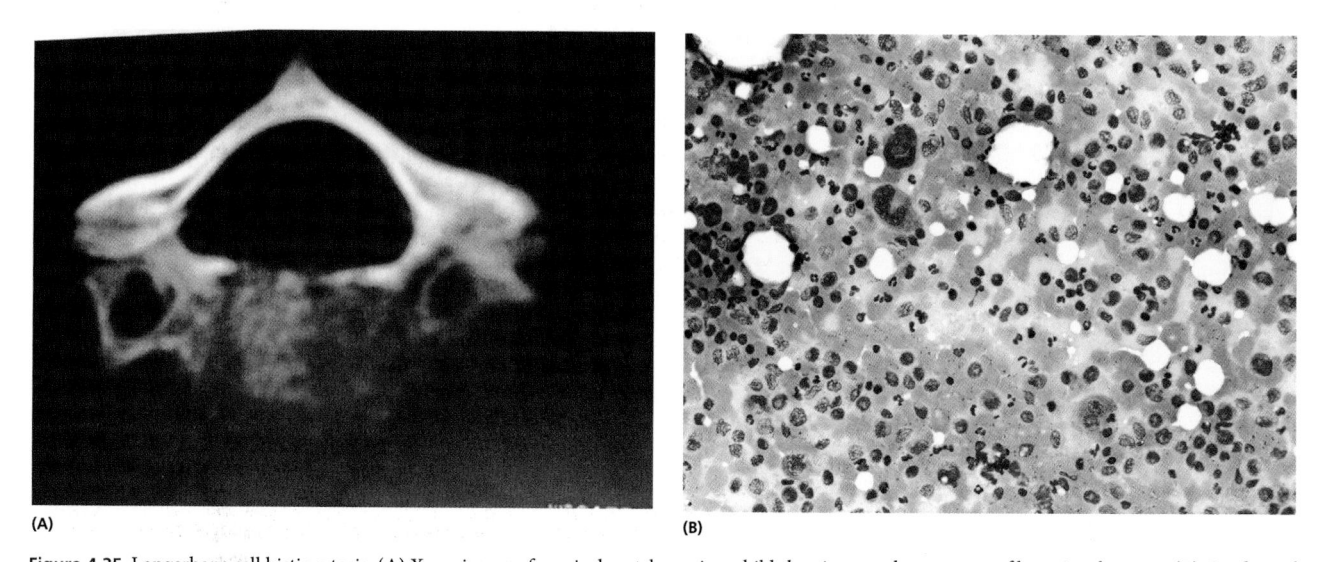

(A)

(B)

(C)

(D)

Figure 4.34 Castleman's disease. (A) 29-year-old patient presented with a painless diffuse swelling of the right side of the neck of some weeks' duration. (B) Hypercellular smear with mature small lymphoid population traversed with numerous blood vessels (×200); (C) Small lymphocytes and follicular dendritic cells (MGG ×600, oil immersion); (D) CD21 staining of follicular dendritic cells. In the clinical context of orophranygeal and mediastinal mass, these findings can be suggestive of Castleman's disease. Biopsy was performed and diagnosis confirmed.

(A)

(B)

Figure 4.35 Langerhans cell histiocytosis. (A) X-ray image of cervical vertebrum in a child showing translucent areas of bone involvement. (B) Cytological appearance of LCH. Numerous Langerhans cells admixed with eosinophils, neutrophils, lymphocytes, macrophages and multinucleated giant cells.

grooved nuclei (Fig. 4.36) [140]. Immunocytochemistry shows positivity of these cells for the S100, CD1a (leu 6) and HLA-DR antibody [141]. They are generally negative for LCA, lysosyme, Leu-M1, LN1 and epithelial membrane antigen. Electron microscopy of the aspiration-derived specimen reveals Birbeck granules [132, 142]. Patterns of cytological presentation may vary from Langerhans cell predominant, eosinophil predominant and macrophage predominant [143]. Failure to recognise the diversity of presentations of disease may result in diagnostic errors. Differential diagnosis includes sinus histiocytosis with massive lymphadenopathy but the presence of characteristic cells and abundance of eosinophils is helpful in distinguishing the two conditions.

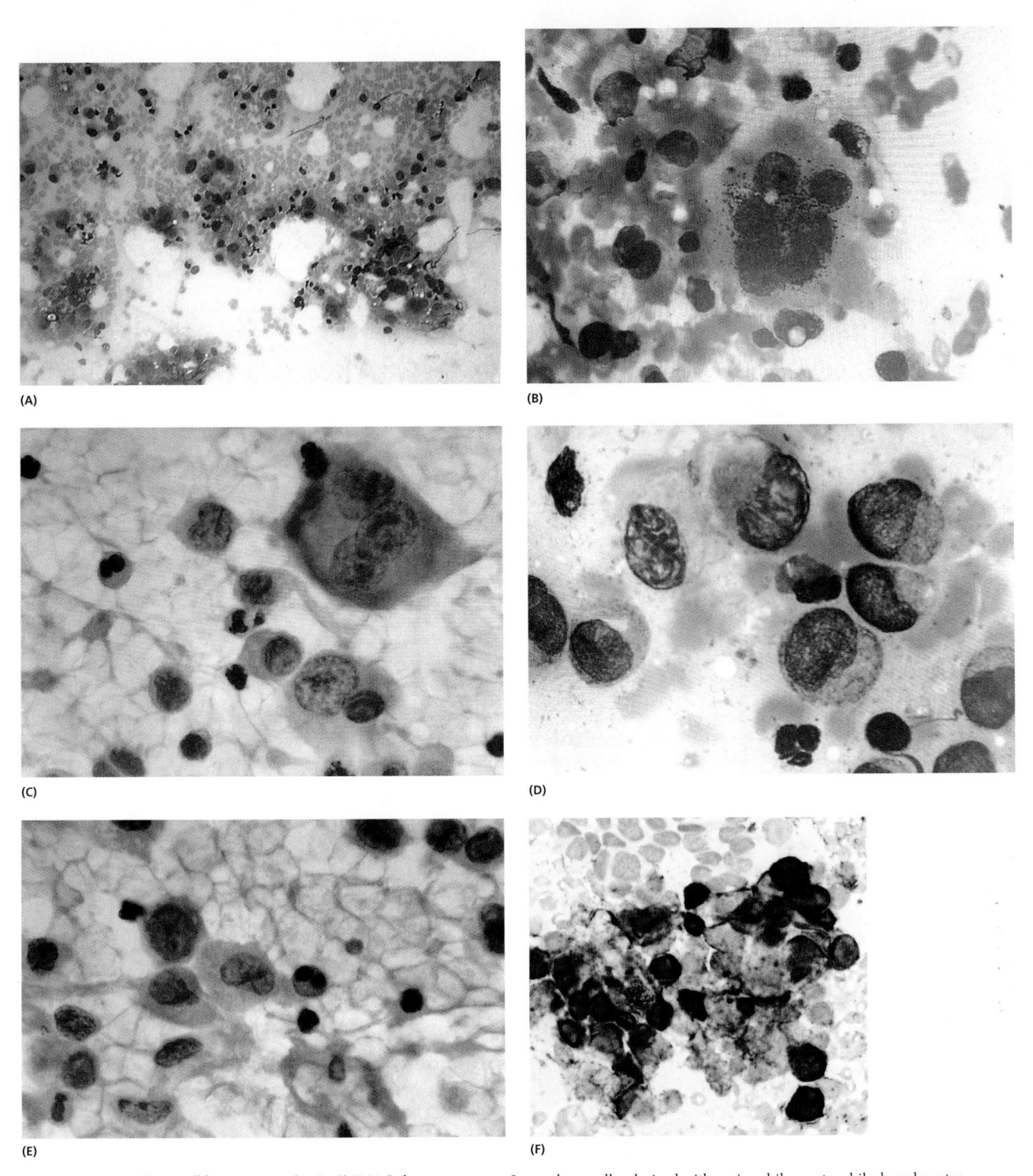

Figure 4.36 Langerhans cell histiocytosis. (A, B, C) FNAC shows numerous Langerhans cells admixed with eosinophils, neutrophils, lymphocytes, macrophages and multinucleated giant cells (MGG ×200, MGG ×1000, oil, PAP ×1000, oil). (D, E) Characteristic Langerhans cells have abundant pale non-phagocytic cytoplasm and somewhat irregular, folded or grooved nuclei]. Immunocytochemistry shows positivity of these cells for S100, CD1a (leu 6) and HLA-DR antibody (MGG, PAP ×1000, oil immersion). (F) CD1 positive Langerhans cells (×400, APAAP).

In the largest series of cases diagnosed on FNAC, Pohar Marinsek et al. determined diagnostic accuracy in recognising Langerhans cell histiocytosis in cytological smears. They diagnosed the condition in 27 out of 28 adequate FNAC samples with only one case suspected of malignancy [144]. The cytomorphological pattern of Langerhans Cell Histiocytosis in FNAC smears is usually characteristic, and a correct diagnosis is possible, especially with the aid of electron microscopy and immunocytochemistry.

4.2.6.3 Post-transplant lymphadenopathy

Post-transplant lymphoproliferative disorder (PTLD) constitutes a heterogenous spectrum of Epstein–Barr virus (EBV)-associated lymphoid proliferations that affect 2–4% of organ allograft recipients [145, 146]. Histological features of PTLD vary from polymorphic to monomorphic, often requiring a combination of morphological and ancillary studies to gain diagnostic and prognostic information (Table 4.4). No reliable morphological, immunophenotypic or genotypic criteria unequivocally distinguish between a monomorphic or monoclonal PTLD and malignant lymphoma. This distinction rests on the biological response of the individual. If withdrawal of immunosuppression fails to result in reduction in the size of the mass, the process is best considered malignant, requiring appropriate treatment.

Table 4.4 WHO categories of post-transplant lymphoproliferative disorders (PTLD).

1. Early lesions
Reactive plasmacytic hyperplasia
Infectious mononucleosis-like

2. PTLD – polymorphic
Polyclonal (rare)
Monoclonal

3. PTLD monomorphic (classify according to lymphoma classification)
• B-cell lymphomas
Diffuse large B-cell lymphoma (immunoblastic, centroblastic, anaplastic)
Burkitt/Burkitt-like lymphoma
Plasma cell myeloma

• T-cell lymphomas
Peripheral T-cell lymphoma, not otherwise categorized
Other types (hepatosplenic, gamma-delta, T/NK)

4. Other types (rare)
Hodgkin's disease-like lesions (associated with methotrexate therapy)
Plasmacytoma-like lesions

Source: [46] Swerdlow SH, Campo E, Harris NL, Jaffe ES, Pileri SA, Stein H, et al., eds. *WHO Classification of Tumors of Haemotopoietic and Lymphoid Tissue*, 4th edn. Lyon: IARC, 2008.

PTLD have been described only rarely in cytological specimens [145–147]. However, cytological samples may provide the initial diagnosis of this potentially fatal disease and allow appropriate intervention.

Cytological features: The diagnosis of PTLD should be suggested when cytological specimens from organ allograft recipients show a polymorphous atypical lymphoid proliferation, frequently with plasmacytoid differentiation and necrosis (Fig. 4.37 and Chapter 3, Fig. 3.33). Morphological presentations of PTLD range from plasmacytoid lymphoproliferative disease to those of an immunoblastic or large-cell lymphoma [147, 148]. Plasmacytoid lymphoproliferative disease is characterised by a mostly polymorphous population of lymphoid cells containing many large transformed lymphocytes, occasional immunoblast-like atypical lymphocytes, necrosis and, frequently, obvious plasmacytoid differentiation. Immunoblastic or large-cell lymphoma cytological presentation may be a monotonous population of large lymphoid cells consistent with malignant lymphoma, large-cell type [146]. The presence of EBV can be documented in the majority of cases by in situ hybridisation, PCR or Southern blot. Although this generally establishes a causal relationship of the tumour to EBV, it rarely provides useful diagnostic information [149]. In addition to morphology, flow cytometric immunophenotyping and, in selected cases, the DNA PCR can be performed on FNAC material to show monoclonal or polyclonal rearrangement of the immunoglobulin heavy chain gene [149].

Differential diagnosis of a mass developing in a post-transplant immunosuppressed patient includes localised infections, malignant neoplasms and EBV related neoplasms, in particular PTLD. The presence of PTLD in a body fluid specimen is a poor prognostic indicator [145, 150].

4.2.6.4 Kimura's disease

Kimura's disease (Table 4.3) is a chronic angioproliferative disorder of unknown aetiology. Patients usually present with a painless mass involving a major salivary gland with lymphadenopathy (Fig. 4.38). Current studies suggest an immunologic mechanism for the pathogenesis of this disease entity. The immunohistochemical findings are usually nonspecific but might help in eliminating malignancies. The role of FNAC and biopsy procedure appears to be limited in making the diagnosis of Kimura disease. Peripheral blood eosinophilia and raised serum IgE levels are features of the condition. It occurs endemically in the Far East and sporadically in the West.

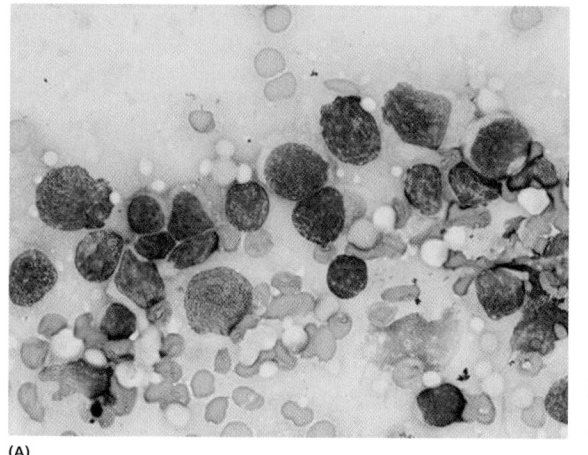 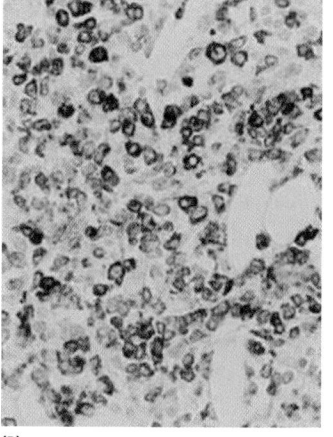 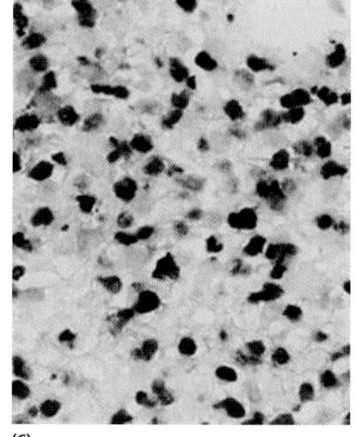

(A) (B) (C)

Figure 4.37 Post-transplant lymphadenopathy. (A) Polymorphous atypical lymphoid proliferation, frequently with plasmacytoid differentiation. No necrosis (MGG ×600, oil). (B) CD79A positivity in large transformed lymphocytes and atypical immunoblasts. (C) FISH for EBV shows strong nuclear staining.

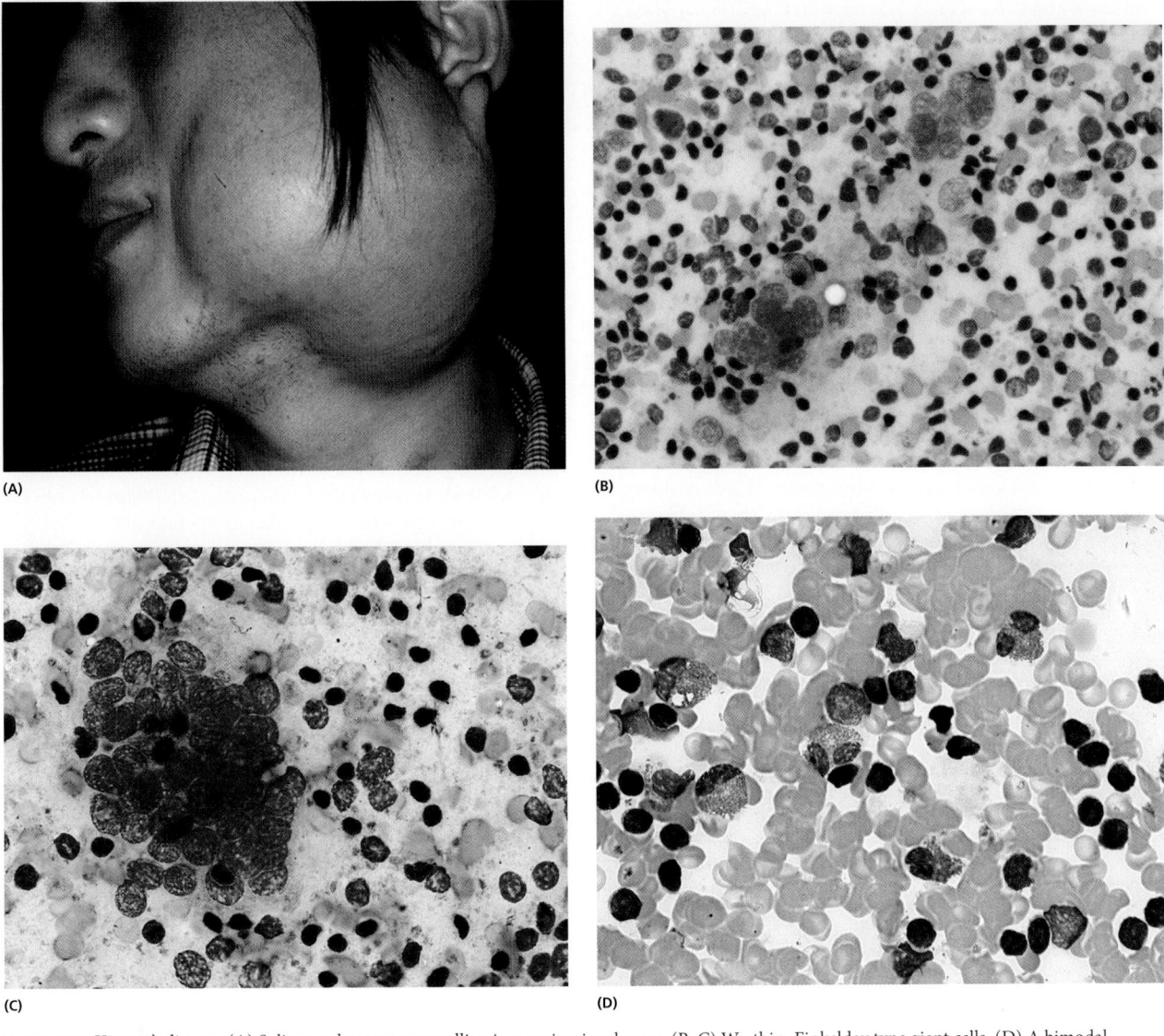

(A)

(B)

(C)

(D)

Figure 4.38 Kimura's disease. (A) Solitary subcutaneous swelling in a periauricualr area. (B, C) Warthin–Finkeldey type giant cells. (D) A bimodal population of lymphocytes and eosinophils.

The overall prognosis is good. The natural history of the disease appears to be indolent, without any malignant transformation reported, although recurrence can be frequent. Treatment is surgery or, conservative treatment with either corticosteroids or radiation [151]. Complete surgical excision whenever feasible is the preferred treatment despite a high recurrence rate.

Histologically, the lesions are characterised by proliferating blood vessels with rich eosinophilic infiltrate. Hyperplastic lymph nodes show prominent germinal centres surrounded by concentrically arranged small lymphocytes. In the interfollicular areas there is a marked small vessel proliferation, presence of plasma cells, mast cells, lymphoid cells and eosinophils, occasionally forming eosinophilic microabscesses. Plump endothelial cells are seen.

Cytological features are characterised by the Warthin–Finkeldey type giant cells against a background of a bimodal population of lymphocytes and eosinophils [152, 153]. The prominent feature is the presence of significant numbers of eosinophils in a background of lymphoid cells [154].

Differential diagnosis includes haemangioma, histiocytosis, schwannoma, angiosarcoma, Hodgkin's lymphoma, angioimmunoblastic lymphadenopathy (AILD) and AILD-like T-cell lymphoma, lymphoepithelioid T-cell lymphoma, Langerhans Cell Histiocytosis (LCH), angiolymphoid hyperplasia with eosinophilia, angiofollicular lymph node hyperplasia (Castleman's disease) and other reactive lymphadenopathies [151, 154]. Angiolymphoid hyperplasia with eosinophilia (ALHE) shares similar histological features with Kimura disease, however, is believed to be a more superficial, vascular lesion with the absence of lymphadenopathy or peripheral eosinophilia. Cytologically, Kimura's disease shares some of the morphological and clinical features of all of these diseases. The cytological features therefore are characteristic but not specific. Imaging can further help delineate Kimura disease from malignant tumours. Computed tomographic scans may show poor to moderate enhancement of the lesion. Lymphadenopathy is characteristically not cystic or necrotic in appearance, as it might be in malignancy. Magnetic resonance imaging can show hyperintense signal on T2-weighted images [155]. A primary diagnosis of Kimura's disease may need to be confirmed by a biopsy. FNAC may be valuable in the diagnosis of recurrent lesions and may spare the patient from repeated biopsies.

4.3 Hodgkin's lymphoma

Hodgkin's lymphoma (disease) is a clonal proliferation of (in most cases) B-cells. The Rye classification postulated four subtypes of Hodgkin's disease and these are virtually unchanged until today. The majority of classical Hodgkin's falls into three categories and an additional 'lymphocyte rich' classical Hodgkin's of the current WHO classification (Table 4.5) (Fig 4.39). The lymphocyte predominant type is classified separately [156].

Lymphocyte Rich, Nodular Sclerosis, Mixed Cellularity and *Lymphocyte Depletion* types of Hodgkin's disease all contain binuclear or mulinucleate Reed–Sternberg (RS) cells and mononuclear Hodgkin cells with a cellular infiltrate of lymphoid cells, eosinophils and other inflammatory cells in various proportions [157, 158]. RS cells are typically CD30 and CD15 positive (Table 4.6). The grading system adopted in nodular sclerosis has not been upheld by the WHO classification since it has not shown clinical relevance so far [159].

The *Nodular Lymphocyte Predominance* type of Hodgkin's disease is, both clinically and immunophenotypically, a distinct entity from

Table 4.5 WHO classification of lymphoid neoplasms.

B-cell neoplasms

Precursor B-cell neoplasm
- Precursor B-lymphoblastic leukaemia/lymphoma (precursor B-cell acute lymphoblastic leukaemia)

Mature (peripheral) B-cell neoplasms
- B-cell chronic lymphocytic leukaemia/small lymphocytic lymphoma
- B-cell prolymphocytic leukaemia
- Lymphoplasmacytic lymphoma
- Splenic marginal zone B-cell lymphoma (+/– villous lymphocytes)
- Hairy cell leukaemia
- Plasma cell myeloma/plasmacytoma
- Extranodal marginal zone B-cell lymphoma of MALT type
- Nodal marginal zone B-cell lymphoma (+/– monocytoid B-cells)
- Follicular lymphoma
- Mantle cell lymphoma
- Diffuse large B-cell lymphoma
- Mediastinal large B-cell lymphoma
- Primary effusion lymphoma
- Burkitt lymphoma/Burkitt cell leukaemia

T and NK-cell neoplasms

Precursor T-cell neoplasm
- Precursor T-lymphoblastic lymphoma/leukaemia (precursor T-cell acute lymphoblastic leukaemia)

Mature (peripheral) T-cell neoplasms
- T-cell prolymphocytic leukaemia
- T-cell granular lymphocytic leukaemia
- Aggressive NK-cell leukaemia
- Adult T-cell lymphoma/leukaemia (HTLV1+)
- Extranodal NK/T-cell lymphoma, nasal type
- Enteropathy-type T-cell lymphoma
- Hepatosplenic γδ T-cell lymphoma
- Subcutaneous panniculitis-like T-cell lymphoma
- Mycosis fungoides/Sezary syndrome
- Anaplastic large cell lymphoma, T-/null cell, primary cutaneous type
- Peripheral T-cell lymphoma, not otherwise characterised
- Angioimmunoblastic T-cell lymphoma
- Anaplastic large cell lymphoma, T-/null cell, primary systemic type

Hodgkin's lymphoma (Hodgkin's disease)
- Nodular lymphocyte predominance Hodgkin's lymphoma
- Classical Hodgkin's lymphoma
  Nodular sclerosis Hodgkin's lymphoma (Grades 1 and 2)
  Lymphocyte-rich classical Hodgkin's lymphoma
  Mixed cellularity Hodgkin's lymphoma
  Lymphocyte depletion Hodgkin's lymphoma

* More common entities are underlined. † B- and T/NK-cell neoplasms are grouped according to major clinical presentations (predominantly disseminated/leukaemic, primary extranodal, predominantly nodal).
* Only major categories are included. Subtypes and variants will be discussed in the text and in other tables.
Source: [46] Swerdlow SH, Campo E, Harris NL, Jaffe ES, Pileri SA, Stein H, et al., eds. *WHO Classification of Tumors of Haemotopoietic and Lymphoid Tissue*, 4th edn. Lyon: IARC, 2008.

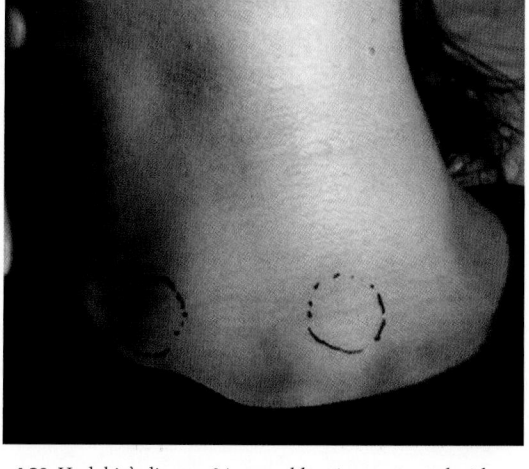

Figure 4.39 Hodgkin's disease. 34-year-old patient presented with clinically unexplained cervical lymphadenopathy. Nodes were soft, mobile and painless. There was no history of skin itchung, temperature or night sweats. FNAC was performed and Hodgkin's disease diagnosed. Patient was referred for biopsy prior to treatment.

Lymphocyte Rich Hodgkin's lymphoma. In the nodular lymphocyte predominance type of Hodgkin's disease, scattered neoplastic 'L&H' (lymphocytic and histiocytic) or 'popcorn' cells lie within large nodular areas made up of small lymphoid cells. Nodules contain extensive meshwork of follicular dendritic cells and lymphoid cells are polyclonal small B-cell lymphocytes expressing both IgM and IgD. T-cells are found around 'L&H' cells and are sparse. This background distinguishes nodular lymphocyte predominance from other types, which have backgrounds rich in T-cells. 'L&H' cells express B-cell markers and J chain, a protein associated with B-cells but not present in RS cells. Unlike classical RS cells, 'L&H' cells express CD 45(LCA), EMA (often), CDw75 (LN1), CD30 is positive sometimes, CD3 is negative (Table 4.6). Nodular lymphocyte predominance Hodgkin's disease shows male predominance and an indolent course although they may progress to a large B-cell lymphoma (See section 4.3.1).

The cytological diagnosis of classical Hodgkin's disease depends upon demonstration of RS or Hodgkin's cells amongst appropriate reactive cell components. However, RS-like cells have been reported in benign lympho-proliferative conditions like reactive hyperplasia and infectious mononucleosis, and certain non-Hodgkin's lymphoma subtypes as well as non-lymphoid malignancies like metastatic carcinoma, melanoma, sarcomas and germ cell tumours. Non-Hodgkin's lymphoma subtypes, for example anaplastic large cell lymphoma, T-cell-histiocytic-rich B-cell lymphoma and pleomorphic peripheral T-cell lymphoma, which can be misdiagnosed as Hodgkin's lymphoma, need immunohistochemical studies to be differentiated [160].

Despite this, diagnostic accuracy of FNAC for HD has been invariably high (>85%) [10, 161]. However, due to the lack of architectural features included in the subtyping, FNAC has limited value in the primary diagnosis and sub-classification of Hodgkin's disease but is very useful in diagnosing recurrent disease [162–168]. At present, when Hodgkin's disease is suspected morphologically or immunophenotypically, a biopsy must be performed.

Classic RS cells are easily identified in FNAC preparations. They have bi-lobed or poly-lobed nuclei with prominent nucleoli and moderately abundant cytoplasm. These cells are scattered among the background of small lymphocytes admixed with other inflammatory cells, particularly eosinophils (Fig. 4.40).

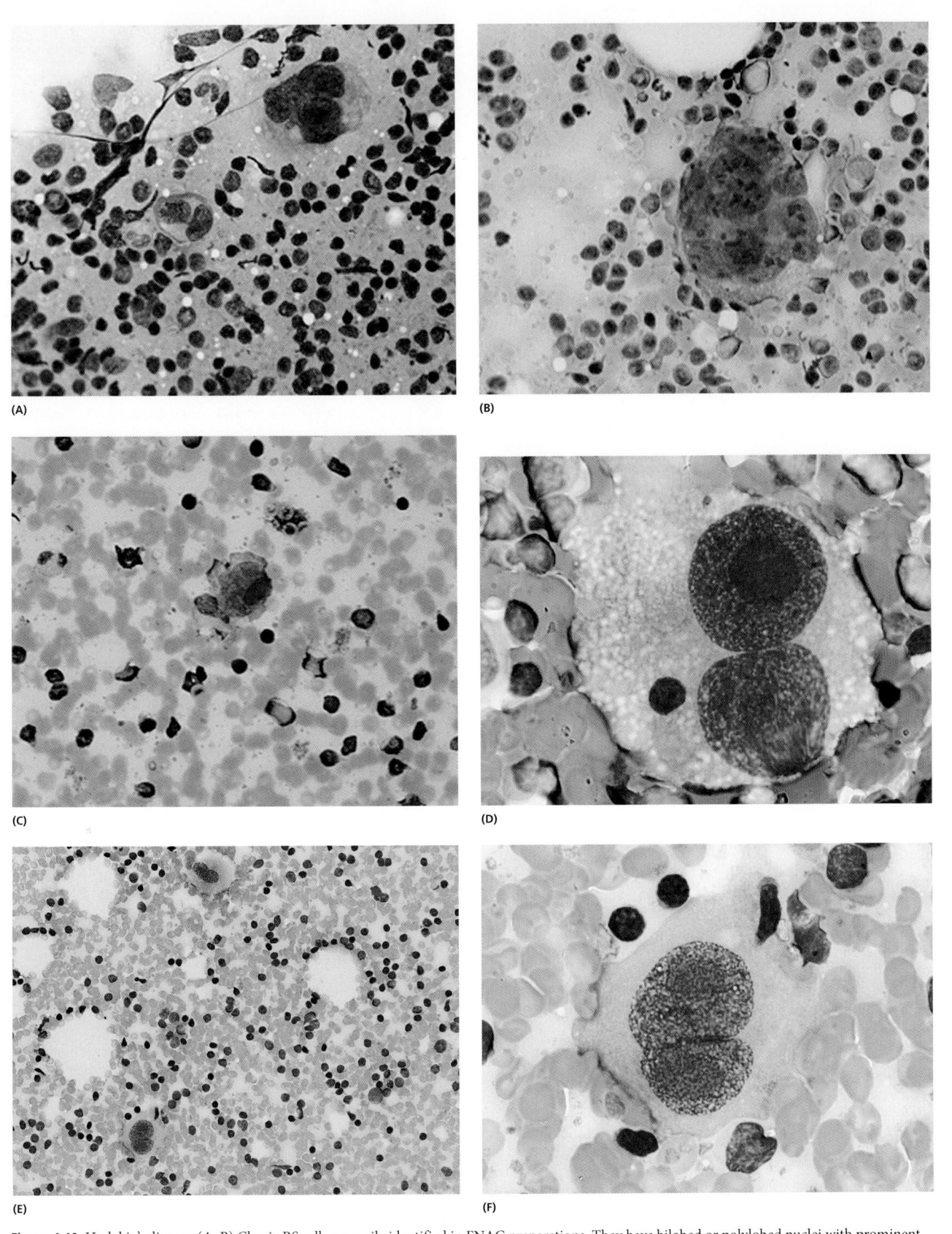

Figure 4.40 Hodgkin's disease. (A, B) Classic RS cells are easily identified in FNAC preparations. They have bilobed or polylobed nuclei with prominent nucleoli and moderately abundant cytoplasm. These cells are scattered among the background of small lymphocytes admixed with other inflammatory cells, particularly eosinophils (MGG ×400, ×1000, oil immersion). (C, D, E, F) Different appearance of mononuclear Hodgkin and RS cells. The prominent basophilic nucleoli with a well-defined nucleolar margin are characteristic. Epitheliod cells, reflecting granulomatous reaction, may be seen (MGG ×100, oil immersion).

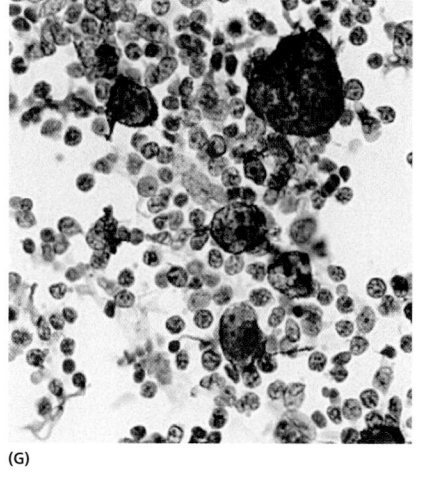
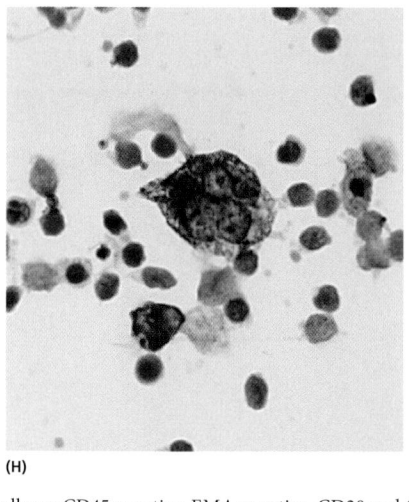

(G) (H)

Figure 4.40 (*Continued*) (G, H) CD30 and CD15 positive staining. Hodgkin's cells are CD45 negative, EMA negative, CD20 and CD3 negative, although in 25% of cases they stain with CD20.

Table 4.6 Cell phenotype in Hodgkin's disease.

	Classical R-S cells	L and H cells
CD3/TCRP	Occasionally positive	Negative
CDIS	Usually positive	Usually negative
CD20	Occasionally positive	Usually positive
Other B markers	Rarely positive	Frequently positive
CD30 (Ki- 1)	Positive	Sometimes positive
CD45 (LCA)	Usually negative	Often positive
CDw75 (LN 1)	Usually negative	Usually positive
EMA	Usually negative	Often positive
Ig	Polytypic or negative	Negative or monotypic
J chain	Negative	Positive
EBV genome	Frequently positive	Infrequently positive

Source: Mason D, Gatter K, *Lymphoma Classification*. Blackwell Science, 1998.

Immunophenotype: (Table 4.6) Hodgkin and classical RS cells are CD45 negative, EMA negative, CD30 positive and CD15 positive. Usually they are CD20 and CD3 negative although in 25% of cases they stain with CD20. Cases of Epstein–Barr virus associated Hodgkin's will be positive for the EBV latent membrane protein [169].

Pitfalls in diagnosis include peripheral T-cell lymphoma and anaplastic large cell lymphomas (ALCL). EMA and T-cell antigen activity favours ALCL, whereas CD15 positivity favours Hodgkin's disease. In difficult cases T-cell receptor gene rearrangement and t(2;5) translocation can help diagnose peripheral T-cell lymphoma and ALCL, respectively. A Hodgkin's-like variant of Richter syndrome is another pitfall [170] (Chapter 5, Fig. 5.16). Suppurative type of Hodgkin's disease is another unusual FNAC presentation that can be diagnosed on FNAC. Smears are dominated by neutrophils, macrophages, and cellular debris. Only a few large, atypical cells of the Hodgkin's and RS type are observed [171–173].

4.3.1 Nodular Lymphocyte Predominant Hodgkin's lymphoma

Lymphocyte predominant Hodgkin's disease is now recognised as a separate entity from classical Hodgkin's disease and may be closer to peripheral B-cell lymphoma. It involves peripheral lymph nodes sparing the mediastinum.

Cytological features: Classic RS cells are not present, instead L&H cells may be present in the background of epithelioid cells and mature lymphocytes. The L&H cells vary from polypoid cells with large nucleoli to cells with features of RS cells and their variants.

Immunophenotype: L&H cells are B-cells (CD20 and CD45 positive), Ig negative, CD15 negative CD30+/– and EMA negative. Numerous CD57 T-cells may be present (Fig. 4.41).

Cytological diagnosis may be difficult and the entity has to be borne in mind when encountering FNAC samples from persistent lymphadenopathy without classical RS cells.

4.4 Non-Hodgkin's lymphoma

4.4.1 Introduction

With the advances in molecular pathology, the cell as a morphological and functional unit has become essential in the diagnosis of lymphoma. Conventional staining, preparation and interpretation of cells, as seen in FNAC, often used as a first line investigation of lymphadenopathy, is being supplemented with an array of immunocytochemical and molecular analyses, aimed not only at a more precise disease definition, but also at recognising factors that can predict prognosis and response to treatment [3a, 174]. Recent changes in the classification of non-Hodgkin's lymphoma (NHL), in particular the new WHO classification based on the principles of the REAL classification, emphasise the diagnostic importance of individual cell cytomorphology, immunophenotyping, genotyping and clinical findings in addition to histology [46, 156, 175] (Table 4.5). These changes have allowed for a greater role of FNAC in the diagnosis of NHL [169] (Table 4.1 and 4.2).

[See BOX 4.3. Summary of ultrasound features: Lymphoma on www.wiley.com/go/kocjan/clinical_cytopathology_head_neck2e]

The FNAC diagnosis of NHL relies on cell morphology as well as finding of a relatively monotonous population of lymphoid cells in smears [176]. This may sometimes prove difficult, particularly in low grade NHL with polymorphous cell population. Despite the difficulties, the evidence shows that a large percentage of NHL cases can be recognised and correctly classified using FNAC. This is particularly true of recurrences of lymphoma that amount to up to more than 50% of all lymphomas diagnosed on FNAC (Fig. 4.42) [177]. Diagnostic sensitivity of FNAC is dependent on several factors including the type of NHL and is reported in the literature to be 61–100%. Specificity of most studies is >90% [7, 11, 27, 29, 30, 44, 178–196].

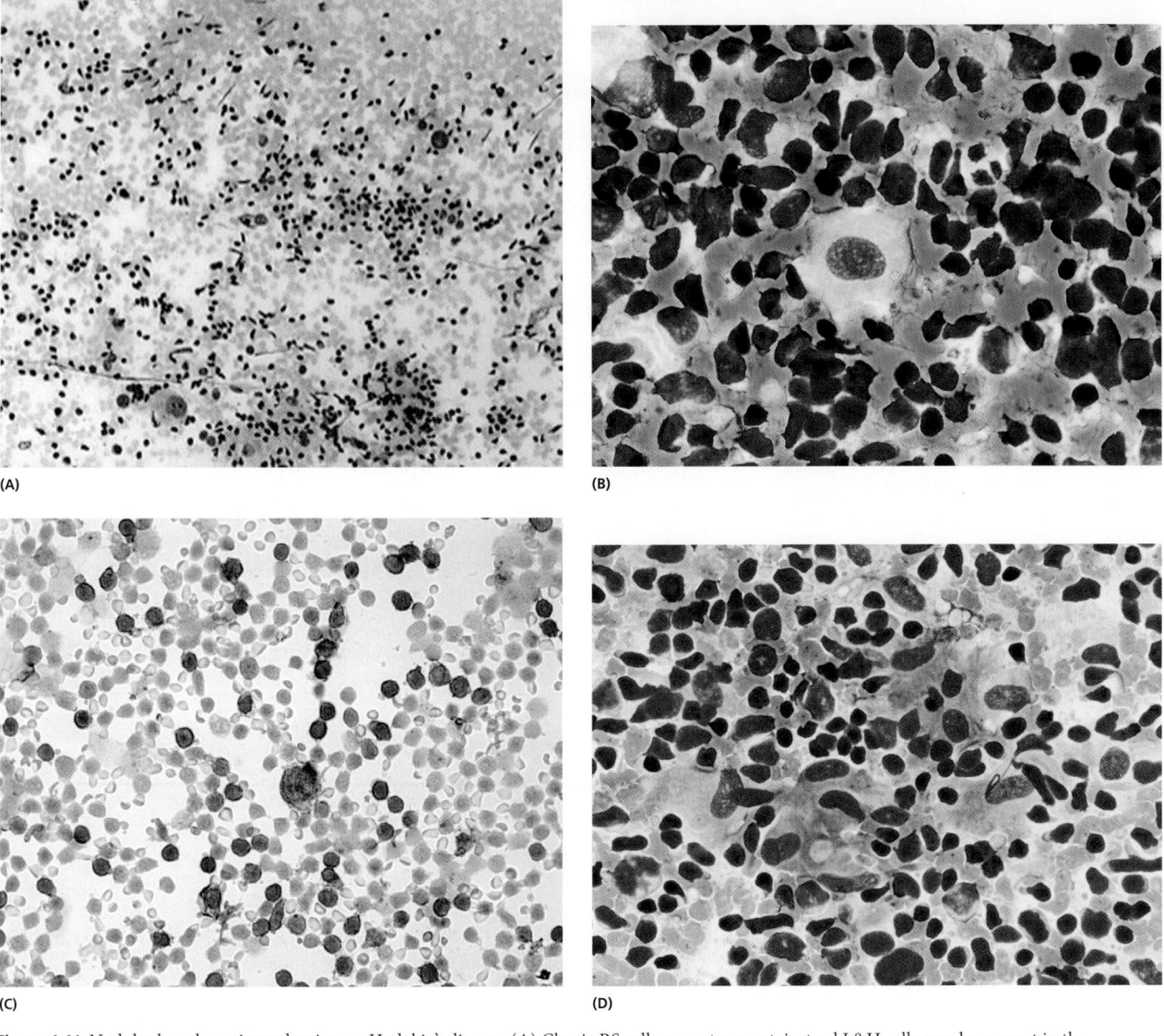

Figure 4.41 Nodular lymphocytic predominance Hodgkin's disease. (A) Classic RS cells are not present, instead L&H cells may be present in the background of epithelioid cells and mature lymphocytes (MGG ×200). (B) The L&H cells vary from polypoid cells with large nucleoli to cells with features of RS cells and their variants. (C) L&H cells are CD20 positive. Immunoprophile of this type of Hodgkin's disease is CD30−, CD15−, ALK−, CD45+, CD20+ and EMA+/−. (D) A granulomatous background with aggregates of epithelioid cells is frequently associated with HD.

There are recognised difficulties in separating florid reactive hyperplasia and atypical non-neoplastic lymphoid proliferations from low-grade malignant lymphoma on FNAC [44]. The reported cytodiagnostic accuracy of FNAC in diagnosis of follicular lymphomas and nodular sclerosis type of Hodgkin's disease is less compared to other subtypes of NHL and HD, respectively [12]. Similar difficulties exist in diagnosis of marginal zone lymphoma MALT (where the helpful lymphoepithelial lesions are absent in the smears), T-cell rich B-cell lymphoma [197], immunoglobulin negative malignant lymphoma, composite lymphoma and peripheral T-cell lymphomas. Differential diagnostic problems also include a group of small round cell tumours and non-lymphoid acute leukaemia. These can be overcome by the use of ancillary techniques.

Currently, the role of FNAC in management of lymphomas is evolving [1, 12, 20, 51, 198–202]. Whilst it remains the first line of investigation of most lymphadenopathies, excision biopsy may be required for confirmation only in certain lymphomas, such as follicle centre, mantle zone, MALT/marginal zone lymphoma and

Hodgkin's disease. In other disorders, where the diagnosis is not based on architecture and where cytomorphology, immunocytochemistry and molecular techniques complement the clinical setting, excision may not be necessary. These include reactive lymphoid hyperplasia, small lymphocytic lymphoma, anaplastic large cell (Ki-1) lymphoma, diffuse large B-cell lymphoma and Burkitt's lymphoma [198]. Even the subclassification of follicle-derived low grade NHL (follicle centre and mantle zone), can now be established with high accuracy on FNAC material if cytomorphology is corroborated by a complete immunophenotypic analysis [200]. Biopsy can be avoided also in detecting residual disease, recurrences and progression of low-grade to high-grade lymphoma and staging of lymphomas. Biopsy of difficult intra-abdominal sites may also be avoided by using the FNAC [33].

With these management principles in mind, the *ancillary techniques* play an important part of FNAC diagnosis of NHL (see Section 4.1). Routine samples requiring molecular analysis are equally relevant to histopathologists and cytopathologists, and

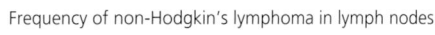

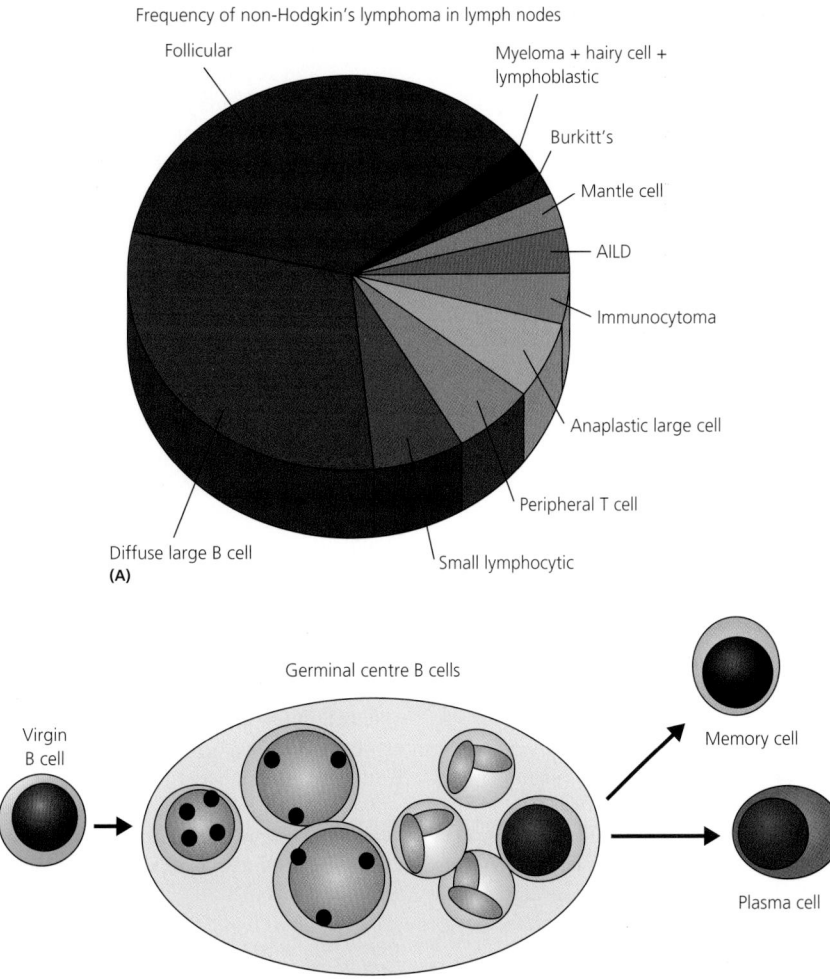

(A)

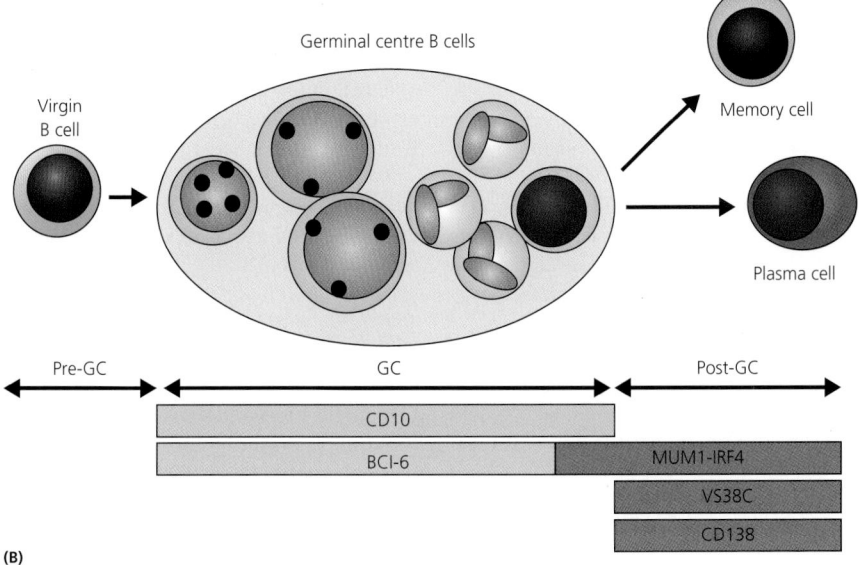

(B)

Figure 4.42 (A) Frequency of non-Hodgkin's lymphoma in lymph nodes (Source: Mason D, Gatter K. *Lymphoma Classification*, 1998). Follicular and Diffuse Large Cell lymphoma are by far the most frequent NH lymphomas in the USA and Europe accounting for 2/3 of cases. (B) This scheme depicts expression of stage-specific differentiation antigens in relation to normal B-cell differentiation, that is pre-germinal centre (GC), GC and post-GC stages. (Source: [220] De Leval L, Harris NL. *Histopathology* 2003; 43: 509–28.)

molecular biology laboratories are now using cytological as well as histological material for diagnostic testing, allowing different specimen types to be used as and when they are most appropriate [203]. The commonly used ancillary techniques in lymphomas are immunocytochemistry (IC), flow cytometry, Southern blot (SB) technique, polymerase chain reaction (PCR) and fluorescent in situ hybridisation (FISH). In addition, laser scanning cytometry (LSC) and DNA microarray technologies are in the research phase. These various laboratory techniques are used for immunophenotyping, demonstration of monoclonality, identification of chromosomal translocation, assessment of cell kinetics and expression of mRNA in the tumour cells. Flow cytometry helps in rapid immunophenotyping of NHL and it has an added advantage over IC in recognizing the co-expression of CD markers [204]. (See section 4.1.4.1).

Ancillary techniques contribute to the correct distinction between reactive and neoplastic lymphoid proliferation in 97% of cases [205]. Combination of flow cytometry (FC) and morphology helps diagnose 80% of NHL (69% of the primary lymphomas and 88% of the recurrent lymphomas) without the need for histological sampling [29, 195, 206, 207]. Combined FNAC and FC show sensitivity of 98% and a specificity of 100% for diagnosis of lymphoma [44, 208–210]. In using the ancillary studies, several authors recommend a multiparameter approach ('triple test'), that is, the importance of interpretation of ancillary techniques in conjunction with cytomorphology and clinical information [19, 43, 179]. PCR amplification of the complementarity-determining region (CDR)3 of the T-cell receptor (TCR) gamma gene can be used to assess clonality of T-cell populations as a supportive diagnostic tool for

T-cell neoplasms [211]. Whilst ancillary techniques have made significant contributions to the identification and typing of lymphomas, there is still a requirement for a simple and rapid diagnostic procedure for the patient who presents with persistent lymphadenopathy. Light microscopic examination of FNAC smears fulfils this role, provided its limitations and pitfalls are recognised [92]. The selective separation of cytology specimens allows the application of immunophenotypic analysis including flow cytometry and immunohistochemistry as well as molecular analyses, such as fluorescence in situ hybridisation (FISH) and PCR strategies. With the integrative procedure presented, cytology offers an excellent cost-effective tool for the diagnostic approach of patients with suspected hematopathological malignancies allowing a high diagnostic accuracy, ideal for initial diagnosis or follow-up [212].

4.4.2 Obtaining appropriate material

Cytopathologists should be familiar with the possibilities opened to them in handling the FNAC material. With training, it is simple to obtain an average of 20 million cells per procedure without much discomfort for the patient [198]. Use of very fine gauge (25 or higher) heparinised needles, aspiration without suction and rapid movement whilst within the node usually produces sufficient cell yield. Less material is needed if a single Feulgen stained slide is used for image analysis for DNA ploidy and proliferation and if marker studies are performed on cytospin preparations instead of flow cytometry. PCR detection of gene rearrangement requires much less cells than Southern blot studies [42]. Recently, a laser scanning cytometer (Compucyte, Cambridge, MA) has evolved as a hybrid between a flow cytometer and an image analyser that requires only a small quantity of cells (about 50 000). Cells may be placed on a specially configured slide for multiparameter immunophenotyping, which can obtain results within 2 hours [199].

4.4.3 Classification of Non-Hodgkin's lymphoma

The history of lymphoma classification has been long and controversial (Table 4.5). However, within the last 30 years much has been learned about the biology of lymphoma. The concept of classifying malignant lymphoma according to the (proposed) normal counterpart was developed in the Kiel classification [213]. In 1994, the International Lymphoma Study Group (ILSG) developed a consensus list of lymphoid neoplasms, which was published as the 'Revised European-American Classification of Lymphoid Neoplasms' (REAL) and consisted of a clinicopathological entities recognised at the time [214]. These tumours were divided into three major categories: B-cell neoplasms, T-cell and postulated natural killer cell neoplasms and Hodgkin's disease. The classification was based on the principle that a classification is a list of 'REAL' disease entities, which are defined by a combination of morphology, immunophenotype, genetic features and clinical features. The relative importance of each of these features varies among diseases and there is no one 'gold standard'. In some tumours morphology is paramount, in others it is immunophenotype, a specific genetic abnormality or clinical features [156, 215]. Each distinct disease may have a range of histological grade and clinical aggressiveness. Prognostic factors can be defined within an entity, on a clinical, morphological, immunohistochemical or genetic basis. Although many distinct diseases can now be recognised, three of them (follicular lymphoma, diffuse large B-cell lymphoma and Hodgkin's disease) account for the majority of the cases seen in Europe and the USA [216] (Fig. 4.42A). Recognition of distinct disease entities

is essential in order to develop and test effective therapies [217]. The International Lymphoma Study showed that the REAL classification could be used by pathologists, with inter-observer reproducibility better than for other classifications (>85%) [156]. The WHO classification for lymphomas is similar, based on the principle to define disease entities that can be recognised by the pathologists and are of clinical relevance [46, 156, 176, 218].

The changes in the classification of NHL emphasise the diagnostic importance of cytomorphology, immunophenotyping and molecular findings in addition to histology [17]. These changes have allowed for a greater role of FNAC in the diagnosis of NHL [169]. The REAL classification of lymphoid neoplasms was reviewed in the context of its adaptability to the cytological diagnosis of lymphoid neoplasms and it was concluded that FNAC is being used more frequently in the diagnosis, staging and follow-up of lymphoma whenever supportive studies are readily available [169]. Many cases of NHL can be diagnosed and sub-classified by FNAC when there is adequate immunophenotypic information [219]. Figure 4.42B depicts the expression of stage-specific differentiation antigens in relation to normal B-cell differentiation, that is pre-germinal centre (GC), GC and post-GC stages. Pre-GC B-cells are virgin B-cells, cells comprising the GC consist of small blast cells, centroblasts, centrocytes and occasional plasma cells (from left to right). B-cells exiting the GC differentiate either towards memory cells or immunoglobulin-secreting plasma cells. Normal GC B-cells express CD10 and Bcl-6. The latter antigen may be lost by late GC B-cells, which in turn acquire MUM-1 expression. MUM-1, VS38c and CD138 are expressed by post-GC B-cells. While MUM-1 may be acquired late in the GC reaction, VS38c and CD138 expression is usually restricted to cells exhibiting plasmacytic differentiation and to plasma cells [220].

4.4.4 Precursor lesions

4.4.4.1 Lymphoblastic leukaemia/lymphoma

Lymphoblastic neoplasms, of B- or T-cell type, present either as localised solid tumours in lymph nodes or, more usually, as a leukaemia [156] (Table 4.3). Disease affects all ages although it is more common in older children and young adults. It usually presents as a symptomatic mediastinal mass with pleural or pericardial effusion and will progress rapidly to involve blood, bone marrow, CNS and gonads. Lymphoblastic lymphoma/leukaemia is an aggressive but curable disease, particularly in children [221].

Cytological features: Lymphoblastic lymphomas are composed of medium sized lymphoid cells, which are oval or rounded or highly convoluted, have pale staining nuclei with fine blast-like chromatin and inconspicuous nucleoli (except in 10% of cases where they are prominent) (Fig. 4.43) [187]. The size of the cells and lack of prominent nucleoli may be misleading into calling the lesion a low-grade lymphoma. Unlike low-grade lymphoma, there are usually many mitoses and blast like chromatin is apparent. Differentiation from diffuse large cell lymphoma or transformed mantle zone lymphoma and histiocytic lymphoma may be a morphological pitfall that has to be resolved with immunocytochemistry [192].

Immunophenotypically, lymphoblasts express TdT. All other lymphomas are negative for TdT. CD45 is positive only in 80% of cases. The majority of lymphoblastic lymphomas (85%) are of T-cell lineage and they nearly always express surface or intracytoplasmic CD3. This is important for excluding all other B-cell lymphomas. If lymphoblastic lymphoma is of B-cell lineage it expresses CD 10 (CALLA) and CD19. Only about 50% of B-cell lymphoblastic lymphomas express CD20 because of their immaturity. Genotyping

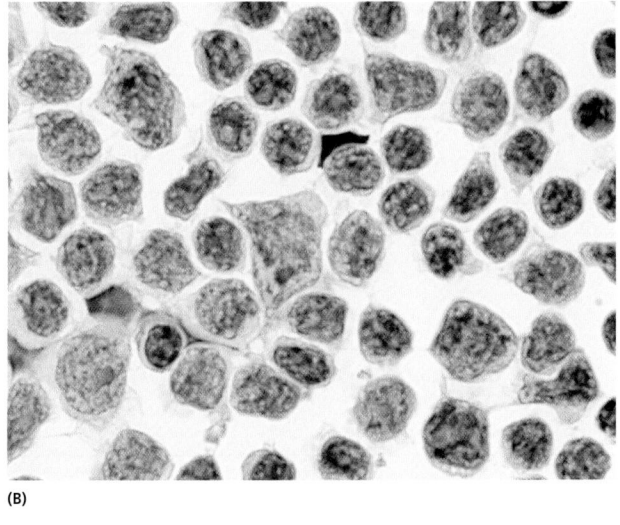

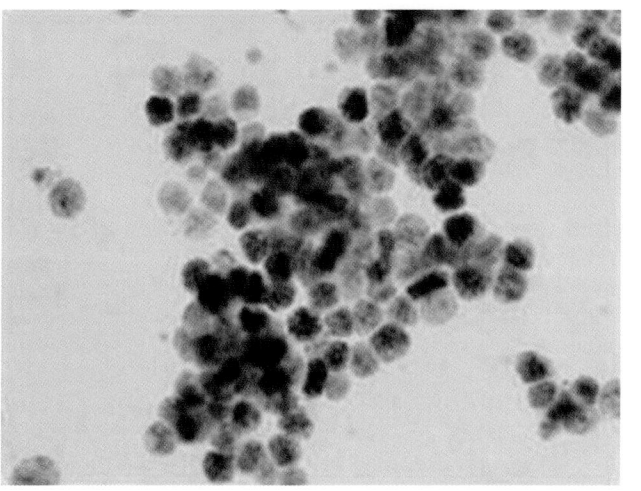

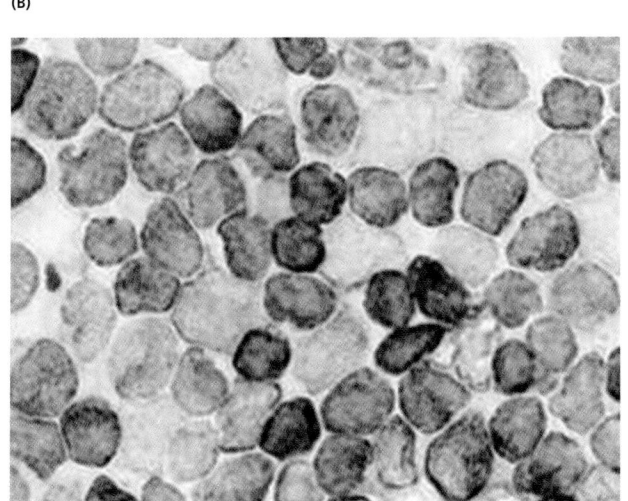

Figure 4.43 Lymphoblastic lymphoma, Precurosor T-ALL. A 16-year-old boy presented with a short history of shortness of breath. Chest X-ray revealed mediastinal mass. FNAC was requested for urgent diagnosis. (A) Smears are composed of small and medium sized lymphoid cells, with oval nuclei, fine blast-like chromatin and inconspicuous nucleoli. The size of the cells and lack of prominent nucleoli may be misleading into calling the lesion a low grade lymphoma (MGG ×100, oil). (B) Pap staining show blast chromatin pattern. (C) TDT positivity in all cells. (D) CD3 positivity in all cells (APAAP, ×1000, oil).

for lineage assignment and/or clonality be performed in cases of equivocal markers [47].

FNAC samples are adequate for accurate characterisation of lymphoblastic lymphomas and may obviate the need for surgical biopsy [186, 191]. When combined with immunological phenotyping, definitive initial pathologic diagnosis of lymphoblastic lymphoma and recurrent ALL is possible and preferable using only FNAC. It should be considered as part of the initial evaluation and management whenever a mass lesion appears in a child with a suspected lymphoblastic neoplasm. It can preclude the need for a surgical biopsy in those with a mediastinal mass and the superior mediastinal syndrome [193].

4.4.5 B-cell lymphomas

4.4.5.1 B-cell small lymphocytic lymphoma

The 2008 WHO classification of tumours of hematopoietic and lymphoid tissues has adopted consensus guidelines for the definition of well-defined entities [46].

The major principle of the classification is the recognition of distinct diseases according to a combination of morphology,

immunophenotype, genetic, molecular and clinical features. These disease entities are stratified according to their cell lineage and their derivation from precursor or mature lymphoid cells. Although the 2008 WHO classification intentionally does not divide lymphomas by grade, traditionally mature B-cell lymphomas composed mainly of small lymphocytes have been called low-grade lymphomas. These small B-cell lymphomas include chronic lymphocytic leukemia/small lymphocytic lymphoma (CLL), follicular lymphoma (FL), nodal marginal zone lymphoma (MZL), MALT lymphoma, hairy cell leukaemia and lymphoplasmacytic lymphoma (LPL). An entity that should be included in the differential diagnosis of lymphomas composed mainly by small lymphocytes but with a rather aggressive behaviour is mantle cell lymphoma (MCL) (Tables 4.7 and 4.8).

As a consequence of new and better available techniques in routine diagnosis, an increased recognition of early and precursor lesions of lymphoid neoplasms has emerged. The emerging concepts such as, BCL2 negative FL, grading of FL, paediatric FL and indolent and cyclin D1 negative MCL, CD5þ low-grade lymphomas are beyond the scope of this book [221].

Table 4.7 Immunophenotype of low grade lymphomas.

	B-CLL Small lymphocytic lymphoma	Lymphoplasmacytic lymphoma	Mantle zone lymphoma	Follicular lymphoma	MALT lymphoma
CD20	pos	pos	pos	pos	pos
CD79a	pos	pos	pos	pos	pos
CD10	neg	neg	neg/pos	pos/neg	neg
CD23	neg	neg	neg	neg/pos	neg
CD5	pos	neg	pos	neg	neg
CD43	pos	pos/neg	pos	neg	neg/pos
DBA44	neg	pos/neg	pos/neg	neg	neg
TRAP	neg	N/A	neg	neg	neg
bcl-2	pos	pos	pos	pos	pos
Cyclin D1	neg	neg	pos	neg	neg

Source: [222] Wotherspoon A. Immunocytochemistry of low grade B-cell lymphomas. *CPD Bulletin Cellular Pathology* 1999;1: 158–61.

Table 4.8 Comparative cytomorphology of small cell lymphomas.

Follicular	Mixture of small and large cleaved cells (centrocytes as well as centroblasts
Mantle cell	Monomorphic, irregular, small/medium size, clumped chromatin, occasional 'blastoid' cells
Marginal zone/MALT	Small, round with scattered immunoblast like nucleolated large cells+/– plasmacytoid
Small lymphocytic/CLL	Small, round, occasional prolymphocytes and 'paraimmunoblasts', clumped chromatin
Lymphoblastic	Small, blast like fine chromatin, inconspicuous nucleoli, mitoses
Burkitt	Small. Round, coarse chromatin, multiple small nucleoli, abundant vacuolated cytoplasm, mitoses, apoptoses, tingible body macrophages.

Source: [46] Swerdlow SH, Campo E, Harris NL, Jaffe ES, Pileri SA, Stein H, et al., eds. *WHO Classification of Tumors of Haemotopoietic and Lymphoid Tissue*, 4th edn. Lyon: IARC, 2008.

Lymphocytic lymphoma is a neoplasm composed of small lymphocytes and may present as lymphoma or leukaemia (chronic lymphocytic leukaemia and prolymphocytic leukaemia) (Table 4.5) [156]. Histologically, there is an infiltrate of small cells with clusters of larger cells ('proliferation centres'). Disease runs an indolent course but in a percentage of cases may undergo transformation into a high grade lymphoma (Richter syndrome) (see Fig 4.44e and Chapter 5 Fig. 5.16).

Cytological features: Small lymphocytic lymphoma (SLL) is composed of small lymphoid cells with round, regular nuclear membranes and coarsely clumped chromatin. Apart from small cells, SLL contains also a population of larger cells, representing prolymphocytes and 'paraimmunoblasts' (Fig. 4.44). These larger cells are observed in aggregates in the proliferation centres that resemble pale areas or pseudofollicles in histological sections. When paraimmunoblasts/prolymphocytes dominate, a paraimmunoblstic variant may be suspected. This has worse prognosis than SLL but better than diffuse large cell lymphoma.

Immunophenotype: (Table 4.7) IgM, CD 5 and CD 23 positive in addition to 'pan B panel' (CD19, CD20, CD79a, CVd22, CD23) (Table 4.5). Both SLL and mantle zone lymphoma are CD5 positive and CD10 negative. SLL is, however, CD23 positive. SLL shows weak Ig and CD20 positivity whilst mantle zone lymphoma shows strong positivity. Mantle zone lymphoma is also positive for Cyclin D1 (bcl-1) and has a t(11;14). Genetically, SLL show trisomy 12 or 13Q in some cases [223].

4.4.5.2 Lymphoplasmacytic lymphoma (immunocytoma)
Lymphoplasmacytic lymphoma is an uncommon type of NHL comprising only 2–3% of NHL (Fig. 4.42). Lymphocytes in lymphoplasmacytic lymphoma show plasma cell differentiation. Plasmacytoid cells contain IgM, sometimes as intranuclear inclusions (Dutcher bodies). MALT lymphoma and SLL may show plasmacytoid features so the diagnosis should be made by exclusion of other entities [224]. Disease may present as Waldonström's Macroglobulinaemia with IgM detectable in the serum, as nodal or extranodal lymphoma [225]. Immunocytoma has generally an indolent course but transformation into large cell lymphoma occurs in approximately 5–10% of cases.

Cytological features: Lymphoplasmacytic lymphoma is composed of a mixed population of small lymphocytes, plasmacytoid lymphocytes, plasma cells and scattered plasmacytoid immunoblasts (Fig. 4.45). Intranuclear inclusions (Dutcher bodies) and intacytoplasmic inclusions (Russel bodies) are usually numerous. If there is predominance of immunoblasts, the disease may be labelled as polymorphous immunocytoma indicating a possible more aggressive course. Epithelioid cells and mast cell infiltration has been reported, the former may cause confusion with T-cell lymphomas (Table 4.5).

Immunophenotype and molecular: (Table 4.7) Surface IgM, Cytoplasmic Ig, CD19, 20, 22 and 79a positive; CD5, CD10 and CD23 negative. Combination of morphology and immunophenotype is useful in separating the lymphoplasamcytic from small lymphocytic and mantle zone lymphoma (Table 4.8) [224]. The absence of t(1;14)(p22;q32) and t(11;18)(q21;q21) is useful in the differential diagnosis between lymphoplasmacytic lymphoma and MALT.

4.4.6 Mantle zone lymphoma
Mantle-cell lymphoma is a lymphoproliferative disorder derived from a subset of naive pregerminal centre cells characterised by a nodular or diffuse proliferation of atypical lymphoid cells with a monoclonal B-cell phenotype and co-expression of CD5 (Tables 4.5, 4.7 and 4.8) [156]. Clinically, mantle cell lymphoma presents as advanced disease with frequent extranodal involvement, particularly with involvement of bone marrow, gastrointestinal tract and spleen. Disease usually presents with lymphadenopathy but may be present in extranodal sites, particularly gastrointestinal tract. Histologically, the growth pattern is often nodular and the cells tend to converge ('home') to the mantle zones of lymphoid follicles. Mantle zone lymphoma has distinct clinical, immunological and genetic characteristics and has been shown to have worse survival than other lymphomas previously grouped as follicle centre derived. The clinical evolution is relatively aggressive, with poor response to conventional therapeutic regimens and a median survival duration of 3–4 years.

Cytological features: (Table 4.8) Two cytological variants have been identified, typical and blastic. Typical cases show a monotonous population of small to intermediately sized lymphoid cells with irregular nuclei, coarse chromatin, small nucleoli and scarce

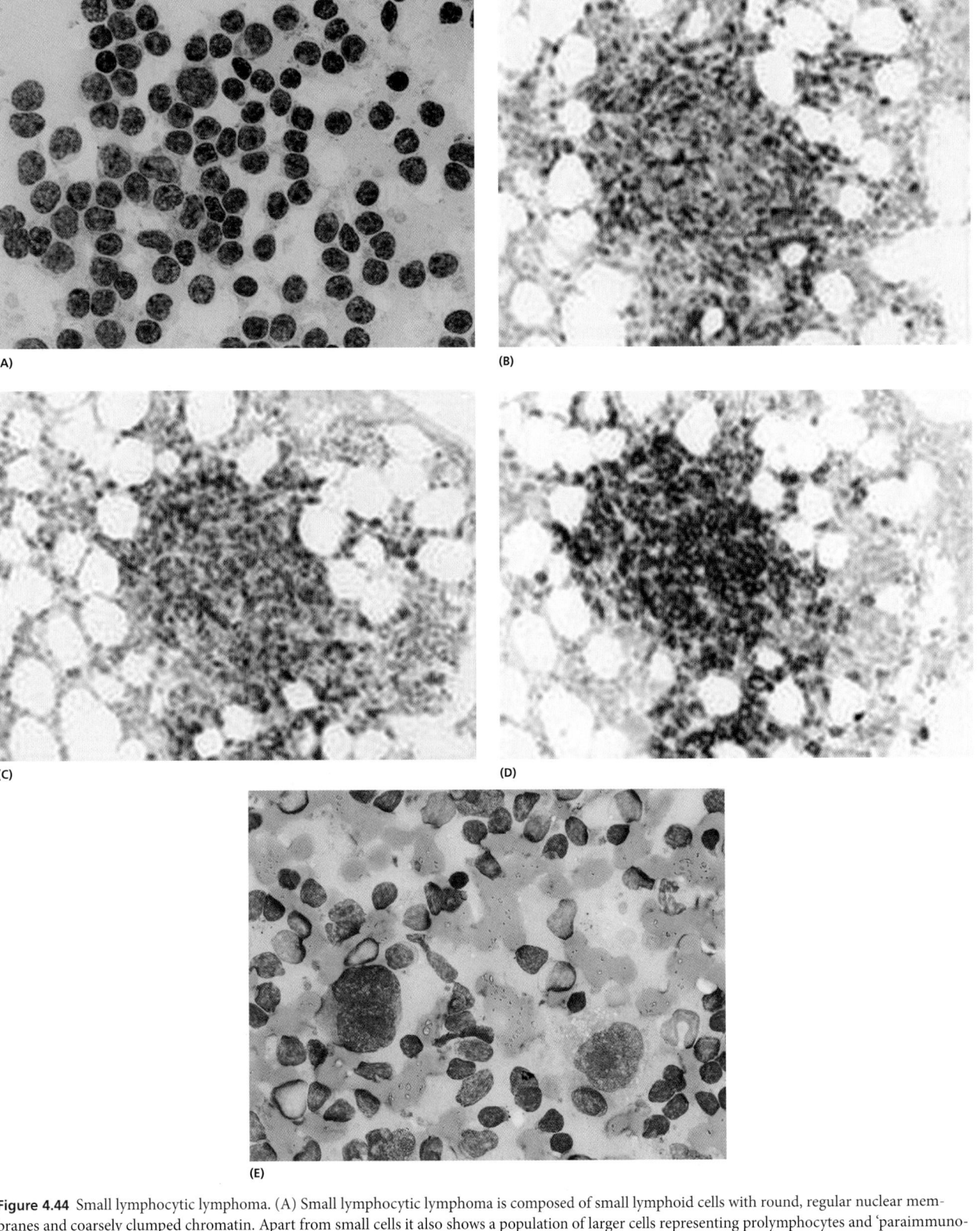

(A)

(B)

(C)

(D)

(E)

Figure 4.44 Small lymphocytic lymphoma. (A) Small lymphocytic lymphoma is composed of small lymphoid cells with round, regular nuclear membranes and coarsely clumped chromatin. Apart from small cells it also shows a population of larger cells representing prolymphocytes and 'paraimmunoblasts'. These larger cells are observed in aggregate reflecting proliferation centres (MGG ×1000, oil immersion). (B) CD5 positivity. (C) CD20 positivity. (D) CD23 positivity. (E) Richter syndrome. CLL recurrence can sometimes show cells resembling Hodgkin's cells.

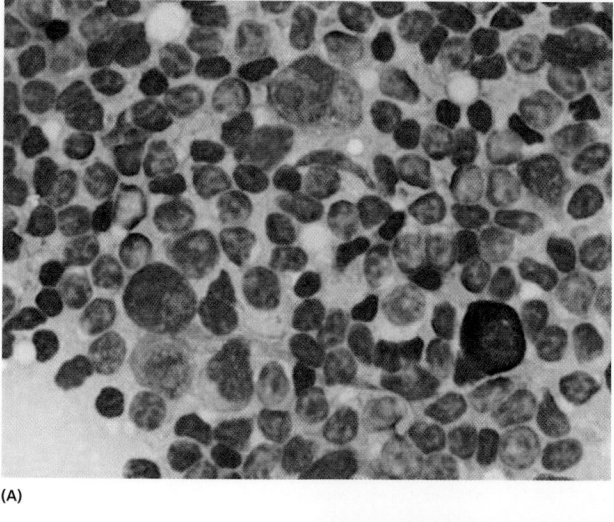

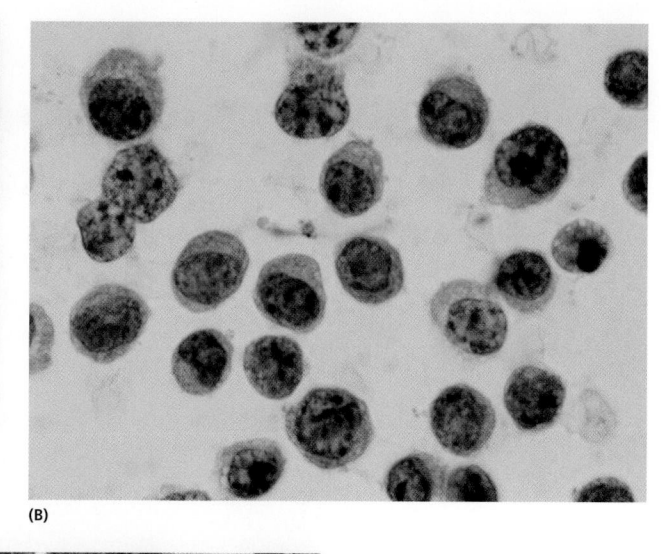

(A)

(B)

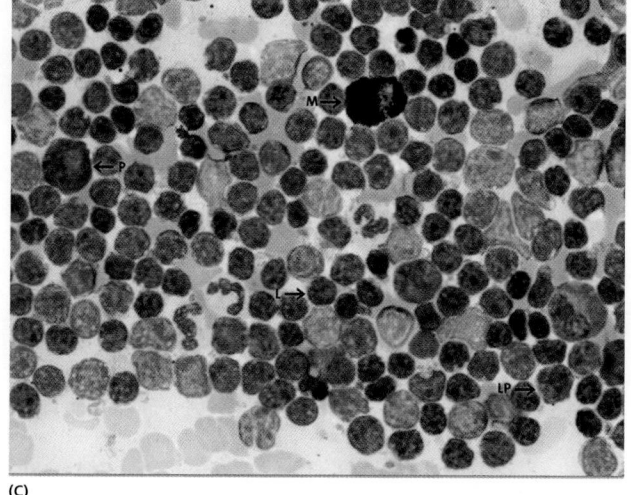

(C)

Figure 4.45 Lymphoplasmacytic lymphoma. (A) FNAC is composed of mixed population of small lymphocytes, plasmacytoid lymphocytes, plasma cells and scattered plasmacytoid mmunoblasts (MGG ×600, oil immersion). (B) Pap staining shows chromatin pattern of plasmacytoid lymphoid cells. (C) Bone marrow cytology (May-Grünwald-Giemsa stain) of a patient with immunocytoma showing a dense infiltration of small lymphocytes (L), lymphoplasmacytic cells (LP), a few plasma cells (P) and mast cells (M). The cells produce monoclonal IgM, characterising it as a Waldenström's disease (Courtesy of Sysmex).

cytoplasm (centrocytes) (Fig. 4.46). Blastic variants include a spectrum of intermediate to large cells with round or irregular nuclei and finely dispersed chromatin. These cases have a higher proliferative activity and a more aggressive clinical evolution [184, 194, 226]. Chromatin is not clumped as in small lymphocytic lymphoma. There are no larger cells admixed in the tumour as in the marginal zone lymphoma or follicular lymphoma. If present, the large cells represent cells from residual follicles which are overrun by tumour. The blastic variant resembles lymphoblastic lymphoma. The FNAC smears show a monotonous population of intermediate-sized lymphocytes with irregular nuclear contours, finely dispersed nuclear chromatin and inconspicuous nucleoli [227]. The clinical history and the absence of TdT helps to differentiate the two. *Immunophenotypically*, mantle zone lymphoma is surface Ig, CD5, CD19, 20, 22 and 79a and Cyclin D1 positive, CD23 and CD10 negative.

Cyclin D1 positivity reflects genetic abnormality t(11;14), reciprocal chromosomal translocation, which causes overexpression of bcl-1 or PRAD-1 gene which encodes cyclin D1. It is present in 50–67% of mantle zone lymphomas. CD5 is commonly present in other lymphomas but it differs from other CD5 positive diseases by being CD23 negative (Table 4.7). Cyclin D1 is present in only a few reported cases of aggressive variants of chronic lymphocytic leukaemia/small lymphocytic lymphoma and a small percentage of cases of multiple myeloma. Aggressive variants of mantle zone lymphoma have additional genetic alterations, including inactivation of p53 and p16INK4a tumour-suppressor genes [226]. Recently, other markers, such as SOX11 immunostaining on FNAC samples have been shown to be highly sensitive and specific for MCL and can be used as a reliable adjunct to confirm MCL, especially in a recurrent setting [223]. Positive Bcl-1 gene rearrangement helps distinction of blastic variant of mantle zone lymphoma from Diffuse Large B cell Lymphoma.

Sub-classification of follicle-derived low grade NHL can be established with high accuracy on FNAC material if cytomorphology is corroborated by a complete immunophenotypic analysis, which can be performed on both fresh and frozen material. The currently used criteria can be applied to aspirated cells for a conclusive cytopathological diagnosis of mantle zone lymphoma, which is of great clinical importance [200, 226] (Table 4.9).

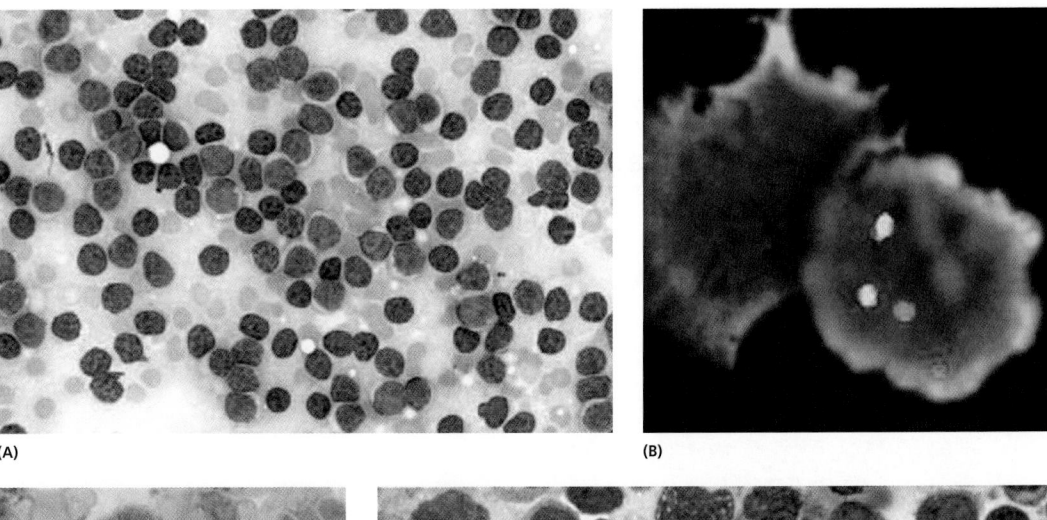

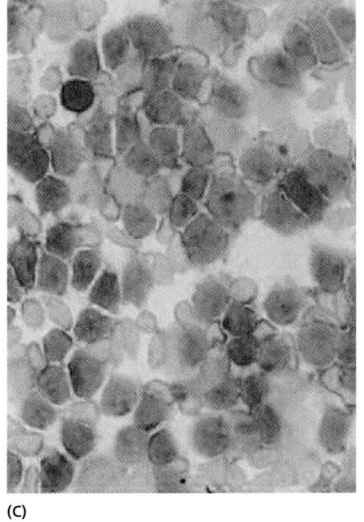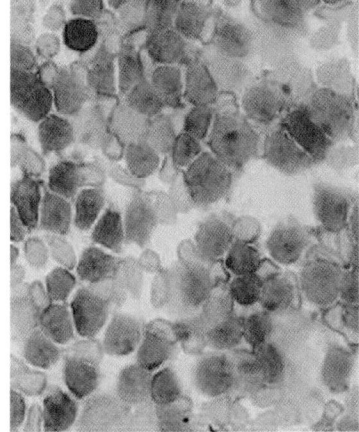

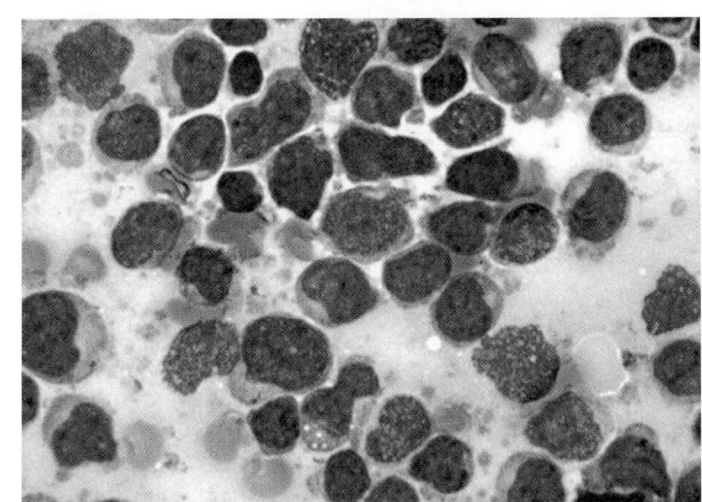

Figure 4.46 Mantle zone lymphoma. (A) Monotonous population of small to intermediate sized lymphoid cells with irregular nuclei, coarse chromatin, small nucleoli and scarce cytoplasm (centrocytes). Chromatin is not clumped as in small lymphocytic lymphoma. There are no larger cells admixed in the tumour as in the marginal zone lymphoma or follicular lymphoma (MGG ×600; ×600; ×1000 oil immersion). (B) Immunofluorescence highlights the t;(11, 14). (C) CD5 positivity in tumour cells. (D) Blastic variant includes a spectrum of intermediate to large cells with round or irregular nuclei and finely dispersed chromatin. These cases have a higher proliferative activity and a more aggressive clinical evolution. Features may resemble lymphoblastic lymphoma.

4.4.7 Follicular lymphoma

According to WHO classification follicular lymphoma (FL) is a neoplasm composed of follicle centre (germinal centre) B-cells, which usually has a partially follicular pattern at least. This is one of the most common lymphomas in Europe and America (Fig. 4.42). The characteristic chromosomal translocation of follicular lymphoma is t(14;18)(q32;q21) with transposition of BCL2 onco-gene to the regulatory region of immunoglobulin heavy chain gene IgH. Histological grading is proposed according to the number of centroblasts/high power field, for example grade 1 (1–5 CB/hpf), grade 2 (6–15 CB/hpf) and grade 3 (>15 CB/hpf) (Tables 4.5, 4.7, 4.8 and 4.9) [156].

Disease affects adults and, although it has an indolent course with median survival of 7–9 years, it is incurable.

Cytological features: The cells of follicular lymphoma are composed of variable mix of small (small cleaved) and large (large cleaved) lymphoid cells that are commonly found in follicle centre (Fig. 4.47). The small cells (cleaved cells, centrocytes) are slightly larger than mature lymphocytes, have condensed chromatin, irregular nuclear outline and lack prominent nucleoli. The large cells

Table 4.9 WHO classification of follicular lymphoma and mantle cell lymphoma grading and variants.

Follicular lymphoma
Grades:
Grade 1: 0-5 centroblasts/hpf
Grade 2: 6-15 centroblasts/hpf
Grade 3: >15 centroblastslhpf
3a: >15 centroblasts, but centrocytes are still present
3b. Centroblasts form solid sheets with no residual centrocytes
Variants:
Cutaneous follicle centre lymphoma
Diffuse follicle centre lymphoma
   Grade 1: 0-5 CB/hpf
   Grade 2: 6-15 CB/hpf
Mantle cell lymphoma
   Variant: blastoid

Source: [46] Swerdlow SH, Campo E, Harris NL, Jaffe ES, Pileri SA, Stein H, et al., eds. *WHO Classification of Tumors of Haemotopoietic and Lymphoid Tissue*, 4th edn. Lyon: IARC, 2008.

(large cleaved cells) are two to three times the size of small cleaved cells. The large non-cleaved cells, centroblasts, have round nuclei and prominent nucleoli. CD21, which stains follicular dendritic cells, can be used to outline the nodular, follicular pattern, of the

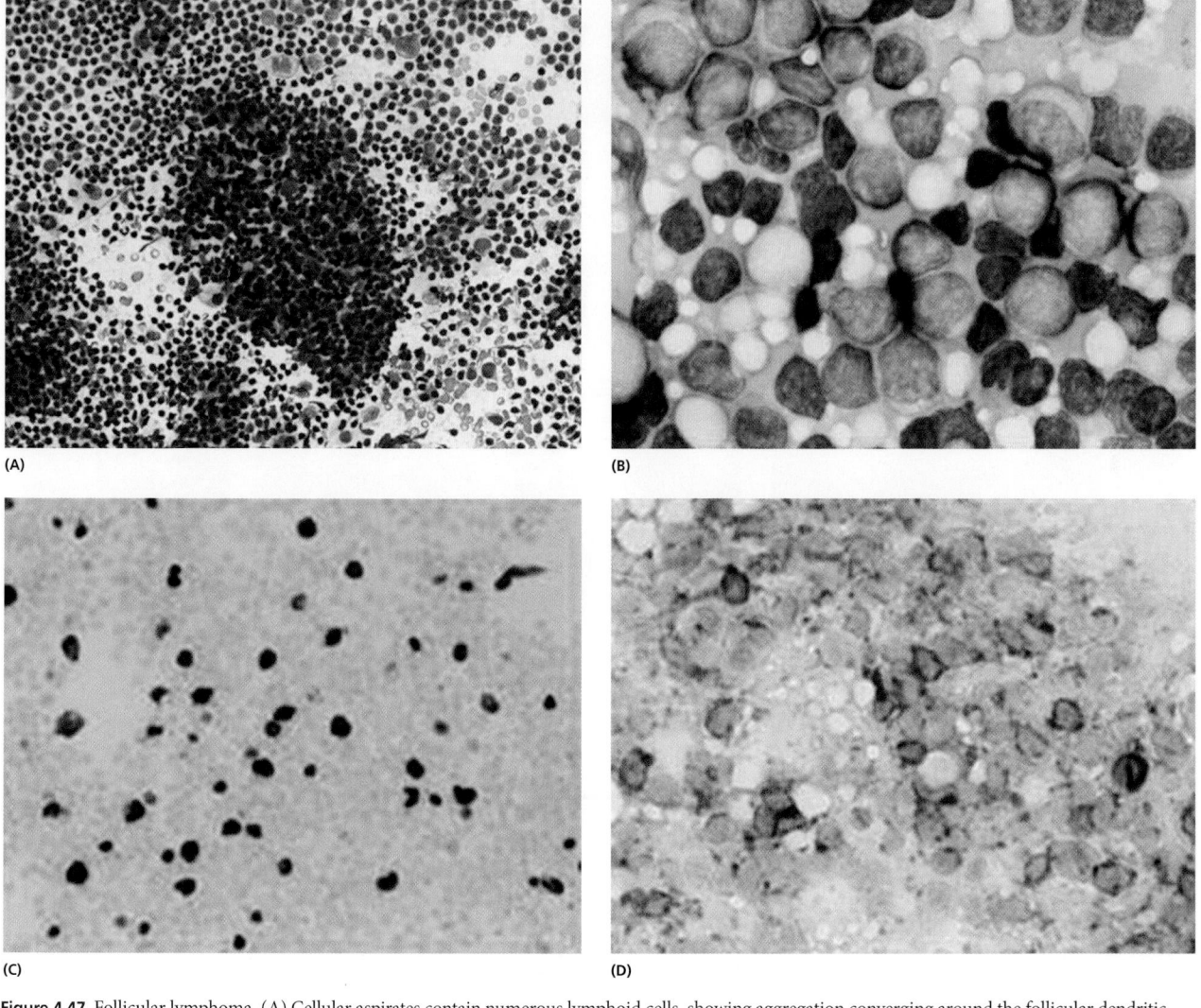

(A)

(B)

(C)

(D)

Figure 4.47 Follicular lymphoma. (A) Cellular aspirates contain numerous lymphoid cells, showing aggregation converging around the follicular dendritic cells. (B) A mixture of small cells (cleaved cells, centrocytes) which are slightly larger than mature lymphocytes, have condensed chromatin, irregular nuclear outline and lack prominent nucleoli and the large non-cleaved cells, centroblasts, have round nuclei and prominent nucleoli. (C) A low proliferation index highlighted by Ki67. (D) CD10 highlights cells of follicle centre origin.

lesion. The presence of 'aggregation' of uniform lymphoid cells, probably due to cell adhesions with the support of dendritic reticulum cells, is seen in follicular lymphomas [228].

The grading of follicular lymphomas endorsed by the WHO classification can be applied to cytological preparations (Table 4.9). Grade 1 corresponds to predominantly small cleaved cell population, Grade 2 to mixed small and large cleaved cells and Grade 3 corresponds to follicular large cell. Follicular large cell is difficult to differentiate from diffuse large cell lymphoma. The distinction is not critical since both lymphomas are treated aggressively. The aggressive lymphomas usually have >20% of centroblasts.

Diagnosis of follicular lymphoma without the aid of ancillary techniques may be difficult and the most frequent false negative diagnoses of non-Hodgkin's lymphoma, prior to the advent of immunocytochemistry and other ancillary techniques, relate to this category [229].

Immunophenotypically, cells show surface Ig, CD10, CD19, 20, 22, 79a and BCL-2 positivity and is CD5 negative (Table 4.7). The 14;18 translocation is present in the majority of cases (80–90%). This causes expression of bcl-2 protein, which is normally not expressed by the follicle centre cells that are bcl-2 negative. Bcl-2 is expressed even in cases, which lack translocation. The expression of bcl-2 is

not useful in cytological preparations because of lack of architecture. It is present also in hyperplasia, marginal zone lymphoma small B-cell follicular lymphoma. Bcl-6 expression is common in low-grade FCL but is rare in other indolent B-cell lymphoid disorders, and may be a useful adjunct in classification of indolent lymphomas [230]. The May–Grunwald–Giemsa stain routine and archival cytological smears can be used for PCR-based ancillary methods and the rate of detection of IgH/BCL2 rearrangement is similar to results reported for paraffin-embedded tissues (Fig. 4.61). For patients with detectable baseline molecular marker, PCR is a highly suitable method for detection of bone marrow involvement and monitoring minimal residual disease (MRD) [231].

4.4.8 Marginal zone lymphoma (MALT type)

Marginal zone B-cell lymphomas represent 8% of non-Hodgkin's lymphoma that may arise in a wide variety of extranodal organs where they are termed low grade B-cell lymphomas of mucosa-associated lymphoid tissue (MALT) (Fig. 2.21, Chapter 2). Marginal zone lymphomas may involve primarily lymph nodes and or spleen where they are designated monocytoid B-cell lymphoma or splenic

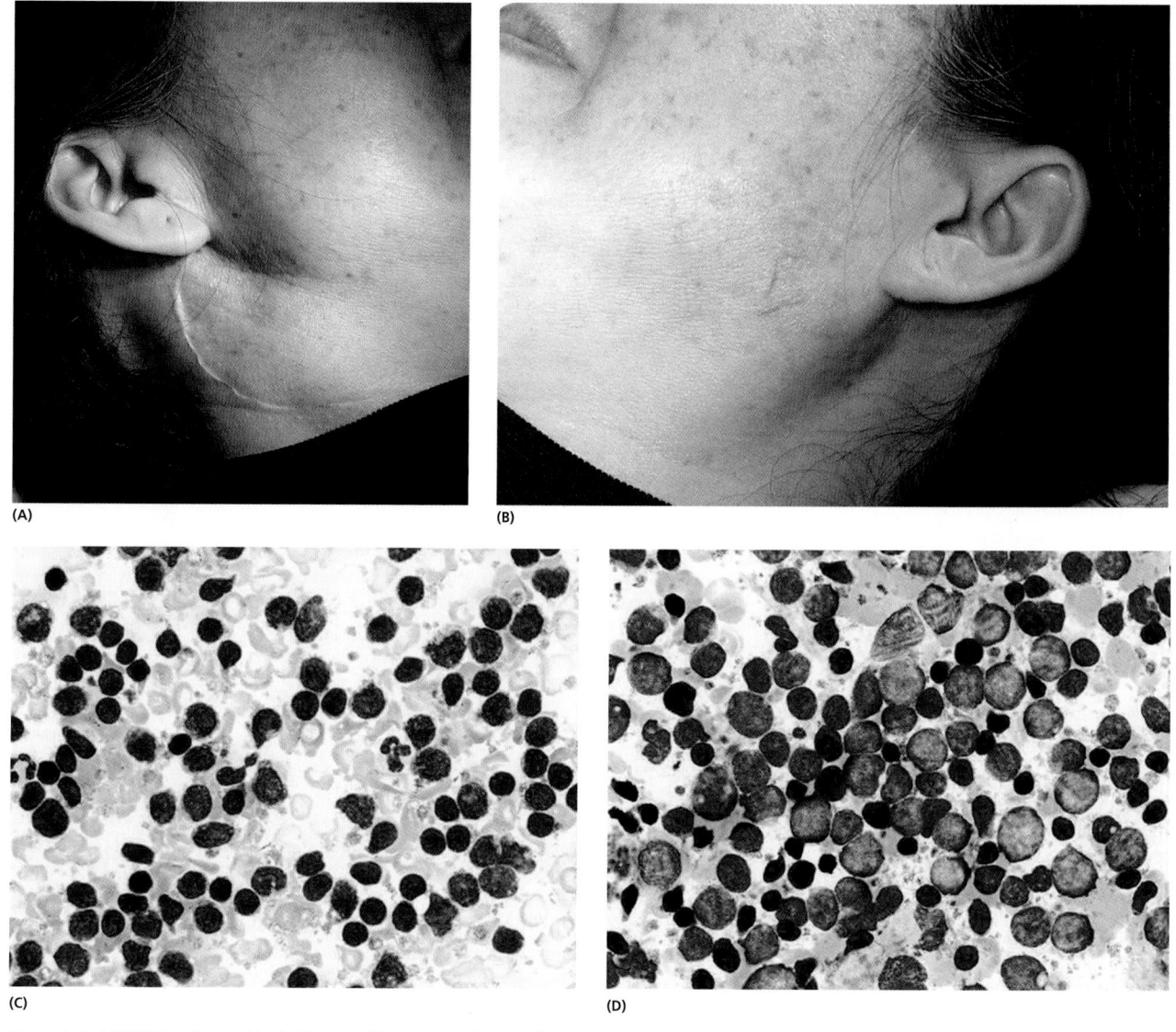

Figure 4.48 MALT lymphoma. (A) A 53-year-old woman with a scar from the excision of MALT lymphoma 7 years previously. (B) Now presents with a painless diffuse swelling of the contralateral side. (C,D) Polymorphous proliferation comprising a predominant population of intermediate sized lymphoid cells with round-to-irregular nuclear outline (centrocyte-like or monocytoid features), chromatin slightly paler and less clumped than in small mature lymphocytes, small inconspicuous nucleolus and a distinct pale cytoplasm. In addition, there are small mature round lymphocytes, transformed cells, and variable numbers of immunoblasts.

marginal zone lymphoma, respectively. The small cell type of marginal zone lymphoma (MALT lymphoma) derives from B-cells associated with epithelial tissues [232–234]. They tend to remain localised with good prognosis but can undergo blastic transformation to a large B-cell lymphoma. Recent data show that primary large cell lymphomas, of mucosa associated tissues, differ cytogenetically from low-grade MALT lymphomas. If found, areas of large cell lymphoma within MALT should be diagnosed as diffuse B-cell lymphoma (and not high grade MALT) not to confuse the management of otherwise indolent low-grade MALT lymphomas. The WHO classification proposes grading according to the number of blasts, for example >5%, thought to confer worse prognosis (Table 4.5).

Cytological features: specimens show a polymorphous proliferation comprising a predominant population of intermediate sized lymphoid cells with round-to-irregular nuclear outline (centrocyte-like or monocytoid features), chromatin slightly paler and less clumped than in small mature lymphocytes, small

inconspicuous nucleolus and a distinct pale cytoplasm. In addition, there are small mature round lymphocytes, transformed cells, and variable numbers of immunoblasts (Fig. 4.48 and Fig. 2.24, Chapter 2) [234]. These findings, while highly suggestive of MALT lymphoma in extranodal proliferations, may be more difficult to distinguish from reactive conditions in lymph nodes [188]. In 10% of cases, marginal zone lymphoma transforms into large cell lymphoma. The nuclei of marginal zone lymphoma are usually round or only slightly irregular in contrast to the small-cleaved cells of follicular lymphoma and mantle zone lymphoma. Lymphoid cells may have plasmacytoid features. Mature plasma cells may be seen. Morphologically, follicular lymphomas differ from marginal zone lymphomas in that they have a range of nuclear sizes ranging from small to large. On the other hand, mantle zone lymphoma has monotonous cell population of irregularly shaped small to medium sized cells. These contrast with marginal zone lymphoma that has predominantly small cells with a few large lymphoid cells without transitional forms (Table 4.8).

Immunophenotype: Nearly all marginal zone lymphomas express surface immunoglobulin. Approximately 50% express intracytoplasmic Ig. CD5, CD10 and CD23 are negative.

Molecular markers: There are four main recurrent chromosomal translocations associated with MALT lymphomas: t(1;14)(p22;q32), t(11;18)(q21;q21), t(14;18)(q32;q21), and t(3;14)(p14.1;q32) [15–18]. Translocation t(11;18)(q21;q21) is the most common (15-40%) and was mainly found in pulmonary and gastric tumors, whereas t(14;18)(q32;q21) was most detected in ocular adnexal, orbit, skin, and salivary gland MALT lymphoma [188a] other genetic alterations have been described [188b].

4.4.9 Diffuse large B-cell lymphoma

DLBCL is the most common lymphoid malignancy worldwide. It includes tumours that cannot be morphologically classified (NOS) and clinico-pathological variants characterised by specific features (e.g. age, primary site, immunodeficiency and/or relationship with infectious agents) (Table 4.10) [235]. Nowadays, the cell of origin (COO) and complex cytogenetic alterations deserve great attention by affecting the disease behaviour and therapeutic decisions. Next generation sequencing has highlighted a series of mutations that might represent the rationale for innovative-targeted therapies.

Gene expression profiling (GEP) studies, based on the COO, have subdivided DLBCL/NOS into three main molecular subtypes: the activated B-cell-like (ABC), the germinal center B-cell-like (GCB) group and Type-III, with ABC-DLBCL characterized by a poor prognosis and constitutive NF-κB activation. The "gold standard" methods for COO are based on GEP of RNA from fresh frozen tissue using microarray technology, which is an impractical solution if formalin-fixed paraffin-embedded tissue (FFPET) is used. Reflecting the importance of reliably assigning COO in the clinic, considerable efforts have been made to approximate the results of the gold standard method using practical technology platforms including IHC and quantitative Rt PCR using RNA derived from FFPET [235a,b].

Immunohistochemistry, a more practical method can be performed with antibodies against CD10, BCL6, MUM1, CCND2, and FOXP1—five proteins that are highly differentially expressed between the two COO groups. However, no one single IHC stain was sufficient to accurately assign COO [235c,d]. Similarly, MiRNAs qualify as potential diagnostic and prognostic biomarkers in DLBCL [235b].

Previously called 'centroblastic' lymphoma, it was thought to be different from 'immunoblastic' lymphoma and therefore

listed separately (Kiel classification). However, there is no evidence as to the validity of this distinction, no survival advantage, specific genetic abnormality or definite morphological distinction (Table 4.5) [156]. Diffuse large cell lymphoma therefore combines characteristics of both of these previously separate entities (Table 4.10). It can arise *de novo* or can be a result of transformation of other lymphomas. Clinically, there are multiple distinct presentations e.g. mediastinal/thymic large cell lymphoma, primary CNS lymphoma and primary effusion lymphoma (Figs 4.49, 4.50) [236]. *Cutaneous B-cell lymphoma* is a separate entity, the morphology of which can range from low grade follicular lymphoma to diffuse large B-cell lymphoma (Fig. 4.51). However, disease has indolent clinical course and should not be treated aggressively like other systemic large cell lymphomas. Systemic disease requires aggressive treatment and may respond well [221].

Cytological features: Diffuse large cell lymphoma has a monomorphous population of large cells with prominent nucleoli and basophilic cytoplasm. Diffuse large B-cell lymphoma represents heterogenous group of entities, all of which have a significant component of large cells (Fig. 1.9, Chapter 1). Immunoblasts are large cells with eccentric nuclei, prominent, usually single large nucleolus and basophilic cytoplasm. Centroblasts are smaller than immunoblasts, round, with central nucleus, evenly distributed basophilic cytoplasm and usually multiple nucleoli. Pleomorphic poly-lobed cells, signet ring cells and spindle cells can all be seen in different types of large cell lymphoma [237] (Figs 4.50–4.53).

Immunophenotype: Surface Ig +/−, Cytoplasmic Ig +/−, CD 5, CD10 +/−, CD19, CD20, 22, 79a, CD45 positive and EMA negative. Large B-cell lymphoma may contain a mixture of other cell types, for example T-cell rich B-cell lymphoma or histiocyte rich B-cell lymphoma [197]. A minority of cases (30%) show t(14–18). Nearly all cases have detectable immunoglobulin light chain or heavy chain rearrangements (Fig. 4.52). Bcl-1 gene rearrangement is generally not found. This helps distinction from blastic variant of mantle zone lymphoma, which frequently demonstrates this rearrangement.

Table 4.10 WHO classification of diffuse large B-cell lymphoma, morphological variants and subtypes.

Diffuse large B-cell lymphoma, morphological variants:
- Centroblastic
- Immunoblastic
- T-cell/histiocyte-rich
- Lymphomatoid granulomatosis type
- Anaplastic large B-cell
- Plasmablastic

Diffuse large B-cell lymphoma, subtypes:
- Mediastinal (thymic) large B-cell lymphoma
- Primary effusion lymphoma
- Intravascular large B-cell lymphoma

Source: [46] Swerdlow SH, Campo E, Harris NL, Jaffe ES, Pileri SA, Stein H, et al., eds. *WHO Classification of Tumors of Haemotopoietic and Lymphoid Tissue*, 4th edn. Lyon: IARC, 2008.

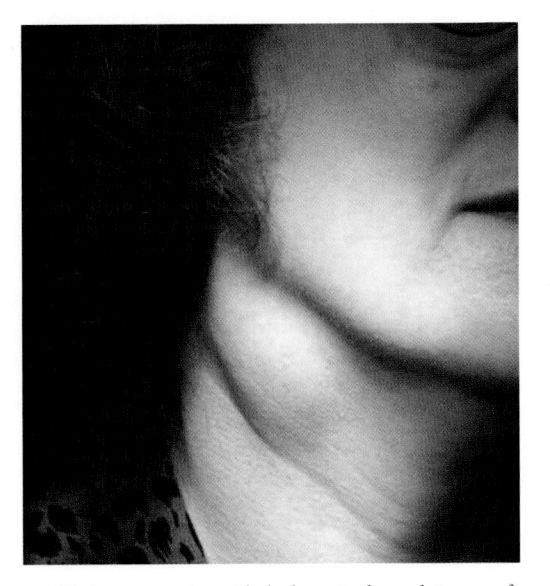

Figure 4.49 Patient presenting with the lump in the neck 5 years after treatment of carcinoma of the breast. Clinically, a metastasis was suspected. FNAC findings in Figure 4.50.

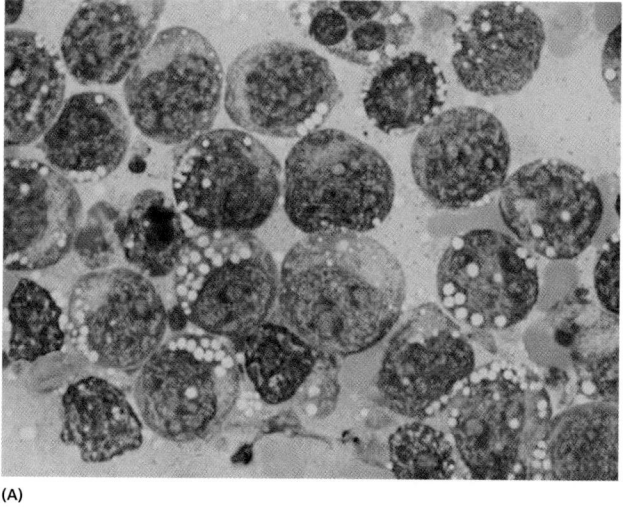
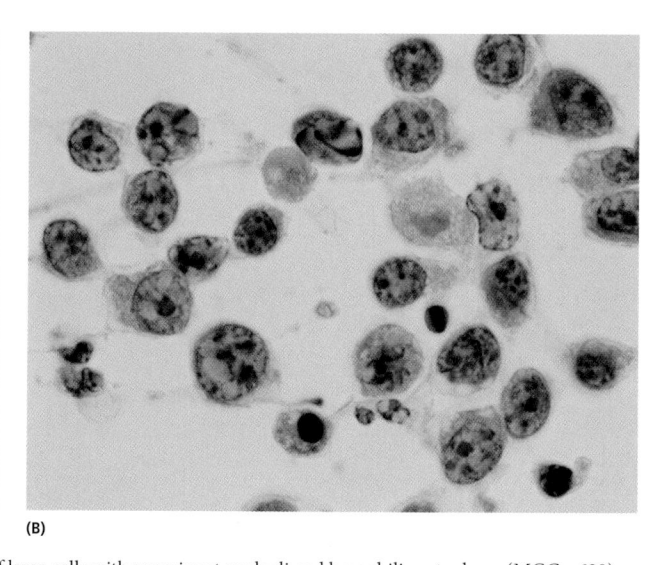

Figure 4.50 Diffuse large cell lymphoma. (A) Monomorphous population of large cells with prominent nucleoli and basophilic cytoplasm (MGG ×600). (B) Immunoblasts are large cells with eccentric nuclei, prominent, usually single large nucleolus and basophilic cytoplasm. Centroblasts are smaller than immunoblasts, round, with central nucleus, evenly distributed basophilic cytoplasm and usually multiple nucleoli. Pleomorphic polilobated cells, signet ring cells and spindle cells can all be seen in different types of large cell lymphoma (MGG ×1000, oil immersion).

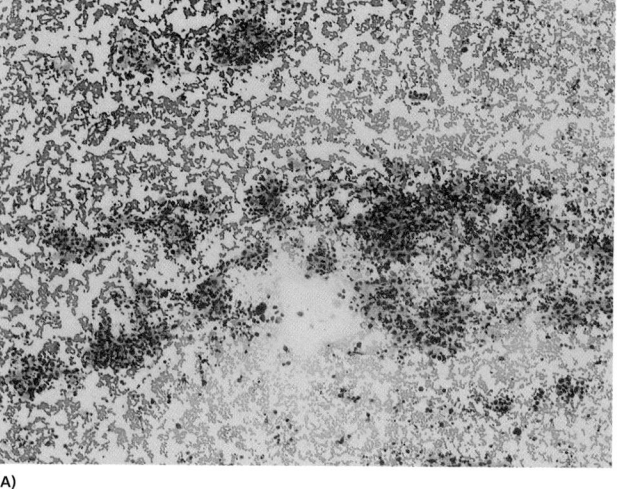
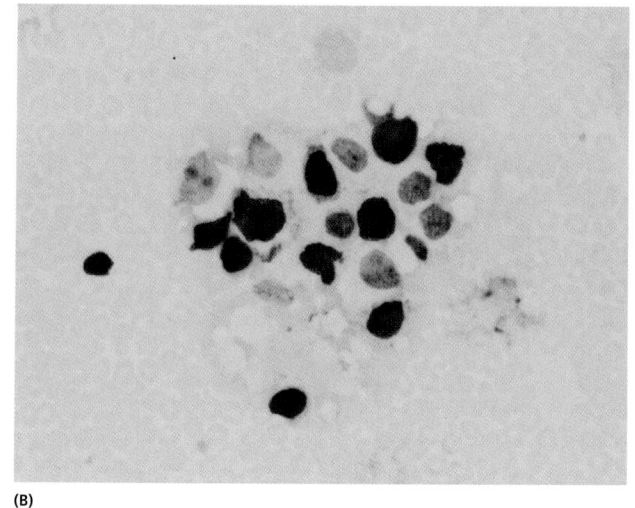

Figure 4.51 Diffuse large B-cell lymphoma. (A) Low power view shows pleomorphic cells with abundant cytoplasm and are arranged in aggregates resembling carcinoma. (B) MIB1 (Ki67) staining positive in the majority of cells.

4.4.10 Primary effusion lymphoma

Primary effusion lymphoma (PEL) is a subtype of B-cell lymphomas and has been recognized as a body-cavity-based lymphoma that was originally reported to be associated with human herpesvirus 8 (HHV8) infection and was frequently found in human immunodeficiency virus-positive (HIV) patients. However, there are case reports of PEL in immunocompetent patients [156, 238]. On the other hand, HHV-8 negative effusion lymphoma, which is different from PEL in many ways, has also been reported and is referred to as HHV8-unrelated PEL-like lymphoma [197a]. Since the effusion is often the first and only site of presentation, disease has special significance for cytopathologists since they are often the first to diagnose, the often unsuspected, disease. PEL, together with Kaposi's sarcoma, multicentric Castleman's disease and others, has been associated with Human herpesvirus-8 infection (HHV-8) [239]. It arises in a body cavity or space without an associated tumour mass, displays the cytomorphology of anaplastic large cell lymphoma, is a clonal B-cell neoplasm, and contains KSHV as well as EBV. Kaposi's sarcoma and multicentric Castleman's disease patients may develop body cavity effusions that, unlike primary effusion lymphoma, are poorly characterised. In the setting of HHV-8 infection, two effusion types may occur. One fulfils the criteria for HHV-8-positive PEL (lymphoma-morphology, HHV-8-DNA(+), IgH rearrangement). The other seems more reminiscent of an HHV-8-associated non-neoplastic process (monocyte-macrophage morphology, HHV-8-DNA(+/−), germline IgH) [240]. A single case of the latter effusion type harboured a B-cell monoclonal proliferation, which suggests the hypothesis that a pre-lymphomatous effusion may precede overt body cavity lymphoma. Primary effusion lymphoma has been limited almost entirely to the pleural, peritoneal, pericardial cavities and in the subarachnoid space (Fig. 4.53) [241].

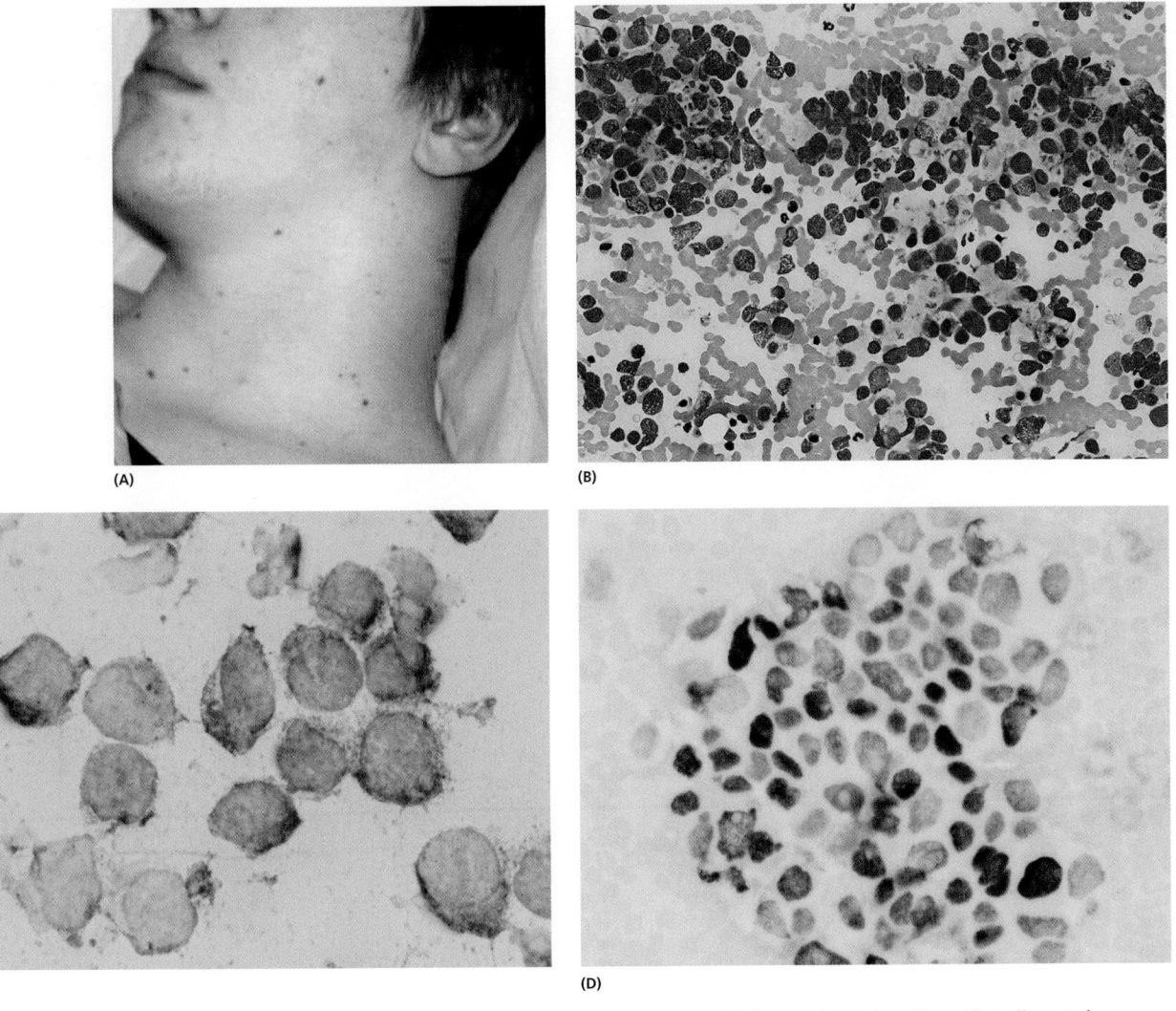

Figure 4.52 Diffuse large cell lymphoma. (A) Adolescent patient presented with a short history of diffuse tender neck swelling. Clinically, an infection was suspected. (B) FNAC shows a lymphoid cell population with predominance of large blasts (MGG ×600, ×1000, oil immersion). (C) Lymphoid cells are B marker positive (CD20, IP, ×1000, oil immersion). (D) BCL6 positivity confirms follicle centre origin.

4.4.11 Burkitt's lymphoma

For Burkitt's lymphoma WHO classification proposes two morphological variants, 'Burkitt-like' and 'with plasmacytoid differentiation (AIDS associated)', and three subtypes: 'endemic', 'sporadic' and 'immunodeficiency-associated' (Table 4.11) [156]. In most 'endemic' African cases, which affect the jaw or extranodal sites of children, Epstein–Barr viral DNA is found in malignant cells. Histologically and phenotypically identical cases are seen in the West. These may be associated with immunosuppression and about half of the cases have EB virus detectable. Non-African 'sporadic' cases affect children and adults and present most commonly in the abdomen. They show EB in about 25% of cases. Histologically, the tumour is made of medium sized B-cells interspersed with macrophages containing karyorrhectic debris ('starry sky' appearance in sections). Disease affects children more than adults. Treatment is aggressive but curable in children.

Cytological features: FNAC smears from Burkitt's lymphoma show high cellularity and an individual cell pattern (Fig. 4.54). Extracellular 'lymphoglandular' bodies are abundant and tingible body macrophages are prominent. Nuclei are intermediate in size (8–25 μm,

with an average of 10–12 μm) and round with a finely dispersed chromatin on May–Grunwald–Giemsa stained smears. Cytoplasm is basophilic and scant with prominent vacuoles. Extracellular vacuoles and vacuoles within 'lymphoglandular' bodies are also seen [190]. Papanicolaou stain shows coarse chromatin and 2–5 prominent nucleoli. 'Burkitt-like' lymphoma represents morphological appearance with more pleomorphism and larger cells than Burkitt's but is probably best managed as a variant of Burkitt's lymphoma, that is very high grade tumour with a proliferation fraction >99%, and not as diffuse large B-cell lymphoma. International panel review of mature B-cell lymphoma/leukaemia in children and adolescents highlighted difficulties in sub-classification, particularly with Burkitt-like lymphoma, which is a 'provisional entity' in the REAL Classification. Morphology needs to be complemented by other studies, such as molecular genetics and cytogenetics, to discriminate between the B-cell lymphomas.

Immunophenotype: Surface IgM positive, CD5, BCl2, CD23 negative, CD10 positive, CD19, 20, 22 and 79a positive, Ki67 > 90% of cells. Almost all cases show chromosomal translocation involving the cMYC gene on chromosome 8 and the gene for Ig heavy chain or, less commonly, one of the two light chain genes. The gold

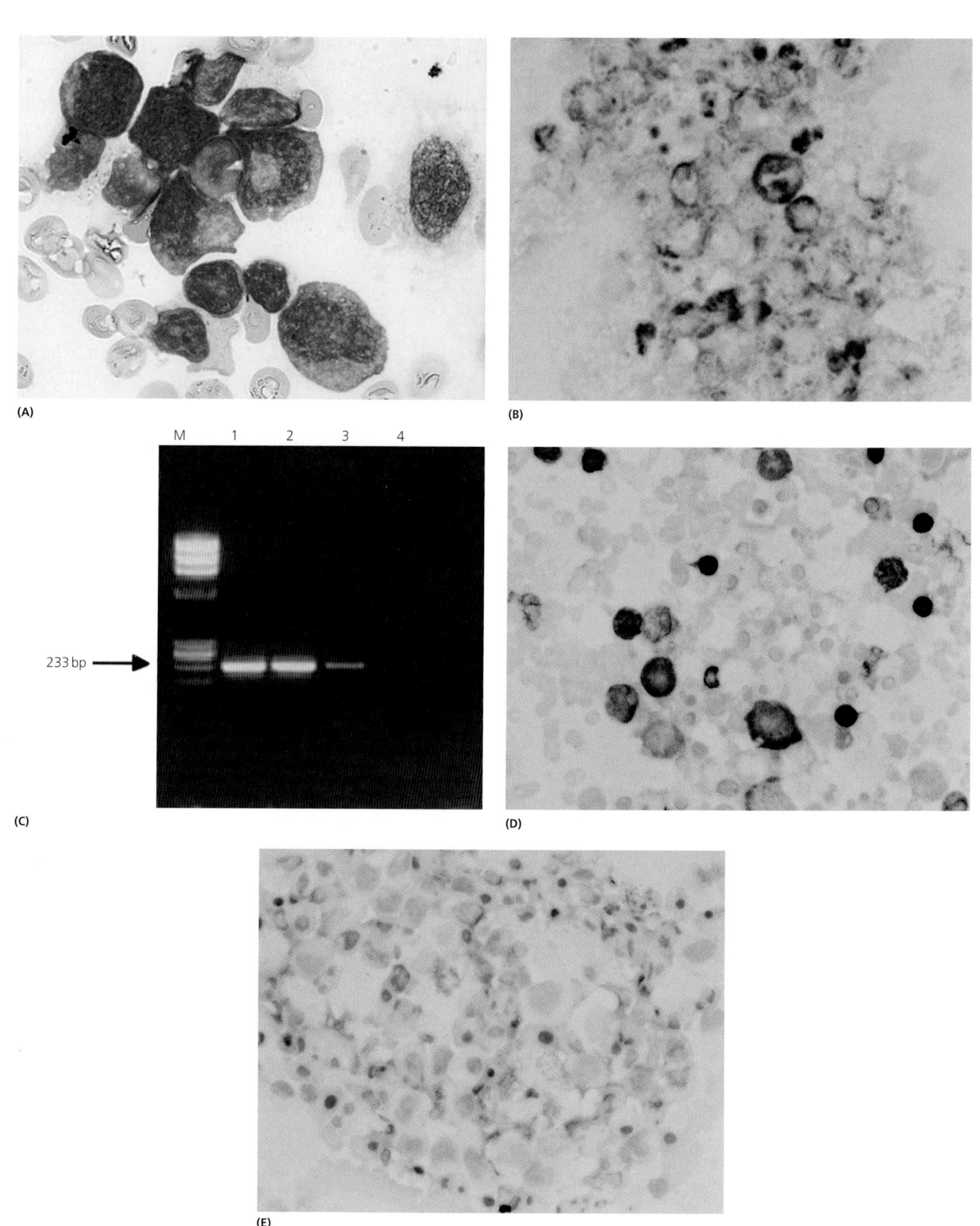

Figure 4.53 Primary effusion lymphoma. (A) Pleural effusion containing numerous lymphoid cells with features of high grade lymphoma. Cells are variably large, immunoblastic or have anaplastic features ('horseshoe nuclei'). They show numerous mitoses (MGG, PAP ×600, oil immersion). (B) PEL cells are KSHV positive (APAAP, ×600). (C) PCR confirms a monoclonal band. (D) CD3 positive cells. (E) CD20 negative cells.

Table 4.11 WHO classification of Burkitt's lymphoma, morphological variants and subtypes.

Burkitt lymphoma, morphological variants
- Burkitt-like
- With Plasmacytoid differentiation (AIDS-associated)

Burkitt lymphoma, subtypes (clinical and genetic)
    Endemic
    Sporadic
    Immunodeficiency-associated

Source: [46] Swerdlow SH, Campo E, Harris NL, Jaffe ES, Pileri SA, Stein H, et al., eds. *WHO Classification of Tumors of Haemotopoietic and Lymphoid Tissue*, 4th edn. Lyon: IARC, 2008.

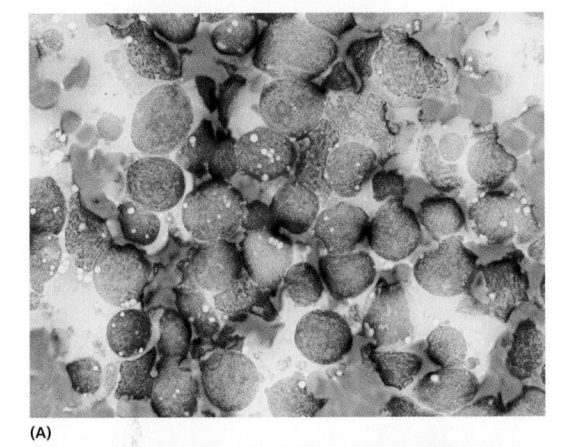

(A)

(B)

Figure 4.54 Burkitt's lymphoma. (A) FNAC smears from Burkitt's lymphoma of the jaw show high cellularity and an individual cell pattern. Extracellular lymphoglandular bodies are abundant and tingible body macrophages are prominent (MGG ×600, oil). (B) FISH investigation confirms Burkitt's lymphoma.

standard for diagnosis of Burkitt's lymphoma is either cytogenetic analysis or, if not available, proliferation fraction. This should be >99%. In the case of suspected Burkitt's lymphoma, the finding of a translocation (8;14) or associated variant translocation, along with the characteristic cytomorphology and proliferation fraction allows a definitive diagnosis by FNAC and may alleviate the need for biopsy [190].

4.4.12 T/NK-cell lymphomas

4.4.12.1 Peripheral T-cell lymphoma

T cell lymphomas are rare (10% of all lymphomas) in the Western world although there are more common in the Far East [242]. Peripheral T-cell lymphoma (PTCL) does not have a common

cytological composition, immunophenotype or cytogenetic characteristics. Instead, the disease(s) are defined by clinical syndromes and location (nodal vs extranodal and specific extranodal sites) which are important in determining biological behaviour (Table 4.5) [156, 156a]. Given the difference in clinical behaviour between nodal and extranodal sites, WHO classification suggests separating the lymphomas into nodal and extranodal types. Cytological sub-classification of peripheral T-cell lymphomas is not necessary for clinical purposes.

Cytological features: The most prominent cytological features of PTCL are a variable combination of small, intermediate and large lymphoid cells with irregular nuclei, presence of epithelioid histiocytes and atypical mononuclear cells (Fig. 4.55) [187]. The small cells have very irregular nuclei with condensed chromatin. Large cells may have prominent nucleoli and abundant, usually pale cytoplasm. An infiltrate of host cells is common in T-cell lymphomas. This includes small lymphocytes, polymorphs, epithelioid and non-epithelioid histiocytes and plasma cells. Cytological grading using large B-cells as internal yardsticks, as well as molecular genotypic measures of lymphoma cell burden, have prognostic value [243]. The diagnosis of PTCL is difficult. This entity can be misdiagnosed as Hodgkin's disease or a reactive process such as non-necrotising granulomatous lymphadenitis or it can present a problem in lymphoma classification [187]. Cases of skin and extracutaneous involvement of mycosis fungoides contain atypical small and large lymphocytes with cerebriform appearance (Fig. 4.56) [244–247].

FNAC of high grade PTCL from human T-lymphotropic virus-1 (HTLV-1) positive patients show a distinctive cytological pattern with a dominance of rounded cells with irregular nuclei and a moderately basophilic cytoplasm (Fig. 4.57). Irregular cells with a pale abundant cytoplasm are present in varying amounts. Giant cells with cerebriform nuclei, plasma cells and eosinophils are also seen. Epithelioid cells are an inconstant finding. PTCL from HTLV-1 positive patients have cytological patterns that are distinctive enough to allow a conclusive diagnosis of high grade T-cell lymphoma [248].

Immunophenotype: Unless there is history or a suspicion of T-cell lymphoma, the first line of investigation will be to exclude B-cell lymphoma which are more common. To establish a diagnosis of T-cell lymphoma, all B-cell markers must be negative and at least one of the pan T-cell markers positive (Figs 4.58, 4.59). T-cell panel includes CD1a, CD2, CD3, CD4, CD5, CD7 and CD8. Detection of T-cell gene rearrangement may be helpful in diagnosis of difficult cases. The failure to demonstrate this rearrangement does not rule out diagnosis of T-cell lymphoma. Many of the cases of T-cell lymphoma are mixed small and large cell, and in Korea, where the incidence of extranodal and T-cell lymphoma is high, the usefulness of FNAC for the initial diagnosis of malignant lymphoma is limited. For a definitive diagnosis, biopsy is required [242].

4.4.13 Anaplastic large cell lymphoma

Anaplastic large cell lymphoma (ALCL) was first recognised as a neoplasm, which was positive for the Ki-1 or CD30 antigen and also found on Reed–Sternberg cells. Tumour presents in children or young adults and can have two different patterns of presentation: systemic type with widespread involvement of lymph nodes or localised form that is confined to skin (Figs 4.60, 4.61). The two types have very different prognosis, the cutaneous type is usually indolent but resistant to cure whilst systemic type is aggressive but

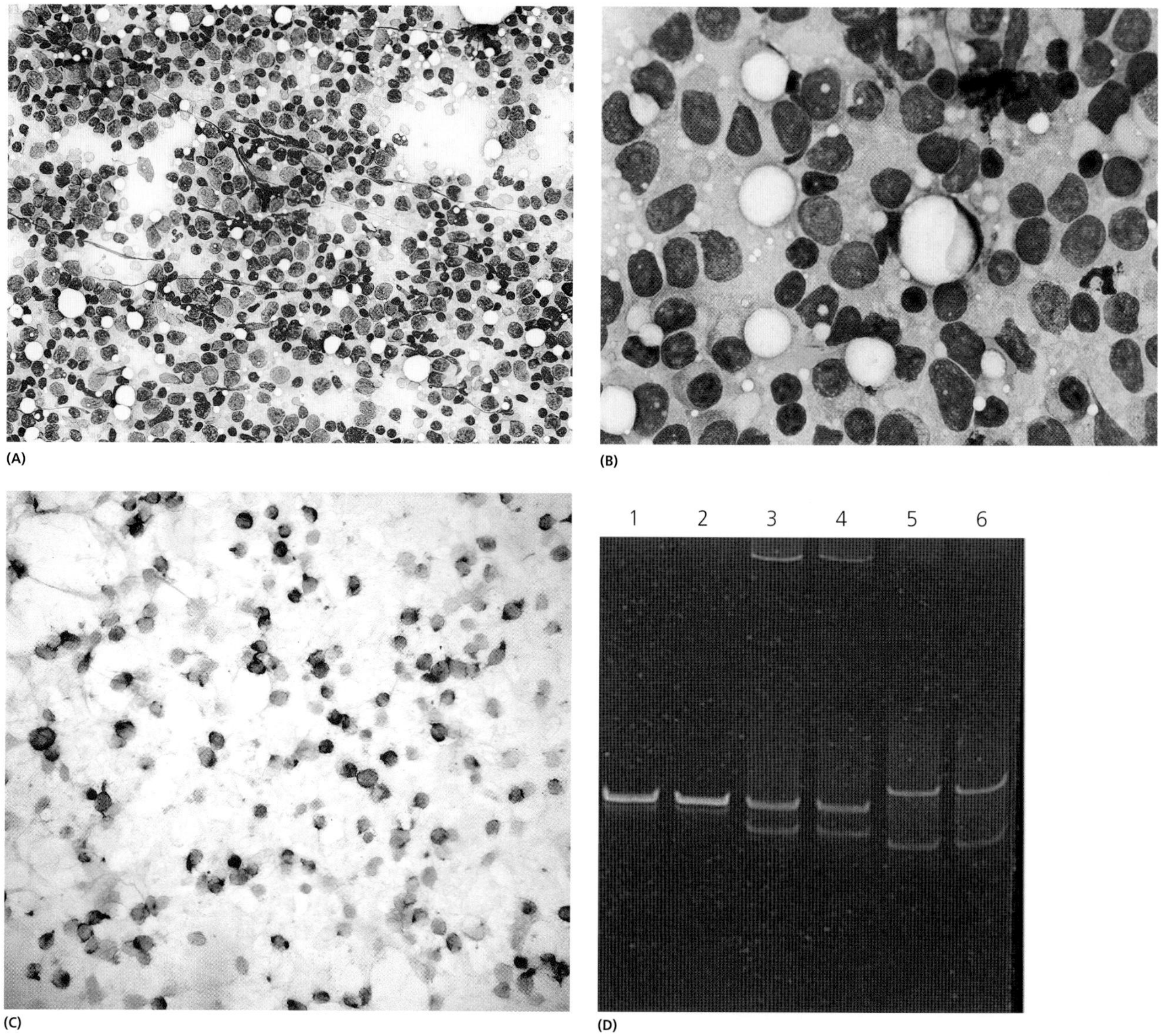

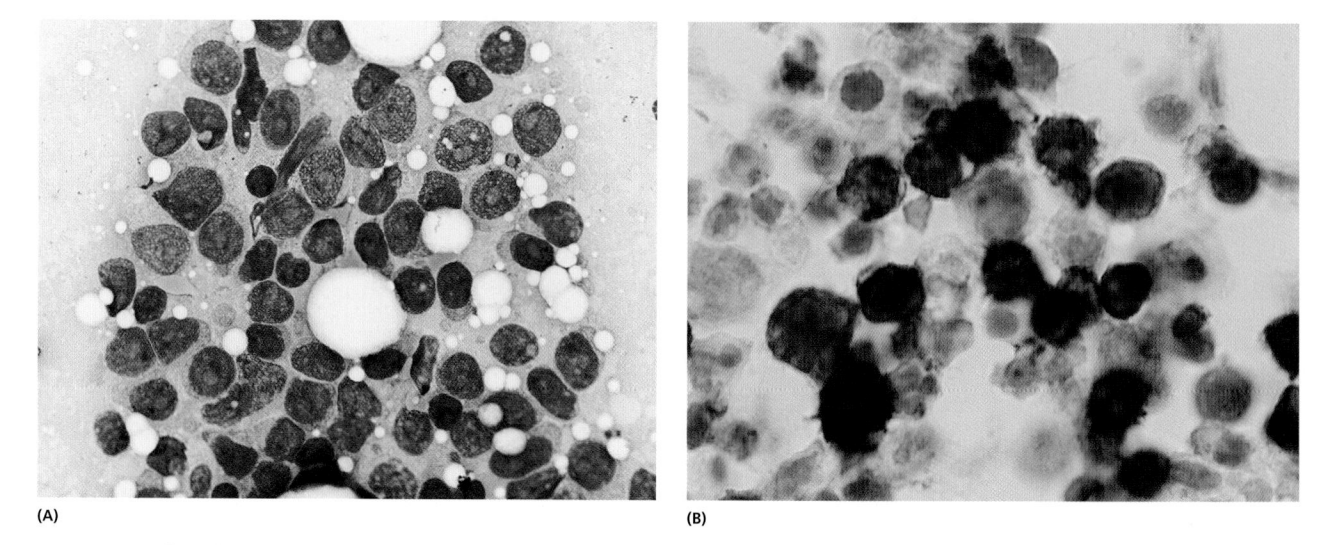

Figure 4.55 Peripheral T-cell lymphoma. FNAC of parotid. (A) Low power view reveals a dense lymphoid infiltrate of parotid gland (MGG ×200). (B) Variable combination of small, intermediate, and large lymphoid cells with irregular nuclei, epithelioid histiocytes and atypical mononuclear cells (MGG ×600, oil immersion). (C) CD3 positive cells confirm a T-cell lymphoma. (D) PCR in a patient. The patient had a history of T-cell cutaneous NHL, now nodule in the buttock and forearm. PCR, lanes 3 and 4, shows amplification of TCR-gamma chain gene with biallelic rearrangement.

Figure 4.56 High grade peripheral T-cell lymphoma. (A) FNAC of a skin nodule contains atypical small and large lymphocytes with cerebriform appearance (MGG ×1000, oil). (B) Cells are strongly CD3 positive. Note cerebriform outline of the nucleus (CD3, APAAp, ×1000, oil immersion).

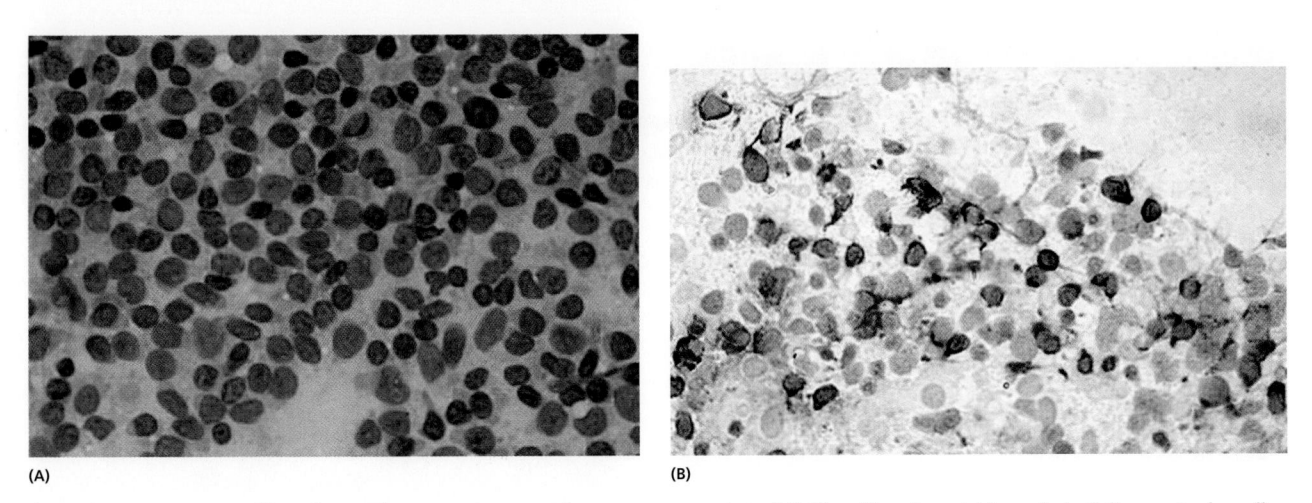

(A)

(B)

Figure 4.57 Cutaneous T-cell lymphoma. This is a separate entity from cutaneous variant of ALCL and lymphomatoid papulosis. Cells are mixed, small and medium sized, some with cerebriform nuclei (A, B).

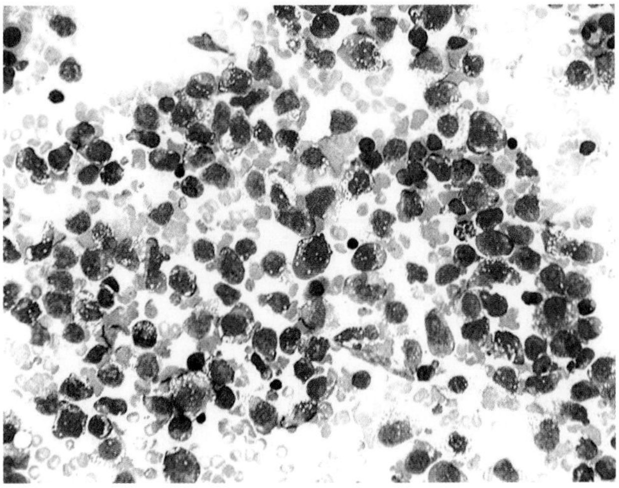

(A)

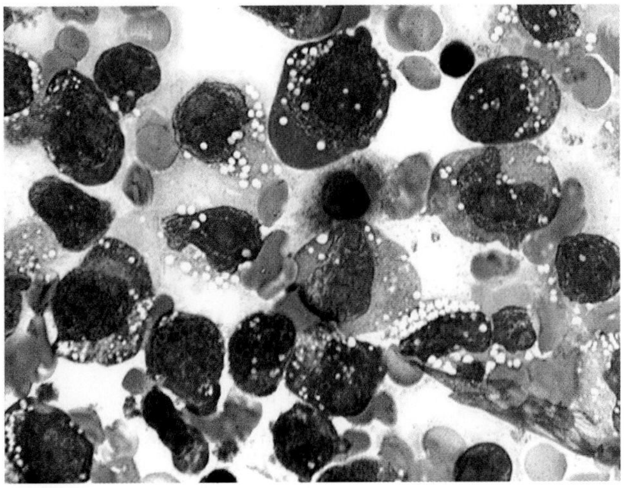

(B)

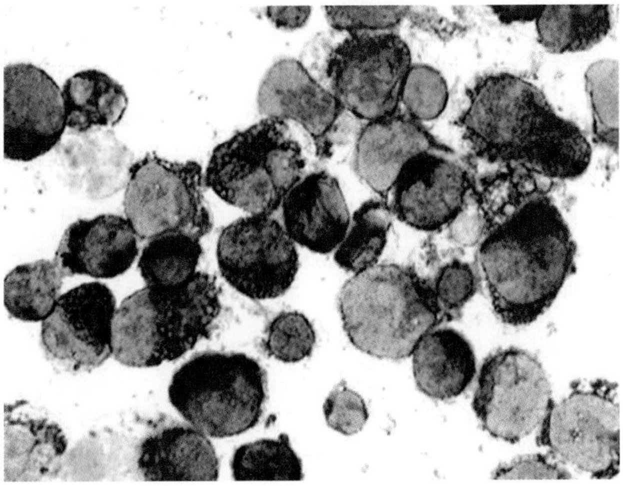

(C)

Figure 4.58 Large cell T-cell lymphoma. (A) FNAC smears show a high grade lymphoma with immunoblastic features (MGG ×400). (B) Individual cells show pleomorphism (MGG ×1000, oil immersion). (C) CD3 positive staining confirms the lymphoma to be T cell (CD3, APAAP, ×600, oil immersion).

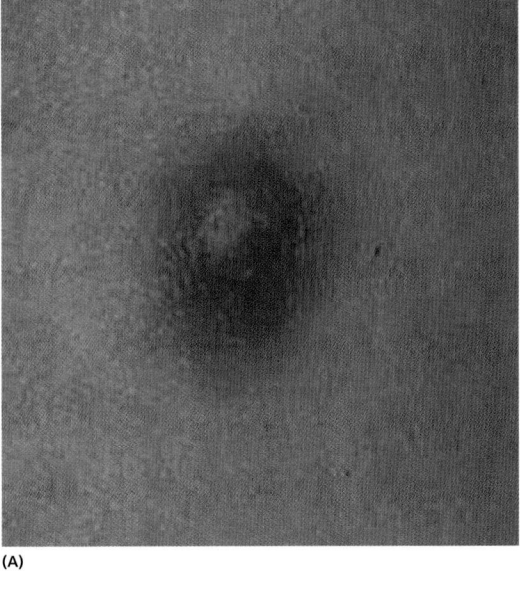

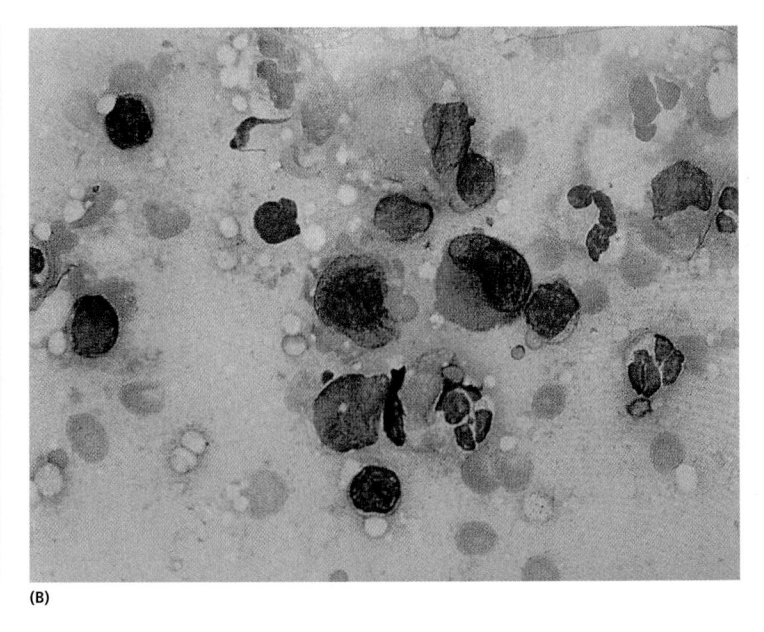

(A)　　　　　　　　　　　　　　　　　　　　　　(B)

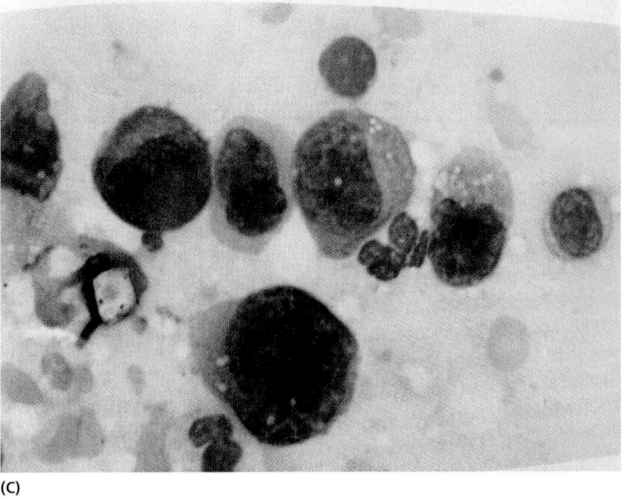

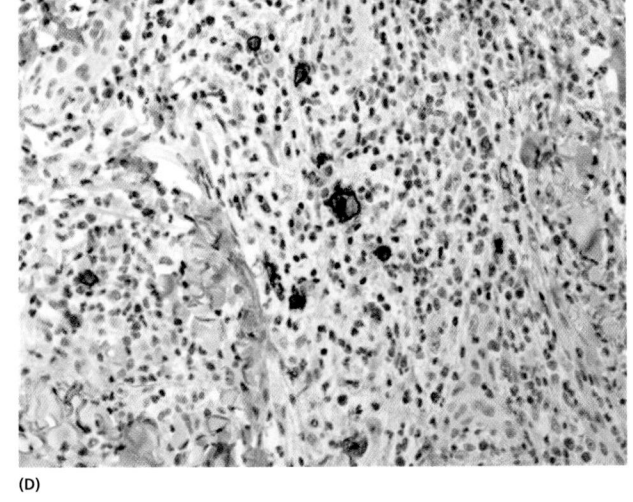

(C)　　　　　　　　　　　　　　　　　　　　　　(D)

Figure 4.59 CD30 positive lymphoproliferative conditions of the skin. (A) Lymphomatoid papulosis is a lymphoid infiltrate of the skin. (B, C) FNAC shows a mixture of large atypical lymphoid cells, histiocytes and inflammatory cells. Some of the cells have bizarre features tempting a diagnosis of malignancy. Disease is self-limiting and morphologically difficult to distinguish from cutaneous variant of ALCL (MGG ×1000, oil immersion). (D) CD30 positive cells on histological section.

potentially curable [221]. Cutaneous type also lacks t(2;5) (p23;q35) and is ALK protein negative. However, it shows FISH positivity for an IRF4 translocation which is highly specific for primary cutaneous ALCL (99% specificity) (Table 4.12) [156a]. This entity should be regarded separate from the systemic type. Cutaneous ALCL is part of the 'CD30 positive lymphoproliferative skin conditions' that also includes lymphomatoid papulosis and CD30+ cutaneous T-cell lymphomas that do not have typical 'anaplastic' morphology [156, 249].

Cytological features: Systemic ALCL has neoplastic cells larger than any other type of lymphoma and can be misdiagnosed as malignant histiocytosis or Hodgkin's lymphoma. The most common phenotype is that of pleomorphic cells with multilobated and multinucleated cells although a monomorphic variant exists. ALCL is a cytologically undifferentiated malignant lymphoma that needs to be distinguished from a variety of other neoplasms using immunohistochemistry. It is composed of single cells and poorly cohesive groups of cells with large, pleomorphic nuclei, many containing prominent nucleoli and a moderate amount of cytoplasm (Fig. 4.62). Many binucleate and multinucleate tumour cells are present (average size 42 μm), some with a 'wreath-like' arrangement of nuclei [250]. Cells have a 'ropey' chromatin pattern and deeply basophilic, variably vacuolated cytoplasm. Necrosis is frequent. A proteinaceous background is prominent in cellular samples. 'Lymphoglandular' bodies and lymphoid tangles are not prominent [251]. Cytological features may suggest metastatic anaplastic carcinoma since anaplastic cells may be admixed with mature lymphocytes and follicle centre cells, reflecting the histological features of malignant cells in ALCL often being confined to subcapsular and medullary sinuses resembling metastatic carcinoma [252]: ALCL may sometimes be composed mainly of spindle-shaped and strap cells, mimicking sarcoma [253].

Immunocytochemistry is essential in distinguishing ALCL from metastatic carcinoma, melanoma and Hodgkin's disease. ALCL is

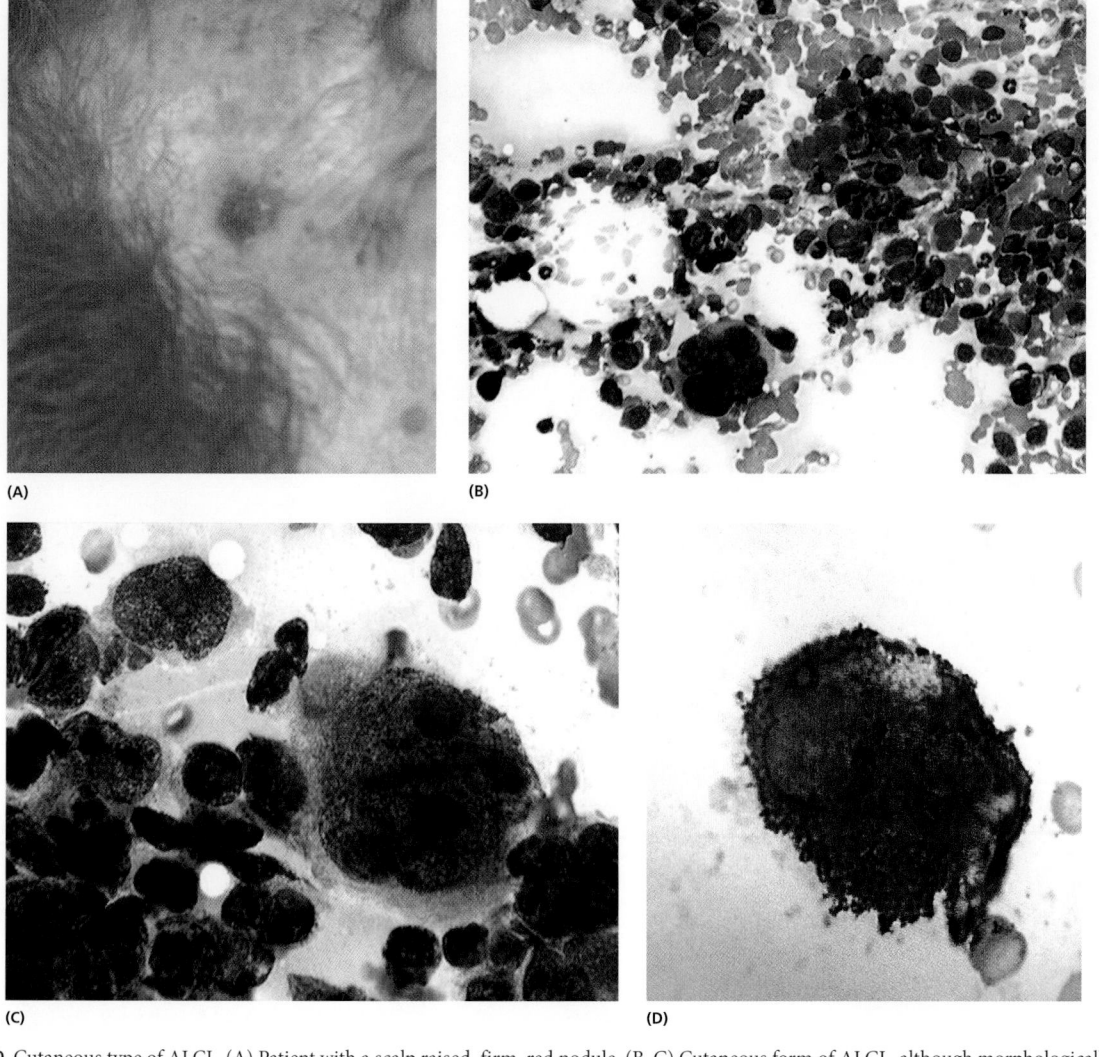

Figure 4.60 Cutaneous type of ALCL. (A) Patient with a scalp raised, firm, red nodule. (B, C) Cutaneous form of ALCL, although morphologically similar to systemic ALCL, is a defined clinical entity (see text) which cytopathologists should be aware of because its anaplastic features are indistinguishable from the systemic type of ALCL (Figure 4.62) and yet its management and prognosis are different (MGG ×200, ×600, ×1000, oil immersion). (D) CD30 positive cells.

positive for CD45 (LCA) in only 67% of cases. It is nearly always negative for cytokeratin but positive for EMA in systemic cases (75%) [251]. Nearly all malignant cells express CD30 positivity (surface membrane and cytoplasmic paranuclear dot-like staining) [254]. CD125 is usually negative in ALCL. When cell lineage markers are present, they show T-cell origins.

The cytogenetic abnormality in ALCL, t(2;5)(p23;q35), can be successfully detected with antibodies against ALK protein in 65% of classical nodal ALCL [255]. The ALK positive group seems to have a good prognosis. Given the importance of ALK protein, WHO classification recommends that all ALCL be classified as ALK positive or ALK negative. The presence of severe pleomorphism and anaplasia was found to correlate with ALK-negative status [256]. However, ALK translocations and overexpression are not specific for ALCL, because tumors other than ALCL can express ALK either as fusion proteins or as full-length proteins [156a].

HHV-8 can associate with solid lymphomas and take ALCL morphology. The recently described HHV-8 associated lymphomas in HIV positive patients may exhibit anaplastic large cell morphology

and express CD30. However, the chromosomal translocation t(2;5)-associated chimeric protein p80NPM/ALK is not observed in any of these cases [255, 257]. This suggests that ALCL is not pathogenetically related to the majority of other types of aggressive T-NHL. Those lymphomas should be distinguished from the classical ALCL as were defined by the REAL and WHO classifications of lymphoid neoplasms even though morphology and a part of immunophenotype mimic that of classical ALCL. Lymphomas developing as a sequel to Post Transplant Lymphadenopathy may exceptionally also have ALCL phenotype [258].

The FNAC diagnosis of ALCL should be considered in the cytological differential diagnosis of anaplastic tumour within a lymph node or extranodal sites [254, 259, 260]. The differential diagnosis may include anaplastic carcinoma, malignant melanoma, sarcoma, Hodgkin's disease and histiocytic lymphoma (Fig. 4.68, next section) [261]. Immunostaining of FNAC is necessary for confirmation of the diagnosis. ALCL has a distinct cytomorphologic appearance and molecular, and cytogenetic prophile such that a reliable diagnosis can be made on cytological material [252, 253, 262, 263, 263a].

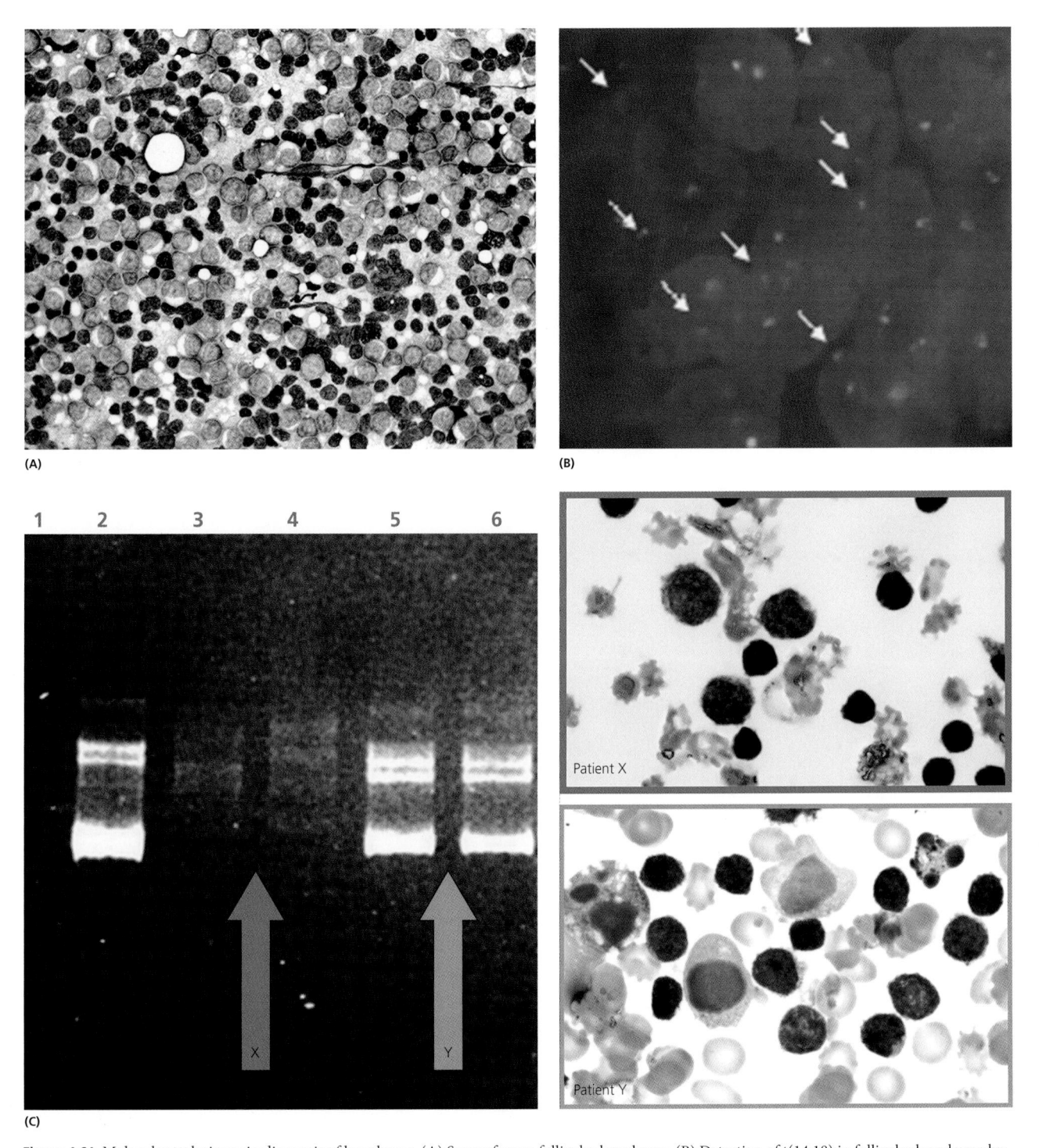

Figure 4.61 Molecular techniques in diagnosis of lymphoma. (A) Smear from a follicular lymphoma. (B) Detection of t(14;18) in follicular lymphoma by dual-colour FISH. FISH demonstrated BCL2/IGH fusion in nuclei of neoplastic follicles. Green signals represent 14q32, whereas orange ones represent 18q21. Arrows indicate colocalised signals. (C) Two patients with pleural effusions, both with previous dg of follicular lymphoma. Lane 1 negative control, Lane 2 Monoclonal control, Lane 3 and 4: patient X, no bands. Lane 5 and 6: Patient Y, dominant bands suggesting a clonal expansion. PCR amplification of IgH confirms the presence of lymphoma in Patient Y.

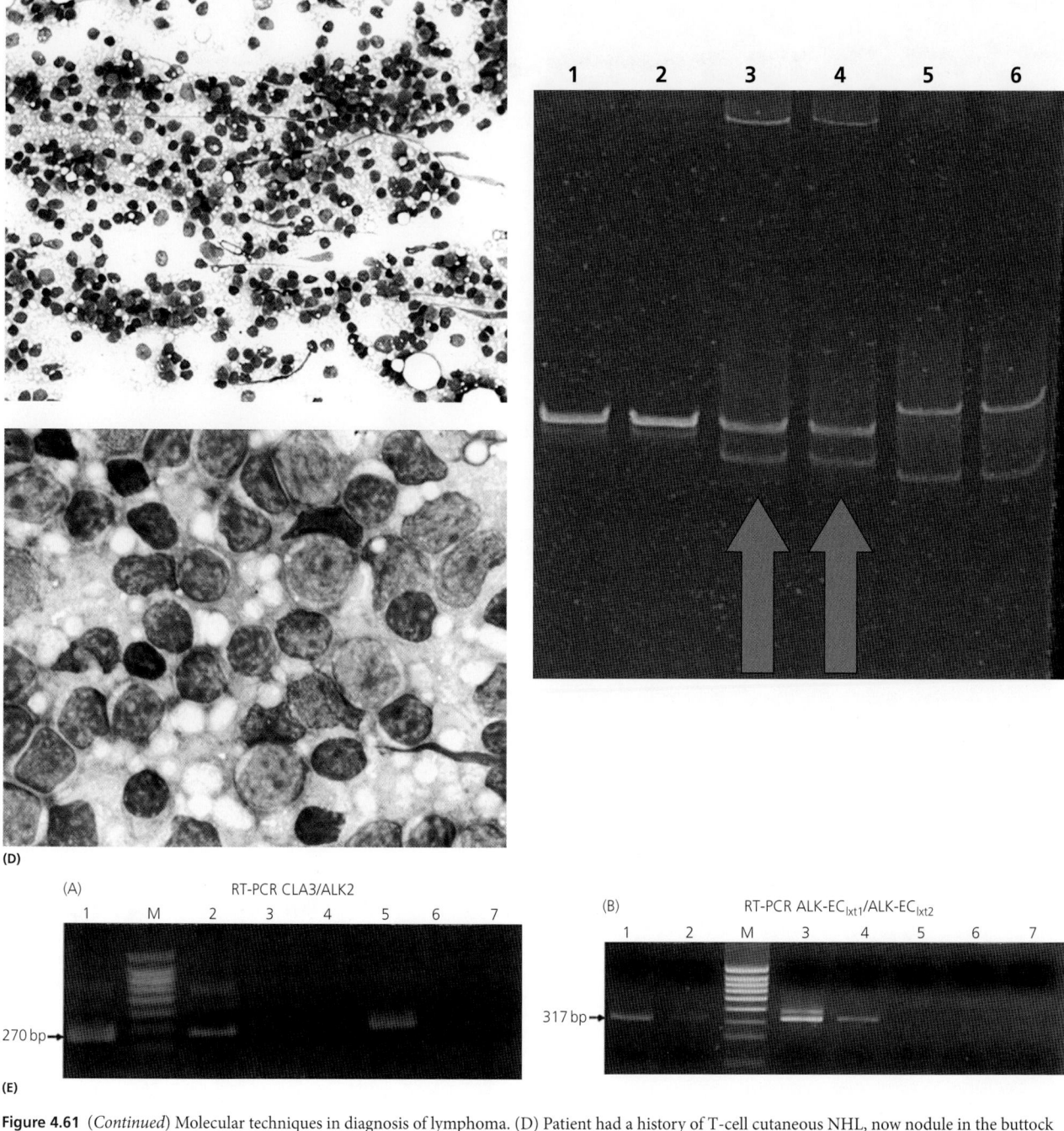

Figure 4.61 (*Continued*) Molecular techniques in diagnosis of lymphoma. (D) Patient had a history of T-cell cutaneous NHL, now nodule in the buttock and forearm. PCR amplification of TCR-gamma chain gene show biallelic rearrangement in Lanes 3 and 4 confirming that the lesion in the buttock is a lymphoma. (E) RT PCR detection of ALK protein in anaplastic large cell lymphoma.

4.5 Metastatic carcinoma in lymph nodes

Metastatic carcinoma represents the most commonly diagnosed condition in the FNAC of lymph nodes in our practice (Fig. 4.2). Sometimes, a lymph node enlargement is the first manifestation of cancer. FNAC is usually used to confirm malignancy, identify histological type of tumour and possibly establish primary site of carcinoma (Figs 4.63–4.74). If the primary tumour remains unknown, diagnostic imaging of the neck, chest, abdomen and

pelvis is the most appropriate initial investigation following a FNAC diagnosis of metastatic adenocarcinoma [264].

[See BOX 4.4. Summary of ultrasound features: Metastatic lymph node on www.wiley.com/go/kocjan/clinical_cytopathology_head_neck2e]

The most common primary sites of metastatic carcinoma in the neck nodes is from the perioral area. They include cancers

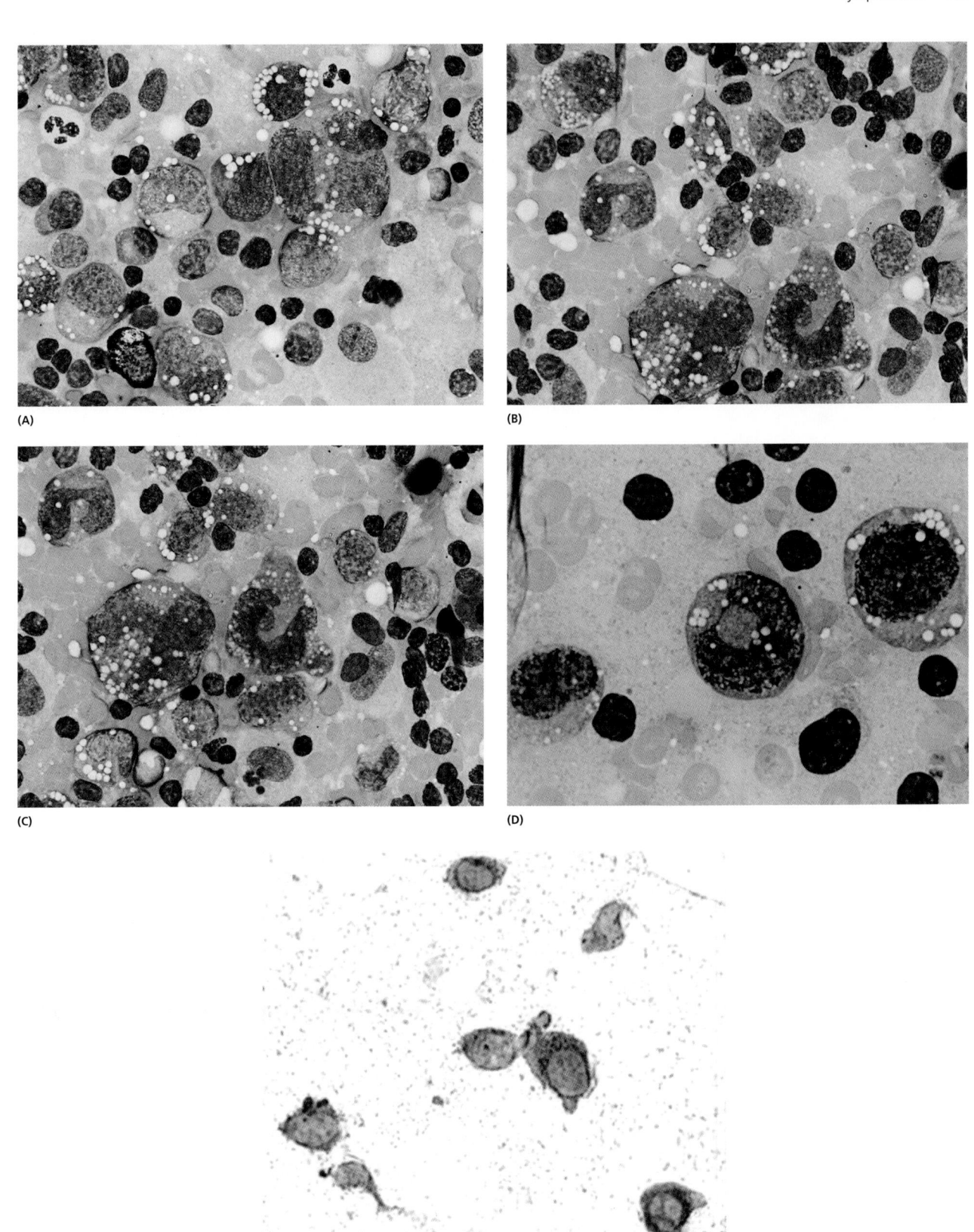

Figure 4.62 Anaplastic large cell lymphoma. A 25-year-old patient was referred for the suprasternal swelling thought to be thyroid gland. (A) FNAC shows a population of large pleomorphic cells against a background of mature lymphocytes (MGG ×400). (B, C, D) High power view shows cells with large, pleomorphic nuclei, many containing prominent nucleoli, and a moderate amount of cytoplasm. Many binucleate and multinucleate tumour cells are present (average size 42 μm), some with a 'wreath-like' arrangement of nuclei (D). Cells have a coarse chromatin pattern and deeply basophilic, variably vacuolated cytoplasm (MGG ×100, oil immersion). (E) Lymphoma cells are CD30 positive.

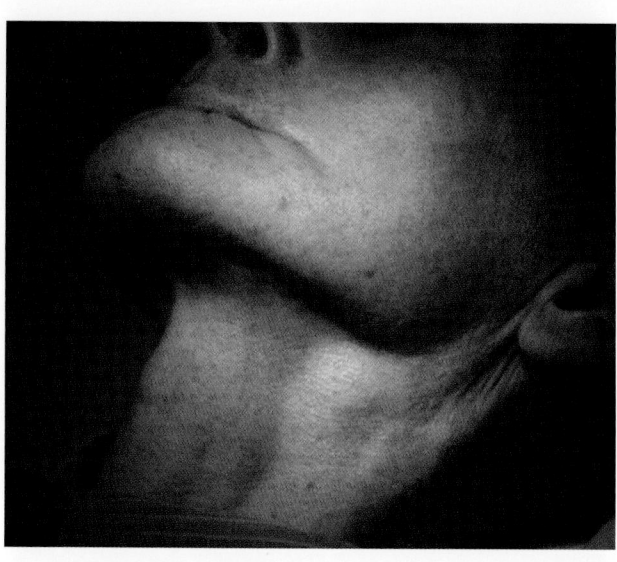

Figure 4.63 This 63-year-old patient was referred to the FNAC clinic for an enlarged cervical lymph node. He had a history of squamous cell carcinoma in the oropharynx. FNAC revealed reactive changes only. There was no evidence of metastases.

of the lip, buccal mucosa, tongue, larynx, nasopharynx and hypopharynx. These are followed by the metastases from the lung, breast, GI tract, urinary bladder, cervix and thyroid. Some cytomorphological characteristics are useful for presumption of primary sites, such as: monolayered papillary fronds with intranuclear cytoplasmic inclusions in thyroid papillary carcinoma; large, polygonal, keratinised cells with a low nuclear/cytoplasmic ratio and anucleate squames in perioral cancers; and numerous naked nuclei, destroyed nuclei and marked lymphocytic infiltrates in nasopharyngeal carcinoma. The accuracy rate of presumption of primary sites is 100% in thyroid papillary carcinoma, 83% in perioral cancer and 77% in nasopharyngeal carcinoma but low in other malignancies [265]. The measurement of thyroglobulin (Tg) in the FNAC washout fluid increases the diagnostic performance of cytology [266]. HPV status of squamous cell carcinoma of the head and neck may be established by various methods including immunohistochemistry for p16, HPV-in situ hybridization, and HPV-Polymerase chain reaction. Its application may help localize the primary site during the diagnostic work-up [267, 267a,b]. The occurrence of both, carcinoma and lymphoma, in the same lymph node is extremely rare and may be diagnosed on FNAC [268].

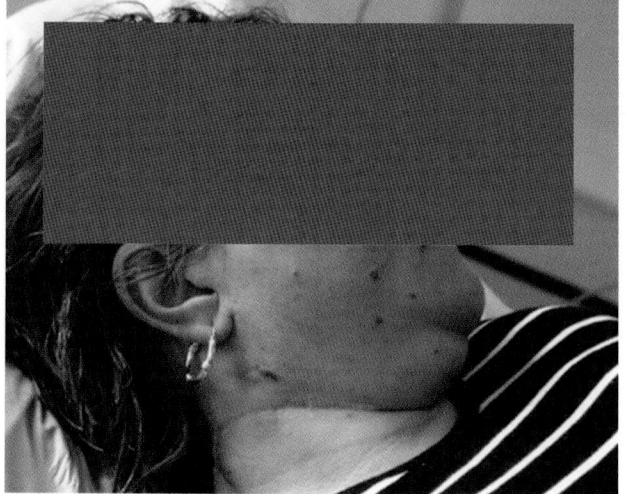

(A)

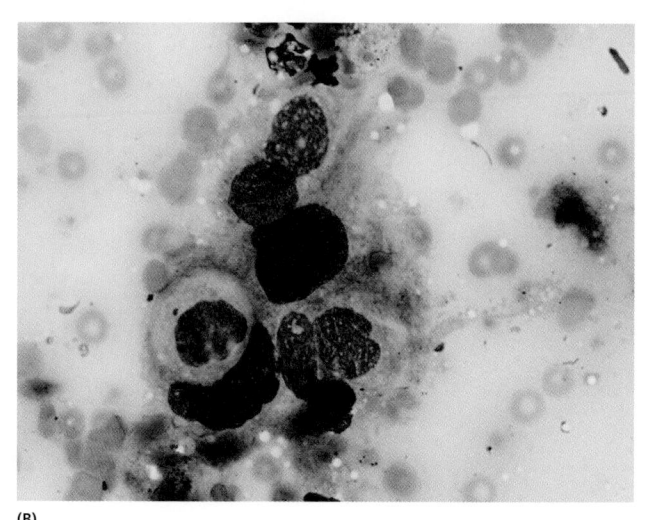

(B)

Figure 4.64 Metastatic squamous cell carcinoma. (A) This 33-year-old patient has had ethmoid adenocarcinoma treated and the skin grafted. She was referred for investigation of enlarged lymph node at the angle of mandible. (B) Regional lymph node contained mature squamous epithelium consistent with metastatic carcinoma (MGG V6900, oil).

Table 4.12 ALK translocations and overexpression.

Lymphoid neoplasms		
ALK-positive ALCL	t(2;5)	NPM1-ALK
ALK-positive diffuse large B-cell lymphoma	t(2;17)	CLTC-ALK
Nonlymphoid neoplasms		
Inflammatory myofibroblastic tumor	t(1;2)	TPM3-ALK
Lung adenocarcinoma	inv(2)(p21p23)	EML4-ALK
Rhabdomyosarcoma		native ALK
Neuroblastoma		native ALK

ALK are not specific for ALCL, because tumors other than ALCL can express ALK either as fusion proteins or as full-length proteins (Modified from de Leval L, Gaulard P. Tricky and terrible T-cell tumors: these are thrilling times for testing: molecular pathology of peripheral T-cell lymphomas. *Hematology Am Soc Hematol Educ Program.* 2011; 2011: 336–43) [156a].

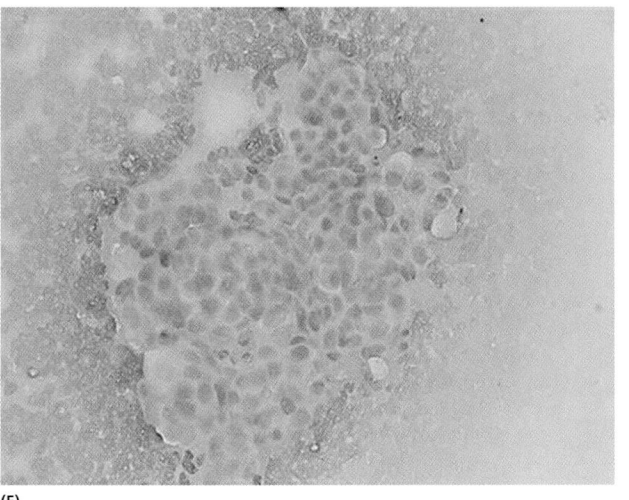

Figure 4.65 Metastatic carcinoma. (A) This 75-year-old patient was referred to FNAC clinic for a swelling in the left supraclavicular fossa near the SC joint. There was no previous history. (B) Metastatic carcinoma. Clusters and single epithelial cells with features of malignancy against a background of lymphoid cells. (C) CK7 positive. (D) ER positive. (E) TTF1 negative tumour cells. The immunoprofile suggests breast as a primary site. The tumour was subsequently found in the breast.

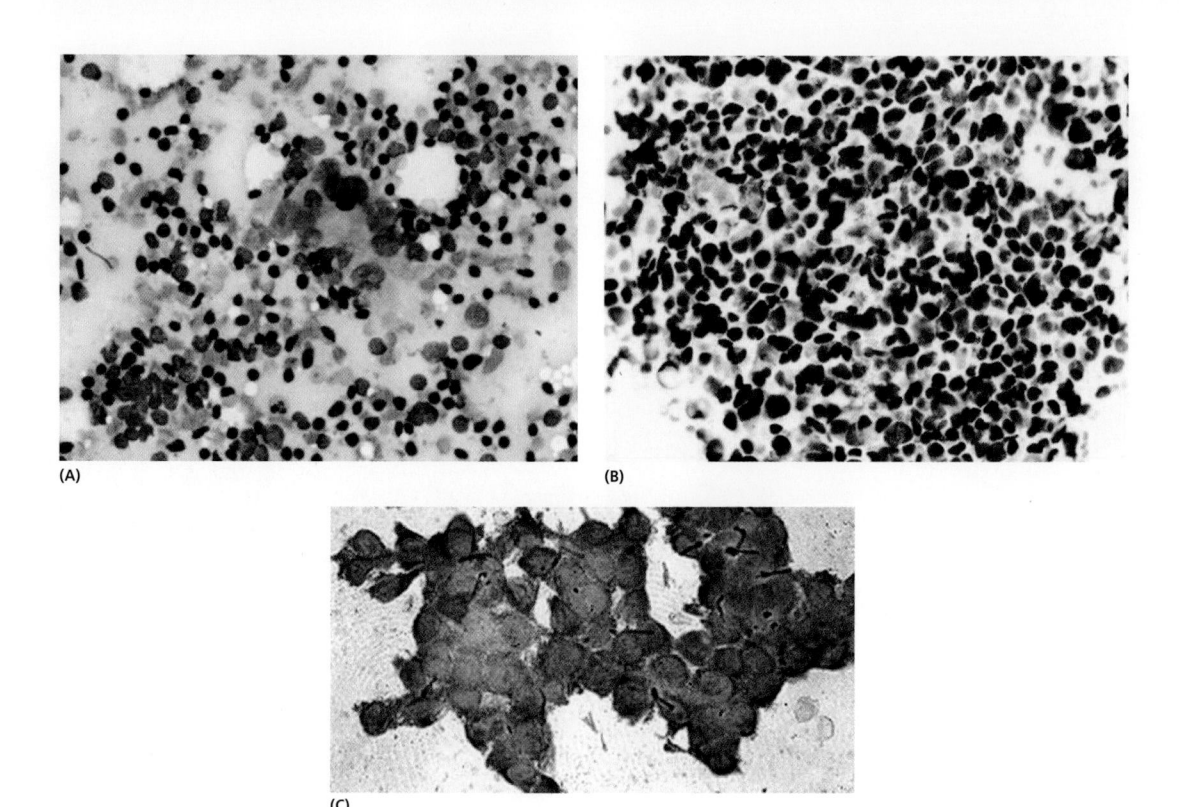

Figure 4.66 FNA lymph node with metastatic tumour. (A) A focus of adenocarcinoma cells in a lymph node. (B) CDX positive cells indicate stomach or colon as possible primary sites. A tumour was found in the stomach. (C) Another case with thyroglobulin positive cells in the FNA of a lymph node which is indicative of a metastatic papillary carcinoma of the thyroid.

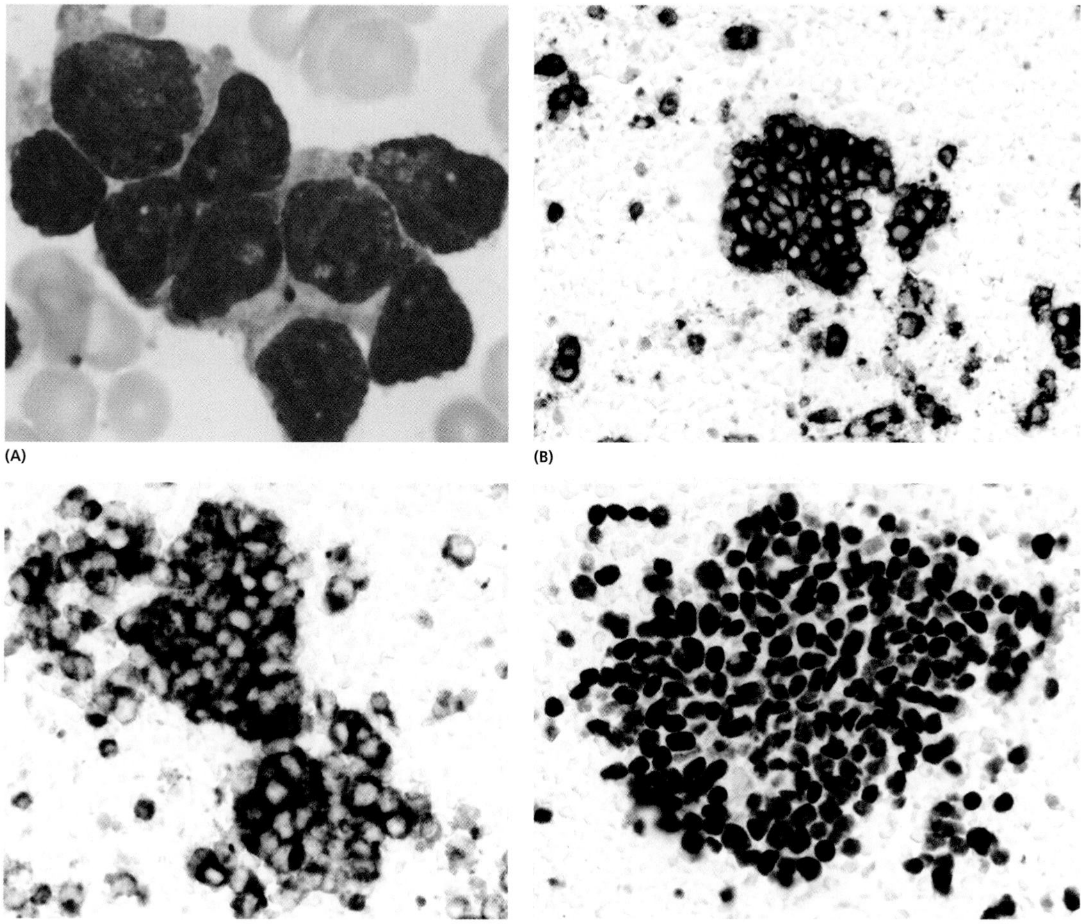

Figure 4.67 Metastatic small cell carcinoma of the lung. This 70-year-old man with SVC obstruction was referred for urgent FNAC of his bilateral supraclavicular swellings. (A) FNAC smear shows a cluster of small to medium sized cells with fine granular chromatin pattern, inconspicuous nucleoli and scant basophilic cytoplasm. Cells show nuclear moulding (MGG ×600, oil immersion). (B) CD56 positive, (C) CAM5.2 positive, dot like and (D) TTF1 positive.

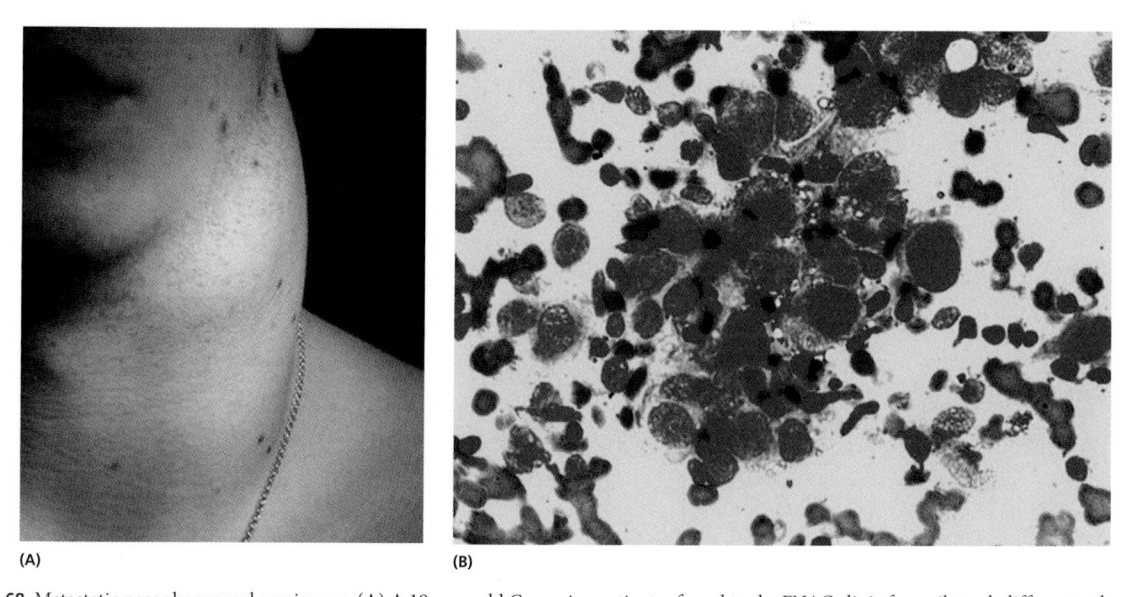

Figure 4.68 Metastatic nasopharyngeal carcinoma. (A) A 19-year-old Caucasian patient referred to the FNAC clinic for unilateral, diffuse, tender swelling of the neck preventing the head movement. On examination, the mass was hard and fixed with no definite edge to it. Clinically it was thought to be an infection. (B) FNAC smears reveal a malignant tumour with large anaplastic nuclei and prominent nucleoli. Some bizarre, Hodgkin-like cells were noted. Morphologically, tumour was thought to be a lymphoma (Hodgkin's or ALCL). Immunocytochemistry showed positive epithelial markers and FISH showed EBV confirming nasopharyngeal carcinoma.

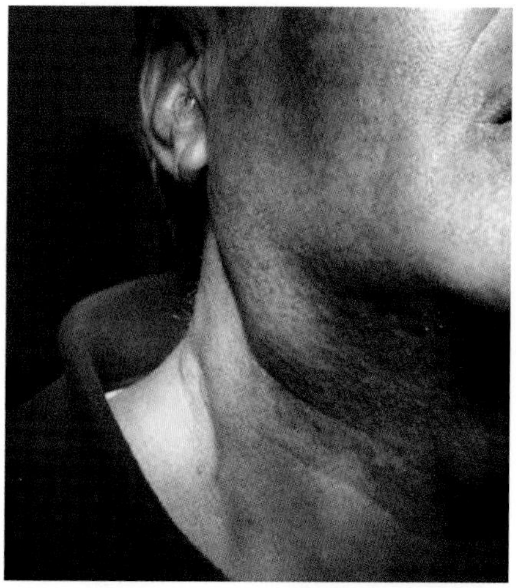

(A) 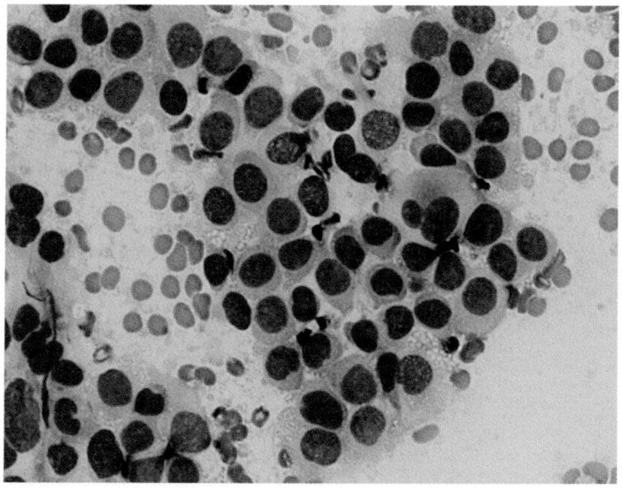   (B)

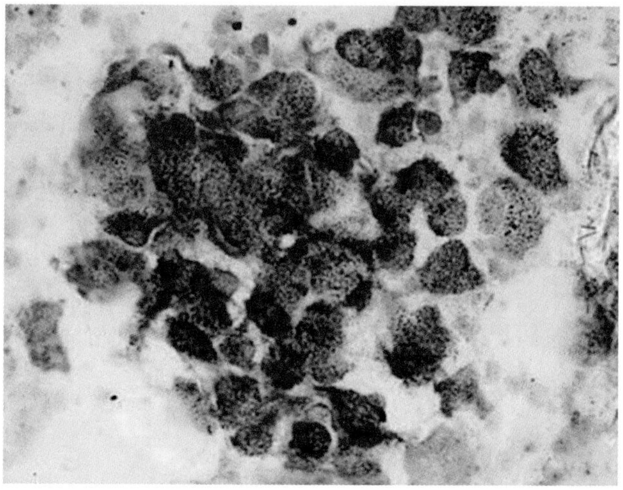

(C)

Figure 4.69 Metastatic malignant melanoma. (A) Patient presented with cervical lymphadenopathy. Clinical history revealed previous melanoma of the skin of the face. (B) Large, mainly single cells with eccentric round or oval nuclei, prominent nucleoli and grey, finely vacuolated cytoplasm. No pigment was seen (MGG ×600, oil immersion). (C) HMB 45, melanoma marker positivity confirms the diagnosis (APAAP, ×600, oil immersion).

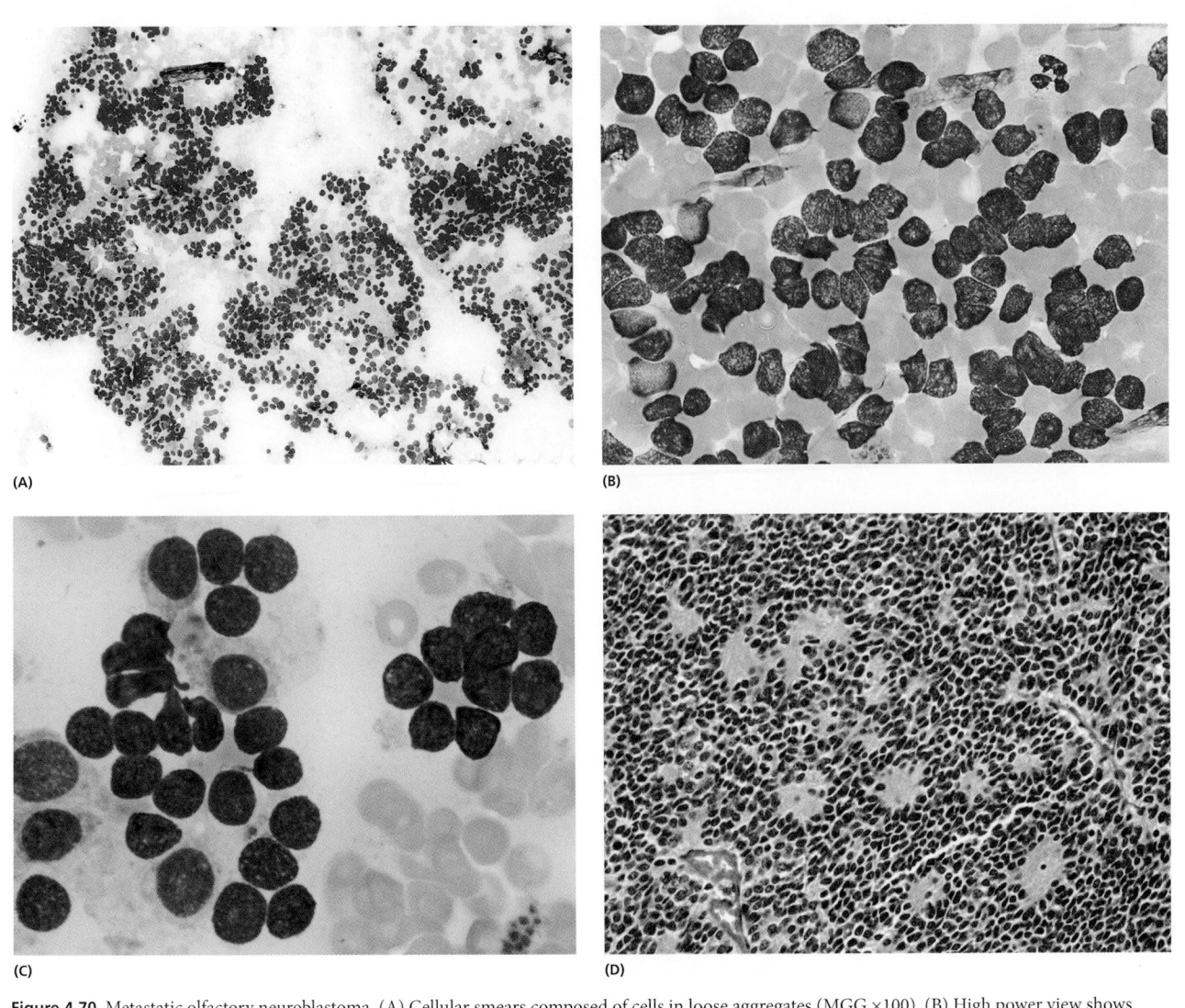

Figure 4.70 Metastatic olfactory neuroblastoma. (A) Cellular smears composed of cells in loose aggregates (MGG ×100). (B) High power view shows small to medium size cells with fine chromatin pattern, inconspicuous nucleoli and finely vacuolated cytoplasm resembling lymphoblasts (MGG ×600, oil immersion). (C) Cells occasionally form rosettes. (MGG ×600, oil immersion). (D) Histology of olfactory neuroblastoma shows prominent rosettes.

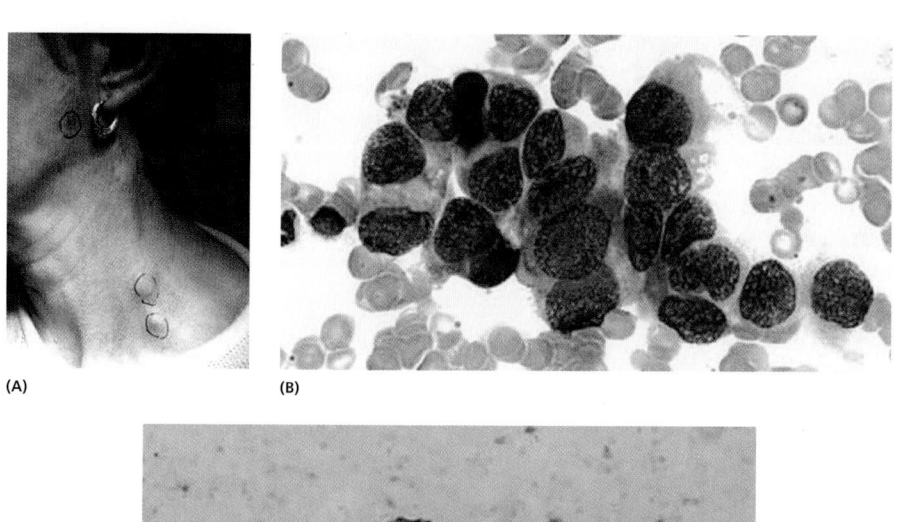

(A)   (B)

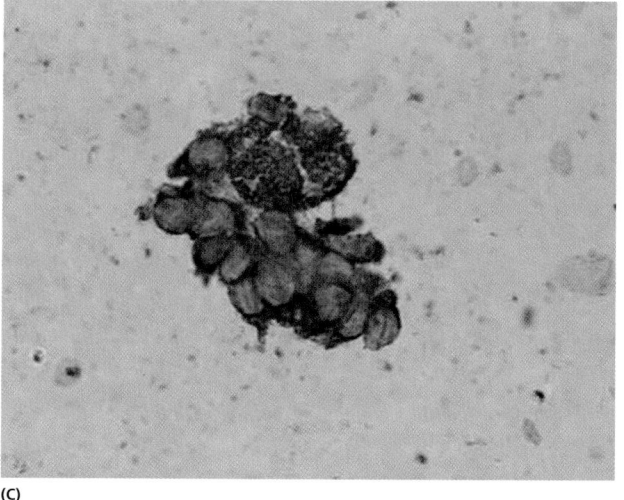

(C)

Figure 4.71 Metastatic angiosarcoma. (A) This patient had radiotherapy for angiosarcoma of the scalp. She presented to the FNAC clinic with two enlarged lymph nodes in the posterior triangle. There was also a hardening of the preauricular area outside the radiation field. (B) FNAC of lymph nodes was cellular, composed of clusters forming occasional acini (MGG ×400). Individual cells were oval, round or spindle with eccentric nuclei, visible nucleoli and moderate to abundant amount of pale blue grey, vacuolated cytoplasm. The cells were 2–9 times larger than the red cells (MGG ×600, oil immersion). (C) Immunocytochemistry is positive for endothelial marker CD31.

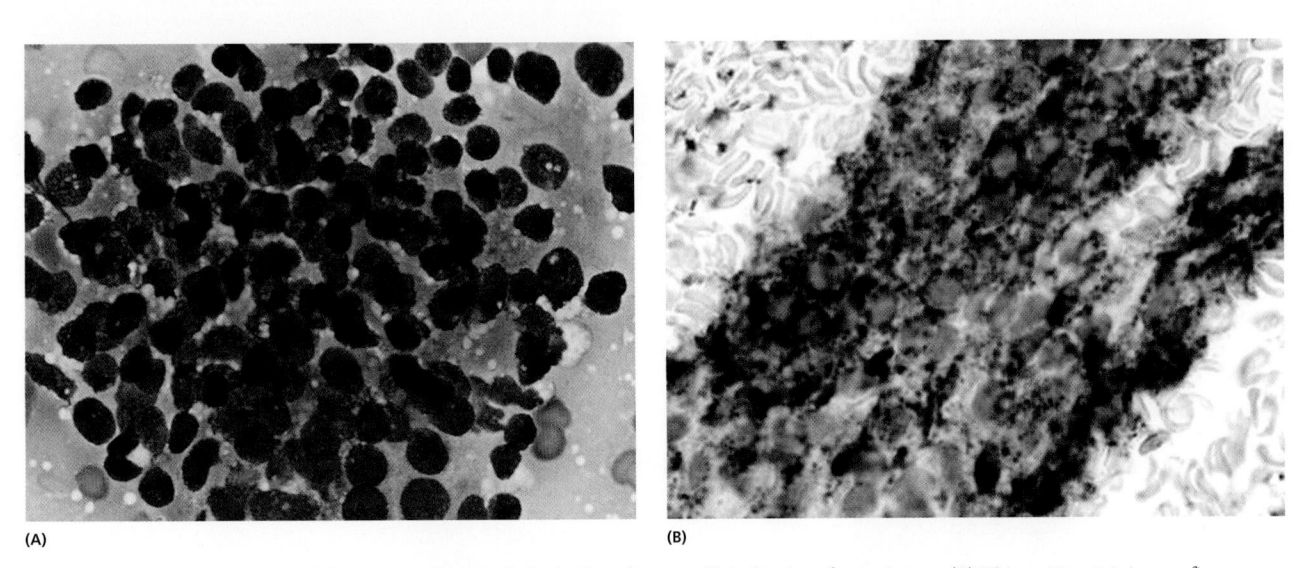

(A)

(B)

Figure 4.72 Metastatic carcinoma of the prostate. (A) Morphologically malignant cells indicative of a carcinoma. (B) PSA positive staining confirms prostate as the primary site.

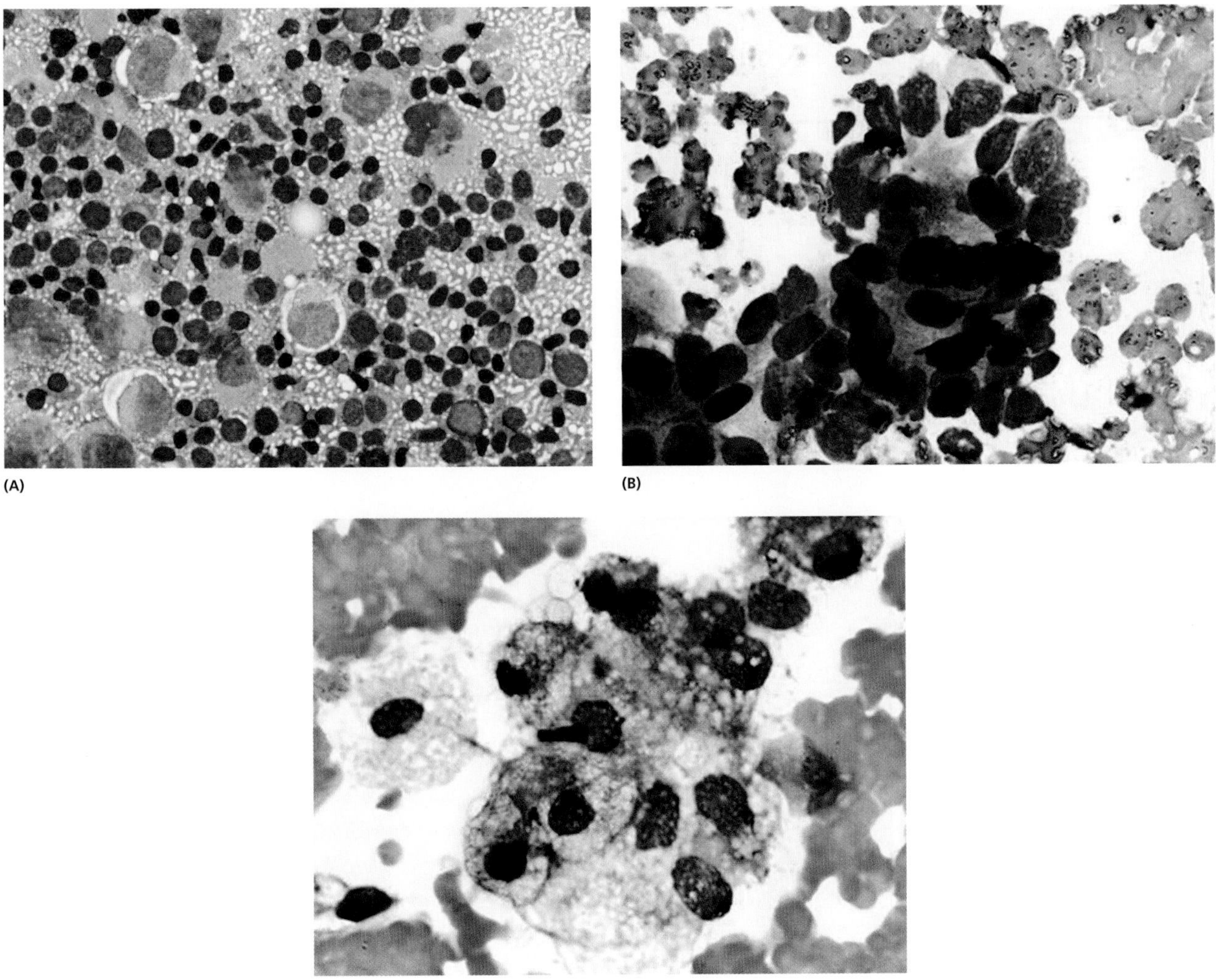

(A)

(B)

(C)

Figure 4.73 Metastatic tumours in the lymph node: (A) seminoma, (B) rectal carcinoma and (C) renal cell carcinoma.

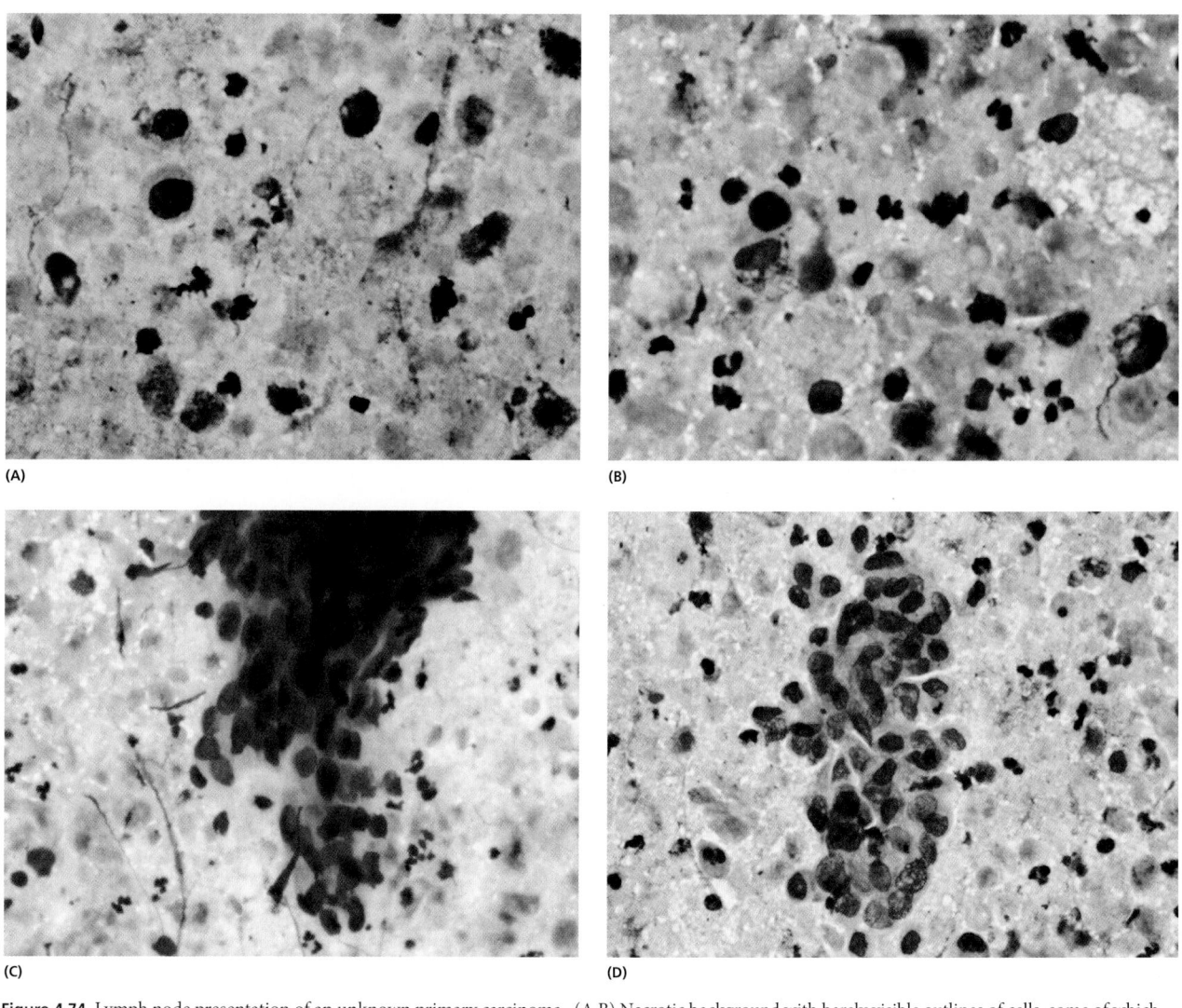

(A)

(B)

(C)

(D)

Figure 4.74 Lymph node presentation of an unknown primary carcinoma. (A,B) Necrotic background with barely visible outlines of cells, some of which have dense piknotic nuclei. (C,D) Microbiospy fragments and aggregates of cells which appear epithelial and show squamous differentiation. The diagnosis was metastatic squamous cell carcinoma.

This chapter also has online only material. Ultrasound Summary boxes, which have been cited throughout the chapter text as 'Summary of ultrasound features', are available on www.wiley.com/go/kocjan/clinical_cytopathology_head_neck2e for the following diseases

Box 4.1   Summary of ultrasound features: Normal (reactive) lymph node

Box 4.2   Summary of ultrasound features: Tuberculous (TB) lymph node

Box 4.3   Summary of ultrasound features: Lymphoma

Box 4.4   Summary of ultrasound features: Metastatic lymph node

References

1. Lopes Cardozo P. The significance of fine needle aspiration cytology for the diagnosis and treatment of malignant lymphomas. *Folia Haematol Int Mag Klin Morphol Blutforsch* 1980; **107**(4): 601–20.

2. Layfield LJ. Fine-needle aspiration of the head and neck. *Pathology (Phila)* 1996; **4**(2): 409–38.

3. Nasuti JF, Yu G, Boudousquie A, Gupta P. Diagnostic value of lymph node fine needle aspiration cytology: an institutional experience of 387 cases observed over a 5-year period. *Cytopathology* 2000 Feb; **11**(1): 18–31.

3a. Kocjan G. Best Practice No 185. Cytological and molecular diagnosis of lymphoma. *J Clin Pathol.* 2005; **58**(6): 561–7.

4. Proctor I, Edmunds L, Falzon M et al. The role of Fine Needle Aspiration Cytology in the diagnosis of patients with lymphadenopathy. *Acta Cytol* 2013: **57**(suppl) P-297: 126.

5. Thomas JO, Adeyi D, Amanguno H. Fine-needle aspiration in the management of peripheral lymphadenopathy in a developing country. *Diagn Cytopathol* 1999; **21**(3): 159–62.

6. Mitra S, Ray S, Mitra PK. Analysis of FNAC of cervical lymph nodes: experience over a three-year period. *J Indian Med Assoc* 2013; **111**(9): 599–602.

7. Pilotti S, Di Palma S, Alasio L et al. Diagnostic assessment of enlarged superficial lymph nodes by fine needle aspiration. *Acta Cytol* 1993; **37**(6): 853–66.

8. Steel BL, Schwartz MR, Ramzy I. Fine needle aspiration biopsy in the diagnosis of lymphadenopathy in 1,103 patients. Role, limitations and analysis of diagnostic pitfalls. *Acta Cytol* 1995; **39**(1): 76–81.

9. Schoengen A, Binder T, Fembacher P, Zeelen U. The fine-needle aspiration cytology of lymph nodes suspected of malignancy. Its diagnostic value and capacity to predict the histogenesis. *Dtsch Med Wochenschr* 1995; **120**(16): 549–54.

10. Poorey VK, Tyagi A. Accuracy of fine needle aspiration cytology in head and neck masses. *Indian J Otolaryngol Head Neck Surg* 2014; **66**(2): 182–6.

11. Sneige N, Dekmezian RH, Katz RL, et al. Morphologic and immunocytochemical evaluation of 220 fine needle aspirates of malignant lymphoma and lymphoid hyperplasia. *Acta Cytol* 1990; **34**(3): 311–22.

12. Das DK. Value and limitations of fine-needle aspiration cytology in diagnosis and classification of lymphomas: A review. *Diagn Cytopathol* 1999; **21**(4): 240–9.

13. Lee DH, Baek HJ, Kook H et al. Clinical value of fine needle aspiration cytology in pediatric cervical lymphadenopathy patients under 12-years-of-age. *Int J Pediatr Otorhinolaryngol* 2014; **78**(1): 79–81.

14. Lioe TF, Elliott H, Allen DC, Spence RA. The role of fine needle aspiration cytology (FNAC) in the investigation of superficial lymphadenopathy; uses and limitations of the technique. *Cytopathology* 1999; **10**(5): 291–7.

15. Katz RL. Pitfalls in the diagnosis of fine-needle aspiration of lymph nodes. *Monogr Pathol* 1997; **39**: 118–33.

16. Tani EM, Christensson B, Porwit A, Skoog L. Immunocytochemical analysis and cytomorphologic diagnosis on fine needle aspirates of lymphoproliferative disease. *Acta Cytol* 1988; **32**(2): 209–15.

17. Katz RL, Wojcik EM, el-Naggar AK et al. Proliferation markers in non-Hodgkin's lymphoma. A comparative study between cytophotometric quantitation of Ki-67 and flow cytometric proliferation index on fine needle aspirates. *Anal Quant Cytol Histol* 1993; **15**(3):179–86.

18. Brown DC, Gatter KC, Mason DY. Proliferation in non-Hodgkin's lymphoma: a comparison of Ki-67 staining on fine needle aspiration and cryostat sections. *J Clin Pathol* 1990; **43**(4): 325–8.

19. Reid MM. Fine needle aspiration and the diagnosis of non-Hodgkin's lymphoma [letter; comment]. *J Clin Pathol* 1998; **51**(9): 712.

20. Simsir A, Fetsch P, Stetler-Stevenson M, Abati A. Immunophenotypic analysis of non-Hodgkin's lymphomas in cytologic specimens: a correlative study of immunocytochemical and flow cytometric techniques. *Diagn Cytopathol* 1999; **20**(5): 278–84.

21. Cha I, Goates JJ. Fine-needle aspiration of lymph nodes: use of flow cytometry immunophenotyping. *Pathology (Phila)* 1996; **4**(2): 337–64.

22. Ravinsky E, Morales C, Kutryk E et al. Cytodiagnosis of lymphoid proliferations by fine needle aspiration biopsy. Adjunctive value of flow cytometry. *Acta Cytol* 1999; **43**(6): 1070–8.

23. Henrique RM, Sousa ME, Godinho MI et al. Immunophenotyping by flow cytometry of fine needle aspirates in the diagnosis of lymphoproliferative disorders: A retrospective study. *J Clin Lab Anal* 1999; **13**(5): 224–8.

24. Zeppa P, Vigliar E, Cozzolino I et al. Fine needle aspiration cytology and flow cytometry immunophenotyping of non-Hodgkin lymphoma: can we do better? *Cytopathology*. 2010; **21**(5): 300–10.

25. Ensani F, Mehravaran S, Irvanlou G et al. Fine-needle aspiration cytology and flow cytometric immunophenotyping in diagnosis and classification of non-Hodgkin lymphoma in comparison to histopathology. *Diagn Cytopathol*. 2012; **40**(4): 305–10.

26. Stacchini A, Aliberti S, Pacchioni D et al. Flow cytometry significantly improves the diagnostic value of fine needle aspiration cytology of lymphoproliferative lesions of salivary glands. *Cytopathology*. 2014; **25**(4): 231–40.

27. Jeffers MD, Milton J, Herriot R, McKean M. Fine needle aspiration cytology in the investigation on non-Hodgkin's lymphoma. *J Clin Pathol* 1998; **51**(3): 189–96.

27a. Barroca H, Marques C, Candeias J. Fine needle aspiration cytology diagnosis, flow cytometry immunophenotyping and histology in clinically suspected lymphoproliferative disorder: a comparative study. *Acta Cytol.* 2008; **52**(2): 124–32.

27b. Ho AK, Hill S, Preobrazhensky SN, Miller ME, Chen Z, Bahler DW. Small B-cell neoplasms with typical mantle cell lymphoma immunophenotypes often include chronic lymphocytic leukemias. *Am J Clin Pathol.* 2009 Jan; **131**(1): 27–32.

27c. Paul T, Gautam U, Rajwanshi A, Das A, Trehan A, Malhotra P, Srinivasan R. Flow cytometric immunophenotyping and cell block immunocytochemistry in the diagnosis of primary Non-Hodgkin's Lymphoma by fine-needle aspiration: Experience from a tertiary care center. *J Cytol.* 2014 Jul; **31**(3): 123–30.

28. Chernoff WG, Lampe HB, Cramer H, Banerjee D. The potential clinical impact of the fine needle aspiration/flow cytometric diagnosis of malignant lymphoma. *J Otolaryngol* 1992; **21**(Suppl 1): 1–15.

29. Dunphy CH, Ramos R. Combining fine-needle aspiration and flow cytometric immunophenotyping in evaluation of nodal and extranodal sites for possible lymphoma: a retrospective review. *Diagn Cytopathol* 1997; **16**(3): 200–6.

30. Robins DB, Katz RL, Swan F, Jr. et al. Immunotyping of lymphoma by fine-needle aspiration. A comparative study of cytospin preparations and flow cytometry. *Am J Clin Pathol* 1994; **101**(5): 569–76.

31. Lima CE, Mizushima Y, Masuda S, Kitagawa M. Comparison of DNA flow cytometric analysis of body cavity fluids with conventional cytology. *In Vivo* 1994; **8**(3): 359–62.

32. Saikia UN, Dey P, Vohra H, Gupta SK. DNA flow cytometry of non-Hodgkin's lymphomas: correlation with cytologic grade and clinical relapse. *Diagn Cytopathol* 2000 Mar; **22**(3): 142–6.

33. Liu K, Mann KP, Vitellas KM et al. Fine-needle aspiration with flow cytometric immunophenotyping for primary diagnosis of intra-abdominal lymphomas. *Diagn Cytopathol* 1999; **21**(2): 98–104.

34. Jeffers MD, McCorriston J, Farquharson MA et al. Analysis of clonality in cytologic material using the polymerase chain reaction (PCR). *Cytopathology* 1997; **8**(2): 114–21.

35. Alkan S, Lehman C, Sarago C et al. Polymerase chain reaction detection of immunoglobulin gene rearrangement and bcl-2 translocation in archival glass slides of cytologic material. *Diagn Mol Pathol* 1995; **4**(1): 25–31.

36. Shivnarain D, Ladanyi M, Zakowski MF. Detection of BCL2 rearrangement in archival cytological smears of B-cell lymphomas. *Mod Pathol* 1994; **7**(9): 915–9.

37. Kube MJ, McDonald DA, Quin JW, Greenberg ML. Use of archival and fresh cytologic material for the polymerase chain reaction. Detection of the bcl-2 oncogene in lymphoid tissue obtained by fine needle biopsy. *Anal Quant Cytol Histol* 1994; **16**(3): 174–82.

38. Aiello A, Delia D, Giardini R et al. PCR analysis of IgH and BCL2 gene rearrangement in the diagnosis of follicular lymphoma in lymph node fine-needle aspiration. A critical appraisal. *Diagn Mol Pathol* 1997; **6**(3): 154–60.

39. Grosso LE, Collins BT. DNA polymerase chain reaction using fine needle aspiration biopsy smears to evaluate non-Hodgkin's lymphoma. *Acta Cytol* 1999; **43**(5): 837–41.

39a. Bogdanic M, Ostojic Kolonic S, Kaic G, Kardum Paro MM, Lasan Trcic R, Kardum-Skelin I. Fine-needle aspiration cytology yield as a basis for morphological, molecular, and cytogenetic diagnosis in alk-positive anaplastic large cell lymphoma with a typical clinical presentation. *Diagn Cytopathol.* 2016 Jul 29. doi: 10.1002/dc.23542.

40. Katz RL, Hirsch-Ginsberg C, Childs C et al. The role of gene rearrangements for antigen receptors in the diagnosis of lymphoma obtained by fine-needle aspiration. A study of 63 cases with concomitant immunophenotyping. *Am J Clin Pathol* 1991; **96**(4): 479–90.

41. Alkan S, Eltoum IA, Tabbara S et al. Usefulness of molecular detection of human herpesvirus-8 in the diagnosis of Kaposi sarcoma by fine-needle aspiration. *Am J Clin Pathol* 1999; **111**(1): 91–6.

42. Williams ME, Frierson HF, Jr., Tabbarah S, Ennis PS. Fine-needle aspiration of non-Hodgkin's lymphoma. Southern blot analysis for antigen receptor, bcl-2, and c-myc gene rearrangements. *Am J Clin Pathol* 1990; **93**(6): 754–9.

43. Stewart CJ, Farquharson MA, Kerr T, McCorriston J. Immunoglobulin light chain mRNA detected by in situ hybridisation in diagnostic fine needle aspiration cytology specimens. *J Clin Pathol* 1996; **49**(9): 749–54.

44. Stewart CJ, Duncan JA, Farquharson M, Richmond J. Fine needle aspiration cytology diagnosis of malignant lymphoma and reactive lymphoid hyperplasia. *J Clin Pathol* 1998; **51**(3): 197–203.

45. Vianello F, Tison T, Radossi P et al. Detection of B-cell monoclonality in fine needle aspiration by PCR analysis. *Leuk Lymphoma* 1998; **29**(1–2): 179–85.

46. Swerdlow SH, Campo E, Harris NL et al., eds. *WHO classification of tumors of haemotopoietic and lymphoid tissue*, 4th edn. Lyon: IARC, 2008.

47. Frederiksen JK, Sharma M, Casulo C, Burack WR. Systematic review of the effectiveness of fine-needle aspiration and/or core needle biopsy for subclassifying lymphoma. *Arch Pathol Lab Med*. 2015; **139**: 245–51; doi: 10.5858/arpa.2013-0674-RA.

48. Liliemark J, Tani E, Christensson B, Svedmyr E, Skoog L. Fine-needle aspiration cytology and immunocytochemistry of abdominal non-Hodgkin's lymphomas. *Leuk Lymphoma*. 1989; **1**(1): 65–69.

49. Sneige N, Dekmezian RH, Katz RL, et al. Morphologic and immunocytochemical evaluation of 220 fine needle aspirates of malignant lymphoma and lymphoid hyperplasia. *Acta Cytol*. 1990; **34**(3): 311–322.

50. Sneige N, Dekmezian R, el-Naggar A, Manning J. Cytomorphologic, immunocytochemical, and nucleic acid flow cytometric study of 50 lymph nodes by fine-needle aspiration: comparison with results obtained by subsequent excisional biopsy. *Cancer*. 1991; **67**(4): 1003–1007.

51. Sapia S, Sanchez Avalos JC, Monreal M, et al. Fine needle aspiration for flow cytometry immunophenotyping of non Hodgkin lymphoma. *Medicina (B Aires)*. 1995; **55**(6): 675–680.

52. Ben-Yehuda D, Polliack A, Okon E, et al. Image-guided core-needle biopsy in malignant lymphoma: experience with 100 patients that suggests the technique is reliable. *J Clin Oncol*. 1996; **14**(9): 2431–2434.

53. Hughes JH, Katz RL, Fonseca GA, Cabanillas FF. Fine-needle aspiration cytology of mediastinal non-Hodgkin's nonlymphoblastic lymphoma. *Cancer*. 1998; **84**(1): 26–35.

54. Jeffers MD, Milton J, Herriot R, McKean M. Fine needle aspiration cytology in the investigation on non-Hodgkin's lymphoma. *J Clin Pathol*. 1998; **51**(3): 189–196.

55. Young NA, Al-Saleem TI, Ehya H, Smith MR. Utilization of fine-needle aspiration cytology and flow cytometry in the diagnosis and subclassification of primary and recurrent lymphoma. *Cancer*. 1998; **84**(4): 252–261.

56. Ravinsky E, Morales C, Kutryk E, Chrobak A, Paraskevas F. Cytodiagnosis of lymphoid proliferations by fine needle aspiration biopsy: adjunctive value of flow cytometry. *Acta Cytol*. 1999; **43**(6): 1070–1078.

57. Mayall F, Dray M, Stanley D, Harrison B, Allen R. Immunoflow cytometry and cell block immunohistochemistry in the FNA diagnosis of lymphoma: a review of 73 consecutive cases. *J Clin Pathol*. 2000; **53**(6): 451–457.

58. Meda BA, Buss DH, Woodruff RD, et al. Diagnosis and subclassification of primary and recurrent lymphoma: the usefulness and limitations of combined fine-needle aspiration cytomorphology and flow cytometry. *Am J Clin Pathol*. 2000; **113**(5): 688–699.

59. Siebert JD, Weeks LM, List LW, et al. Utility of flow cytometry immunophenotyping for the diagnosis and classification of lymphoma in community hospital clinical needle aspiration/biopsies. *Arch Pathol Lab Med*. 2000; **124**(12): 1792–1799.

60. Demharter J, Muller P, Wagner T, Schlimok G, Haude K, Bohndorf K. Percutaneous core-needle biopsy of enlarged lymph nodes in the diagnosis and subclassification of malignant lymphomas. *Eur Radiol*. 2001; **11**(2): 276–283.

61. Dong HY, Harris NL, Preffer FI, Pitman MB. Fine-needle aspiration biopsy in the diagnosis and classification of primary and recurrent lymphoma: a retrospective analysis of the utility of cytomorphology and flow cytometry. *Mod Pathol*. 2001; **14**(5): 472–481.

62. Liu K, Stern RC, Rogers RT, Dodd LG, Mann KP. Diagnosis of hematopoietic processes by fine-needle aspiration in conjunction with flow cytometry: a review of 127 cases. *Diagn Cytopathol*. 2001; **24**(1): 1–10.

63. Ribeiro A, Vazquez-Sequeiros E, Wiersema LM, Wang KK, Clain JE, Wiersema MJ. EUS-guided fine-needle aspiration combined with flow cytometry and immunocytochemistry in the diagnosis of lymphoma. *Gastrointest Endosc* 2001; **53**(4): 485–491.

64. Mourad WA, Tulbah A, Shoukri M, et al. Primary diagnosis and REAL/WHO classification of non-Hodgkin's lymphoma by fine-needle aspiration: cytomorphologic and immunophenotypic approach. *Diagn Cytopathol*. 2003; **28**(4): 191–195.

65. Zeppa P, Marino G, Troncone G, et al. Fine-needle cytology and flow cytometry immunophenotyping and subclassification of non-Hodgkin lymphoma: a critical review of 307 cases with technical suggestions. *Cancer*. 2004;**102**(1): 55–65.

66. Landgren O, Porwit MacDonald A, Tani E, et al. A prospective comparison of fine-needle aspiration cytology and histopathology in the diagnosis and classification of lymphomas. *Hematol J*. 2004; **5**(1): 69–76.

67. Hehn ST, Grogan TM, Miller TP. Utility of fine-needle aspiration as a diagnostic technique in lymphoma. *J Clin Oncol*. 2004; **22**(15): 3046–3052.

68. Gong JZ, Snyder MJ, Lagoo AS, et al. Diagnostic impact of core-needle biopsy on fine-needle aspiration of non-Hodgkin lymphoma. *Diagn Cytopathol*. 2004; **31**(1): 23–30.

69. Ravinsky E, Morales C. Diagnosis of lymphoma by image-guided needle biopsies: fine needle aspiration biopsy, core biopsy or both? *Acta Cytol*. 2005; **49**(1): 51–57.

70. Li L, Wu QL, Liu LZ, et al. Value of CT-guided core-needle biopsy in diagnosis and classification of malignant lymphomas using automated biopsy gun. *World J Gastroenterol*. 2005; **11**(31): 4843–4847.

71. Dey P, Amir T, Al Jassar A, et al. Combined applications of fine needle aspiration cytology and flow cytometric immunphenotyping for diagnosis and classification of non Hodgkin lymphoma. *Cytojournal*. 2006; **3**:24.

72. Mathiot C, Decaudin D, Klijanienko J, et al. Fine-needle aspiration cytology combined with flow cytometry immunophenotyping is a rapid and accurate approach for the evaluation of suspicious superficial lymphoid lesions. *Diagn Cytopathol*. 2006; **34**(7): 472–478.

73. Venkatraman L, Catherwood MA, Patterson A, Lioe TF, McCluggage WG, Anderson NH. Role of polymerase chain reaction and immunocytochemistry in the cytological assessment of lymphoid proliferations. *J Clin Pathol*. 2006; **59**(11): 1160–1165.

74. de Kerviler E, de Bazelaire C, Mounier N, et al. Image-guided core-needle biopsy of peripheral lymph nodes allows the diagnosis of lymphomas. *Eur Radiol*. 2007; **17**(3): 843–849.

75. de Larrinoa AF, del Cura J, Zabala R, Fuertes E, Bilbao F, Lopez JI. Value of ultrasound-guided core biopsy in the diagnosis of malignant lymphoma. *J Clin Ultrasound*. 2007; **35**(6): 295–301.

76. Lachar WA, Shahab I, Saad AJ. Accuracy and cost-effectiveness of core needle biopsy in the evaluation of suspected lymphoma: a study of 101 cases. *Arch Pathol Lab Med*. 2007; **131**(7): 1033–1039.

77. Loubeyre P, McKee TA, Copercini M, Rosset A, Dietrich PY. Diagnostic precision of image-guided multisampling core needle biopsy of suspected lymphomas in a primary care hospital. *Br J Cancer*. 2009; **100**(11): 1771–1776.

78. Pfeiffer J, Kayser G, Ridder GJ. Sonography-assisted cutting needle biopsy in the head and neck for the diagnosis of lymphoma: can it replace lymph node extirpation? *Laryngoscope*. 2009; **119**(4): 689–695.

79. Huang PC, Liu CY, Chuang WY, Shih LY, Wan YL. Ultrasound-guided core needle biopsy of cervical lymphadenopathy in patients with lymphoma: the clinical efficacy and factors associated with unsuccessful diagnosis. *Ultrasound Med Biol*. 2010; **36**(9): 1431–1436.

80. Kuveždić KG, Aurer I, Ries S, et al. FNA based diagnosis of head and neck nodal lymphoma. *Coll Antropol*. 2010; **34**(1): 7–12.

81. Pedote P, Gaudio F, Moschetta M, Cimmino A, Specchia G, Angelelli G. CT-guided needle biopsy performed with modified coaxial technique in the diagnosis of malignant lymphomas. *Radiol Med*. 2010; **115**(8): 1292–1303.

82. Senjug P, Ostovic KT, Miletic Z, et al. The accuracy of fine needle aspiration cytology and flow cytometry in evaluation of nodal and extranodal sites in patients with suspicion of lymphoma. *Coll Antropol*. 2010; **34**(1): 131–137.

83. Yuan J, Li XH. Evaluation of pathological diagnosis using ultrasonography-guided lymph node core-needle biopsy. *Chin Med J (Engl)*. 2010; **123**(6): 690–694.

84. Amador-Ortiz C, Chen L, Hassan A, et al. Combined core needle biopsy and fine-needle aspiration with ancillary studies correlate highly with traditional techniques in the diagnosis of nodal-based lymphoma. *Am J Clin Pathol*. 2011; **135**(4): 516–524.

85. Burke C, Thomas R, Inglis C, et al. Ultrasound-guided core biopsy in the diagnosis of lymphoma of the head and neck: a 9 year experience. *Br J Radiol*. 2011; **84**(1004): 727–732.

86. Metzgeroth G, Schneider S, Walz C, et al. Fine needle aspiration and core needle biopsy in the diagnosis of lymphadenopathy of unknown aetiology. *Ann Hematol*. 2012; **91**(9): 1477–1484.

87. Stacchini A, Carucci P, Pacchioni D, et al. Diagnosis of deep-seated lymphomas by endoscopic ultrasound-guided fine needle aspiration combined with flow cytometry. *Cytopathology*. 2012; **23**(1): 50–56.

88. Thierauf J, Lindemann J, Bommer M et al. Value of fine needle aspiration cytology and core needle biopsy in the head and neck region. *Laryngorhinootologie. J Pathol Transl Med*. 2015; **49**(2): 136–43.

89. Volmar KE, Singh HK, Gong JZ. The advantages and limitations of the role of core needle and fine-needle aspiration biopsy of lymph nodes in the modern era. *Pathology Case Reviews*. 2007; **12**: 10–26.

90. Popescu A, Saftoiu A. Can elastography replace fine needle aspiration? *Endosc Ultrasound* 2014; **3**: 109–17.

91. Leong AS, Stevens M. Fine-needle aspiration biopsy for the diagnosis of lymphoma: a perspective. *Diagn Cytopathol* 1996; **15**(4): 352–7.

92. Pontifex AH, Haley L. Fine-needle aspiration cytology in lymphomas and related disorders. *Diagn Cytopathol* 1989; **5**(4): 432–5.

93. Layfield LJ. Fine needle aspiration cytologic findings in a case of sinus histiocytosis with massive lymphadenopathy (Rosai-Dorfman syndrome). *Acta Cytol* 1990; **34**(6): 767–70.

93a. Monaco SE, Khalbuss WE, Pantanowitz L. Benign non-infectious causes of lymphadenopathy. *Diagn Cytopathol* 2012; **40**: 925–38.

94. Gupta S, Gupta DC. Cytologic appearance of sinus histiocytosis with massive lymphadenopathy: a case report. *Acta Cytol* 1996; **40**(3): 595–8.

95. Trautman BC, Stanley MW, Goding GS, Rosai J. Sinus histiocytosis with massive lymphadenopathy (Rosai-Dorfman disease): diagnosis by fine-needle aspiration. *Diagn Cytopathol* 1991; **7**(5): 513–6.

96. Schmitt FC. Sinus histiocytosis with massive lymphadenopathy (Rosai-Dorfman disease): cytomorphologic analysis on fine-needle aspirates. *Diagn Cytopathol* 1992; **8**(6): 596–9.

97. Alvarez Alegret R, Martinez Tello A, Ramirez T et al. Sinus histiocytosis with massive lymphadenopathy (Rosai-Dorfman disease): diagnosis with fine-needle aspiration in a case with nodal and nasal involvement. *Diagn Cytopathol* 1995; **13**(4): 333–5.

98. Chang YW. Sinus histiocytosis with massive lymphadenopathy. Report of a case with fine needle aspiration cytology. *Acta Cytol* 1993; **37**(2): 186–90.

99. Stastny JF, Wilkerson ML, Hamati HF, Kornstein MJ. Cytologic features of sinus histiocytosis with massive lymphadenopathy. A report of three cases. *Acta Cytol* 1997; **41**(3): 871–6.

100. Viguer JM, Jimenez-Heffernan JA, Lopez-Ferrer P, Vicandi B. Importance of Papanicolaou-stained smears and immunocytochemistry in the diagnosis of Rosai-Dorfman disease [letter]. *Acta Cytol* 1999; **43**(2): 328–30.

101. Pettinato G, Manivel JC, d'Amore ES, Petrella G. Fine needle aspiration cytology and immunocytochemical characterization of the histiocytes in sinus histiocytosis with massive lymphadenopathy (Rosai-Dorfman syndrome). *Acta Cytol* 1990; **34**(6): 771–7.

102. Deshpande V, Verma K. Fine needle aspiration (FNAC) cytology of Rosai Dorfman disease. *Cytopathology* 1998; **9**(5): 329–35.

103. Suh KW, Park CS, Lee JT, Lee KG. Diagnosis of cervical tuberculous lymphadenitis with fine needle aspiration biopsy and cytologic examination under ultrasonographic guides. *Yonsei Med J* 1993; **34**(4): 328–33.

104. Chatterjee D, Dey P. Tuberculosis revisited: Cytological perspective. *Diagn Cytopathol.* 2014; **42**(11): 993–1001.

105. Chand P, Dogra R, Chauhan N et al. (2014). Cytopathological Pattern of Tubercular Lymphadenopathy on FNAC: Analysis of 550 Consecutive Cases. *J Clin Diagn Res* **8**(9): FC16–9.

106. Lapuerta P, Martin SE, Ellison E. Fine needle aspiration of peripheral lymph nodes in patients with tuberculosis and HIV. *Am J Clin Pathol* 1997; **107**(3): 317–20.

107. Khurana KK, Stanley MW, Powers CN, Pitman MB. Aspiration cytology of malignant neoplasms associated with granulomas and granuloma-like features. *Cancer* 1998; **84**: 84–9.

108. Donnelly A, Hendricks G, Martens S et al. Cytologic diagnosis of cat scratch disease (CSD) by fine-needle aspiration. *Diagn Cytopathol* 1995; **13**(2): 103–6.

109. Kojima M, Nakamura S, Koshikawa T et al. Imprint cytology of cat scratch disease. A report of eight cases. *Apmis* 1996; **104**(5): 389–94.

110. Silverman JF. Fine needle aspiration cytology of cat scratch disease. *Acta Cytol* 1985; **29**(4): 542–7.

111. Christ ML, Feltes-Kennedy M. Fine needle aspiration cytology of toxoplasmic lymphadenitis. *Acta Cytol* 1982; **26**(4): 425–8.

112. Macey-Dare LV, Kocjan G, Goodman JR. Acquired toxoplasmosis of a submandibular lymph node in a 9-year-old boy diagnosed by fine-needle aspiration cytology. *Int J Paediatr Dent* 1996; **6**(4): 265–9.

113. Zaharopoulos P. Demonstration of parasites in toxoplasma lymphadenitis by fine-needle aspiration cytology: report of two cases. *Diagn Cytopathol* 2000 Jan; **22**(1): 11–5.

114. al-Jitawi SA, Farraj SE, Ramahi SA. Conventional scraping versus fine needle aspiration cytology in the diagnosis of cutaneous leishmaniasis. *Acta Cytol* 1995; **39**(1): 82–4.

115. Perez-Guillermo M, Hernandez-Gil A, Bonmati C. Diagnosis of cutaneous leishmaniasis by fine needle aspiration cytology. Report of a case. *Acta Cytol* 1988; **32**(4): 485–8.

116. Tallada N, Raventos A, Martinez S et al. Leishmania lymphadenitis diagnosed by fine-needle aspiration biopsy. *Diagn Cytopathol* 1993; **9**(6): 673–6.

117. Tsang WY, Chan JK. Fine-needle aspiration cytologic diagnosis of Kikuchi's lymphadenitis. A report of 27 cases. *Am J Clin Pathol* 1994; **102**(4): 454–8.

118. Hong L, Wang X, Huang Z et al. Histiocytic necrotizing lymphadenitis diagnosed by conventional cytology and liquid based cytology. *Int J Clin Exp Pathol.* 2014 Aug 15; **7**(9): 6186–90

119. Mannara GM, Boccato P, Rinaldo A et al. Histiocytic necrotizing lymphadenitis (Kikuchi-Fujimoto disease) diagnosed by fine needle aspiration biopsy. *ORL J Otorhinolaryngol Relat Spec* 1999; **61**(6): 367–71.

120. Stanley MW, Steeper TA, Horwitz CA et al. Fine-needle aspiration of lymph nodes in patients with acute infectious mononucleosis. *Diagn Cytopathol* 1990; **6**(5): 323–9.

121. Hanks D, Bhargava V. Fine-needle aspiration diagnosis of HIV-related conditions. *Pathology (Phila)* 1996; **4**(2): 221–52.

122. Reid AJ, Miller RF, Kocjan GI. Diagnostic utility of fine needle aspiration (FNAC) cytology in HIV-infected patients with lymphadenopathy. *Cytopathology* 1998; **9**(4): 230–9.

123. Strigle SM, Rarick MU, Cosgrove MM, Martin SE. A review of the fine-needle aspiration cytology findings in human immunodeficiency virus infection. *Diagn Cytopathol* 1992; **8**(1): 41–52.

124. Ellison E, Lapuerta P, Martin SE. Fine needle aspiration (FNAC) in HIV+ patients: results from a series of 655 aspirates. *Cytopathology* 1998; **9**(4): 222–9.

125. Shapiro AL, Pincus RL. Fine-needle aspiration of diffuse cervical lymphadenopathy in patients with acquired immunodeficiency syndrome. *Otolaryngol Head Neck Surg* 1991; **105**(3): 419–21.

126. Burton F, Patete ML, Goodwin WJ, Jr. Indications for open cervical node biopsy in HIV-positive patients. *Otolaryngol Head Neck Surg* 1992; **107**(3): 367–9.

127. Nathan DL, Belsito DV. Carbamazepine-induced pseudolymphoma with CD-30 positive cells. *J Am Acad Dermatol* 1998; **38**(5 Pt 2): 806–9.

128. Abbondazo SL, Irey NS, Frizzera G. Dilantin-associated lymphadenopathy. Spectrum of histopathologic patterns. *Am J Surg Pathol* 1995; **19**(6): 675–86.

129. Meyer L, Gibbons D, Ashfaq R et al. Fine-needle aspiration findings in Castleman's disease. *Diagn Cytopathol* 1999; **21**(1): 57–60.

129a. Castleman B, Iverson L, Menendez VP. Localized mediastinal lymphnode hyperplasia resembling thymoma. *Cancer.* 1956;**9**(4):822–30.

130. Kirchgraber PR, Weaver MG, Arafah BM, Abdul-Karim FW. Fine needle aspiration cytology of Langerhans cell histiocytosis involving the thyroid. A case report. *Acta Cytol* 1994; **38**(1): 101–6.

131. Dey P, Luthra UK, Sheikh ZA. Fine needle aspiration cytology of Langerhans cell histiocytosis of the thyroid. A case report. *Acta Cytol* 1999; **43**(3): 429–31.

132. Sahoo M, Karak AK, Bhatnagar D, Bal CS. Fine-needle aspiration cytology in a case of isolated involvement of thyroid with Langerhans cell histiocytosis. *Diagn Cytopathol* 1998; **19**(1): 33–7.

133. Nagaoka S, Maruyama R, Koike M et al. Cytology of Langerhans cell histiocytosis in effusions: a case report. *Acta Cytol* 1996; **40**(3): 563–6.

134. Elsheikh T, Silverman JF, Wakely PE, Jr. et al. Fine-needle aspiration cytology of Langerhans' cell histiocytosis (eosinophilic granuloma) of bone in children. *Diagn Cytopathol* 1991; **7**(3): 261–6.

135. Shabb N, Fanning CV, Carrasco CH et al. Diagnosis of eosinophilic granuloma of bone by fine-needle aspiration with concurrent institution of therapy: a cytologic, histologic, clinical, and radiologic study of 27 cases. *Diagn Cytopathol* 1993; **9**(1): 3–12.

136. Katz RL, Silva EG, deSantos LA, Lukeman JM. Diagnosis of eosinophilic granuloma of bone by cytology, histology, and electron microscopy of transcutaneous bone-aspiration biopsy. *J Bone Joint Surg [Am]* 1980; **62**(8): 1284–90.

137. Musy JP, Ruf L, Ernerup I, Baltisser-Bielecka I. Cytopathologic diagnosis of an eosinophilic granuloma of bone by needle aspiration biopsy [letter]. *Acta Cytol* 1989; **33**(5): 683–5.

138. Yasko AW, Fanning CV, Ayala AG et al. Percutaneous techniques for the diagnosis and treatment of localized Langerhans-cell histiocytosis (eosinophilic granuloma of bone). *J Bone Joint Surg Am* 1998; **80**(2): 219–28.

139. Lee JS, Lee MC, Park CS, Juhng SW. Fine needle aspiration cytology of Langerhans cell histiocytosis confined to lymph nodes. A case report. *Acta Cytol* 1997; **41**(6): 1793–6.

140. Das DK, Nayak NC. Diagnosis of Langerhans cell histiocytosis by fine needle aspiration cytology [letter]. *Acta Cytol* 1995; **39**(6): 1260–3.

141. Van Heerde P, Maarten Egeler R. The cytology of Langerhans cell histiocytosis (histiocytosis X). *Cytopathology* 1991; **2**(3): 149–58.

142. Layfield LJ, Bhuta S. Fine-needle aspiration cytology of histiocytosis X: a case report. *Diagn Cytopathol* 1988; **4**(2): 140–3.

143. Akhtar M, Ali MA, Bakry M et al. Fine-needle aspiration biopsy of Langerhans histiocytosis (histiocytosis-X). *Diagn Cytopathol* 1993; **9**(5): 527–33.

144. Pohar-Marinsek Z, Us-Krasovec M. Cytomorphology of Langerhans cell histiocytosis. *Acta Cytol* 1996; **40**(6): 1257–64.

145. Dusenbery D, Nalesnik MA, Locker J, Swerdlow SH. Cytologic features of post-transplant lymphoproliferative disorder. *Diagn Cytopathol* 1997; **16**(6): 489–96.

146. Gattuso P, Castelli MJ, Peng Y, Reddy VB. Posttransplant lymphoproliferative disorders: a fine-needle aspiration biopsy study. *Diagn Cytopathol* 1997; **16**(5): 392–5.

147. Davey DD, Gulley ML, Walker WP, Zaleski S. Cytologic findings in posttransplant lymphoproliferative disease. *Acta Cytol* 1990; **34**(3): 304–10.

148. Reyes CV, Jensen JA, Chinoy M. Pulmonary lymphoma in cardiac transplant patients treated with OKT3 for rejection: diagnosis by fine-needle aspiration. *Diagn Cytopathol* 1995; **12**(1): 32–6.

149. Collins BT, Ramos RR, Grosso LE. Combined fine needle aspiration biopsy, and immunophenotypic and genotypic approach to posttransplantation lymphoproliferative disorders. *Acta Cytol* 1998; **42**(4): 869–74.

150. Haddad MG, Silverman JF, Joshi VV, Geisinger KR. Effusion cytology in Burkitt's lymphoma. *Diagn Cytopathol* 1995; **12**(1): 3–7.

151. Gumbs MA, Pai NB, Saraiya RJ et al. Kimura's disease: a case report and literature review. *J Surg Oncol* 1999; **70**(3): 190–3.

152. Kini U, Shariff S. Cytodiagnosis of Kimura's disease. *Indian J Pathol Microbiol* 1998; **41**(4): 473–7.

153. Jayaram G, Peh KB. Fine-needle aspiration cytology in Kimura's disease. *Diagn Cytopathol* 1995; **13**(4): 295–9.

154. Chow LT, Yuen RW, Tsui WM et al. Cytologic features of Kimura's disease in fine-needle aspirates. A study of eight cases. *Am J Clin Pathol* 1994; **102**(3): 316–21.

155. Kapoor NS, O'Neill JP, Katabi N et al. Kimura disease: diagnostic challenges and clinical management. *Am J Otolaryngol* 2012; **33**(2): 259–62.

156. Harris NL, Jaffe ES, Diebold J et al. The World Health Organization classification of neoplastic diseases of the haematopoietic and lymphoid tissues: Report of the Clinical Advisory Committee Meeting, Airlie House, Virginia, November 1997. *Histopathology* 2000 Jan; **36**(1): 69–86.

156a. de Leval L, Gaulard P. Tricky and terrible T-cell tumors: these are thrilling times for testing: molecular pathology of peripheral T-cell lymphomas. *Hematology Am Soc Hematol Educ Program* 2011; 2011: 336–43.

157. Grosso LE, Collins BT, Dunphy CH, Ramos RR. Lymphocyte-depleted Hodgkin's disease: diagnostic challenges by fine-needle aspiration. *Diagn Cytopathol* 1998; **19**(1): 66–9.

158. Das DK, Gupta SK. Fine needle aspiration cytodiagnosis of Hodgkin's disease and its subtypes. II. Subtyping by differential cell counts. *Acta Cytol* 1990; **34**(3): 337–41.

159. Stanley MW, Powers CN. Syncytial variant of nodular sclerosing Hodgkin's disease: fine-needle aspiration findings in two cases. *Diagn Cytopathol* 1997; **17**(6): 477–9.

160. Das DK, Francis IM, Sharma PN et al. Hodgkin's lymphoma: diagnostic difficulties in fine-needle aspiration cytology. *Diagn Cytopathol* 2009; **37**(8): 564–73.

161. Kardos TF, Vinson JH, Behm FG et al. Hodgkin's disease: diagnosis by fine-needle aspiration biopsy. Analysis of cytologic criteria from a selected series. *Am J Clin Pathol* 1986; **86**(3): 286–91.

162. Das DK, Gupta SK, Datta BN, Sharma SC. Fine needle aspiration cytodiagnosis of Hodgkin's disease and its subtypes. I. Scope and limitations. *Acta Cytol* 1990; **34**(3): 329–36.

163. Daskalopoulou D, Tamiolakis D, Tsousis S et al. Sources of discrepancies in the diagnosis of Hodgkin's disease by fine needle aspiration. *Arch Anat Cytol Pathol* 1996; **44**(4): 166–73.

164. Fulciniti F, Vetrani A, Zeppa P et al. Hodgkin's disease: diagnostic accuracy of fine needle aspiration; a report based on 62 consecutive cases. *Cytopathology* 1994; **5**(4): 226–33.

165. Krasne DL, Naritoku WY, Cosgrove MM. Diagnosis of syncytial (lacunar cell-predominant) nodular sclerosing Hodgkin's disease by fine needle aspiration. A case report. *Acta Cytol* 1993; **37**(3): 418–22.

166. Spina M, Sandri S, Tirelli U. Hodgkin's disease in HIV-infected individuals. *Curr Opin Oncol* 1999; **11**(6): 522–6.

167. Stephen MR, Mallon EA. An unusual presentation of fine needle aspiration (FNAC) cytology from the syncytial variant of nodular sclerosing Hodgkin's disease. *Cytopathology* 1998; **9**(4): 271–6.

168. Boudjerra N, Hamladji R, Abdennebi A, Colonna P. Value and limits of fine needle aspiration biopsy in Hodgkin disease. Usefulness in developing countries. *Bull Cancer* 1993; **80**(4): 339–44.

169. Young NA, Al-Saleem T. Diagnosis of lymphoma by fine-needle aspiration cytology using the revised European-American classification of lymphoid neoplasms. *Cancer* 1999; **87**(6): 325–45.

170. Simpson JL, Moriarty AT, Earls J et al. Hodgkin's disease variant of Richter's syndrome. Report of a case with diagnosis by fine needle biopsy. *Acta Cytol* 1997; **41**(3): 823–9.

171. Tani E, Ersoz C, Svedmyr E, Skoog L. Fine-needle aspiration cytology and immunocytochemistry of Hodgkin's disease, suppurative type. *Diagn Cytopathol* 1998; **18**(6): 437–40.

172. Fulciniti F, Zeppa P, Vetrani A et al. Hodgkin's disease mimicking suppurative lymphadenitis: a possible pitfall in fine-needle aspiration biopsy cytology. *Diagn Cytopathol* 1989; **5**(3): 282–5.

173. Vicandi B, Jimenez-Heffernan JA, Lopez-Ferrer P et al. Hodgkin's disease mimicking suppurative lymphadenitis: a fine-needle aspiration report of five cases. *Diagn Cytopathol* 1999; **20**(5): 302–6.

174. Wakely PE, Jr. Fine-needle aspiration cytopathology in diagnosis and classification of malignant lymphoma: accurate and reliable? *Diagn Cytopathol* 2000 Feb; **22**(2): 120–5.

175. Jaffe ES, Harris NL, Diebold J, Muller-Hermelink HK. World Health Organization classification of neoplastic diseases of the hematopoietic and lymphoid tissues. A progress report. *Am J Clin Pathol* 1999; **111**(1 Suppl 1): S8–12.

176. Suhrland MJ, Wieczorek R. Fine needle aspiration biopsy in the diagnosis of lymphoma. *Cancer Invest* 1991; **9**(1): 61–8.

177. Carrasco CH, Richli WR, Lawrence D et al. Fine needle aspiration biopsy in lymphoma. *Radiol Clin North Am* 1990; **28**(4): 879–83.

178. Akhtar M, Ali MA, Haider A et al. Fine-needle aspiration biopsy of Ki-1-positive anaplastic large-cell lymphoma. *Diagn Cytopathol* 1992; **8**(3): 242–7.

179. Cartagena N, Jr., Katz RL, Hirsch-Ginsberg C et al. Accuracy of diagnosis of malignant lymphoma by combining fine-needle aspiration cytomorphology with immunocytochemistry and in selected cases, Southern blotting of aspirated cells: a tissue-controlled study of 86 patients. *Diagn Cytopathol* 1992; **8**(5): 456–64.

180. Cafferty LL, Katz RL, Ordonez NG et al. Fine needle aspiration diagnosis of intraabdominal and retroperitoneal lymphomas by a morphologic and immunocytochemical approach. *Cancer* 1990; **65**(1): 72–7.

181. Carter TR, Feldman PS, Innes DJ, Jr. et al. The role of fine needle aspiration cytology in the diagnosis of lymphoma [published erratum appears in Acta Cytol 1989 Nov-Dec;33(6):951]. *Acta Cytol* 1988; **32**(6): 848–53.

182. Das DK, Gupta SK, Pathak IC et al. Burkitt-type lymphoma. Diagnosis by fine needle aspiration cytology. *Acta Cytol* 1987; **31**(1): 1–7.

183. Daskalopoulou D, Harhalakis N, Maouni N, Markidou SG. Fine needle aspiration cytology of non-Hodgkin's lymphomas. A morphologic and immunophenotypic study. *Acta Cytol* 1995; **39**(2): 180–6.

184. Gagneten D, Hijazi YM, Jaffe ES, Solomon D. Mantle cell lymphoma: a cytopathological and immunocytochemical study. *Diagn Cytopathol* 1996; **14**(1): 32–7.

185. Jacobs JC, Katz RL, Shabb N et al. Fine needle aspiration of lymphoblastic lymphoma. A multiparameter diagnostic approach. *Acta Cytol* 1992; **36**(6): 887–94.

186. Kardos TF, Sprague RI, Wakely PE, Jr., Frable WJ. Fine-needle aspiration biopsy of lymphoblastic lymphoma and leukemia. A clinical, cytologic, and immunologic study. *Cancer* 1987; **60**(10): 2448–53.

187. Katz RL, Gritsman A, Cabanillas F et al. Fine-needle aspiration cytology of peripheral T-cell lymphoma. A cytologic, immunologic, and cytometric study. *Am J Clin Pathol* 1989; **91**(2): 120–31.

188. Matsushima AY, Hamele-Bena D, Osborne BM. Fine-needle aspiration biopsy findings in marginal zone B-cell lymphoma. *Diagn Cytopathol* 1999; **20**(4): 190–8.

188a. B. Streubel, I. Simonitsch-Klupp, L. Müllauer et al., "Variable frequencies of MALT lymphoma-associated genetic aberrations in MALT lymphomas of different sites," *Leukemia*, vol. 18, no. 10, pp. 1722–1726, 2004.

188b. Troppan K, Wenzl K, Neumeister P, Deutsch A. Molecular Pathogenesis of MALT Lymphoma. *Gastroenterol Res Pract* 2015; 2015: 102656. doi: 10.1155/2015/102656. Epub 2015 Apr 1.

189. Sneige N, Dekmezian R, el-Naggar A, Manning J. Cytomorphologic, immunocytochemical, and nucleic acid flow cytometric study of 50 lymph nodes by fine-needle aspiration. Comparison with results obtained by subsequent excisional biopsy. *Cancer* 1991; **67**(4): 1003–7.

190. Stastny JF, Almeida MM, Wakely PE, Jr. et al. Fine-needle aspiration biopsy and imprint cytology of small non-cleaved cell (Burkitt's) lymphoma. *Diagn Cytopathol* 1995; **12**(3): 201–7.

191. Tani E, Liliemark J, Svedmyr E et al. Cytomorphology and immunocytochemistry of fine needle aspirates from blastic non-Hodgkin's lymphomas. *Acta Cytol* 1989; **33**(3): 363–71.

192. Tarantino DR, McHenry CR, Strickland T, Khiyami A. The role of fine-needle aspiration biopsy and flow cytometry in the evaluation of persistent neck adenopathy. *Am J Surg* 1998; **176**(5): 413–7.

193. Wakely PE, Jr., Kornstein MJ. Aspiration cytopathology of lymphoblastic lymphoma and leukemia: the MCV experience. *Pediatr Pathol Lab Med* 1996; **16**(2): 243–52.

194. Wojcik EM, Katz RL, Fanning TV et al. Diagnosis of mantle cell lymphoma on tissue acquired by fine needle aspiration in conjunction with immunocytochemistry and cytokinetic studies. Possibilities and limitations. *Acta Cytol* 1995; **39**(5): 909–15.

195. Young NA, Al-Saleem TI, Ehya H, Smith MR. Utilization of fine-needle aspiration cytology and flow cytometry in the diagnosis and subclassification of primary and recurrent lymphoma. *Cancer* 1998; **84**(4): 252–61.

196. Liliemark J, Tani E, Mellstedt H, Skoog L. Fine-needle aspiration cytology and immunocytochemistry of malignant non-Hodgkin's lymphoma in the oral cavity. *Oral Surg Oral Med Oral Pathol* 1989; **68**(5): 599–603.

197.   Galindo LM, Havlioglu N, Grosso LE. Cytologic findings in a case of T-cell rich B-cell lymphoma: potential diagnostic pitfall in FNAC of lymph nodes. *Diagn Cytopathol* 1996; **14**(3): 253–7; discussion 257–8.

197a. Ogasawara Y, Machishima T, Shimada T, Takahashi H, Fukunaga M, Mizoroki F, Dobashi N, Usui N, Aiba K. [Human herpesvirus 8-negative primary effusion lymphoma-like lymphoma with t(8;14)(q24;q32)]. *Rinsho Ketsueki* 2015 Aug; **56**(8): 1082–8.

198.   Katz RL, Caraway NP. FNAC lymphoproliferative diseases: myths and legends. *Diagn Cytopathol* 1995; **12**(2): 99–100.

199.   Katz RL. Controversy in fine-needle aspiration of lymph nodes. A territorial imperative? [editorial]. *Am J Clin Pathol* 1997; **108**(4 Suppl 1): S3–5.

200.   Rassidakis GZ, Tani E, Svedmyr E et al. Diagnosis and subclassification of follicle center and mantle cell lymphomas on fine-needle aspirates: A cytologic and immunocytochemical approach based on the Revised European-American Lymphoma (REAL) classification. *Cancer* 1999; **87**(4): 216–23.

201.   Wakely PE, Jr. Fine needle aspiration cytopathology of malignant lymphoma. *Clin Lab Med* 1998; **18**(3): 541–59, vi-vii.

202.   Wakely PE, Jr. Aspiration cytopathology of malignant lymphoma: coming of age [editorial; comment]. *Cancer* 1999; **87**(6): 322–4.

203.   Boyd C, Boyle DP. Molecular diagnosis on tissues and cells: how it affects training and will affect practice in the future. *Cytopathology* 2012; **23**(5): 286–94.

204.   Dey P. Role of ancillary techniques in diagnosing and subclassifying non-Hodgkin's lymphomas on fine needle aspiration cytology. *Cytopathology* 2006; **17**(5): 275–87.

205.   Stewart CJ, Jackson R, Farquharson M, Richmond J. Fine-needle aspiration cytology of extranodal lymphoma. *Diagn Cytopathol* 1998; **19**(4): 260–6.

206.   Sapia S, Sanchez Avalos JC, Monreal M et al. Fine needle aspiration for flow cytometry immunophenotyping of non Hodgkin lymphoma. *Medicina (B Aires)* 1995; **55**(6): 675–80.

207.   Zander DS, Iturraspe JA, Everett ET et al. Flow cytometry. *In vitro* assessment of its potential application for diagnosis and classification of lymphoid processes in cytologic preparations from fine-needle aspirates. *Am J Clin Pathol* 1994; **101**(5): 577–86.

208.   Schmid S, Tinguely M, Cione P et al. Flow cytometry as an accurate tool to complement fine needle aspiration cytology in the diagnosis of low grade malignant lymphomas. *Cytopathology* 2011; **22**(6): 397–406.

209.   Senjug P, Ostovic KT, Miletic Z et al. The accuracy of fine needle aspiration cytology and flow cytometry in evaluation of nodal and extranodal sites in patients with suspicion of lymphoma. *Coll Antropol* 2010; **34**(1): 131–7.

210.   Stacchini A, D Pacchioni, Demurtas A et al. Utility of flow cytometry as ancillary study to improve the cytologic diagnosis of thyroid lymphomas. *Cytometry B Clin Cytom.* 2014; **88**(5): 320–9.

211.   Mochizuki H, Nakamura K, Sato H et al. Multiplex PCR and Genescan analysis to detect immunoglobulin heavy chain gene rearrangement in feline B-cell neoplasms. *Vet Immunol Immunopathol* 2011; **143**(1–2): 38–45.

212.   Bode B, Tinguely M. Role of cytology in hematopathological diagnostics. *Pathologe* 2012; **33**(4): 316–23.

213.   Muller-Hermelink HK. Worldwide consensus: the way from the KIEL classification to the REAL classification to the WHO classification. *Verh Dtsch Ges Pathol* 1999; **83**: 155–61.

214.   Chan JK, Banks PM, Cleary ML et al. A proposal for classification of lymphoid neoplasms (by the International Lymphoma Study Group). *Histopathology* 1994; **25**(6): 517–36.

215.   Harris NL, Jaffe ES, Diebold J et al. Lymphoma classification--from controversy to consensus: The R.E.A.L. and WHO Classification of lymphoid neoplasms. *Ann Oncol* 2000; **11**(Suppl 1): 3–10.

216.   Siebert JD, Mulvaney DA, Potter KL et al. Relative frequencies and sites of presentation of lymphoid neoplasms in a community hospital according to the revised European-American classification. *Am J Clin Pathol* 1999; **111**(3): 379–86.

217.   Harris NL. Principles of the revised European-American Lymphoma Classification (from the International Lymphoma Study Group). *Ann Oncol* 1997; **8**(Suppl 2): 11–6.

218.   Harris NL, Jaffe ES, Diebold J et al. World Health Organization classification of neoplastic diseases of the hematopoietic and lymphoid tissues: report of the Clinical Advisory Committee Meeting, Airlie House, Virginia, November 1997. *J Neurooncol* 1999; **43**(3): 203–8.

219.   Young NA, Al-Saleem T. Hematopathologists and cytopathologists: enemies or allies? [editorial]. *Diagn Cytopathol* 1999; **21**(5): 305–6.

220.   De Leval L, Harris NL. Variability in immunophenotype in diffuse large B-cell lymphoma and its clinical relevance. *Histopathology* 2003; **43**: 509–28.

221.   Quintanilla-Fend L. *Hematopathology: LC14–1 SMALL B-CELL lymphomas. diagnosis of malignant lymphomas in 2014.* (IAP 2014 Abstracts).

222.   Wotherspoon A. Immunocytochemistry of low grade B-cell lymphomas. *CPD Bulletin Cellular Pathology* 1999;**1**: 158–61.

223.   Zhang YH, Liu J, Dawlett M et al. The role of SOX11 immunostaining in confirming the diagnosis of mantle cell lymphoma on fine-needle aspiration samples. *Cancer Cytopathol.* 2014; **122**(12): 892–7.

224.   Tworek JA, Singleton TP, Schnitzer B et al. Flow cytometric and immunohisto-chemical analysis of small lymphocytic lymphoma, mantle cell lymphoma, and plasmacytoid small lymphocytic lymphoma. *Am J Clin Pathol* 1998; **110**(5): 582–9.

225.   Kuruvilla S, Gomathy DV, Shanthi AV et al. Primary pulmonary lymphoma. Report of a case diagnosed by fine needle aspiration cytology. *Acta Cytol* 1994; **38**(4): 601–4.

226.   Campo E, Raffeld M, Jaffe ES. Mantle-cell lymphoma. *Semin Hematol* 1999; **36**(2): 115–27.

227.   Hughes JH, Caraway NP, Katz RL. Blastic variant of mantle-cell lymphoma: cytomorphologic, immunocytochemical, and molecular genetic features of tissue obtained by fine-needle aspiration biopsy. *Diagn Cytopathol* 1998; **19**(1): 59–62.

228.   Suh YK, Shabaik A, Meurer WT, Shin SS. Lymphoid cell aggregates: a useful clue in the fine-needle aspiration diagnosis of follicular lymphomas. *Diagn Cytopathol* 1997; **17**(6): 467–71.

229.   McNeely TB. Diagnosis of follicular lymphoma by fine needle aspiration biopsy. *Acta Cytol* 1992; **36**(6): 866–8.

230.   Raible MD, Hsi ED, Alkan S. Bcl-6 protein expression by follicle center lymphomas. A marker for differentiating follicle center lymphomas from other low-grade lymphoproliferative disorders. *Am J Clin Pathol* 1999; **112**(1): 101–7.

231.   Stoos-Veic T, Livun A, Ajdukovic R et al. Detection of t(14;18) by PCR of IgH/BCL2 fusion gene in follicular lymphoma from archived cytological smears. *Coll Antropol* 2010; **34**(2): 425–9.

232.   Allen EA, Ali SZ, Mathew S. Lymphoid lesions of the parotid. *Diagn Cytopathol* 1999; **21**(3): 170–3.

233.   MacCallum PL, Lampe HB, Cramer H, Matthews TW. Fine-needle aspiration cytology of lymphoid lesions of the salivary gland: a review of 35 cases. *J Otolaryngol* 1996; **25**(5): 300–4.

234.   Cha I, Long SR, Ljung BM, Miller TR. Low-grade lymphoma of mucosa-associated tissue in the parotid gland: a case report of fine-needle aspiration cytology diagnosis using flow cytometric immunophenotyping. *Diagn Cytopathol* 1997; **16**(4): 345–9.

235.   Pileri SA. *Diffuse Large B-cell Lymphoma (DLBCL): Still a Pandora's box?* (IAP 2014 Abstracts LC14–1).

235a. Scott DW. Cell-of-Origin in Diffuse Large B-Cell Lymphoma: Are the Assays Ready for the Clinic? *Am Soc Clin Oncol Educ Book* 2015:e458-66. doi:10.14694/EdBook_AM.2015.35.e458.

235b. Xue X, Zeng N, Gao Z, Du MQ. Diffuse large B-cell lymphoma: sub-classification by massive parallel quantitative RT-PCR. *Lab Invest* 2015 Jan; **95**(1): 113–20. doi:10.1038/labinvest.2014.136. Epub 2014 Nov 24.

235c. Jørgensen LK, Poulsen MØ, Laursen MB, Marques SC, Johnsen HE, Bøgsted M, Dybkær K. MicroRNAs as novel biomarkers in diffuse large B-cell lymphoma–a systematic review. *Dan Med J* 2015 May; **62**(5).

235d. Hans CP, Weisenburger DD, Greiner TC, et al. Confirmation of the molecular classification of diffuse large B-cell lymphoma by immunohistochemistry using a tissue microarray. *Blood* 2004; **103**: 275-282.

236.   Hughes JH, Katz RL, Fonseca GA, Cabanillas FF. Fine-needle aspiration cytology of mediastinal non-Hodgkin's nonlymphoblastic lymphoma. *Cancer* 1998; **84**(1): 26–35.

237.   Yu GH, Shin HJ, Santos-Ocampo R, Katz RL. Fine-needle aspiration of a case of non-Hodgkin's lymphoma containing signet ring cells [letter]. *Diagn Cytopathol* 1995; **13**(2): 183–5.

238.   Tanaka S, Katano H, Tsukamoto K et al. HHV8-negative primary effusion lymphoma of the peritoneal cavity presenting with a distinct immunohistochemical phenotype. *Pathol Int* 2001; **51**(4): 293–300.

239.   Ascoli V, Sirianni MC, Mezzaroma I et al. Human herpesvirus-8 in lymphomatous and nonlymphomatous body cavity effusions developing in Kaposi's sarcoma and multicentric Castleman's disease. *Ann Diagn Pathol* 1999; **3**(6): 357–63.

240.   Lobo C, Amin S, Ramsay A et al. Serous fluid cytology of multicentric Castleman's disease and other lymphoproliferative disorders associated with Kaposi sarcoma-associated herpes virus: a review with case reports. *Cytopathology* 2012; **23**(2): 76–85.

241.   Ely SA, Powers J, Lewis D et al. Kaposi's sarcoma-associated herpesvirus-positive primary effusion lymphoma arising in the subarachnoid space. *Hum Pathol* 1999; **30**(8): 981–4.

242.   Park IA, Kim CW. FNAC of malignant lymphoma in an area with a high incidence of T-cell lymphoma. Correlation of accuracy of cytologic diagnosis with histologic subtype and immunophenotype. *Acta Cytol* 1999; **43**(6): 1059–69.

243. Tan LH, Tan SY, Tang T et al. Relationship between atypical T- and B-cell size predicts survival in peripheral T-cell lymphomas with large B-cells. *Pathology* 2013; **45**(1): 28–37.

244. Laforga JB, Chorda D, Sevilla F. Intramammary lymph node involvement by mycosis fungoides diagnosed by fine-needle aspiration biopsy. *Diagn Cytopathol* 1998; **19**(2): 124–6.

245. Ludwig RA, Balachandran I. Mycosis fungoides. The importance of pulmonary cytology in the diagnosis of a case with systemic involvement. *Acta Cytol* 1983; **27**(2): 198–201.

246. Rosen SE, Koprowska I, Vonderheid EC. Skin imprint cytology in the diagnosis of cutaneous T-cell lymphomas. A preliminary report. *Acta Cytol* 1982; **26**(6): 819–22.

247. Rosen SE, Vonderheid EC, Koprowska I. Mycosis fungoides with pulmonary involvement. Cytopathologic findings. *Acta Cytol* 1984; **28**(1): 51–7.

248. Oshima K, Tani E, Masuda Y et al. Fine needle aspiration cytology of high grade T-cell lymphomas in human T-lymphotropic virus type 1 carriers. *Cytopathology* 1992; **3**(6): 365–72.

249. Pileri A, Bacci F, Neri I et al. Persistent agmination of lymphomatoid papulosis: an ongoing debate. *Dermatology* 2012; **225**(2): 131–4.

250. Jayaram G, Abdul Rahman N. Cytology of Ki-1-positive anaplastic large cell lymphoma. A report of two cases. *Acta Cytol* 1997; **41**(4 Suppl): 1253–60.

251. Sgrignoli A, Abati A. Cytologic diagnosis of anaplastic large cell lymphoma. *Acta Cytol* 1997; **41**(4): 1048–52.

252. McCluggage WG, Anderson N, Herron B, Caughley L. Fine needle aspiration cytology, histology and immunohistochemistry of anaplastic large cell Ki-1-positive lymphoma. A report of three cases. *Acta Cytol* 1996; **40**(4): 779–85.

253. Vij M, Dhir B, Verma R et al. Cytomorphology of ALK+ anaplastic large cell lymphoma displaying spindle cells mimicking a sarcomatous tumor: report of a case. *Diagn Cytopathol* 2011; **39**(10): 775–9.

254. Zakowski MF, Feiner H, Finfer M et al. Cytology of extranodal Ki-1 anaplastic large cell lymphoma. *Diagn Cytopathol* 1996; **14**(2): 155–61.

255. Wellmann A, Otsuki T, Vogelbruch M et al. Analysis of the t(2;5)(p23;q35) translocation by reverse transcription-polymerase chain reaction in CD30+ anaplastic large-cell lymphomas, in other non-Hodgkin's lymphomas of T-cell phenotype, and in Hodgkin's disease. *Blood* 1995; **86**(6): 2321–8.

256. Rapkiewicz A, Wen H, Sen F, Das K. Cytomorphologic examination of anaplastic large cell lymphoma by fine-needle aspiration cytology. *Cancer* 2007; **111**(6): 499–507.

257. Katano H, Suda T, Morishita Y et al. Human herpesvirus 8-associated solid lymphomas that occur in AIDS patients take anaplastic large cell morphology. *Mod Pathol* 2000 Jan; **13**(1): 77–85.

258. Jimenez-Heffernan JA, Viguer JM, Vicandi B et al. Posttransplant CD30 (Ki-1)-positive anaplastic large cell lymphoma. Report of a case with presentation as a pleural effusion. *Acta Cytol* 1997; **41**(5): 1519–24.

259. Das DK, Chowdhury V, Kishore B. CD-30(Ki-1)-positive anaplastic large cell lymphoma in a pleural effusion. A case report with diagnosis by cytomorphologic and immunocytochemical studies. *Acta Cytol* 1999; **43**(3): 498–502.

260. Liu K, Dodd LG, Osborne BM et al. Diagnosis of anaplastic large-cell lymphoma, including multifocal osseous KI-1 lymphoma, by fine-needle aspiration biopsy. *Diagn Cytopathol* 1999; **21**(3): 174–9.

261. Bizjak-Schwarzbartl M. Large cell anaplastic Ki-1+ non-Hodgkin's lymphoma vs. Hodgkin's disease in fine needle aspiration biopsy samples. *Acta Cytol* 1997; **41**(2): 351–6.

262. Aljajeh IA, Das DK, Krajci D. Ki-1-positive anaplastic large cell lymphoma initially diagnosed as Hodgkin's disease by fine needle aspiration (FNAC) cytology. *Cytopathology* 1995; **6**(4): 226–35.

263. Yazdi HM, Burns BF. Fine needle aspiration biopsy of Ki-1-positive large-cell 'anaplastic' lymphoma. *Acta Cytol* 1991; **35**(3): 306–10.

263a. Bogdanic M, Ostojic Kolonic S, Kaic G, Kardum Paro MM, Lasan Trcic R, Kardum-Skelin I. Fine-needle aspiration cytology yield as a basis for morphological, molecular, and cytogenetic diagnosis in alk-positive anaplastic large cell lymphoma with atypical clinical presentation. *Diagn Cytopathol.* 2017; **45**(1): 51–54.

264. Pepper C, Pai I, Hay A et al. Investigation strategy in the management of metastatic adenocarcinoma of unknown primary presenting as cervical lymphadenopathy. *Acta Otolaryngol* 2014; **134**(8): 838–42.

265. Liu YJ, Lee YT, Hsieh SW, Kuo SH. Presumption of primary sites of neck lymph node metastases on fine needle aspiration cytology. *Acta Cytol* 1997; **41**(5): 1477–82.

266. Torres MR, Nobrega Neto SH, Rosas RJ et al. Thyroglobulin in the washout fluid. *Thyroid* 2014: **24**: 7–18.

267. Smith DF, Maleki Z, Coughlan D et al. Human papillomavirus status of head and neck cancer as determined in cytologic specimens using the hybrid-capture 2 assay. *Oral Oncol.* 2014; **50**(6): 600–4.

267a. Hakima L, Adler E, Prystowsky M et al. Hybrid Capture 2 human papillomavirus testing of fine needle aspiration cytology of head and neck squamous cell carcinomas. *Diagn Cytopathol.* 2015; **43**(9): 683–7.

267b. Roy-Chowdhuri S, Krishnamurthy S. The role of cytology in the era of HPV-related head and neck carcinoma. *Semin Diagn Pathol.* 2015; **32**(4): 250–7.

268. Caraway NP, Wojcik EM, Saboorian HM, Katz RL. Concomitant lymphoma and metastatic carcinoma in a lymph node: diagnosis by fine-needle aspiration biopsy in two cases. *Diagn Cytopathol* 1997; **17**(4): 287–91.

CHAPTER 5

Miscellaneous lesions of the head and neck

Chapter contents

5.1 Introduction, 176
5.2 Benign soft tissue lesions, 176
    5.2.1 Lipoma, 176
    5.2.2 Fibromatosis colli, 176
    5.2.3 Nodular fasciitis, 178
    5.2.4 Proliferative fasciitis and proliferative myositis, 178
    5.2.5 Benign nerve sheath tumour (neurilemmoma, schwannoma), 180
5.3 Cysts of the head and neck, 181
    5.3.1 Thyroglossal cysts, 181
    5.3.2 Branchial cyst, 181
    5.3.3 Mucous retention cyst, 182
    5.3.4 Intraosseous cysts and other lesions, 183
    5.3.5 Rare cysts and differential diagnosis of cystic lesions of the head and neck, 183

5.4 Small round cell tumours, 184
    5.4.1 Rhabdomyosarcoma, 185
    5.4.2 Ewing's sarcoma/peripheral neuroectodermal tumour/Askin tumour, 186
    5.4.3 Olfactory neuroblastoma, 187
    5.4.4 Lymphoma, 187
5.5 Locally arising miscellaneous tumours, 189
    5.5.1 Carotid body tumours, 189
    5.5.2 Epithelioid sarcoma-like hemangioendothelioma, 190
    5.5.3 Meningioma, 190
    5.5.4 Ethmoid sinus intestinal type adenocarcinoma, 191
    5.5.5 Granular cell tumour, 192
References, 195

5.1 Introduction

In addition to having specific pathology, head and neck swellings are often a presenting site for more general conditions. In this chapter, we describe pathological and clinical entities encountered in our own practice. As a result, this is not a comprehensive account of all conditions that can be seen in the head and neck, but a selection of clinical cases that illustrate different lesions and groups of lesions.

5.2 Benign soft tissue lesions

5.2.1 Lipoma

Cytological diagnosis of lipoma is one of exclusion. Patients usually present with a soft mobile swelling that has been present for some time and usually does not cause any concern to the patient. Referral for imaging and FNAC is mainly in order to exclude other pathology (Figs 5.1–5.4).

[See BOX 5.1. Summary of ultrasound features: Lipoma on www.wiley.com/go/kocjan/clinical_cytopathology_head_neck2e]

Cytological features: Cytological features of lipoma include sparse microbiopsy fragments of adipose tissue composed of meshwork of delicate capillaries surrounding aggregates of fat cells (Fig. 5.5A). These are univacuolated with nuclei that are small

and inconspicuous. There are often bare nuclei in the background. Capillary endothelium may be seen sometimes. Depending on the type of lipoma, cellular components may be varied, for example, *hybernoma* (Fig. 5.5B), *angiolipoma* or *intramuscular lipoma*. The cytomorphology of *spindle-cell lipoma* (Fig. 5.5C) is often distinct, although proportions of different elements vary from case to case and can sometimes be misleading [1]. The smears contain fat fragments mixed with fascicles of uniform spindle cells with elongated, uniform nuclei and collagen fibres, often in a myxoid background matrix [2]. The characteristic finding of *pleomorphic lipoma* is the presence of floret cells: multinucleated giant cells with hyperchromatic nuclei and a moderate amount of cytoplasm. Since it is not possible to distinguish adipose tissue from a lipoma on FNAC, the diagnosis is made according to clinical circumstances [3]. Provided the FNAC is representative, the diagnosis is made by exclusion of other significant pathology. In atypical lipomatous tumour there are large cells with abundant cytoplasm and hyperchromatic, irregular nuclei, singly and in clusters. Atypical lypomatous tumour may be impossible to distinguish from well differentiated liposarcoma [4].

5.2.2 Fibromatosis colli

Fibromatoses form a spectrum of clinicopathological entities characterised by the infiltrative proliferation of fibroblasts that lack malignant cytological features. Fibromatoses present as nodular soft tissue masses almost anywhere in the body including the

Cytopathology of the Head and Neck: Ultrasound Guided FNAC, Second Edition. Gabrijela Kocjan.
© 2017 John Wiley & Sons Ltd. Published 2017 by John Wiley & Sons Ltd.
Companion website: www.wiley.com/go/kocjan/clinical_cytopathology_head_neck2e

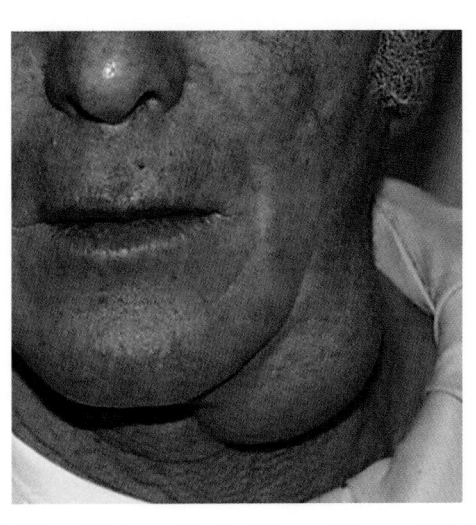

Figure 5.1 Submandibular swelling in a 70-year old man: soft, fluctuant, present for several years and slow growing. Patient was referred to the FNAC clinic where lipoma was confirmed.

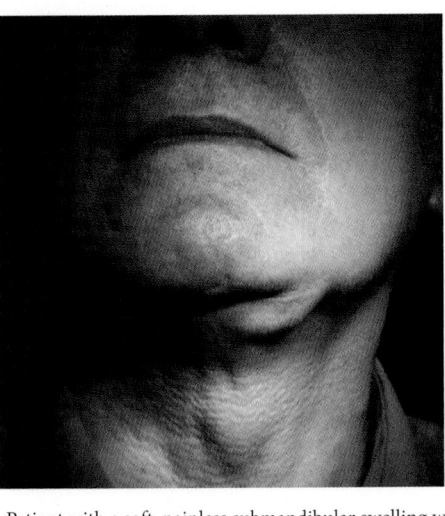

Figure 5.3 Patient with a soft, painless submandibular swelling which was noticed after losing some weight. Clinically, it was thought to be an enlarged submental lymph node. FNAC showed adipose tissue only, consistent with lipoma.

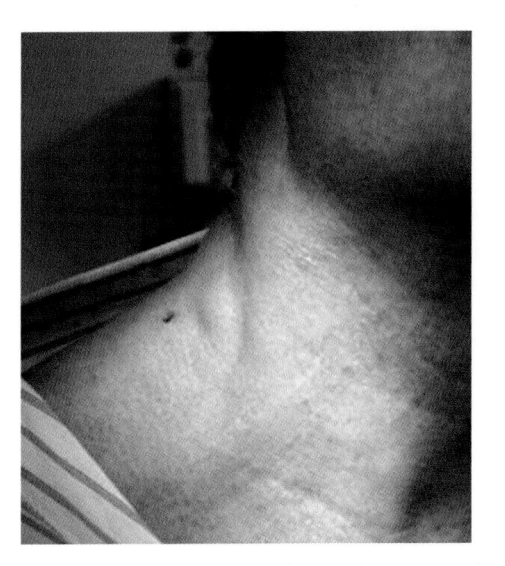

Figure 5.2 Patient with a clinical history of tuberculosis presented with a soft swelling in the posterior triangle, which was thought to be a lymph node. FNAC revealed adipose tissue only, consistent with a lipoma.

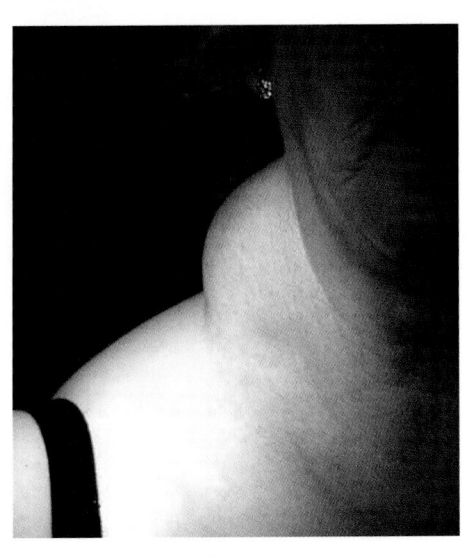
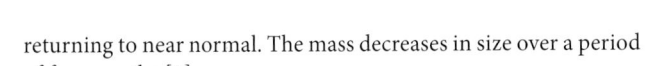

Figure 5.4 Elderly patient with diffuse unilateral soft swelling in the supraclavicular fossa. She was referred for FNAC to exclude lymphadenopathy. FNAC yielded fatty material consistent with a lipoma.

shoulder and the sternocleidomastoid muscle (Fibromatosis colli). Clinical presentation may be of a rapidly growing mass. *Fibromatosis colli* or sternocleidomastoid tumour is a rare cause of benign neck mass in infants. It is a self-limiting fibroblastic lesion usually presenting with torticollis and a history of birth trauma. It mostly appears at 2–4 weeks of age. It is one of the few causes in which FNAC is indicated in a neonate to confirm the diagnosis and to differentiate it from other congenital, inflammatory and neoplastic causes such as branchial cyst, thyroglossal cyst, inflammatory lesions like tuberculous lymphadenitis and neoplastic conditions that could be benign (haemangioma, cystic hygroma) or malignant (neuroblastoma, rhabdomyosarcoma and lymphoma). The condition is generally self-limited. A conservative management in the form of physiotherapy causes swelling to decrease in size after a few weeks, with the neck movements

returning to near normal. The mass decreases in size over a period of few months [5].

Cytological features: FNAC of fibromatosis colli consist of groups of loosely cohesive, bland-appearing, spindle-shaped proliferating fibroblasts with oval to elongated nuclei and cytoplasmic tags. Individual spindle cells and rare inflammatory cells are also present [6].

The aspirate may also contain degenerating skeletal muscle cells including muscle giant cells. A double population of bland spindle cells and muscle giant cells with nuclei showing prominent nucleoli make cause a pitfall in diagnosis by misinterpreting muscle giant cells as malignant cells [7].

FNAC is a useful procedure for the initial and recurrent diagnosis of fibromatoses and in the separation of fibromatoses from other benign and malignant soft tissue lesions. In the initial diagnosis, histological confirmation is recommended [8].

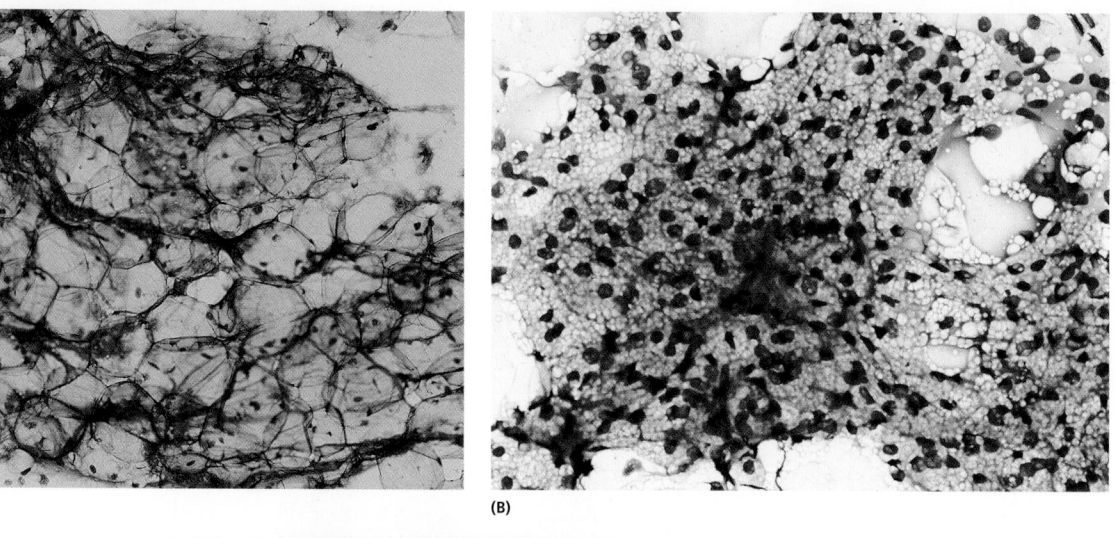

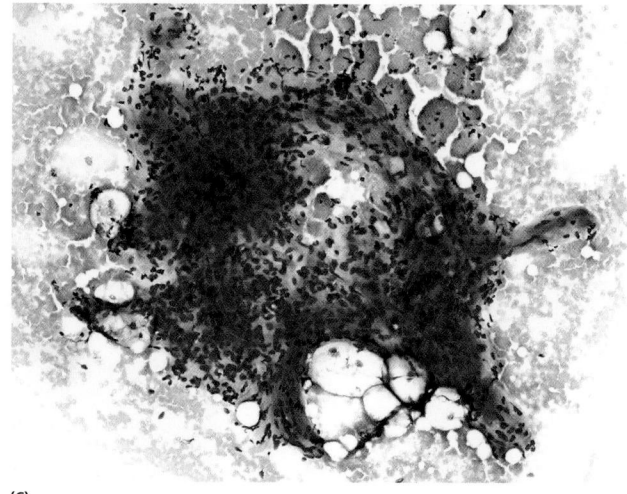

Figure 5.5 Lipoma. (A) Sparse microbiopsy fragments of adipose tissue composed of fat cells in a meshwork of delicate capillaries. The fat cells are univacuolated with nuclei that are small and inconspicuous. It is not possible to distinguish between the lipoma and fat tissue on FNAC. It is therefore important that the FNAC is taken from a representative area under standard conditions, if any conclusions are to be drawn from the material containing fat cells only (MGG × 600). (B) Hybernoma clusters, sheets of round to oval and polygonal cells with abundant microvacuolated or granular cytoplasm, and centrally placed small uniform nuclei, sometimes mimicking a lipoblast. (C) Spindle-cell lipoma. Mixture of loosely cohesive clusters and dispersed bland spindle cells, mature adipose tissue, and fragments of collagen–hyaline fibres. Myxoid background and mast cells are common.

5.2.3 Nodular fasciitis

Nodular fasciitis (NF) is a self-limiting, benign fibroblastic proliferation in soft tissues, which occurs most commonly in the extremities, trunk and head and neck region. Stanley et al. described the cytological features of 11 cases of nodular fasciitis diagnosed by FNAC, including a prominent myxoid background with single cells or cohesive groups of spindle cells ranging from long, slender fibroblast-like forms to plump oval-shaped cells with moderate amounts of basophilic cytoplasm, enlarged nuclei and one or two small nucleoli [9]. However, the authors warn that this cytological picture may be considered non-specific if the clinical features are not evaluated (Figure 5.6) [10].

As such, NF is a well-recognised diagnostic pitfall in Head and Neck FNAC [11–13]. However, the vast majority of lesions regress spontaneously so a conservative management is appropriate.

Cytological features: The lesion is composed of fibroblasts and myofibroblasts showing variable degrees of anisocytosis and anisokaryosis. There is myxoid background substance and tufts of fibrillary myxoid material, more pronounced in the early lesions and giving an impression of a low grade myxoid sarcoma [4] (Fig. 5.6). The smears are, as a rule, hypercellular, composed of haphazardly arranged fibroblast like cells that vary widely from spindle shaped with long cytoplasmic processes to more plump with one or more nuclei with nucleoli. Although there is marked anisokaryosis and prominent nucleoli, the chromatin pattern is finely granular. Collagenous background is noted in more persistent lesions. Ganglion-like cells, admixture of inflammatory cells and histiocytes as well as occasional multinucleated giant cells make cytological appearances of nodular fasciitis fairly characteristic, making it possible to diagnose these lesions in FNAC samples [14, 15].

5.2.4 Proliferative fasciitis and proliferative myositis

Nodular fasciitis (NF), proliferative fasciitis (PF), and proliferative myositis (PM) are pseudosarcomatous lesions that typically resolve spontaneously [16].

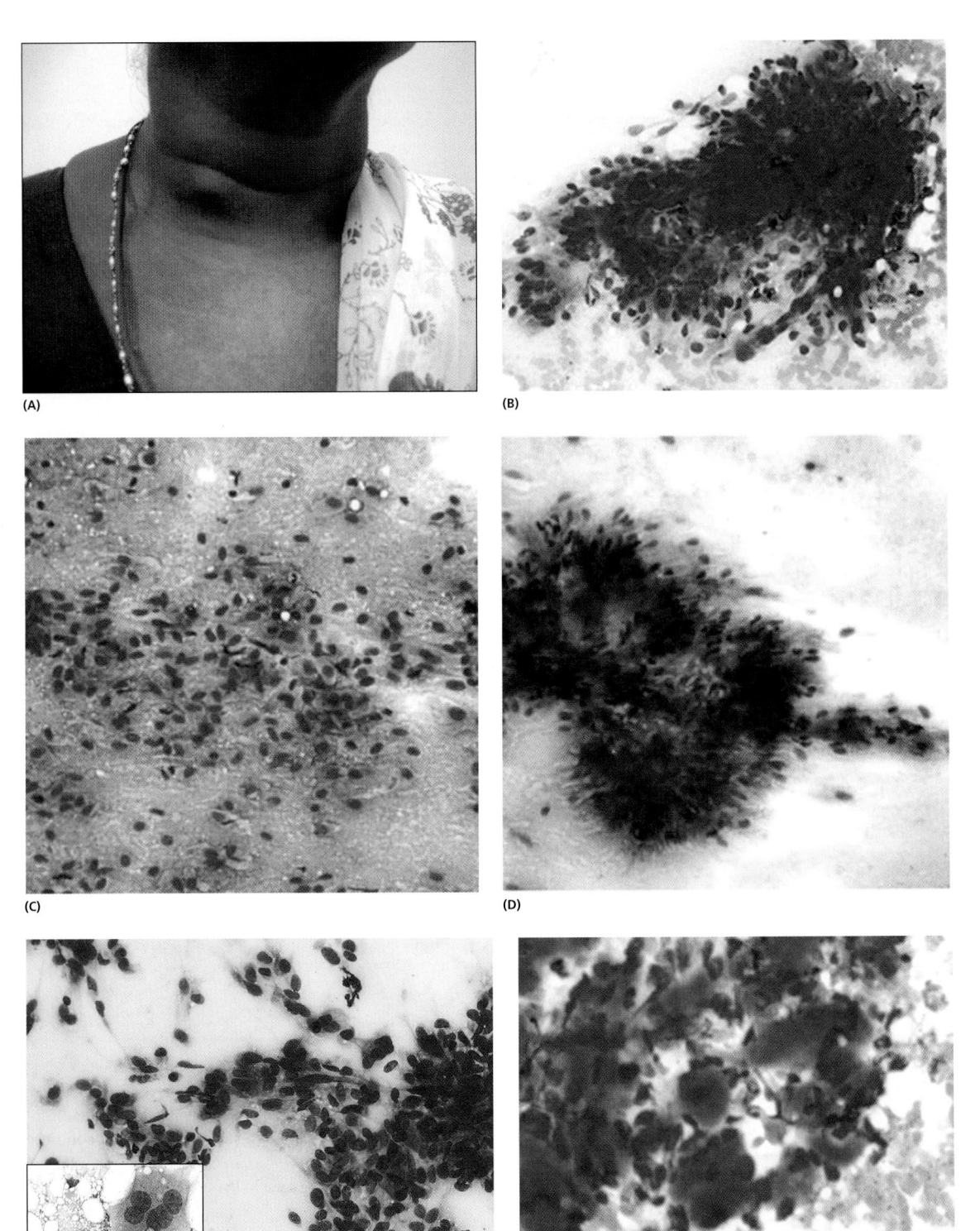

Figure 5.6 Nodular fasciitis. (A) Patient with a slightly tender swelling over right side of neck measuring 3 × 2 cm mimicking origin from right lobe of thyroid. (Source: Reproduced with permission from Articles from Journal of Clinical and Diagnostic Research: courtesy of JCDR Research & Publications Private Limited.) (B) Smears contain myxoid background substance and tufts of fibrillary myxoid material. As a rule, smears are hypercellular (MGG ×400). (C) Myofibroblasts vary widely from spindle shaped with long cytoplasmic processes to more plump with one or more nuclei with nucleoli are seen, a so-called cell culture appearance (MGG ×1000). (D) Spindle and plump cells in a myxoid background of a parotid gland FNAC were misinterpreted as pleomorphic adenoma. (E) Proliferative fasciitis. Loosely cohesive clusters or dispersed relatively pleomorphic cells with round to oval and spindle-shaped nuclei. Admixture of numerous ganglion cell-like cells with binucleation and abundant cytoplasm (inset). (F) Proliferative myositis. Dispersed fibroblastic–myofibroblastic cells with admixture of muscle fragments, multinucleated giant cells, and regenerating muscle fibres. Mitotic figures can be occasionally found in the smears (MGG).

The FNAC diagnosis is therefore even more important in order to avoid surgical intervention. *Proliferative fasciitis* is defined histologically as a spindle-cell lesion containing basophilic giant cells that resemble ganglion cells; the FNAC smears from this lesion are cellular and contain spindle cells as well as numerous large cells with abundant cytoplasm, one to two eccentric nuclei and macronucleoli (Fig. 5.6D). The large cells seen on the aspiration smears correspond well with the classic ganglion-like cells seen on histological sections. Care must be taken so that this distinctive lesion is not misdiagnosed as a malignant soft tissue neoplasm [17]. In FNAC, ganglion cell–like cells are found not only in PF and PM but also in NF. The reported frequency of ganglion cell–like cells is variable in FNAC specimens.

Proliferative myositis shows dispersed fibroblastic–myofibroblastic cells with admixture of muscle fragments, multinucleated giant cells, and regenerating muscle fibres. Mitotic figures can be occasionally found in the smears (MGG) (Fig. 5.6F).

5.2.5 Benign nerve sheath tumour (neurilemmoma, schwannoma)

Benign nerve sheath tumour can occur anywhere in the head and neck and is associated with nerves [18]. Intraparotid facial nerve schwannomas have been documented sporadically throughout the medical literature. These benign tumours of neurogenic origin should be considered in the differential diagnosis of parotid region masses [19–26].

Cytological features: Mainly tumour tissue fragments with sparse dispersed cells and some aggregates against a fibrillary background substance. Smears most often contain a mixture of Antoni A and Antoni B areas and tissue fragments are more common than individual cells. Individual cells have indistinct cell borders, nuclei with pointed ends, occasionally pallisading alternating with more rounded (lymphocytoid) nuclei. Sometimes Verocay body-like structures are seen. Mitoses are not seen [4] (Fig. 5.7). When reviewing a large series of FNAC of neurilemomas, Domansky

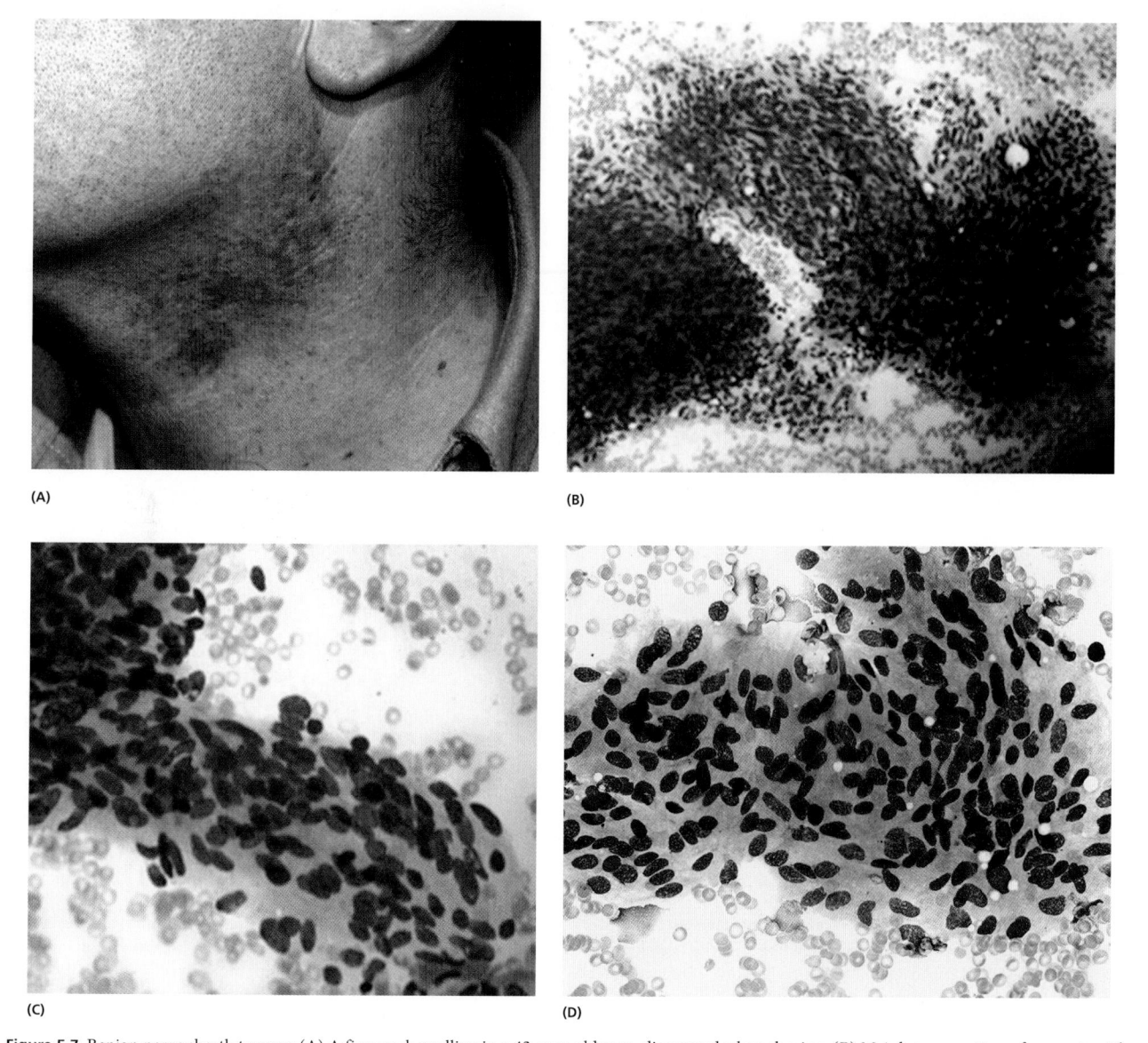

(A)

(B)

(C)

(D)

Figure 5.7 Benign nerve sheath tumour. (A) A firm neck swelling in a 43-year-old man, discovered when shaving. (B) Mainly tumour tissue fragments with sparse dispersed cells and some aggregates against a fibrillary background substance (MGG ×200). (C) Individual cells have indistinct cell borders, nuclei with pointed ends, occasionally pallisading (MGG ×600, oil). (D) Fascicles, clusters and discrete spindle-shaped cells with long wavy nuclei are often seen.

noted that most have distinct cytomorphological features that allow correct diagnosis [27]. A most important diagnostic pitfall in diagnosis of neurilemmoma is leiomyosarcoma. The latter can be misdiagnosed in cases of ancient neurilemmoma. There may be marked cell pleomorphism with large hyperchromatic and bizarre nuclei containing prominent nucleoli. There are no mitoses and intranuclear vacuoles may be seen in ancient neurilemmoma. In the cases of intraparotid neurilemmomas, myoepithelioma of the salivary gland (see Chapter 2, Section 2.3) is a differential diagnosis.

5.3 Cysts of the head and neck

5.3.1 Thyroglossal cysts

Thyroglossal cyst is a congenital cyst. It arises as a rule in the midline of the neck, close to hyoid bone, to which it is usually attached.

[See BOX 5.2. Summary of ultrasound features: Thyroglossal cyst on www.wiley.com/go/kocjan/clinical_cytopathology_head_neck2e]

It arises from the remnants of thyroglossal duct. It is lined with either squamous or columnar epithelium. Clinically, patients present with midline swelling. FNAC yields small amount of fluid. Fluid contains proteinaceous background, macrophages, cholesterol crystals and occasionally some sparse epithelium, either squamous or columnar (Fig. 5.8). There are a number of reports of papillary carcinoma arising in a thyroglossal cyst [28–32].

5.3.2 Branchial cyst

Branchial cysts derive from the second branchial cleft. They may appear in different anatomical positions. As a rule, they are more or less covered by the anterior border of the sternocleidomastoid muscle, but they can occur below and above this position (Figs 5.9a and 5.10a). Clinically, diagnosis of branchial cleft cyst therefore may be more difficult than medial cysts. Lesions of similar appearance in this area include lymph nodes, carotid body tumours, salivary gland tumours, lymphangiomas and lipomas. The reliability of preoperative diagnosis of branchial cleft cyst is between 50–60% [33]. Histologically, the inner layer of the cyst is lined by squamous epithelium with lymphoid cells in the wall of the cyst.

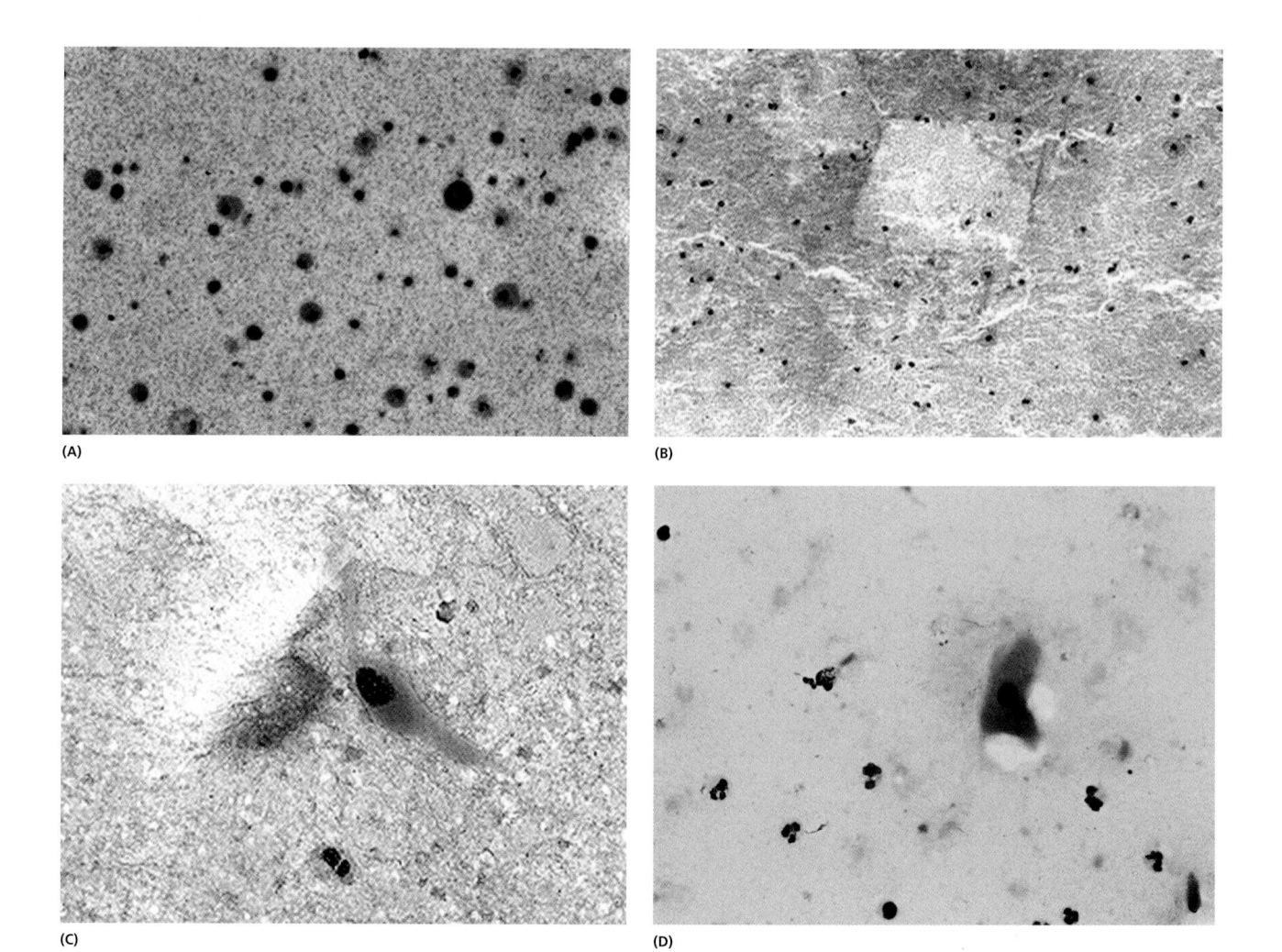

(A) (B) (C) (D)

Figure 5.8 Thyroglossal cyst. (A, B) Fluid from the cyst contains proteinaceous background, debris, macrophages, cholesterol crystals and sparse epithelium (MGG, PAP×200). (C, D) Epithelium of the thyroglossal cyst is inconspicuous and barely noticeable. It is usually squamous, showing marked degenerative changes (MGG×600, oil).

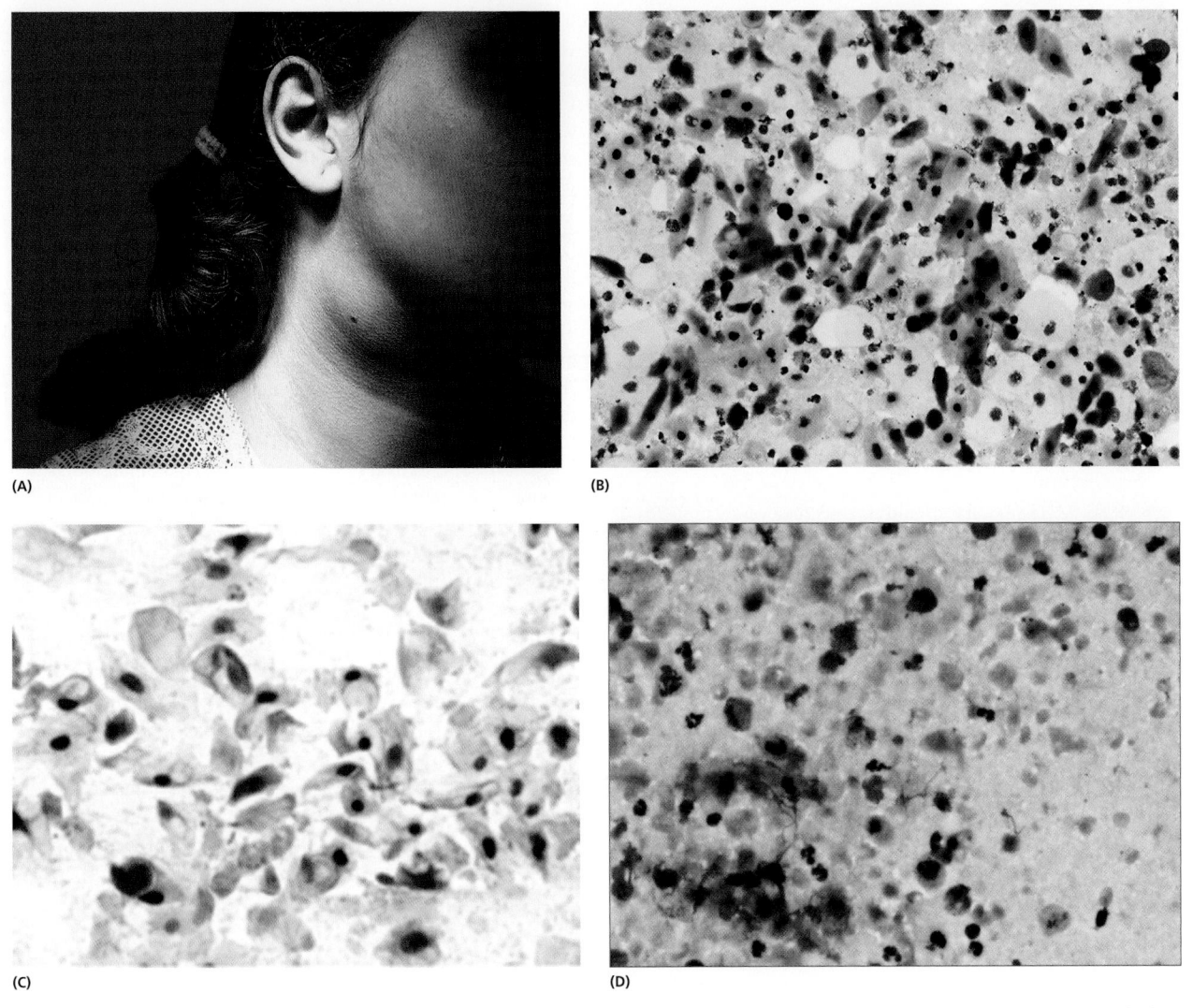

Figure 5.9 Branchial cleft cyst. (A) 26-year-old patient with the a soft, fluctuant swelling in the anterior triangle was subjected to FNAC. (B) Branchial cysts contain epithelial cells and keratinous debris. (C) This is most frequently mature squamous epithelium and anucleate squames, frequently admixed with polymorphs (PAP ×200). (D) Important diagnostic distinction is from a squamous cell carcinoma which shows a necrotic backround with degenerate squamous cells are seen. The material is often difficult to interpret as malignant. An equivocal diagnosis may have to be made.

Cytological features: Branchial cysts contain epithelial cells and keratinous debris. This is most frequently mature squamous epithelium and anucleate squames [34] (Fig. 5.9B; see also Fig. 2.10C, Chapter 2). Inflamed branchial cysts contain polymorphs, macrophages and may contain epithelial atypia that may be mistaken for squamous cell carcinoma [35] (Figs 5.9D and 5.10B). The reverse is also a potential diagnostic pitfall: distinction between branchial cleft cyst and a metastasis of squamous cell carcinoma that may be well differentiated and contain mainly mature squamous epithelial cells. A thorough search for nuclear atypia is suggested. Failing this, the diagnosis of branchial cyst in patients over the age of 30 has to be issued with a degree of caution, allowing for the possibility of a metastasis of a well differentiated squamous cell carcinoma. Confirmation of human papillomavirus (HPV) as a causative agent for a subset of biologically and clinically distinct squamous cell carcinomas of the head and neck (HNSCC) has resulted in a growing need and expectation for HPV testing of head and neck cancers. FNAC of metastatic HNSCC are suitable for standard tissue-based methods of HPV detection such as immunoperoxidase and in situ hybridisation [36]. Different types of cytology specimens including smears, cytospins, cell blocks and aspirated material in the rinse can all be used for different types of HPV testing. The HPV PCR assay on FNAC material showed a high sensitivity 96% and specificity (100%) using the reference standard of HPV PCR analysis on FFPE material of the same patients [36a,b].

Excision biopsy, whilst usually performed on branchial cleft cysts, is not a procedure of choice in the cases of metastatic squamous cell carcinoma. The excision is normally part of a radical neck dissection. Accurate preoperative diagnosis and multidisciplinary discussion are therefore very important.

5.3.3 Mucous retention cyst

Mucous retention cyst is a common submucosal lesion of the oral cavity that, when deeply seated, simulates a neoplasm. Its occurrence within the salivary gland has been described in Section 2.2.3 (Figs 2.8 and 2.9, Chapter 2). Cytological differential diagnosis is from other benign and malignant cystic lesions of the head and neck (see Section 5.2.5) [37].

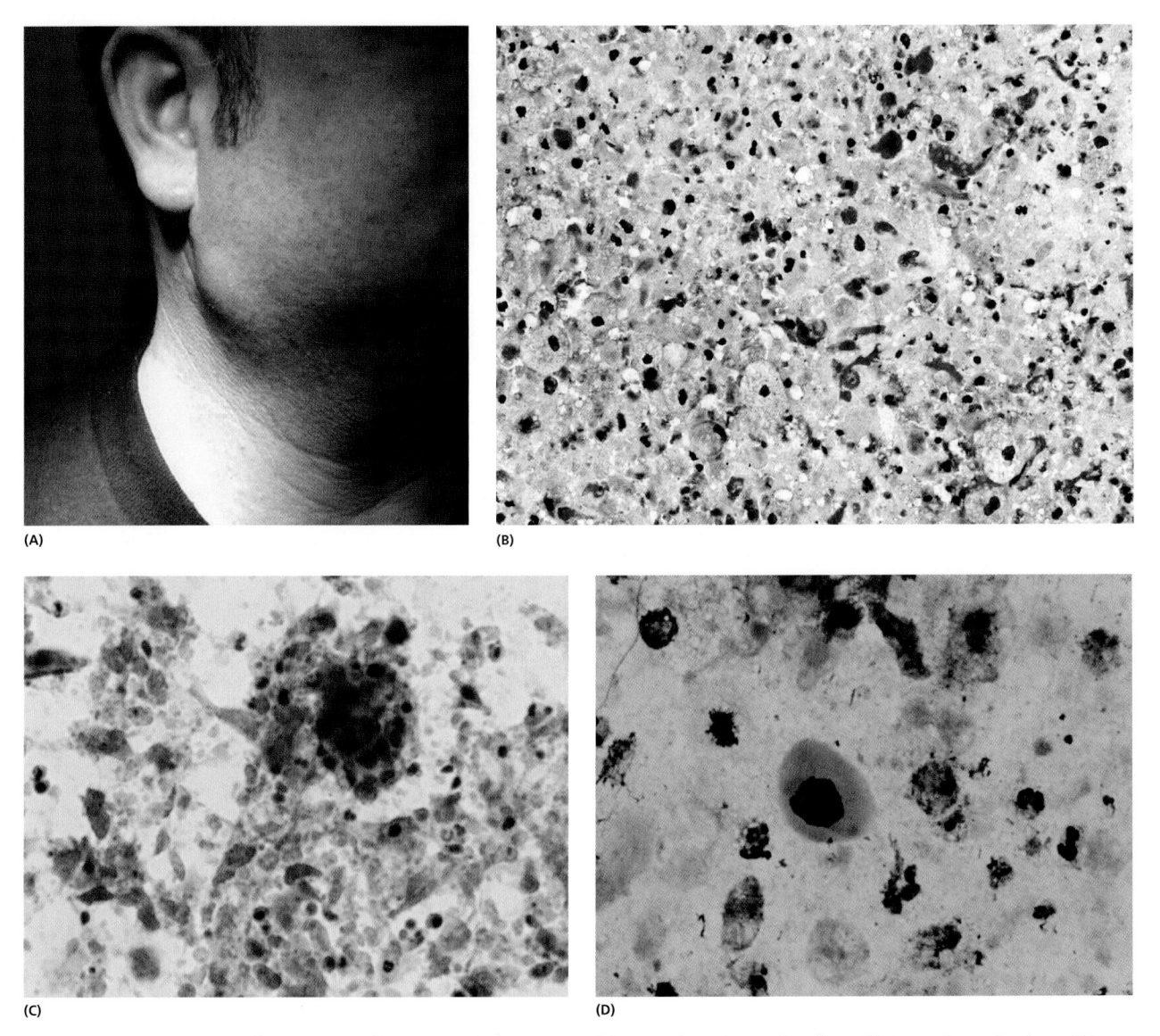

Figure 5.10 Cystic metastasis of a squamous cell carcinoma. (A) A 53-year-old man with an apparently inflamed lesion at the angle of mandible. (B) Inflammatory and necrotic background with very few, poorly preserved squamous cells, some with picnotic, irregular nuclei (MGG, PAP ×600, oil immersion). (C) Irregularly shaped keratin flakes and degenerate cell clusters with hyperchromatic nuclei. (D) Another case. Necrotic background and degenerate cells some of which have large nuclei with irregular nuclear outlines.

5.3.4 Intraosseous cysts and other lesions

The most commonly sampled intraosseous lesions are odontogenic cysts (Fig. 5.11A,B), ameloblastomas (Fig. 5.11C,D,E,F), and fibro-osseous and giant cell lesions [38–43]. *Odontogenic keratocyst (OKC)*, due to its agressive nature and molecular investigations is now considered to be a cystic neoplasm. The combination of FNAC with immunocytochemical determination of CK10 is considered helpful in distinguishing an OKC from a nonkeratinizing odontogenic cyst [43a] (Fig. 5.11A,B). *Dentigerous cyst* is a common cyst of the jaws. It is associated with the crowns of permanent teeth, most frequently associated with impacted mandibular third molars. Bilateral dentigerous cysts are rare and generally occur in association with a developmental syndrome or systemic disease, such as muco-polysaccharidosis and cleidocranial dysplasia. Pathological analysis of the lesion is essential for the definitive diagnosis. Other lesions may share the same radiological features as dentigerous cysts, such as odontogenic keratocysts and unicystic ameloblastoma

(Fig. 5.11C,D,E,F). Radicular cyst is a slow-growing fluid-filled epithelial sac at the apex of a tooth with a nonvital pulp or defective root canal filling. It contains polymorphs and non keratinising squamous epithelium (Fig. 5.12C,D). The interpretation of cystic intraosseous lesions can only be made in conjunction with radiological and clinical appearances in a multidisciplinary setting [44].

5.3.5 Rare cysts and differential diagnosis of cystic lesions of the head and neck

Parathyroid [45, 46], *cervical thymic* [47] and other rare cystic lesions can occasionally be encountered in the head and neck area [48, 48a]. *Epidermoid cyst* of the skin may be mistaken for another lesion (Fig. 5.12).

[See BOX 5.3. Summary of ultrasound features: Epidermoid cyst on www.wiley.com/go/kocjan/clinical_cytopathology_head_neck2e]

Differential diagnosis. Apart from the congenital cysts, other *cystic lesions in the neck* include: lymphangioma, pleomorphic

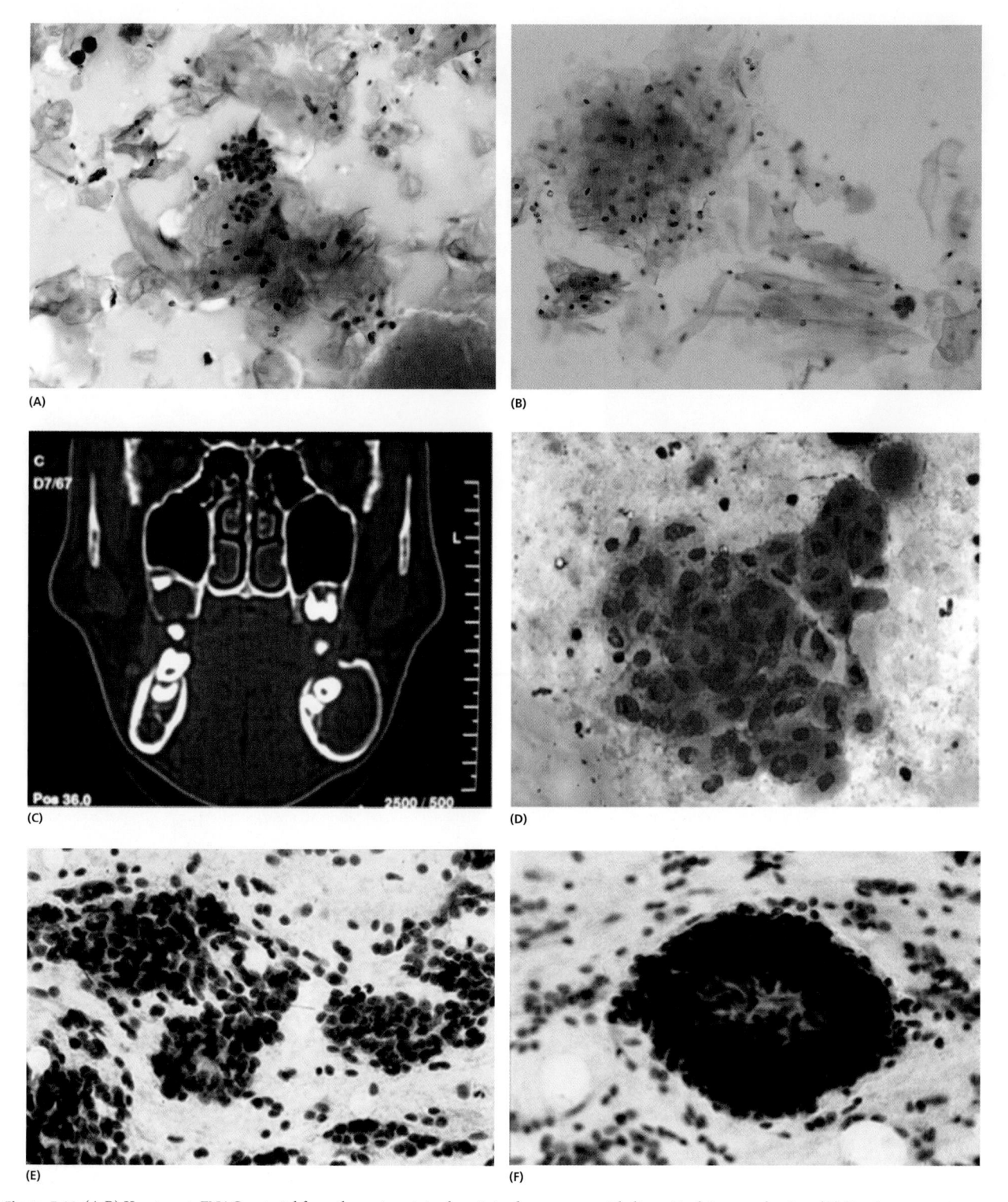

Figure 5.11 (A,B) Keratocyst. FNAC material from the cyst contains keratinised squamous epithelium. Nuclei appear benign. (C) Dentigerous cyst: Radiological appearances. D, It is most frequently associated with impacted third molars. Non keratinising squamous epithelium and debris. (E,F) Ameloblastoma. A patient with a history of resection of ameloblastoma, suspected of recurrence. Smears show tightly cohesive clusters of basaloid ameloblast-like epithelial cells, showing nuclear palisading and resembling odontogenic islands.

adenoma with cystic change, Warthin's tumour, mucoepidermoid carcinoma, squamous cell carcinoma and metastatic papillary carcinoma [49].

[See BOX 5.4. Summary of ultrasound features: Lymphangioma cyst on www.wiley.com/go/kocjan/clinical_cytopathology_head_neck2e]

5.4 Small round cell tumours

A group of malignancies which share similar morphological features are known as 'small round cell tumours'. They commonly occur in childhood and adolescence and include: embryonal and alveolar rhabdomyosarcoma, neuroblastoma, Ewing's sarcoma/

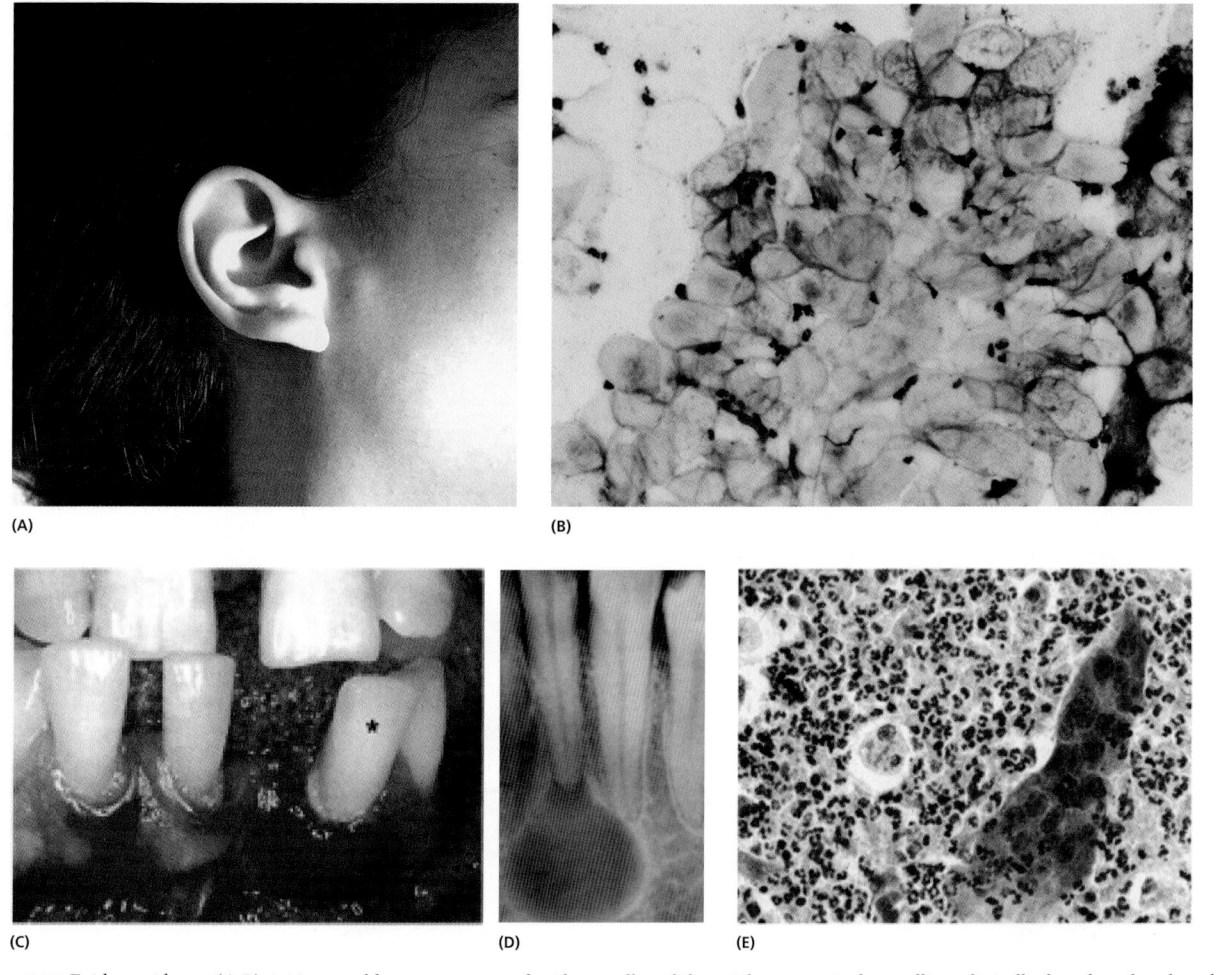

Figure 5.12 Epidermoid cyst. (A,B) A 29-year-old woman presented with a small, mobile, painless preauricular swelling, clinically thought to be a lymph node. MGG stained FNAC smears contain mature squamous cells. (C,D,E) Radicular cyst is a fluid filled sac, radiologically seen at the apex of the tooth. Polymorphs and non kertatinising squamous epithelium in the FNAC sample.

Peripheral Neuroectodermal Tumour (PNET) and lymphoma (usually lymphoblastic). All of these tumours may occur in the head and neck either as primary tumours or metastases. Accurate diagnosis in either of these situations is important to ensure appropriate treatment. Biopsies, particularly in case of secondary deposits, may not be necessary or feasible. FNAC therefore aims to be as diagnostically useful as possible [17, 50–53].

5.4.1 Rhabdomyosarcoma

The head and neck region, including the eye, is one of the most common locations of rhabdomyosarcoma (RMS) [54, 55]. Tumour is common in children and adolescents. Clinically, the enlargement may appear to be inflammatory, and is usually treated unsuccessfully with antibiotics.

Cytological features: Uniform population of primitive, small round cell with scant cytoplasm, arranged as single cells and cohesive aggregates. The smears in embryonal RMS are variably cellular with marked pleomorphism (Fig. 5.13A,B). Alveolar RMS, in contrast, has a more monotonous appearance in cytology with small, more uniform, ovoid or round nuclei and prominent nucleoli (Fig. 5.13C,D). The nuclear chromatin is finely granular and hyperchromatic. Intracytoplasmic vacuoles may be present. The presence of bi/multinucleated rhabdomyoblast-like cells is an important clue for the diagnosis of RMS on FNAC [56–60].

Tumour cells are often enclosed in a background of mucosubstances. The lack of cytological features proving rhabdomyoblastic differentiation, such as cross-striation, requires use of additional methods in the cytological diagnosis [61–63]. An immunoperoxidase stain for the demonstration of intracellular desmin in FNAC smears shows a positive reaction of variable intensity in some of the undifferentiated round cells and in the more mature bipolar sarcomatous elements [64].

Morphological subtyping: RMS is a heterogeneous group of tumours with respect to their molecular basis, degree of differentiation, histology and clinical behaviour. Because of the wide variation of tumour morphology, it is often difficult to distinguish between the distinct subtypes. Differentiation between alveolar and embryonal RMS, although described previously, is not entirely reliable on cytology alone and yet this distinction is very important for further management, not least because the embryonal RMS has a better prognosis than alveolar RMS [65]. The advances in therapeutic approach stress the importance of including molecular diagnostic studies in the routine evaluation of paediatric solid tumours. [66]. Tumour cells of both, embryonal and alveolar RMS express desmin, myogenin and MyoD1 [67]. Aberrant expression of keratins, CD99, S-100 protein, lymphoid markers and NSE poses significant diagnostic challenges and confusion with others mall round blue cell tumours. Most alveolar RMS have either PAX3-FOXO1 or PAX7-FOXO1 gene fusion, which can be detected by FISH [68].

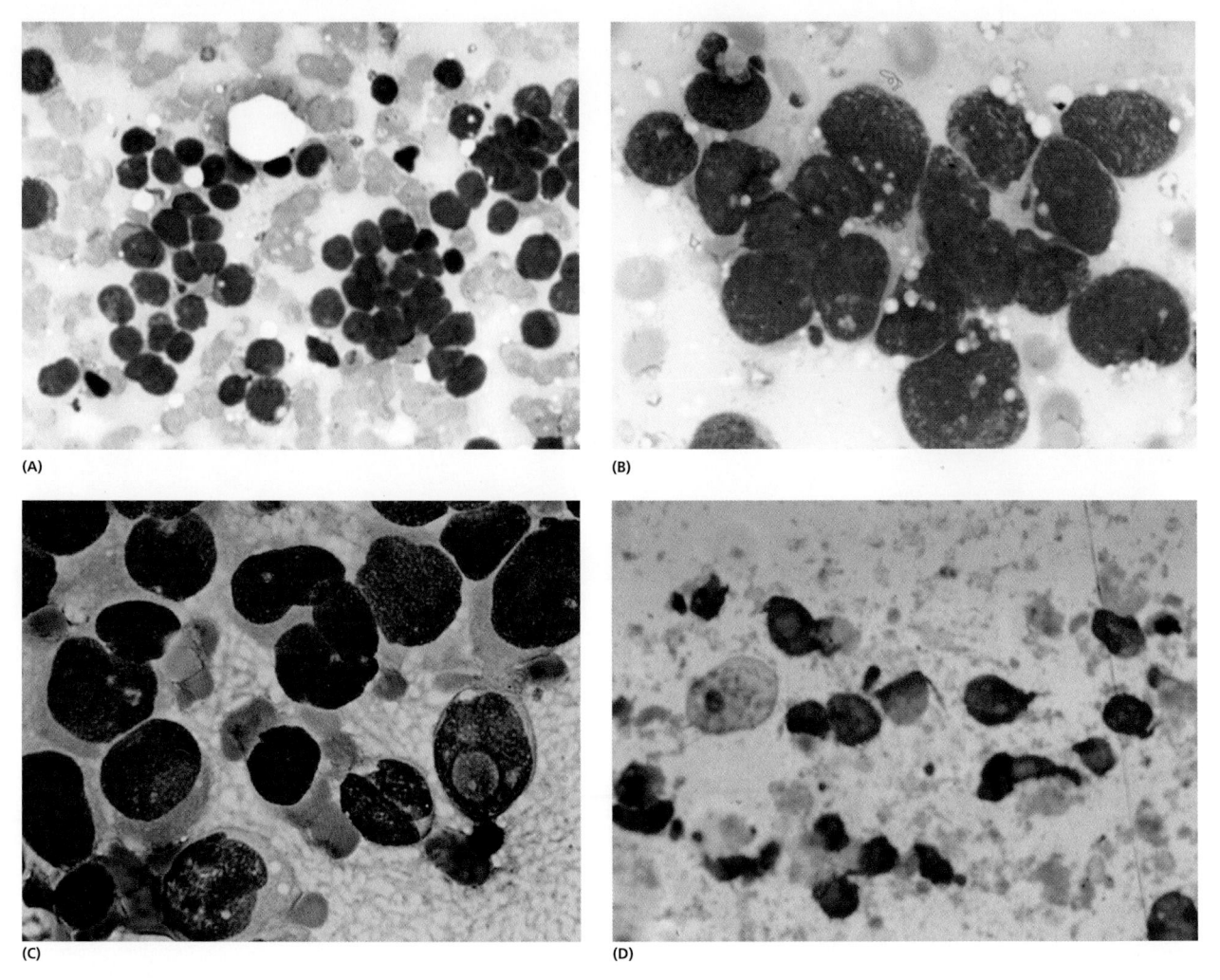

(A) (B) (C) (D)

Figure 5.13 Rhabdomyosarcoma. (A) A case of *embryonal* rhabdomyosaarcoma in a submandibular area of a 9-year-old child. Uniform population of primitive, small round cell with scant cytoplasm, arranged as single cells and cohesive aggregates (MGG, ×200). (B,C) The nuclear chromatin in *alveolar* rhabdomymyosarcoma is finely granular and hyperchromatic, while nucleoli are inconspicuous. Binucleated and multinucleated cells are found in the majority of cases. Intracytoplasmic and intranuclear vacuoles may be present (MGG×600). (D) Desmin in FNAC smears shows a positive reaction in some of the undifferentiated round cells (desmin, APAAP, ×600, oil).

5.4.2 Ewing's sarcoma/peripheral neuroectodermal tumour/Askin tumour

Ewing sarcoma family of tumours (ESFT) are mainly aggressive sarcomas of bone and also arising in soft tissues, which share common features: morphological features of basophilic round cell tumours, immunohistochemical features by expression of membrane CD99 protein and genetic features with a transloca-tion involving EWS and FLI1 in approximately 90% of cases [69]. The discovery of this translocation has made it possible to unify in a single entity several lesions such as PNET, neuropi-theliomas, Askin tumors, Ewing sarcomas.

Extraskeletal Ewing's sarcoma (EES) is a round-cell malignancy that manifests most commonly in the paravertebral and inter-costal regions. It occurs predominantly in adolescents and young adults, between the ages of 10 and 30 years, and follows an aggres-sive course with a high recurrence rate. Distant metastases are common (Fig. 5.14). The tumour is often confused with other round, small-cell neoplasms, including neuroblastoma, embry-onal rhabdomyosarcoma, and lymphoma [70]. The purpose of FNAC is to diagnose these tumours and evaluate metastases in patients with known ES [71].

Cytological features: FNAC smears from ES/PNET show cellular smears with many single cells and focal clustering. Numerous naked nuclei and focal crush artefacts are seen. Mitoses and necrosis are rare. Cells are small with fine chromatin, small inconspicuous but distinct basophilic nucleoli, scanty cytoplasm, cytoplasmic vacuoles and nuclear moulding (the so-called typical variant) [72] (Fig. 5.14). Less common are tumours with cells having abundant eosinophilic cytoplasm, large nuclei, and large eosinophilic nucleoli (atypical or large cell variant). Tumours with features in between, with cells showing abundant cytoplasm, nuclear grooves and medium-sized nucleoli, represent the intermediate variant. Immunocytochemistry (CD99/O13) shows strong membranous reactivity. In addition, cytogenetical (t(11;22) (q24;q12) and/or molecular evidence of ES/PNET specific chromosomal translocation is demonstrated in histo-logical or cytological material [71, 73–78]. Immunocytochemistry with MIC2 (CD99) in FNAC smears can provide initial diagnosis and supportive evidence of ES/PNET in patients with known disease.

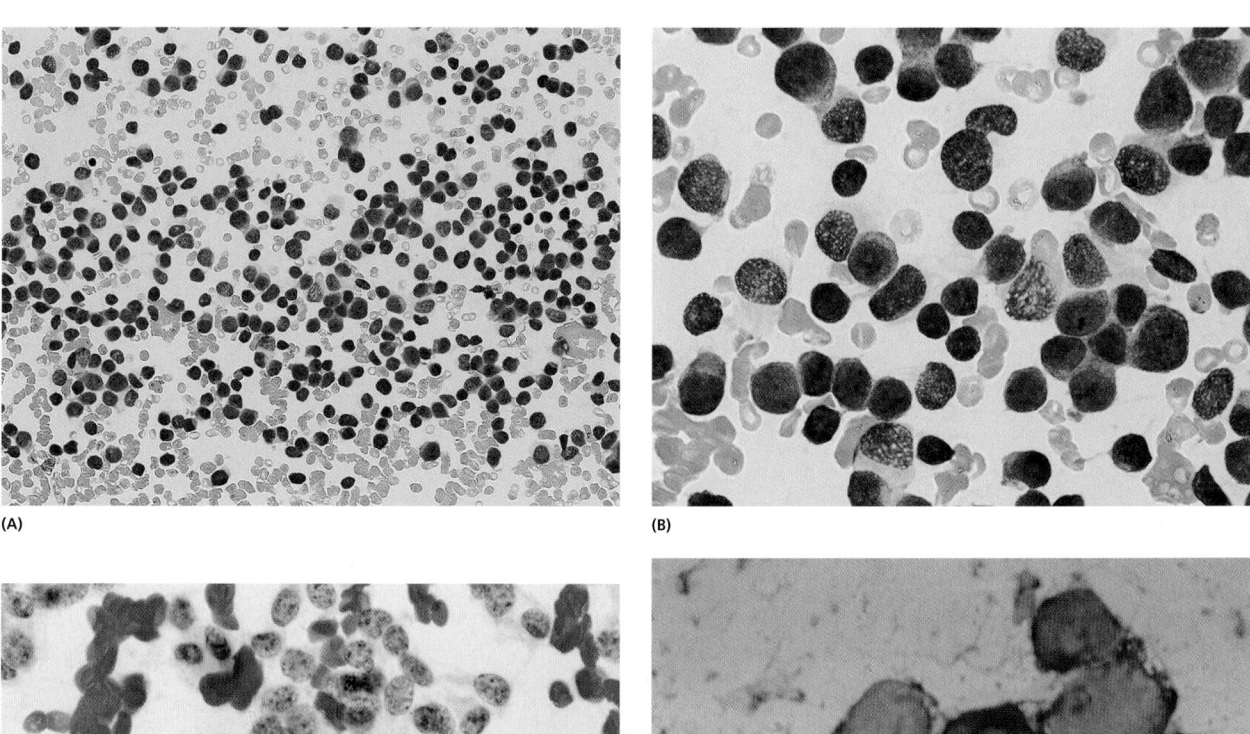

(A)

(B)

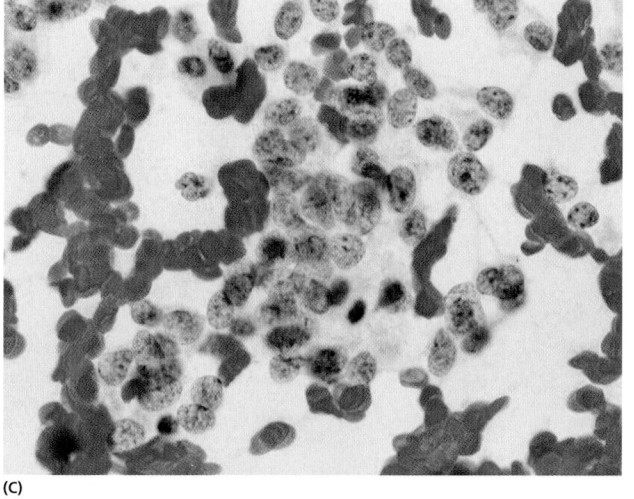

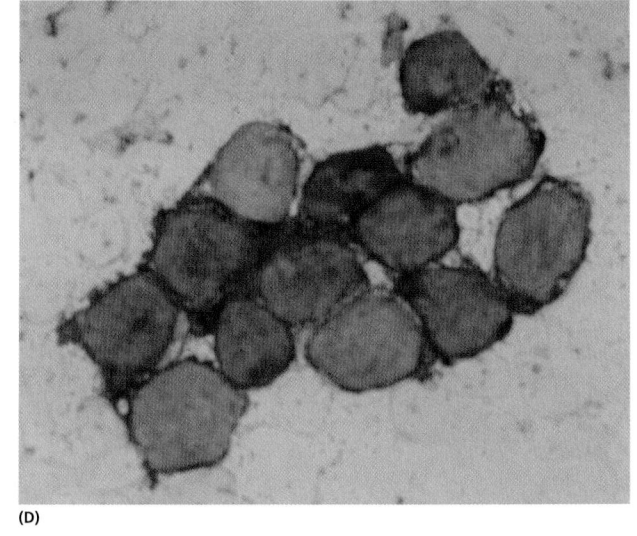

(C)

(D)

Figure 5.14 Ewing's sarcoma. a 14-year-old boy with a subcutaneous deposit of tumour in the scalp. Previous history of Ewing's sarcoma in the forearm. (A) Cellular smears with many single cells and focal clustering. Numerous naked nuclei and focal crush artefacts may be seen (MGG ×200). (B) Cells are small with fine chromatin, small inconspicuous but distinct basophilic nucleoli, scanty cytoplasm, cytoplasmic vacuoles and nuclear moulding (the so-called typical variant). Less common are tumours with cells having abundant eosinophilic cytoplasm, large nuclei, and large eosinophilic nucleoli (atypical or large cell variant). Tumours with features in between, with cells showing abundant cytoplasm, nuclear grooves and medium-sized nucleoli, represent the intermediate variant (MGG ×600, oil immersion). (C) Chromatin structure of this tumour can be seen better on alcohol fixed smears. (D) Immunocytochemistry (CD99/O13) shows strong membranous reactivity (MIC 2, ×1000, oil).

5.4.3 Olfactory neuroblastoma

Oesthesioneuroblastoma (olfactory neuroblastoma) is a rare malignant neoplasm derived from the olfactory epithelium [79]. Although a rare tumour, it is important to recognise because it has a better prognosis than the more commonly encountered malignancies of the nose [80]. It sometimes presents as an orbital lesion causing propotosis [81, 82].

Cytological features: These show very cellular smears with predominance of single cells with intermixed small, loosely cohesive, three-dimensional cell groups. Cell size is small to intermediate, with round nuclei (Fig. 5.15). There is an overall monomorphic appearance, with minimal nuclear pleomorphism. Chromatin is finely granular and stippled, with multiple, small chromocentres. Cytoplasm in the cell groups has a fibrillary quality and is moderate in amount. Single bare nuclei are seen. Occasional pseudorosettes may be noted [83]. Immunocytochemical stains are positive for chromogranin and synaptophysin. Ultrastructural examination shows neuritic cell processes with neurosecretory, membrane-bound, dense-core granules and microtubules. Immunoelectron microscopy shows positive labelling of neurosecretory granules by chromogranin. FNAC morphology, in combination with ancillary studies, can provide an accurate diagnosis of metastatic ONB [84].

5.4.4 Lymphoma

Lymphoma may present as a tumour of the head and neck and its small round cell features may mimic other similar tumours described previously. Cytological and clinical features of lymphomas have been presented in Section 4.4. Occasionally, patients with a known history of lymphoma present with a new mass in the head and neck which needs investigating to exclude other pathology or transformation of the tumour (Fig. 5.16).

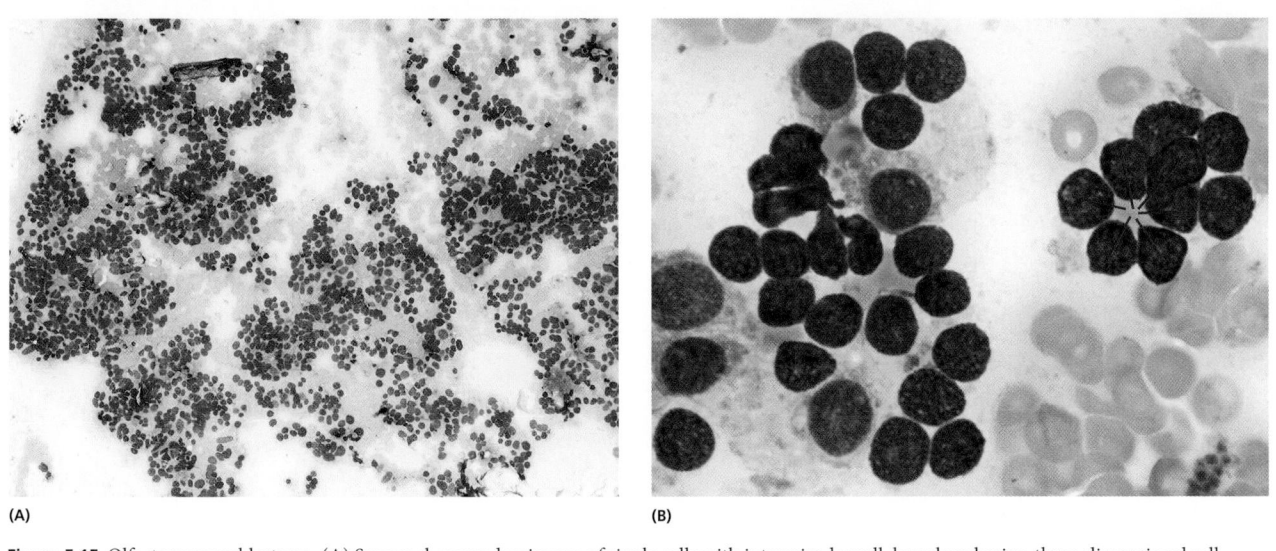

(A)

(B)

Figure 5.15 Olfactory neuroblastoma. (A) Smears show predominance of single cells with intermixed small, loosely cohesive, three-dimensional cell groups (MGG×200). (B) Cell size is small to intermediate, with round nuclei. There is an overall monomorphic appearance, with minimal nuclear pleomorphism. Chromatin is finely granular and stippled, with multiple, small chromocentres. Cytoplasm in the cell groups has a fibrillary quality and is moderate in amount. Single bare nuclei are seen. Occasional pseudorosettes are noted (MGG, PAP ×600, oil immersion).

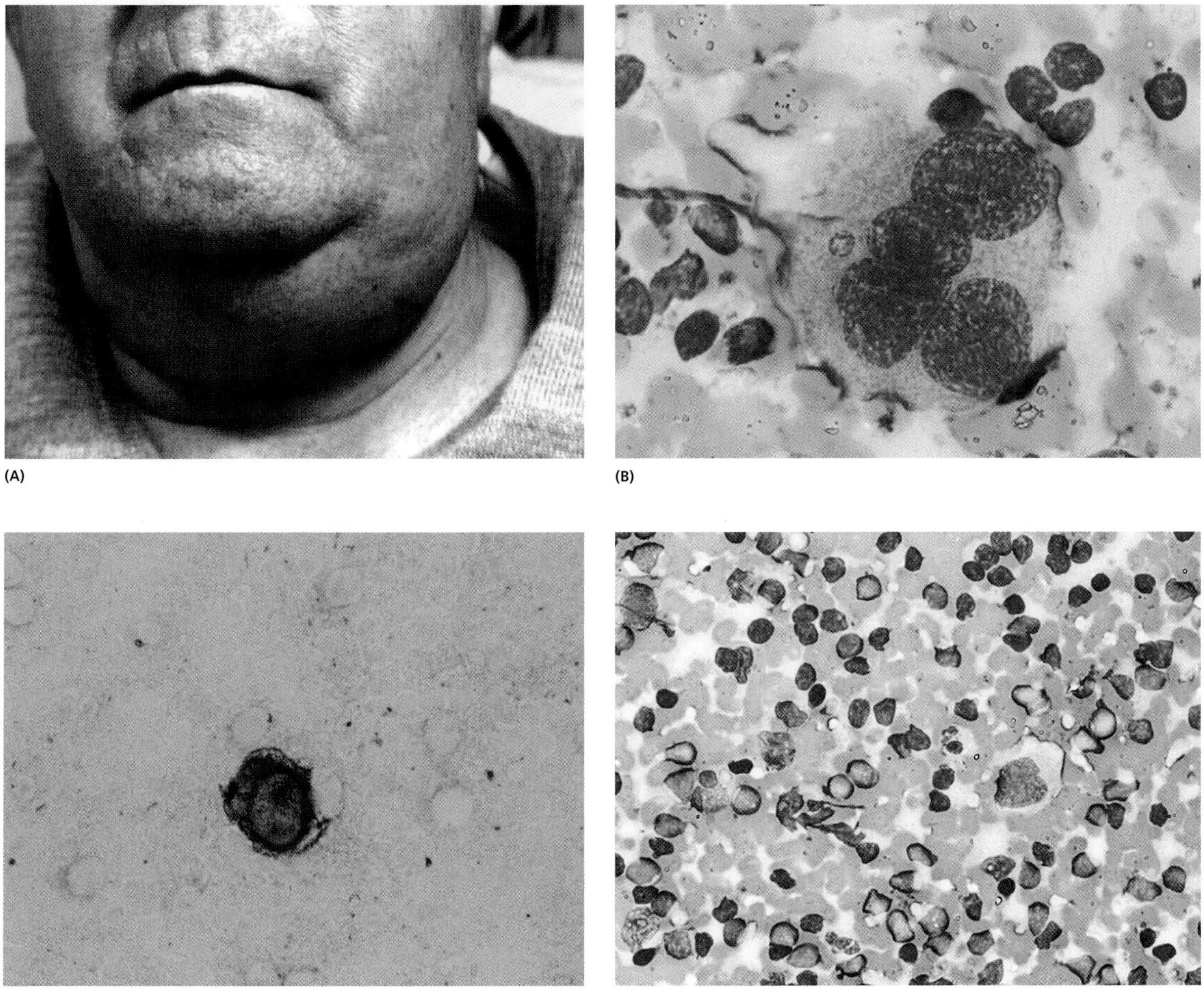

(A)

(B)

(C)

(D)

Figure 5.16 Richter's syndrome. (A) A 64-year-old patient with a history of CLL presented with a large submandibular mass that was clinically thought to be infection. FNAC was performed. (B) Aspirates contain lymphocytes and many large Reed–Sternberg type cells (MGG×1000, oil). (C) Large cells are CD30 positive (CD30, APAAP, ×1000, oil). This phenomenon of Hodgkin-like transformation of CLL has been described and is consistent with disease recurrence and transformation. (D) Background shows small lymphocytes, prolymphocytes and a few eosinophils.

5.5 Locally arising miscellaneous tumours

5.5.1 Carotid body tumours

Carotid body tumours develop from a chemoreceptor organ, which is most often located on the medial aspect of the internal carotid artery close to the bifurcation and is embedded in perivascular connective and fatty tissue. It consists of collections of neuroendocrine cells associated with parasympathetic paraganglion. Clinically, carotid body tumour can be moved horizontally but not vertically, they are vascular and may pulsate. Tumour can be found at any age, predominantly in females and may be bilateral. Patients present with a mass in the neck which may cause symptoms of compression (Fig. 5.17). They are benign tumours although malignant carotid body tumours have been described. Histologically, they are composed of cell nests ('*zellballen*') surrounded by sustentacular cells and stromal septae. The cells contain neurosecretory granules, are argyrophil, but non-chromaffin and only weakly argentaffin [85]. They stain positively with neuroendocrine markers (synaptophysin, chromogranin) [86–88].

Cytological features: Aspirates contain clusters and discretely scattered cells, with occasional acinar/rosette configuration. Cells have round to oval nuclei with moderate to marked anisonucleosis, prominent nucleoli, intranuclear inclusions, abundant, delicate, poorly defined, vacuolated, slightly basophilic cytoplasm. Fine reddish intracytoplasmic granules are also noted [89–97] (Figs. 5.17, 5.18). Striking feature in some of the carotid body tumours may be the presence of capillary endothelium with many spindle shaped cells mixed and wrapping around the epithelium. Fine reddish intracytoplasmic granules are present [98]. Cell pleomorphism, which can be striking and may be misleading, does not imply malignancy. On initial morphological diagnosis, five of the seven paragangliomas diagnosed by Kapila et al., were considered malignant (four undifferentiated and one adenocarcinoma) [99] (Fig. 5.19). Malignant carotid body tumours have been described, presence of mitoses and necrosis is suspicious, but their rarity justifies reporting all carotid body tumours without suggestion of malignancy [89, 100].

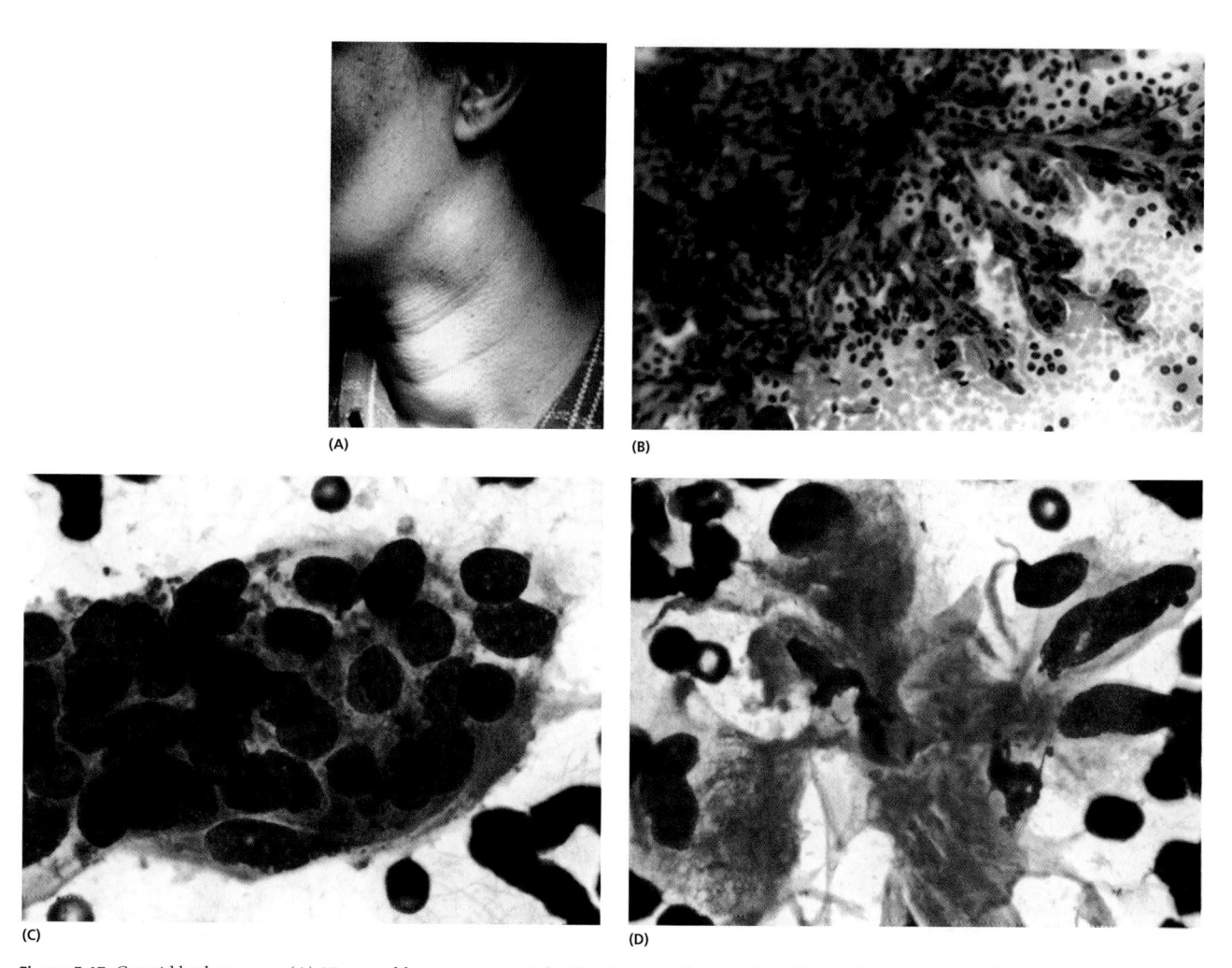

(A)   (B)

(C)   (D)

Figure 5.17 Carotid body tumour. (A) 27-year-old woman presented with a 6 months' history of swelling in the anterior triangle. Mobile in horizontal direction, non-tender, not varying in size. (B) Strikingly vascular lesion with branching capillary meshwork and delicate cells (MGG×200). Oncocytic type cells in cords and nests look monotonously uniform (MGG×200). (C) *Zellballen*, groups of glomus chief cells surrounded by sustentacular cells. (D) Sustentacular cells, when spread may give the lesion a bizarre spindle cell appearance.

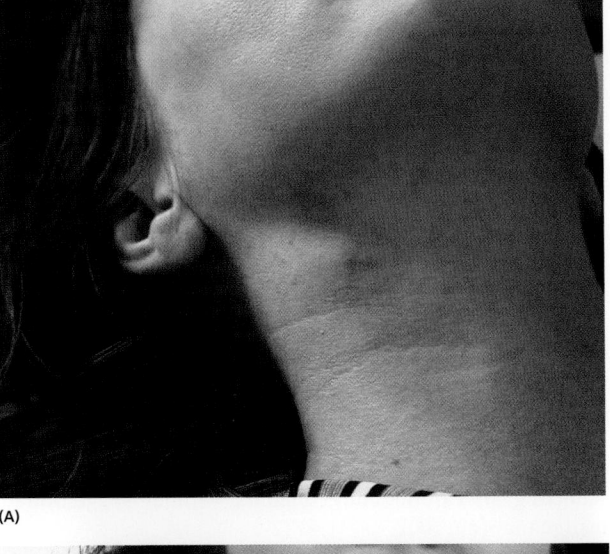

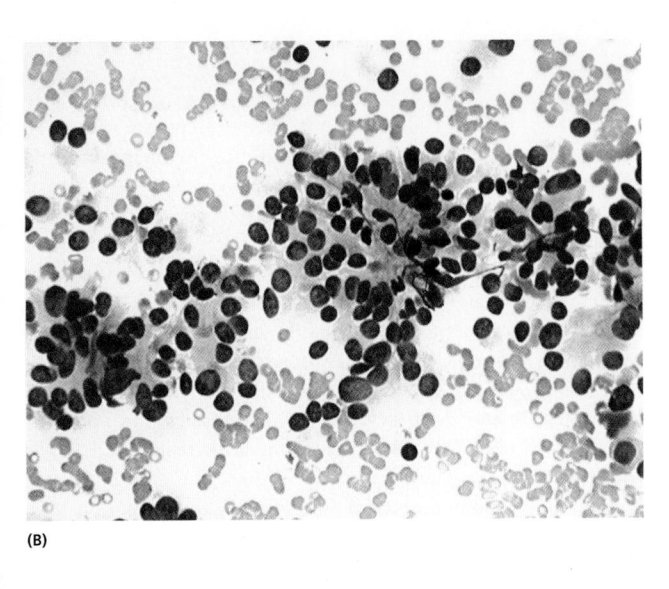

(A)

(B)

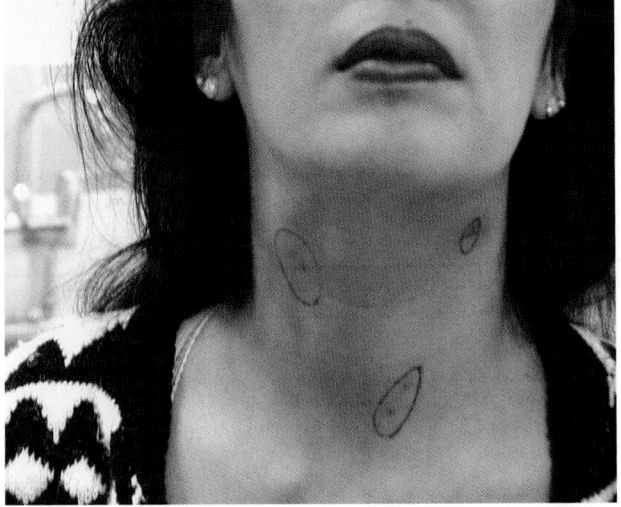

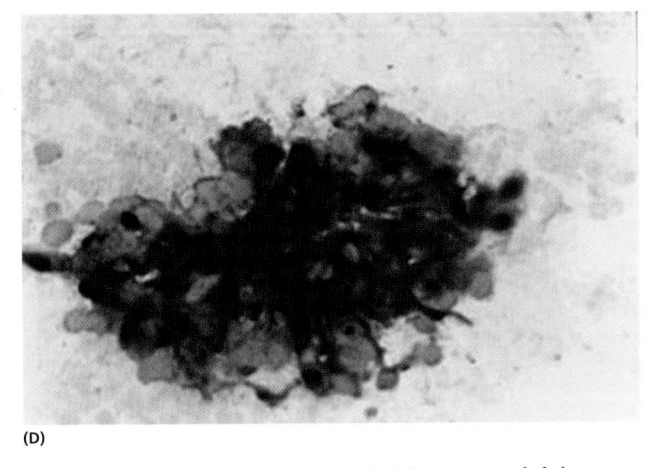

(C)

(D)

Figure 5.18 Carotid body tumour. (A) A 34-year-old patient presented with a painless swelling in the right side of the neck. (B) FNAC revealed clusters and discretely scattered cells, with occasional acinar/rosette configuration. Cells have round to oval nuclei with moderate to marked anisonucleosis, prominent nucleoli, intranuclear inclusions, abundant, delicate, poorly defined, vacuolated, slightly basophilic cytoplasm (MGG×400, ×600, oil immersion). Examination of the material with rapid stain in the clinic raised the suspicion of an endocrine tumour, in a young woman, possibly metastatic from thyroid. (C) Further examination of the patient revealed enlarged right lobe of thyroid and left jugulodigastric lymph node. FNAC were performed of both sites. Thyroid aspirate showed lymphocytic thyroiditis. Jugulodigastric node showed lymph node hyperplasia. Both lesions were unrelated to Carotid body tumour which was diagnosed after immunocytochemistry examination. (D) Synaptophysin positivity in carotid body tumour cells (IP×600, oil).

Differential diagnosis of aspirates of cervical paragangliomas, which may be difficult to interpret due to poor cellularity especially when intranuclear vacuoles are found, is papillary thyroid carcinoma [101] (see Chapter 3, Figs 3.24 and 3.25).

[See BOX 5.5. Summary of ultrasound features: carotid body tumor on www.wiley.com/go/kocjan/clinical_cytopathology_head_neck2e]

5.5.2 Epithelioid sarcoma-like hemangioendothelioma

Epithelioid sarcoma-like hemangioendothelioma is a distinctive, low-grade vascular tumour that closely mimics an epithelioid sarcoma because of growth in solid sheets and nests, the eosinophilia of the rounded to slightly spindled neoplastic cells and the diffuse, strong cytokeratin expression [102].

Cytological features: Oval, round and spindle, mainly discohesive malignant cells of variable size ranging from two to nine times the size of red cells (Fig. 5.20). Nuclei are eccentric, round to spindle shaped with large nucleoli or macronucleoli. Cytoplasm is moderate to abundant pale grey and vacuolated (intracytoplasmic lumina). Microacinar structures lined with abnormal spindle to polygonal cells are noted. The tumours are positive for cytokeratin, vimentin, CD31 and FLI-1, but negative for CD34 [102].

5.5.3 Meningioma

Extracranial extension of meningioma, although rare, is an important differential diagnosis of the head and neck masses [103].

The *cytological appearances* of meningioma in smears are very characteristic [104, 105] (Fig. 5.21). Cellular smears present a

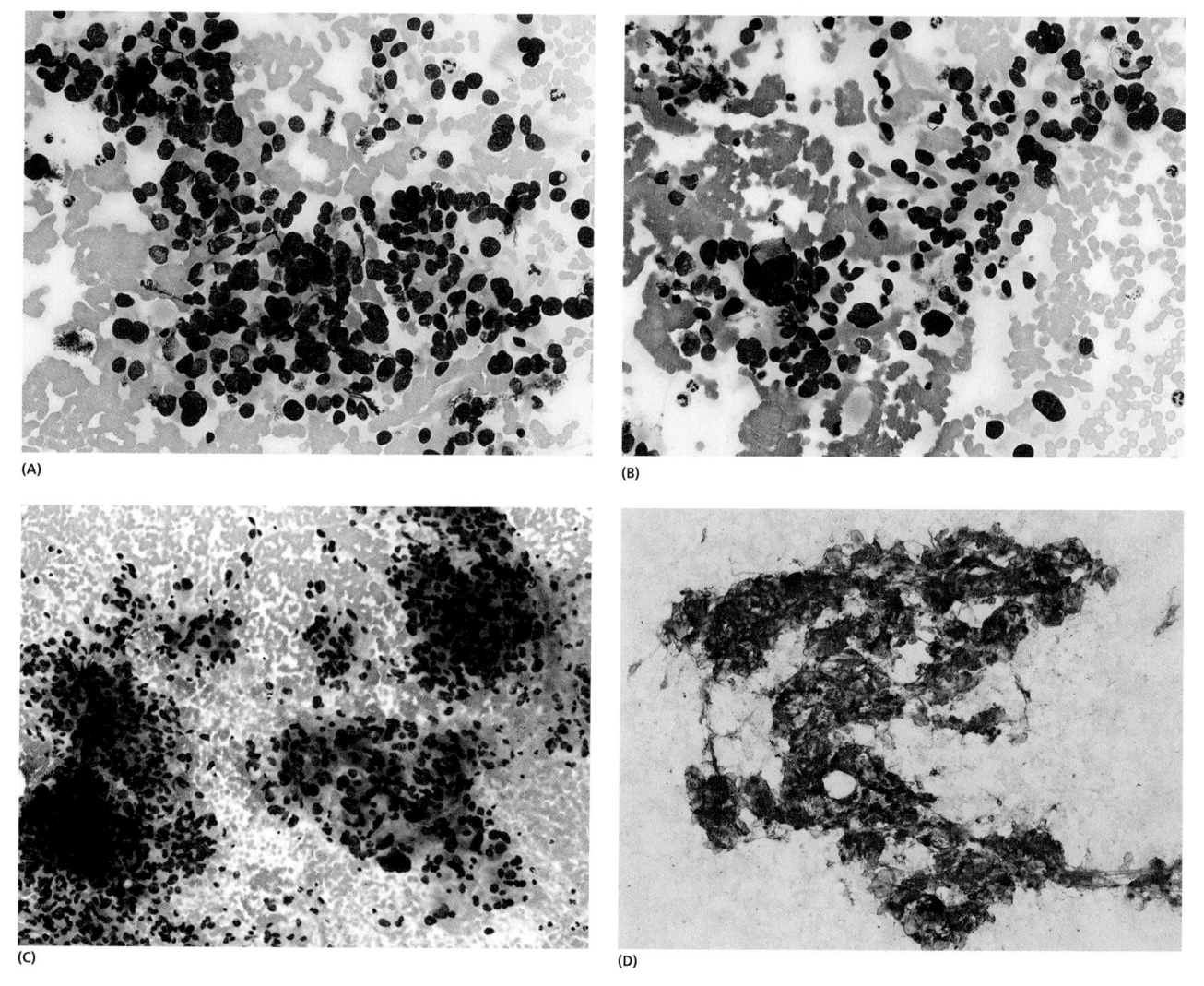

Figure 5.19 Carotid body tumour. (A, B, C) Anisonucleosis, which can be striking, may be mistaken for pleomorphism, and therefore misleading, since it does not imply malignancy. Malignant carotid body tumours have been described, presence of mitoses and necrosis is suspicious, but are extremely rare. (D) Strong chromogranin positivity helps confirm the diagnosis.

uniform appearance with cells appearing as cohesive groups and single discohesive cells in a clean background. Cells have round and oval nuclei and poorly outlined cytoplasm. Nuclei have intranuclear vacuoles [106, 107]. Chromatin is evenly distributed and nucleoli are not prominent. Psammoma bodies, although characteristic, are not always seen [108]. A specific type of meningioma that produces a highly specific appearance on smear is a secretory meningioma. This is characterised by numerous large, round cytoplasmic inclusions that dominate the smear. These inclusions are positive for CEA [109, 110]. Meningiomas frequently show degenerative changes, usually xanthomatous degeneration and may contain foamy macrophages. Fibroblastic meningiomas may show collagen fibres in the background, which may resemble cell processes. Atypical meningiomas are characterised by marked pleomorphism of cells with hyperchromasia and a background of necrosis and haemorrhage [106, 111, 112]. In difficult cases, intranuclear inclusions help differentiate it from other tumours and this is a helpful diagnostic feature. Meningiomas are positive for vimentin and negative for EMA and GFAP (glial fibrillary acid protein).

Differential diagnosis in the neck includes soft tissue tumours and metastatic carcinoma [113, 114].

5.5.4 Ethmoid sinus intestinal type adenocarcinoma

Intestinal-type adenocarcinoma (ITAC) of the ethmoid sinus is a rare, occupational-related tumour showing higher incidence in woodworkers, with frequent local recurrence and invasiveness in the skull base. Histologically, they are peculiar by the predominance of the adenocarcinomas, especially of colonic or enteric type. Squamous carcinoma and adenoid cystic carcinoma are less frequent than in other parts of the sinonasal tract. Rare other tumours, often undifferentiated, include esthesioneuroblastomas, malignant melanomas, neuro-endocrine carcinomas, malignant lymphomas or sarcomas [115].

Ethmoid sinus adenocarcinomas have a tendency for extensive local invasion but a low propensity for lymphatic and hematogenous spread. Hence, local recurrence is the main cause of cancer-related death [116–118]. Direct leptomeningeal spread may occur through

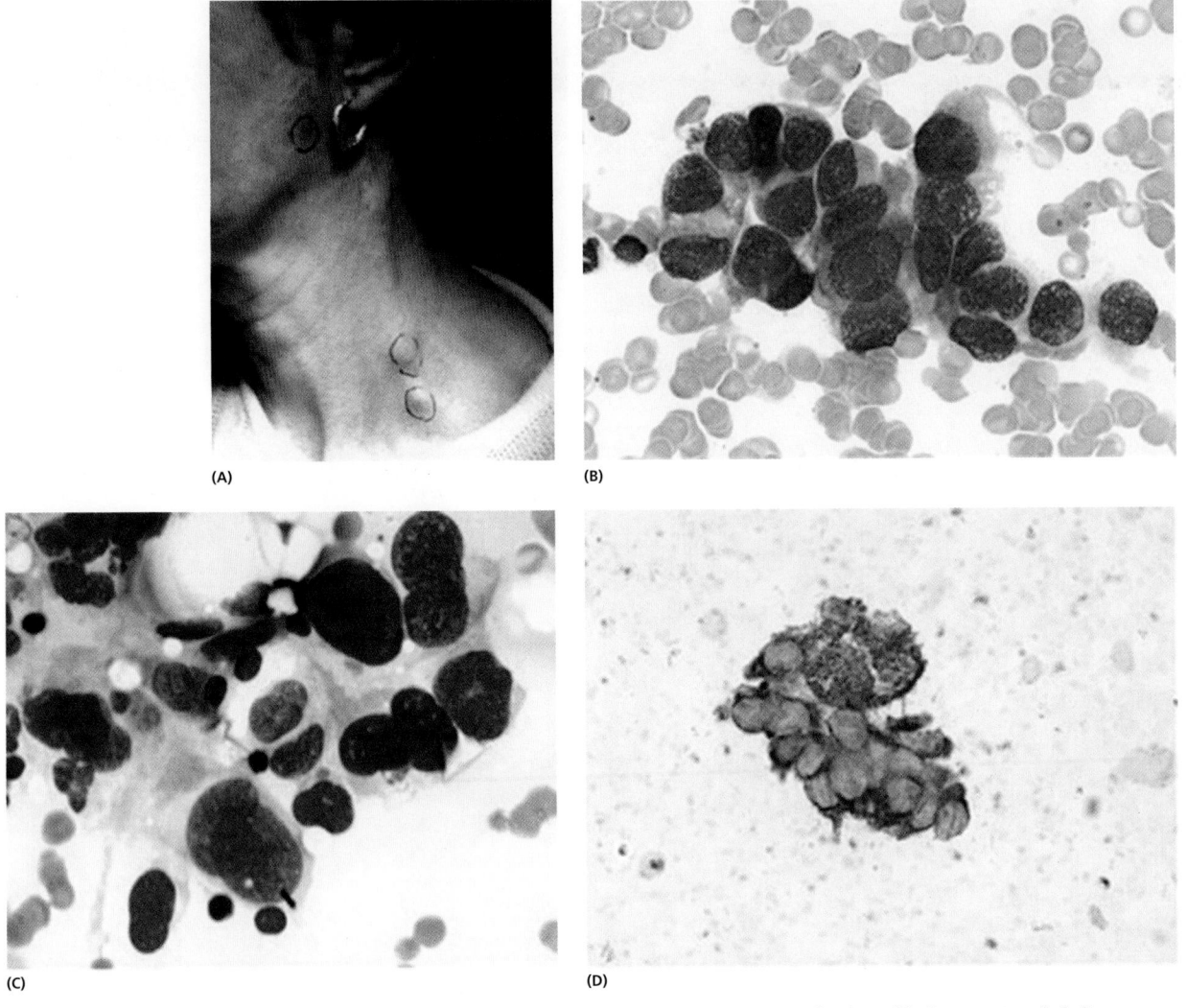

Figure 5.20 Epithelioid sarcoma-like haemangioendothelioma. (A) Patient with neck nodes and history of scalp ES-like haemangioendothelioma. (B) Oval, round and spindle, mainly discohesive cells of variable size ranging from two to nine times the size of red cells. (C) Nuclei are eccentric, round to spindle shaped with large nucleoli or macronucleoli. Cytoplasm is moderate to abundant pale grey and vacuolated (intracytoplasmic lumina). Microacinar structures lined with abnormal spindle to polygonal cells are noted (MGG×600, oil). (D) Immunocytochemistry for KSHV is positive (KS 9.9, IP×600, oil).

the cribriform plate to the CSF [119]. Histologically, the low-grade lesions have a well-developed glandular pattern throughout, very uniform nuclei, and minimal mitotic activity. The high-grade tumours have a less uniform glandular pattern, commonly with solid or sheet-like areas, manifested nuclear pleomorphism, and generally a higher mitotic rate. The low-grade group has a prognosis markedly better than the high-grade group. Since the literature tends to consider all sinonasal adenocarcinomas as relentlessly progressive neoplasms with poor prognosis, it is important to recognise this category of low grade neoplasm in order that treatment and prognosis can be better related to their behaviour [120].

Cytological features: The low grade tumours have relatively uniform large cells arranged in aggregates or singly, with medium-sized, eccentric nuclei, prominent nucleoli and a moderate amount of well-defined cytoplasm (Fig. 5.22). Cytological diagnosis is usually made from cervical lymph node metastases in cases of a known primary tumour. Otherwise, differential diagnosis may include any metastatic adenocarcinoma.

5.5.5 Granular cell tumour

Granular cell tumour is an uncommon benign neoplasm commonly arising in the tongue, gastrointestinal tract, mediastinum, skin and subcutaneous tissue, breast, and other sites in the middle-aged adults. Formerly known as Abrikossoff tumour or granular cell myoblastoma, it is rarely encountered in the FNAC service. However, if recognised, cytology is a good way of diagnosing these unusual and indolent tumours [121, 122].

Cytological features: The tumour cells have round to oval nuclei, inconspicuous nucleoli, and abundant granular cytoplasm (Fig. 5.23). Because of the fragility of tumour cells, smears often contain stripped nuclei in a background of finely granular material. Nuclei are small and dark but occasionally with mild to moderate atypia. The tumour cells stain for S-100 protein, NSE, CD68 and inhibin contain PAS positive diastase-resistant cytoplasmic granules representing the phagolysosomes. Malignant

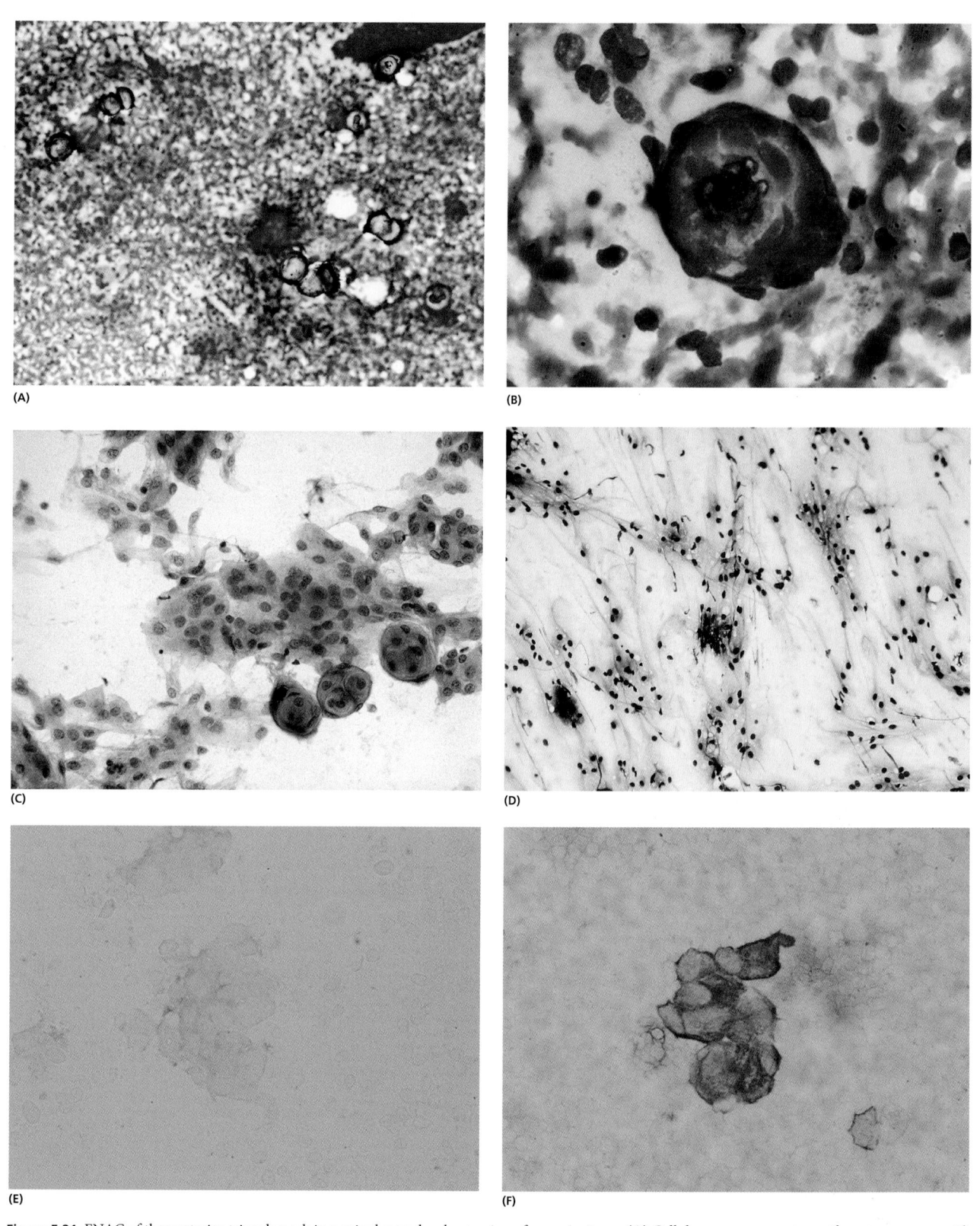

Figure 5.21 FNAC of the posterior triangle neck in a spinal extradural extension of a meningioma. (A) Cellular smears present a uniform appearance with cells appearing as cohesive groups and single discohesive cells in a clean background (×200, MGG). (B) Cells appear to form whorls and concentric laminations of psammoma bodies. Psammoma bodies, although characteristic, are not always seen (MGG ×600). (C) Different case. Intraoperative smear from an intracranial meningioma stained with toluidine blue reveals cell whorls and mast cells. (D) Different case. FNAC of a scalp lesion reveals bland nuclei and numerous cytoplasmic processes. (E) Immunocytochemistry shows meningioma cells to be EMA negative. (F) Vimentin positive cells of meningioma.

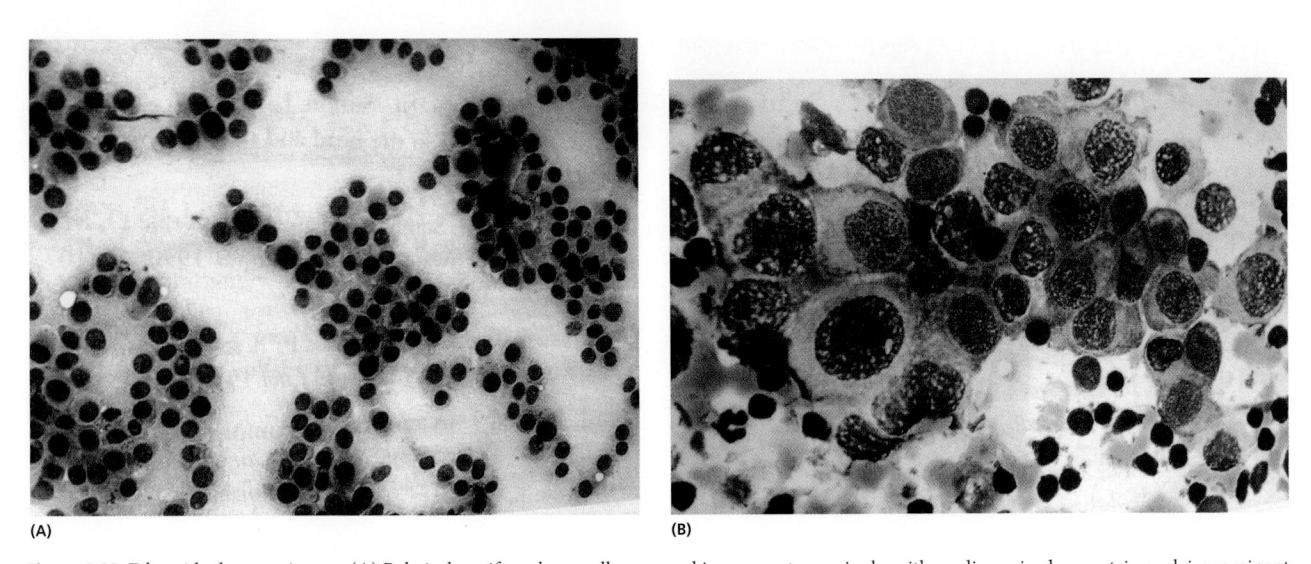

(A)

(B)

Figure 5.22 Ethmoid adenocarcinoma. (A) Relatively uniform large cells arranged in aggregates or singly, with medium-sized, eccentric nuclei, prominent nucleoli and a moderate amount of well-defined cytoplasm against a background of lymphocytes (MGG ×600, oil immersion). (B) Another case of ethmoid adenocarcinoma. High power view. Epithelial cells have a high N/C ratio, eccentric nuclei and prominent nucleoli (MGG ×600 oil immersion). Evidence of attempted gland formation is helpful.

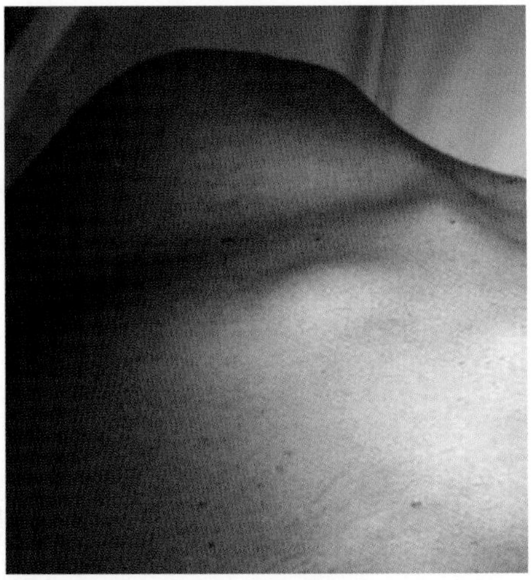

(A)

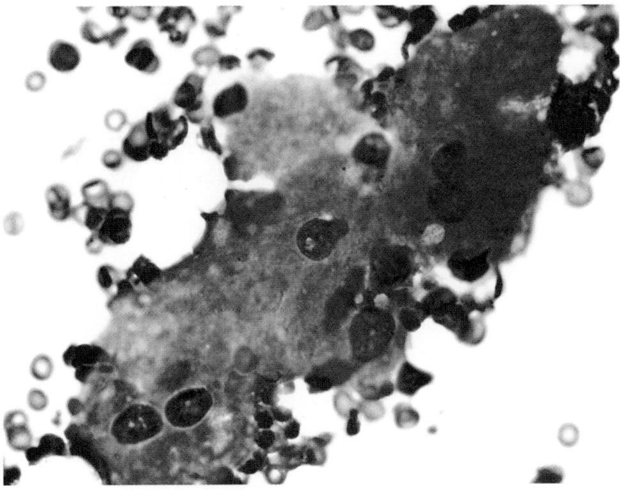

(B)

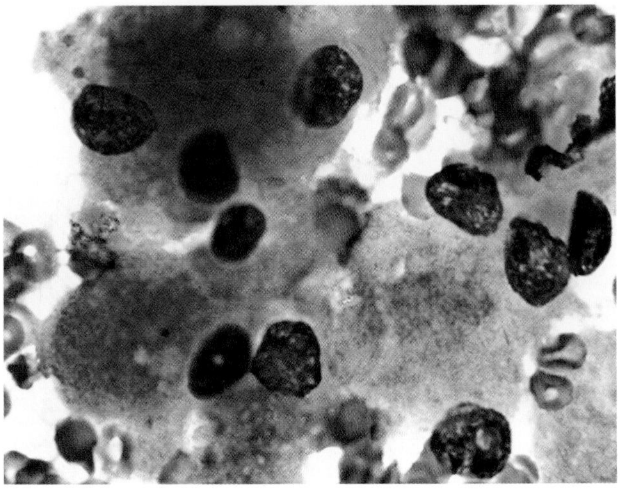

(C)

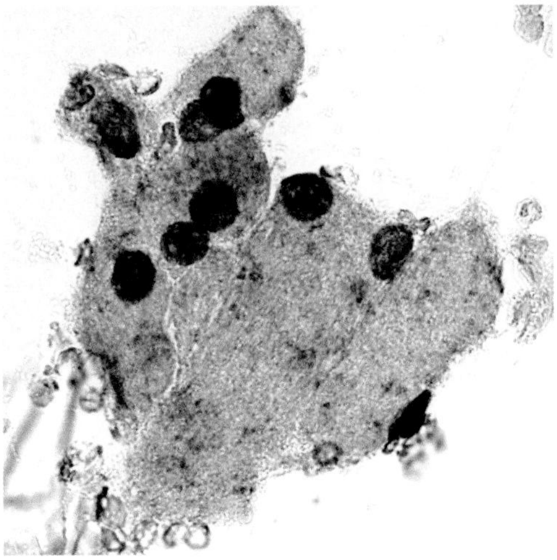

(D)

Figure 5.23 Granular cell tumour. (A) Firm swellings in the subcutaneous tissues. (B) Cells have round to oval nuclei, inconspicuous nucleoli and abundant granular cytoplasm. (C) Smears often contain stripped nuclei in a background of finely granular material. (D) The tumour cells stain for S-100 protein.

granular cell tumours are very rare and smears show morphologic criteria of malignancy such as predominance of pleomorphic spindle cells with large nucleoli, mitoses and necrosis. Differential diagnosis includes hibernoma, adult rhabdomyoma and alveolar soft part sarcoma.

This chapter also has online only material. Ultrasound Summary boxes, which have been cited throughout the chapter text as 'Summary of ultrasound features', are available on www.wiley.com/go/kocjan/clinical_cytopathology_head_neck2e for the following diseases:

Box 5.1 Summary of ultrasound features: **Lipoma**
Box 5.2 Summary of ultrasound features: **Thyroglossal cyst**
Box 5.3 Summary of ultrasound features: **Epidermoid cyst**
Box 5.4 Summary of ultrasound features: **Lymphangioma**
Box 5.5 Summary of ultrasound features: **carotid body tumor**

References

1. Agarwal S, Nangia A, Jyotsna PL, Pujani M. Spindle cell lipoma masquerading as lipomatous pleomorphic adenoma: A diagnostic dilemma on fine needle aspiration cytology. *J Cytol.* 2013 Jan; **30**(1): 55–7.
2. Guo Z, Voytovich M, Kurtycz DF, Hoerl HD. Fine-needle aspiration diagnosis of spindle-cell lipoma: a case report and review of the literature. *Diagn Cytopathol.* 2000 Nov; **23**(5): 362–5.
3. Kapila K, Ghosal N, Gill SS, Verma K. Cytomorphology of lipomatous tumors of soft tissue. *Acta Cytol.* 2003; **47**(4): 555–62.
4. Akerman M. *Fine needle aspiration cytopathology.* 1st edn. Oxford: Blackwell Scientific Publications, 1993.
5. Rajalakshmi V, Selvambigai G, Jaiganesh. Cytomorphology of fibromatosis colli. *J Cytol.* 2009 Jan; **26**(1): 41–2.
6. Khan S, Jetley S, Jairajpuri Z, Husain M. Fibromatosis colli – a rare cytological diagnosis in infantile neck swellings. *J Clin Diagn Res* 2014 Nov; **8**(11): FD08–9. doi: 10.7860/JCDR/2014/10840.5154. Epub 2014 Nov 20.
7. Domanski HA. *Atlas of fine needle aspiration cytology.* Springer, 2014, p. 399.
8. Raab SS, Silverman JF, McLeod DL, et al. Fine needle aspiration biopsy of fibromatoses. *Acta Cytol.* 1993; **37**(3): 323–8.
9. Stanley MW, Skoog L, Tani EM, Horwitz CA. Nodular fasciitis: spontaneous resolution following diagnosis by fine-needle aspiration. *Diagn Cytopathol* 1993; **9**(3): 322–4.
10. Sinhasan SP, Bhat RV KVB, Hartimath BC. Intra–muscular nodular fasciitis presenting as swelling in neck: challenging entity for diagnosis. *Journal of Clinical and Diagnostic Research: JCDR.* 2014; **8**(1): 155–7.
11. Silvanto AM, Melly L, Hannan SA, Kocjan G. FNAC of nodular fasciitis mimicking a pleomorphic adenoma: another diagnostic pitfall. *Cytopathol* 2010; **21**(4): 276–7.
12. Jain D, Khurana N, Jain S. Nodular fasciitis of the external ear masquerading as pleomorphic adenoma: A potential diagnostic pitfall in fine needle aspiration cytology. *Cytojournal.* 2008; **5**: 14.
13. Borumandi F, Cascarini L, Mallawaarachchi R, Sandison A. The chameleon in the neck: Nodular fasciitis mimicking malignant neck mass of unknown primary. *International Journal of Surgery Case Reports.* 2012; **3**(10): 501–3.
14. Stanley MW, Skoog L, Tani EM, Horwitz CA. Nodular fasciitis: spontaneous resolution following diagnosis by fine-needle aspiration. *Diagn Cytopathol* 1993; **9**(3): 322–4.
15. Dahl I, Akerman M. Nodular fasciitis a correlative cytologic and histologic study of 13 cases. *Acta Cytol* 1981; **25**(3): 215–23.
16. Wong NL, Di F. Pseudosarcomatous fasciitis and myositis: diagnosis by fine-needle aspiration cytology. *Am J Clin Pathol.* 2009 Dec; **132**(6): 857–65.
17. Kilpatrick SE, Ward WG, Chauvenet AR, Pettenati MJ. The role of fine-needle aspiration biopsy in the initial diagnosis of pediatric bone and soft tissue tumors: an institutional experience. *Mod Pathol* 1998; **11**(10): 923–8.
18. Samet A, Podoshin L, Fradis M, et al. Unusual sites of schwannoma in the head and neck. *J Laryngol Otol* 1985; **99**(5): 523–8.
19. Bianchini E, Mazzolari MG, Squillaci S, et al. Benign intraparotid schwannoma. *Pathologica* 1990; **82**(1079): 303–7.
20. Helidonis E, Dokianakis G, Pantazopoulos P. A schwannoma of the parotid gland. Report of a case. *J Laryngol Otol* 1978; **92**(9): 833–8.
21. Kuczkowski J, Jagielski J. A case of schwannoma in the parotid gland. *Otolaryngol Pol* 1997; **51**(3): 324–7.
22. Jayaraj SM, Levine T, Frosh AC, Almeyda JS. Ancient schwannoma masquerading as parotid pleomorphic adenoma. *J Laryngol Otol* 1997; **111**(11): 1088–90.
23. Shah HK, Kantharia C, Shenoy AS. Intraparotid facial nerve schwannoma. *J Postgrad Med* 1997; **43**(1): 14–5.
24. Elahi MM, Audet N, Rochon L, Black MJ. Intraparotid facial nerve schwannoma. *J Otolaryngol* 1995; **24**(6): 364–7.
25. Avery AP, Sprinkle PM. Benign intraparotid schwannomas. *Laryngoscope* 1972; **82**(2): 199–203.
26. Claros P, Knaster J, Weinberg P, Claros A. Parotid schwannoma. *Acta Otorrinolaringol Esp* 1994; **45**(4): 295–8.
27. Domanski HA1, Akerman M, Engellau J, et al. Fine-needle aspiration of neurilemoma (schwannoma). A clinicocytopathologic study of 116 patients. *Diagn Cytopathol* 2006 Jun; **34**(6): 403–12.
28. Senthilkumar R, Neville JF, Aravind R. Malignant thyroglossal duct cyst with synchronous occult thyroid gland papillary carcinoma. *Indian J Endocrinol Metab* 2013 Sep; **17**(5): 936–8.
29. Albayrak Y, Albayrak F, Kaya Z, et al. A case of papillary carcinoma in a thyroglossal cyst without a carcinoma in the thyroid gland. *Diagn Cytopathol* 2011 Jan; **39**(1): 38–41.
30. Agarwal K, Puri V, Singh S. Critical appraisal of FNAC in the diagnosis of primary papillary carcinoma arising in thyroglossal cyst: A case report with review of the literature on FNAC and its diagnostic pitfalls. *J Cytol* 2010 Jan; **27**(1): 22–5.
31. Cannizzaro MA, Costanzo M, Fiorenza G, et al. Papillary carcinoma in an isthmic thyroglossal duct cyst: clinical considerations. *Chir Ital* 2006 Jan–Feb; **58**(1): 105–11.
32. Köybaşioğlu F, Simşek GG, Onal BU. Tall cell variant of papillary carcinomaarising from a thyroglossal cyst: report of a case with diagnosis by fine needle aspiration cytology. *Acta Cytol* 2006 Mar–Apr; **50**(2): 221–4.
33. Zajicek J. *Aspiration biopsy cytology.* Stockholm, Sweden, 1974.
34. Ramos-Gabatin A, Watzinger W. Fine needle aspiration and cytology in the preoperative diagnosis of branchial cyst. *South Med J* 1984; **77**(9): 1187–9.
35. Warson F, Blommaert D, De Roy G. Inflamed branchial cyst: a potential pitfall in aspiration cytology [letter]. *Acta Cytol* 1986; **30**(2): 201–2.
36. Holmes BJ, Westra WH. The expanding role of cytopathology in the diagnosis of HPV-related squamous cell carcinoma of the head and neck. *Diagn Cytopathol.* 2014 Jan; **42**(1): 85–93.
36a. Roy-Chowdhuri S, Krishnamurthy S. The role of cytology in the era of HPV-related head and neck carcinoma. *Semin Diagn Pathol.* 2015 Jul; **32**(4): 250–7.
36b. Takes RP, Kaanders JH, van Herpen CM, Merkx MA, Slootweg PJ, Melchers WJ. Human papillomavirus detection in fine needle aspiration cytology of lymph node metastasis of head and neck squamous cell cancer. *J Clin Virol.* 2016; **85**: 22–26.
37. De Las Casas LE, Bardales RH. Fine-needle aspiration cytology of mucous retention cyst of the tongue: distinction from other cystic lesions of the tongue. *Diagn Cytopathol* 2000 May; **22**(5): 308–12.
38. August M, Faquin WC, Ferraro NF, Kaban LB. Fine-needle aspiration biopsy of intraosseous jaw lesions. *J Oral Maxillofac Surg* 1999; **57**(11): 1282–6; discussion 1287.
39. Gunhan O, Demirel D, Sengun O, et al. Cementifying fibroma diagnosed by fine needle aspiration cytology. A case report. *Acta Cytol* 1992; **36**(1): 98–100.
40. Carrillo R, Cuesta C, Rodriguez-Peralto JL, Marin J. Ameloblastic fibroma. Report of a case with fine needle aspiration cytologic findings. *Acta Cytol* 1992; **36**(4): 537–40.
41. Gunhan O, Finci R, Celasun B, Demiriz M. A case of ameloblastoma diagnosed by fine-needle aspiration cytology. *J Nihon Univ Sch Dent* 1989; **31**(4): 565–9.
42. Layfield LJ, Ferreiro JA. Fine-needle aspiration cytology of chondromyoid fibroma: a case report. *Diagn Cytopathol* 1988; **4**(2): 148–51.
43. Chandavarkar V, Uma K, Mishra M, et al. Ameloblastoma: Cytopathologic profile of 12 cases and literature review. *J Cytol.* 2014 Jul; **31**(3): 161–4.
43a. Wang YP. *J Formos Med Assoc.* 2009 Apr; **108**(4): 286–92.
44. Gunhan O, Dogan N, Celasun B, et al. Fine needle aspiration cytology of oral cavity and jaw bone lesions. A report of 102 cases. *Acta Cytol* 1993; **37**(2): 135–41.
45. DeRaimo AJ, Kane RA, Katz JF, Rolla AP. Parathyroid cyst: diagnosis by sonography and needle aspiration. *AJR Am J Roentgenol* 1984; **142**(6): 1227–8.
46. Patel KD, Rege JD, Varthakavi PK, et al. Fine needle aspiration of an unsuspected parathyroid cyst. *J Assoc Physicians India* 1995; **43**(11): 791.
46a. Pontikides N, Karras S, Kaprara A, Cheva A, Doumas A, Botsios D, Moschidis A, Efthimiou E, Wass J, Krassas G. Diagnostic and therapeutic review of cystic parathyroid lesions. *Hormones (Athens).* 2012 Oct–Dec; **11**(4): 410–8.
47. Shepard KA, Miller JD. Cervical thymic cyst. A consideration in the differential diagnosis of neck masses. *J Maine Med Assoc* 1973; **64**(1): 3–4.

48. Engzell U, Zajicek J. Aspiration biopsy of tumors of the neck. I. Aspiration biopsy and cytologic findings in 100 cases of congenital cysts. *Acta Cytol* 1970; **14**(2): 51-7.

49. Frierson HF, Jr. Cysts of the head and neck sampled by fine-needle aspiration: sources of diagnostic difficulty [editorial; comment]. *Am J Clin Pathol* 1996; **106**(5): 559-60.

50. Ravinsky E, Safneck JR, Quinonez G, Yazdi HM. Fine needle aspiration biopsy of a small round cell tumor exhibiting both neural and myogenic differentiation. A case report. *Acta Cytol* 1997; **41**(4 Suppl): 1320-4.

51. Powers CN, Berardo MD, Frable WJ. Fine-needle aspiration biopsy: pitfalls in the diagnosis of spindle-cell lesions. *Diagn Cytopathol* 1994; **10**(3): 232-40; discussion 241.

52. BJ OH, Ehya H, Shields JA, et al. Fine needle aspiration biopsy in pediatric ophthalmic tumors and pseudotumors. *Acta Cytol* 1993; **37**(2):1 25-30.

53. Akhtar M, Ali MA, Sabbah R, et al. Fine-needle aspiration biopsy diagnosis of round cell malignant tumors of childhood. A combined light and electron microscopic approach. *Cancer* 1985; **55**(8): 1805-17.

54. De Lutiis MA, Pizzicannella G, Artese L. Embryonal rhabdomyosarcoma of the eye: cytological diagnosis by fine needle aspiration. *Pathologica* 1991; **83**(1083): 75-9.

55. Salomao DR, Sigman JD, Greenebaum E, Cohen MB. Rhabdomyosarcoma presenting as a parotid gland mass in pediatric patients: fine-needle aspiration biopsy findings. *Cancer* 1998; **84**(4): 245-51.

56. de Almeida M, Stastny JF, Wakely PE, Jr., Frable WJ. Fine-needle aspiration biopsy of childhood rhabdomyosarcoma: reevaluation of the cytologic criteria for diagnosis. *Diagn Cytopathol* 1994; **11**(3): 231-6.

57. Akhtar M, Ali MA, Bakry M, et al. Fine-needle aspiration biopsy diagnosis of rhabdomyosarcoma: cytologic, histologic, and ultrastructural correlations. *Diagn Cytopathol* 1992; **8**(5): 465-74.

58. Henkes DN, Stein N. Fine-needle aspiration cytology of prostatic embryonal rhabdomyosarcoma: a case report. *Diagn Cytopathol* 1987; **3**(2): 163-5.

59. Mazzoleni S, Stellini E, Infantolino D, Favero GA. A case of embryonal rhabdomyosarcoma of the cheek in adolescence. Its cytological diagnosis by fine-needle aspiration via the gingival fornix. *Minerva Stomatol* 1994; **43**(1-2): 43-7.

60. Kumar PV, Kazemi H, Khezri A. Testicular embryonal rhabdomyosarcoma diagnosed by fine needle aspiration cytology. A report of two cases. *Acta Cytol* 1994; **38**(4): 573-6.

61. Seidal T, Walaas L, Kindblom LG, Angervall L. Cytology of embryonal rhabdomyosarcoma: a cytologic, light microscopic, electron microscopic, and immunohistochemical study of seven cases. *Diagn Cytopathol* 1988; **4**(4): 292-9.

62. Agarwal PK, Srivastava A, Mathur N, et al. Fine needle aspiration of poorly differentiated rhabdomyosarcoma presenting with quadriparesis. A case report. *Acta Cytol* 1996; **40**(5): 985-8.

63. Nishikawa A, Tanaka T, Kanai N, et al. Exfoliative cytopathology of alveolar rhabdomyosarcoma. *Acta Pathol Jpn* 1987; **37**(6): 1003-7.

64. Torres V, Ferrer R. Cytology of fine needle aspiration biopsy of primary breast rhabdomyosarcoma in an adolescent girl. *Acta Cytol* 1985; **29**(3): 430-4.

65. Atahan S, Aksu O, Ekinci C. Cytologic diagnosis and subtyping of rhabdomyosarcoma. *Cytopathology* 1998; **9**(6): 389-97.

66. Kushner BH, LaQuaglia MP, Cheung NK, et al. Clinically critical impact of molecular genetic studies in pediatric solid tumors. *Med Pediatr Oncol* 1999; **33**(6): 530-5.

67. Dias P, Chen B, Dilday B, et al. Strong immunostaining for myogenin in rhabdomyosarcoma is significantly associated with tumors of the alveolar subclass. *Am J Pathol* 2000 Feb; **156**(2): 399-408.

68. Dal Cin P, Qian X, Cibas ES. The marriage of cytology and cytogenetics. *Cancer Cytopathol* 2013; **121**: 279-90.

69. Renard C1, Ranchère-Vince D2. Ewing/PNET sarcoma family of tumors: Towards a new paradigm? *Ann Pathol* 2015 Jan; **35**(1): 86-97.

70. Bakhos R, Andrey J, Bhoopalam N, et al. Fine-needle aspiration cytology of extraskeletal Ewing's sarcoma. *Diagn Cytopathol* 1998; **18**(2): 137-40.

71. Collins BT, Cramer HM, Frain BE, Davis MM. Fine-needle aspiration biopsy of metastatic Ewing's sarcoma with MIC2 (CD99) immunocytochemistry. *Diagn Cytopathol* 1998; **19**(5): 382-4.

72. Cohen MC, Pollono D, Tomarchio SA, Drut R. Cytologic characteristics of peripheral neuroectodermal tumors in fine-needle aspiration smears: a retrospective study of three pediatric cases. *Diagn Cytopathol* 1997; **16**(6): 513-7.

73. Guiter GE, Gamboni MM, Zakowski MF. The cytology of extraskeletal Ewing sarcoma. *Cancer* 1999; **87**(3): 141-8.

74. Renshaw AA, Perez-Atayde AR, Fletcher JA, Granter SR. Cytology of typical and atypical Ewing's sarcoma/PNET [see comments]. *Am J Clin Pathol* 1996; **106**(5): 620-4.

75. Kontozoglou T, Krakauer K, Qizilbash AH. Ewing's sarcoma. Cytologic features in fine needle aspirates in two cases. *Acta Cytol* 1986; **30**(5): 513-8.

76. Dahl I, Akerman M, Angervall L. Ewing's sarcoma of bone. A correlative cytological and histological study of 14 cases. *Acta Pathol Microbiol Immunol Scand [A]* 1986; **94**(6): 363-9.

77. Brehaut LE, Anderson LH, Taylor DA. Extraskeletal Ewing's sarcoma. Diagnosis of a case by fine needle aspiration cytology. *Acta Cytol* 1986; **30**(6): 683-7.

78. Meister P, Gokel JM. Extraskeletal Ewing's sarcoma. *Virchows Arch A Pathol Pathol Anat* 1978; **378**(2): 173-9.

79. Jelen M, Wozniak Z, Rak J. Cytologic appearance of esthesioneuroblastoma in a fine needle aspirate. *Acta Cytol* 1988; **32**(3): 377-80.

80. Jobst SB, Ljung BM, Gilkey FN, Rosenthal DL. Cytologic diagnosis of olfactory neuroblastoma. Report of a case with multiple diagnostic parameters. *Acta Cytol* 1983; **27**(3): 299-305.

81. Singhal N, Mundi IK, Handa U, et al. FNA in diagnosis of orbital lesions causing proptosis in adults. *Diagn Cytopathol*. 2012 Oct; **40**(10): 861-4.

82. Akinfolarin J, Jazaerly T, Jones K, et al. Fine needle aspiration cytology of primary sphenoid sinus esthesioneuroblastoma metastatic to the skin. *Avicenna J Med* 2012; Jan; **2**(1): 15-8. doi: 10.4103/2231-0770.94806.

83. Collins BT, Cramer HM, Hearn SA. Fine needle aspiration cytology of metastatic olfactory neuroblastoma. *Acta Cytol* 1997; **41**(3): 802-10.

84. Logrono R, Futoran RM, Hartig G, Inhorn SL. Olfactory neuroblastoma (esthesioneuroblastoma): appearance on fine-needle aspiration: report of a case. *Diagn Cytopathol* 1997; **17**(3): 205-8.

85. Buley I. *Diagnostic cytopathology*. 1st edn. London: Churchill Livingstone, 1995.

86. Masilamani S, Duvuru P, Sundaram S. Fine needle aspiration cytology diagnosis of a case of carotid body tumour. *Singapore Med J* 2012 Feb; **53**(2): e35-7.

87. Rosa M, Sahoo S. Bilateral carotid body tumour: The role of fine-needle aspiration biopsy in the preoperative diagnosis. *Diagn Cytopathol* 2008; **36**: 178-80.

88. Jayaram G, Kaliaperumal S, Kumar G. Bilateral carotid body tumour diagnosed on cytology. *Acta Cytol* 2005; **49**: 690-2.

89. Fleming MV, Oertel YC, Rodriguez ER, Fidler WJ. Fine-needle aspiration of six carotid body paragangliomas. *Diagn Cytopathol* 1993; **9**(5): 510-5.

90. Mincione GP, Urso C. Carotid body paraganglioma (chemodectoma): cytologic remarks. *Pathologica* 1989; **81**(1072): 179-83.

91. Engzell U, Franzen S, Zajicek J. Aspiration biopsy of tumors of the neck. II. Cytologic findings in 13 cases of carotid body tumor. *Acta Cytol* 1971; **15**(1): 25-30.

92. Papanicolaou S, Daskalopoulos Z. Carotid body tumor: report of a case. *J Oral Med* 1986; **41**(3): 204-6, 209.

93. Nickel AA, Jr., Roser SM. Carotid body tumors. *J Oral Med* 1977; **32**(3): 64-6.

94. Krishnamurthy SC, Gopinath KS, Rao RS, Talvalkar GV. Carotid body tumour – a clinicopathologic study of 10 cases. *Indian J Cancer* 1981; **18**(4): 245-9.

95. Kapoor R, Saha MM, Das DK, et al. Carotid body tumor initially diagnosed by fine needle aspiration cytology [letter]. *Acta Cytol* 1989; **33**(5): 682-3.

96. Chen LT, Hwang WS. Fine needle aspiration of carotid body paraganglioma [letter]. *Acta Cytol* 1989; **33**(5): 681-2.

97. Mincione G, Urso C. Fine needle aspiration cytologic findings in a case of carotid body paraganglioma (chemodectoma) [letter]. *Acta Cytol* 1989; **33**(5): 679-81.

98. Rana RS, Dey P, Das A. Fine needle aspiration (FNA) cytology of extra-adrenal paragangliomas. *Cytopathology* 1997; **8**(2): 108-13.

99. Kapila K, Tewari MC, Verma K. Paragangliomas – a diagnostic dilemma on fine needle aspirates. *Indian J Cancer* 1993;3 0(4): 152-7.

100. Rao KS, Prasad AS, Rao AS. Malignant carotid body tumour. *Indian J Pathol Bacteriol* 1968; **11**(3): 207-9.

101. Jacobs DM, Waisman J. Cervical paraganglioma with intranuclear vacuoles in a fine needle aspirate. *Acta Cytol* 1987; **31**(1): 29-32.

102. Billings SD, Folpe AL, Weiss SW. Epithelioid sarcoma-like hemangioendothelioma. *Am J Surg Pathol*. 2003; **27**(1): 48-57.

103. Saade R, Hessel A, Ginsberg L, et al. Primary extradural meningioma presenting as a neck mass: Case report and review of the literature. *Head Neck*. 2015; **37**(8): E92-5.

104. Agrawal M, Chandrakar SK, Lokwani D, Purohit MR. Squash cytology in neurosurgical practice: a useful method in resource-limited setting with lack of frozen section facility. *J Clin Diagn Res*. 2014 Oct; **8**(10): FC09-12.

105. Nguyen GK, Johnson ES, Mielke BW. Cytology of meningiomas and neurilemomas in crush preparations. A useful adjunct to frozen section diagnosis. *Acta Cytol* 1988; **32**(3): 362-6.

106. Vogelsang PJ, Nguyen GK, Mielke BW. Cytology of atypical and malignant meningiomas in intraoperative crush preparations [see comments]. *Acta Cytol* 1993; **37**(6): 884-8.

107. Janisch W, Schreiber D. Morphological findings in the cell nuclei of meningiomas and neurinomas. *Zentralbl Allg Pathol* 1965; **108**(3): 268-76.

108. Cerda-Nicolas M, Piquer J, Peydro A, et al. Cytology of meningiomas. Morphological study of 23 cases. Correlation with the histopathology. *Arch Neurobiol (Madr)* 1988; **51**(6): 342-8.

109. Hinton DR, Kovacs K, Chandrasoma PT. Cytologic features of secretory meningioma. *Acta Cytol* 1999; **43**(2): 121-5.

110. Imlay SP, Snider TE, Raab SS. Clear-cell meningioma: diagnosis by fine-needle aspiration biopsy. *Diagn Cytopathol* 1998; **18**(2): 131-6.

111. Maier H, Ofner D, Hittmair A, et al. Classic, atypical, and anaplastic meningioma: three histopathological subtypes of clinical relevance. *J Neurosurg* 1992; **77**(4): 616–23.

112. Riazmontazer N, Bedayat G. Cytodiagnosis of meningioma with atypical cytologic features. *Acta Cytol* 1991; **35**(5): 501–4.

113. Kobayashi S. Meningioma, neurilemmoma and astrocytoma specimens obtained with the squash method for cytodiagnosis. A cytologic and immunochemical study [see comments]. *Acta Cytol* 1993; **37**(6): 913–22.

114. Kudo M, Mikami T, Maeda Y. Reticulin fiber staining of crush preparations for the rapid differentiation between schwannomas and meningiomas. *Acta Cytol* 1991; **35**(5): 521–3.

115. Carnot F. Histological aspects of naso-ethmoidal tumors. *Neurochirurgie* 1997; **43**(2): 64–7.

116. Gaillard J, Haguenauer JP, Pignat JC, Long C. Plurifocality and concept of recurrence in ethmoido-nasal glandular cancers. *Rev Laryngol Otol Rhinol (Bord)* 1988; **109**(1): 31–3.

117. Jiang GL, Morrison WH, Garden AS, et al. Ethmoid sinus carcinomas: natural history and treatment results. *Radiother Oncol* 1998; **49**(1): 21–7.

118. Harbo G, Grau C, Bundgaard T, et al. Cancer of the nasal cavity and paranasal sinuses. A clinico-pathological study of 277 patients. *Acta Oncol* 1997; **36**(1): 45–50.

119. Devos A, Lemmerling M, Vanrietvelde F, et al. Leptomeningeal metastases from ethmoid sinus adenocarcinoma: clinico-radiological correlation. *Jbr-Btr* 1999; **82**(6): 285–7.

120. Heffner DK, Hyams VJ, Hauck KW, Lingeman C. Low-grade adenocarcinoma of the nasal cavity and paranasal sinuses. *Cancer* 1982; **50**(2): 312–22.

121. Koshy J, Schnadig V, Nawgiri R. Is fine needle aspiration cytology a useful diagnostic tool for granular cell tumors? A cytohistological review with emphasis on pitfalls. *Cytojournal*. 2014 Oct 21; **11**: 28.

122. Chen Q, Li Q, Guo L, et al. Fine needle aspiration cytology of agranular cell tumor arising in the thyroid gland: a case report and review of literature. *Int J Clin Exp Pathol*. 2014 Jul 15; **7**(8): 5186–91.

Index

Note: Page references in *italics* refer to Figures; those in **bold** refer to Tables

acantholysis 58
acinar cells 14, *15*
    mucinous acinar cells 14
    merous acinar cell 14
acinic cell carcinoma 11, 42–3, *44*
    cytological feature 43, *44*
    papillary variant 42
acute sialadenitis *22*
acute (purulent) thyroiditis 85
adenocarcinoma (not otherwise specified) 57, *57*
adenoid cystic carcinoma (AdCC) 11, 33, 45–51, *48*, *49*
adenolymphoma (Warthin's tumour). salivary gland *19*, 29, 35–7, *35*, *36*, *37*
adenomatous nodule 79
alveolar rhabdosarcoma 184, *186*
ameloblastomas 183, *184*
anaplastic large cell 140, 158, 160, *161*
angiolipoma 176
antimalarial drug hypersensitive lymphadenopathy 131
architectural atypia 89, *89*
atypia of uncertain significance (AUS)/Follicular lesion of uncertain significance
    (FLUS) 88–90, 89, 90
    architectural atypia 89, *89*
    atypia secondary to preparation arterfact 90
    atypical cyst-lining cells 90
    nuclear atypia *89*, 90
atypical follicular adenoma, thyroid gland 92
atypical meningioma 191

B-cell lymphoma 114, 143–53
    cutaneous 150, *151*
    diffuse large 140, 145, 150, **150**, *151*
    small lymphocytic 140, 143–4
    see also lymphocytic lymphoma
basal cell adenocarcinoma 53, *53*
basal cell adenoma (BCA) 37–9, *37*
benign nerve sheath tumour 35, 180, 181
benign lymphoepithelial lesion (BLEL) 23
bening neurilemmoma 60
berylliosis 122
biphasic adenosquamous carcinoma 58
biphasic basaloid squamous carcinoma 58
BRAF mutation 78
brachial cleft cyst *19*
branchial cyst 42, 181–2, *182*
brucellosis 122
Burkitt's lymphoma 140, 151–2, *154*
    WHO classification **154**

capillary technique
    salivary gland 3
    thyroid lesions 73
carbamazepine hypersensitive lymphadenopathy 131

carcinoma ex pleomorphic adenoma 57–8, *57*, *58*
carotid body tumours 187, *187*, *188*, *189*
Castleman's disease 131, *133*
cat scratch fever 122–4, *126*
CD30-positive lymphoproliferative conditions of skin *157*
CD31 103, 190
CD34 190
CD44 78
CD45 (LCA)
    anaplastic large cell lymphoma 160
    diffuse large B-cell lymphoma 150
    Hodgkin cells 137
    L&H cells 137, 139
    lymphoblastic leukaemia/lymphoma 142
CD57 (HNK-1)
    L&H cells 139
CD79a
    Burkitt's lymphoma 152
    diffuse large B-cell lymphoma 150
    folliicular lymphoma 148
    lymphocytic lymphoma 144
    mantle zone lymphoma 146
    post-transplant lymphadenopathy *135*
CD99 185
CD99/O13 186
CDw75 (LN1) 137
cell block (CB) 4
centroblastic lymphoma *see* diffuse large-lymphoma
cervical thymic cyst 183
chromogranin 103, 189
clinical history 2, *3*
cMYC 152
colloid (multinodular; non-toxic) goitre 76, 79–81
    adenoma vs adenomatous nodule 79
    cytological features 79–81, *80*
    degenerative changes 81, *82*
    diagnostic evaluation 79
    psammoma bodies 79–81, *81*
    regenerative changes *82*
colour Doppler 14
colour flow Doppler 14
composite lymphoma 140
computed tomography 2
core needle biopsy (CNB) vs FNAC
    lymphoma 117
    thyroid lesions 77
cost effectiveness 13, 77
cribiform adenoma of aminor salivary gland 60
cryptococcosis 125–7, *127*, 131
cutaneous B-cell lymphoma 150, *151*
cutaneous T-cell lymphoma *116*, *156*
cyclin D1 146

cystadenoma, salivary gland 42
cystic lesions
    goitre 76, *82*
    head and neck 181
    salivary gland 11, 17–21, **18**, 23
    thyroid 83, *83*
cystic lymphoid hyperplasia, salivary gland 23
cytological preparation methods **5**
cytomegalovirus sialadenitis 23
cytopathologist 2, *2*
cytopathology report 4, *6*

De Quervain's thyroiditis 85
dermatopathic lymphadenopathy 122
dermoid cyst, salivary gland 19
diffuse large-cell lymphoma 140, 150, *151, 152*
    cytological features 145, 150, *151*
    immunophenotype 150
    WHO classification **150**
diffusion-weighted (DWI) MR techniques 12
DNA microarray technologies
    basal cell adenocarcinoma 53
    lymphoma 141
drug-related lymphadenopathy 131, *132*
Dutcher bodies 144

elastography vs FNAC
    lymphoma 118
embryonal rhabdomyosarcoma 185, *186*
emperipolesis (lymphophagocytosis) 122
eosinophilic granuloma 132
epidermoid cysts 19, 183, *185*
epithelial membrane antigen 39, 57, 60, 99, 134
epithelial--myoepithelial carcinoma 50, 52–3, *52*
    cytological features 52, *53*
    smooth muscle-specific protein immunohistochemistry 52
epithelioid sarcoma-like hemangioendothelioma 190, *192*
Epstein-Barr virus 59, 128, 135, 139, 151
ethmoid sinus intestinal type adenocarcinoma 191–2, *194*
extraskeletal Ewing's sarcoma 186, *187*
    cytological features 186
    immunocytochemistry 186

fibroblastic meningioma 191
fibromatosis colli (sternocleidomastoid tumour) 176–8
fine needle aspiration cystology 1–5
    combined US/FNAC approach 2
    fluids *4*
    rapid staining and examination 4, *4*
    sampling technique 2–5, *2, 3*
    ultrasound guidance 1
flow cytometry 1
    Castleman's disease 131
    diffuse sclerosing variant of papillary carcinoma (DSPC) 99
    lymphoma 114, 141
    clonality analysis 114
    post-transplant lymphoproliferative disorder 135
    lymphoproliferative lesions of salivary glands [49]. 11
    salivary gland tumours 42
follicle centre lymphoma 140, 144
follicular adenoma, thyroid gland *85*, 91–2
    atypical 92
    cytological features 92
follicular carcinoma, thyroid gland 101, *101, 102*
    clear cell variant 101
    cytological features 101
    Hürthle cell variant 101
    insular variant 101, *103*
follicular hyperplasia, lymph node 118–19, *118*
    cytological features 118–19, *119, 120*
    progressive transformation of germinal centres 118
follicular lymphoma 113, *115, 116*, 140, 146–8, *148*
    immunophenotype 148
    WHO classification 146, **147**

frozen section histology
    salivary gland lesions 12–13
    thyroid lesions 77
fungal lymphadenitis 125–6, *127*
'follicular lesions' 90–4

galectin-3 99
GCDFP-15 57
glandular fever (infectious mononucleosis) 128–9, *130*
goitre 79–85
    colloid (multinodular non-toxic) 76, 79–81, *80, 81, 82*
    hyperactive 84–5, *84*
granular cell tumour 192–4, *195*
granulocytic sarcoma, salivary gland 62
granulomatous lymphadenitis 122–7
    mycobacterial infection 122
granulomatous sialadenitis 22–3, *26*
granulomatous thyroiditis 85–6, *86*
Graves' disease 84–5

haemangiopericytoma, salivary gland 61
Hand Schüller-Christian syndrome 132
Hashimoto's thyroiditis *see* lymphocytic thyroiditis
HBME-1 60, 78, 91, 96, 99, 103
heavy chain gene rearrangements 114, 117
    diffuse large-cell lymphoma 150
    marginal zone (MALT type lymphoma) 150
    post-transplant lymphoproliferative disorder 135
hepatitis C 23
histiocytosis X *see* Langerhans' cell histiocytosis
histoplasmosis *126, 127*, 131
    sialadenitis 23
HIV infection/AIDS
    FNAC-detected infections 130–1
    lymph node mass FNAC 131
    mycobacterial granulomatous lymphadenitis 122
    persistent generalised lymphadenopathy 130–1, *131*
    reactoid lymphoid proliferations 23
    salivary gland pathology 18
    salivary lymphepithelial cyst *19*
    p24 marker 19
HLA-DR 134
HNK-1 see CD57
Hodgkin's cells 121, 137, 139
Hodgkin's lymphoma 113, 137–9, *137*
    cell phenotype 137
    cytological diagnosis 139
    diagnostic difficulties 139
    granulomatous reactions *125*
    Hodgkin cells 137, 139
    immunophenotype 139
    L&H (lymphocytic and histiocytic) cells 137, 139
    lymphocyte depletion type 137
    lymphocyte-rich type 137
    mixed cellularity type 137
    nodular lymphocyte predominance type 137, *140*
    nodular sclerosis type 137
    nodular stenosis type 137, 140
    Reed-Sternberg cells 137, 139
    role of FNAC in management 140
    Rye classification 137
human herpesvirus-8 117, 131, 151, 162
human papillomavirus (HPV), squmous cell carcinomas of head and neck (HNSCC) 180
human T-lymphotropic virus-1 (HTLV-1)
    associated T cell lymphoma 154, *156*
Hürthle cell tumour
    adenoma 85
    carcinoma 92–3, *93*
    papillary with lymphoplasmacytic stroma 98
hyalinising trabecular adenoma, thyroid gland 92, 93–4
    immunocytochemistry 94
hybernoma 176, *178*

hydantoin-induced lymphadenopathy 131, *132*
hyperthyroidism, hyperactive goitre 84–5, *84*

immunocytochemistry 1, 4
immunocystoma *see* lymphoplasmacytic lymphoma
immunoglobulin-negative malignant lymphoma 140
immunohistochemistry
    anaplastic thyroid carcinoma 157
    Castleman's disease 131
    cribriform adenocarcinoma of minor salivary gland (CAMSG) 60
    cribriform-morular variant of papillary carcinoma 98–9
    epithelial myoepithelial carcinoma 52
    follicular hyperplasia 118–19, *119*
    hyalinising trabecular adenoma (HTA) 94
    lymphomas 113–14
    MALT lymphoma 23
    mammary analogue secretory carcinoma (MASC) 60
    myoepithelioma, salivary gland 41
    oncocytoma 45
    papillary thyroid carcinoma 99–100
    salivary duct carcinoma 55
    salivary gland lesions 23
    tumour malignancy 45
    small cell carcinoma 59
    thyroid lesions 78, **78**
    see also immunophenotype
immunophenotype 4, 114
    anaplastic large cell lymphoma 158
    Burkitt's lymphoma 151–2
    diffuse large-cell lymphoma 150
    follicular lymphoma 150
    lymphocytic lymphoma 144
    lymphoplastic lymphoma (immunocytoma) 144
    MALT lymphoma 150
    mantle zone lymphoma 144
    peripheral T cell lymphoma 154
    reactive lymphoid hyperplasia 114
immunosuppression
    cryptococcosis 125
    Mycobacterium avium intracellulare lymphadenitis 122
in situ hybridisation 117
    Epstein-Barr virus demonstration 135
infectious mononucleosis (glandular fever) 129–30, *130*
intraductal papillary adenocarcinoma, salivary gland 42
intraductal papilloma, salivary gland 41–2
intramuscular lipoma 176
intraosseous cyst 183, *184*
intraparotid lymphadenitis 35
inverted duct papilloma, salivary gland 42
iodine deficiency 79

Kaposi's sarcoma 131, 151
keratin 57, 59, 103
keratocyst *184*
Ki-67 (MIB-1)
    Burkitt's lymphoma 152
    hyalinising trabecular adenoma, thyroid gland 94
    lymphomas 113
    mammary analogue secretory carcinoma (MASC) 60
    salivary gland lesions 11
    tumour malignancy 42
    parotid gland tumours 11
Kikuchi's lymphadenitis 128
Kimura's disease 135–6, *136*
Kuttner's tumour *see* sialadenitis, chronic

L&H (lymphocytic and histiocytic) cells 137, 139
Langerhans' cell histiocytosis (histiocytosis) 132–5, *133*, *134*
large cell T-cell lymphoma *156*
laser scanning cytometer 141
LCS *see* CD45
leiomyosarcoma, salivary gland 61
Leishman-Donovan bodies 127
leishmaniasis 122, 127

leprosy 122, 127
Letterer-Siwe syndrome 132
leu 6 (CD1a) 134, 154
light chain gene rearrangements 152
light chain ratio (LCR) 114
lipoma 176
    angiolipoma 176
    hybernoma 176, *177*
    intramuscular lipoma 176
    pleomorphic lipoma 176
    spindle-cell lipoma 176, *177*
LN1 (CDw75) 137
local anaesthesia 2, 3
    needle-free system 3, *3*, *4*
lymph node 112–68
    accuracy of FNAC diagnosis 113
    core biopsy vs FBAC 117
    ancillary techniques 113–17
    diagnostic pitfalls 113
    elastography vs FNAC 118
    distribution of pathology 112
    lymphoma *see* lymphoma
    metastatic carcinoma 113, *114*, 160–8
    reactive/inflammatory lesions 112
    role of FNAC 112
lymph node follicular hyperplasia 118–19
lymphadenitis, chronic infective 128–31
lymphadenopathy
    drug reactions 131
    post-transplant 135
lymphoblastic leukaemia/lymphoma 142–3, *144*
lymphocyte-predominant Hodgkin's disease 113, 139–42
lymphocytic lymphoma (B-cell small lymphocytic lymphoma) 113, *115*,
        143–4, **144**
    immunophenotype 144
    role of FNAC in management 140
    transformation of high-grade lymphoma (Richter syndrome 139, 144,
        145, *188*
lymphocytic thyroiditis (Hashimoto's thyroiditis) 76, 85–6, *87*, *88*
    diagnostic problems 76
    differential diagnosis 85
    lymphoma association 103
lymphoepithelial carcinoma 59
lymphoepithelial cyst, salivary gland 19, *19*, *20–1*
lymphoepithelial (nasophryngeal) carcinoma, salivary gland 59
lymphoepithelial sialadenitis (benign lymphoepithelial lesion;
        myoepithelial sialadenitis) 23, *27*
lymphogranuloma venereum 122
lymphoid infiltrate in the parotid *26*
lymphoid proliferations of the salivary gland 23–9, *27*
    neoplastic 23–9
    reactive 23
lymphoma 1, 112, 187
    anaplastic large cell 140, 157–8, *161*
    B-cell 143–53
    cutaneous 150, *151*
    Burkitt's 140, 151–2, **154**, *154*
    composite 140
    diagnosis 112
    core needle biopsy (CNB) vs FNAC 117
    difficulties 113
    elastography vs FNAC 118
    flow cytometry 114, *115*
    immunohistochemistry 113–14
    molecular techniques 113, 114–17, *159–60*
    diffuse large B-cell 140, 146, 150, **150**, *151*
    follicle centre 140
    follicular 140, 144, 146–8, **147**, *148*
    granulomatous reactions 122, *125*
    immunoglobulin negative 140
    immunophenotyping 114, **144**
    lymphocytic (B-cell small lymphocytic) 140, 143–4
    lymphoplasmacytic (immunocytoma) 144
    MALT *see* MALT lymphoma

mantle zone 140, 142, 143, 144–6
    parotid *62*
    peripheral T-cell 139, 154, *155*
    primary effusion 150–1, *153*
    salivary gland 11, 23–5, 62, *62*
    HIV-positive patient 19
    T-cell rich B-cell 140
    T/NK-cell 154–8
    thyroid gland 103–5
    WHO classification 137, **137**, 142, 143
    see also Hodgkin's lymphoma; non-Hodgkin's lymphoma
lymphomatoid papulosis 157, *157*
lymphophagocytosis (emperipolesis) 121
lymphoplasmacytic lymphoma (immunocytoma)
    cytological features 144, *146*
    immunophenotype 144
lymphoproliferative disorders 1
    non-neoplastic 118–36
    salivary gland 11

magnetic resonance imaging (MRI) 1
malignant haemangiopericytoma, salivary gland 61
malignant tumours
    salivary 11, 42–59, 59–64
    thyroid gland 94–106
mammary analogue secretory carcinoma (MASC) 60
MALT lymphoma *116*, 144, 148–50, *149*
    accuracy of FNAC diagnosis 140
    immunophenotype 150
    salivary gland 23, 26, 27, *28–9*, 29, *30*, 62, *62*
    thyroid gland 105
mantle zone lymphoma 113, 114, *115*, 140, 144–6
    blastic variant 146
    immunophenotype 146
marginal zone B-cell lymphoma (MZCL) 23
marginal zone lymphoma 113, 140
    see also MALT lymphoma
medullary carcinoma, thyroid gland 101–3, *104*
meningioma 190–1, *193*
    atypical 191
    fibroblastic 191
    secretory 191
metastatic carcinoma 1
    lymph node 112, 160–8
    salivary gland 64
    HIV-positive patient 19, 23
    thyroid gland 105–6, *106*
methicillin-resistant staphylococcal infection, AIDS patients 131
MIB-1 *see* Ki-67
molecular technique 1, 4
    lymphoma 113, 114–17
    papillary thyroid carcinoma 99–100
    rhabdomyosarcoma 185
monomorphic adenoma, salivary gland 33, 37–8
mucinous adenocarcinoma, salivary gland 54
mucocoele, salivary gland 17, *17*
mucoepidermoid carcinoma (MEC), salivary gland 37, 43–5, *46*, *47*, **48**
    cytological features 45, *46*, *47*
    differential diagnosis 45
    molecular genetics 43
    prognostic features 45
mucus retention cyst 37, 182
multinodular goitre 79, *80*, *81*
    diagnostic problems 79
    non-toxic *see* colloid goitre
    toxic *see* toxic goitre
multiple endocrine neoplasia (MEN) syndrome 103
multiple oncocytic cyst, salivary gland 21
mycobacterial granulomatous lymphadenitis 122
Mycobacterium avium intracellulare lymphadenitis 122, *124*
myoepithelial sialadenitis (MESA) 23, 27, *27*
myoepithelial differentiation, salivary tumour immunohistochemistry 52
myoepithelioma, salivary gland 31, 40–1, *41*
myogenin 185

necrotising sialometaplasia, salivary gland 58
neurilemmoma *see* benign nerve sheath tumour
nodular fasciitis 178, *179*
    salivary gland 41
non-aspiration technique
    salivary gland lesions 10
    thyroid lesions 73
non-Hodgkin's lymphoma 37, *115*
    accuracy of FNAC 140
    ancillary techniques 140–1
    classification 142
    frequency *141*
    obtaining material 142
    precursor lesions 142–3
    handling FNAC material 142
    REAL classification 142
    role of FNAC in management 140–1
non-steroidal anti-inflammatory drugs, hypersensitive lymphadenopathy 131
nuclear grooves 91, 93, 95–6, *95*, *96*, *97*, *98*

odontogenic cysts 183, *184*
odontogenic keratocyst, salivary gland 21
oesthesioneuroblastoma *see* olfactory neuroblastoma
olfactory neuroblastoma 1, 187, *188*
oncocytic change
    thyroid lesions 79, *80*
    colloid goitre 79
    multinodular goitre *80*
    lymphocytic (Hashimoto's) thyroiditis 85, *88*
oncocytic neoplasms
    salivary gland crystalline structures 22
    thyroid gland 79
oncocytoma, salivary gland 35, *35*
    malignant (oncocytic carcinoma) 54–5, *55*
oncogene alterations
    non-Hodgkin's lymphoma 117
One Stop Clinics 4, 13

p16 57, 60
p53 42, 146
p16INK4a 146
paediatric lesions
    cat scratch disease 122–5
    lymphoblastic leukaemia/lymphoma 142
    salivary gland 62
papillary carcinoma, thyroid gland 75, 77, 78, 95–101
    cutaneous needle track metastasis 78
    cytological features 95, *96*
    differential diagnosis 100–1
    FNAC in management 95
    immunohistochemistry 99
    molecular markers 99–100
    nuclear grooves 95–6, *95*, *96*
    psammoma bodies 95, *95*, *97*, *97*, 99, 100
    variants
    columnar cell 97
    cribiform-morular 98–9, *99*
    diffuse sclerosing 99
    follicular 95–6, *98*
    macrofollicular 96
    nodular fasciitis-like stromal component 99
    oncocytic variant of papillary carcinoma (OVPTC) 97–8
    oxyphil cell 98
    papillary Hürthle cell carcinoma with lymphoplasmacytic stroma 98
    tall cell 96, *98*
papillary cystadenocarcinoma, salivary gland 54
papillary Hürthle cell carcinoma with lymphoplasmacytic stroma 98
parathyroid cyst 183
parotid gland 13
    normal appearance 13–14
    pitfalls and scanning issues 14
    ultrasound examination of *10*
parotid lesions, FNAC-related issues 14
parotid lymphoma *62*

parotid tumours 11, 29, 35, 42
    parotid lymphoma *62*
    paediatric lesions *62*
PAX3-FOXO1 or PAX7- FOXO1 gene fusion 185
PC10 *see* proliferating cell nuclear antigen (PCNA)
penicillin, hypersensitive lymphadenopathy 131
peripheral necuroectodermal tumour (PNET) 183, 186
peripheral T-cell lymphoma 140, 154
    cutaneous *156*
    cytological features 154, *155*
    human T-lymphotropic virus-1 (HTLV-1) associated 154, *156*
    immunophenotype 154
    large cell *156*
persistent generalised lymphadenopathy 130-1
physical examination 2, *3*
pleomorphic adenoma 29-35, *31*, *32*, *33*, *34*, *57*
    adenoid cystic carcinoma differentiation 48-50
    cytological features 31-5
    differential diagnosis 31
    paediatric lesions *62*
    salivary gland crystalloid structures 22
pleomorphic lipoma 176
Plummer's disease *see* toxic goitre
polymerase chain reaction (PCR) 4
    human herpesvirus-8 detection 117
    lymphoma 114-17, 141
    post-transplant lymphoproliferative disorder 135
    see also reverse transcriptase polymerase chain reaction (RT-PCR)
polymorphous low grade adenocarcinoma, salivary gland 42, 51-2, *51*, *52*, 60
'Poor Man's cell block' 4
post-transplant lymphoproliferative disorder 135
postirradiation salivary gland changes 11
PRAD-1 146
primary effusion lymphoma 150-1, *153*
    human herpesvirus-8 association 151
primitive neuroectodermal tumour, salivary gland 62-3
primary squamous cell carcinoma
    parotid 58-9, *58*, *60*
    salivary gland 58-9
procedure
    salivary gland lesions 13-14
    thyroid lesions 72-4, *74*
progressive transformation of lymph nodes 113
proliferating cell nuclear antigen (PCNA; PC10) 11, 42
proliferative fasciitis 178-80
proliferative myositis 180
psammoma bodies
    colloid (multinodular non-toxic) goitre 79-81, *81*
    meningioma 191
    papillary thyroid carcinoma 95, *95*, 97, *97*, 99, 100

rapid on site assessment (ROSE) 73-4
rapid reporting system, salivary gland lesion 13
reactive lymphoid hyperplasia
    clonality analysis 114, *115*
    flow cytometry *114*
    immunophenotyping 114
    role of FNAC in management 140
reactive lymphoid proliferations, salivary gland 23
reactive/inflammatory lesions 1
    lymph node 112
Reed-Sternberg cells 130, 137, 139, 157, *188*
referrals *3*
retention cyst, salivary gland 17, *19*
rhabdomyosarcoma 1, 184-5
    alveolar 185, *186*
    cytological features 185
    embryonal 185, *186*
    morphological subtyping 185
    salivary gland 61
rheumatoid arthritis 118
    granulomatous lymphadenitis 122, *125*
Richter's syndrome 139, 144, *145*, *188*

Riedel's thyroiditis 86-7
Rosai Dorfman disorder *see* sinus histiocytosis with massive lymphadenopathy

S-100 protein 60, 121, 122, 134, 185
salivary duct carcinoma 55-6, *56*
salivary gland, cytology of 14-29
    normal 14, *15*
    acinar cells 14, *15*
    ductal cells 14, *15*
salivary gland adenocarcinoma 57
salivary gland crystalloid structures 22, 31
salivary gland cysts 17-21, **18**
    brachial cleft *19*
    dermoid 21
    lymphoepithelial *19*, *20-1*
    mucocoele 17, *17*
    multiple oncocytic 21
    odontogenic keratocysts 21
    retention 17, *19*
salivary gland lesions 9-65
    clinical management 64-5
    cystic *see* salivary gland cysts
    diagnosis 9-10, *10*, 13-14
        accuracy 11, **11**
        difficulties 11-12, 14
        FNAC cost effectiveness 13
        FNAC versus frozen section 12-13
        rapid reporting 13
        ultrasound 12
        ultrasound guided FNAC 10-11
    neoplastic *see* salivary gland tumours
    non-neoplastic/inflammatory 14
    paediatric 62
    ultrasound in 9
    ultrasound-guided FNAC 10-11
salivary gland lymphoid proliferation 23-9
salivary gland tumours 1, 11-12
    benign 11, 29-42
    malignant 11, 42-59, 59-64
    flow cytometry 42
    p53 overexpression marker 42
    smooth muscle-specific proteins 52
    metastatic 63-4
    WHO classification 11
sarcoidosis 23, *25*, 122, *124*
sarcoma, salivary gland 61
schwannoma *see* benign nerve sheath tumour
sclerosing polycystic adenosis 40, *40*
sebaceous adenoma, salivary gland 43
secretory meningioma 191
sensitivity
    non-Hodgkin's lymphoma diagnosis 139, 141
    salivary gland lesions
    FNAC 10
    frozen section 12-13
    thyroid malignancy diagnosis 76
sialadenitis 21-3, *21*, *22*
    acute *22*
    chronic (Kuttner's tumour) 22, *23*, *24*
    crystalloid formation 22, *25*
    cytomegalovirus 23
    granulomatous 22-3
    lymphoepithelial of Sjögren's syndrome 23
    marginal zone B-cell lymphoma (MZCL) 23
    myoepithelial (MESA) 23, *27*
    submandiblular ductal system scanning 21-2
    ultrasound scanning for calculi 21
sialadenoma papilliferum 42
sialadenosis 14-17, *16*
sialectasis 13
sialolithiasis 21
sialography 13
silicone, granulomatous lymphadenitis 122, *125*

sinus histiocystosis with massive lymphadenopathy (Rosai Dorfman)
 119–22, *121*
  cytological features 119–22
  dermatopathic lymphadenopathy 122
  differential diagnosis 122
Sjögren's syndrome, lymphoepithelial sialadenitis 23
  MALT lymphoma 23–5
small cell carcinoma, salivary gland 59
small lymphocytic lymphoma 113, *115*
small round cell tumours 183–8
smooth muscle myosin heavy chains 52, 57
smooth muscle-specific proteins 52
soft tissue lesions, benign 176–81
sonoelastography 12
Southern blot analysis 117
  Epstein-Barr virus demonstration 135
  lymphoma 141
specificity
  non-Hodgkin's lymphoma diagnosis 139, 141
  salivary gland lesions
  FNAC 10
  frozen section 12–13
  thyroid malignancy diagnosis 76, 77
spindle-cell lipoma 176, *177*
spindle cell neoplasm 31
squamous cell carcinoma, primary of salivary gland 58–9
staining methods 4, *4*
sublingual gland tumours 29
submandibular gland tumours
  oncocytoma 35, *35*
  scanning difficulties 14
sulphonamide hypersensitive lymphadenopathy 131
surface Ig
  Burkitt's lymphoma 152
  diffuse large-cell lymphoma 150
  follicular lymphoma 146
  lymphoplasmacytic lymphoma (immunocytoma) 144
  mantle zone lymphoma 146
  marginal zone lymphoma (MALT type) 150
synaptophysin 187
synovial sarcoma, salivary gland 61, *61*
syphilis 122, 127
syringes 3, *4*

t(2;5)(p23;q35), anaplastic large cell lymphoma 158
t(8;14), Burkitt's lymphoma 152
t(11;14), mantle zone lymphoma 146
t(11;22)(q24;q12), extraskeletal Ewing's sarcoma/peripheral
 neuroectodermal tumour (PNET) 186
t(14;18)
  diffuse large B-cell lymphoma 148
  follicular lymphoma 147, 148, *159*
T-cell lymphoma 113
  cutaneous *156*
T-cell receptor gene rearrangements 122, 139
T-cell rich B-cell lymphoma 140
T/NK-cell lymphoma 154–7
TdT 142, 146
telomerase assay 78
thymic, cervical, cyst 183

thyroglobulin 85, 94, 99
thyroglossal cyst 181, *181*
thyroid cyst 83, *83*
thyroid cancer
  incidence 71, 72, **72**
  mortality rate 71
thyroid hyperplasia (goitre) *see* colloid goitre
thyroid lesions 1, 71–106
  classification 74, **75**
  complications of FNAC 78–9
  cost-effectiveness of FNAC 71
  diagnosis **73**
  accuracy 74–6
  FNAC reporting categories 74
  FNAC frozen section and core biopsy histology 77
  physical examination 72
  problems 76
  ultrasound and FNAC 72–4, **73**
  follicular lesions 90–4
  immunocytochemistry 78, **78**
  multinucleate giant cells 85
  non-neoplastic/inflammatory 79–87
  post-FNAC infarction 79
  procedure 72–4, *74*
  ancillary techniques 78
  complications of FNAC 78–9
  ultrasound guidance 72–4, **73**
  role of FNAC 76–7, 78
  sampling technique 4, *4*
thyroid metastatic tumours 105–6, *106*
Thyroid Imaging Reporting and Data System (TIRADS) 76
thyroiditis 76, 85–8
  acute (purulent) 85
  De Quervain's 85
  granulomatous 85, *86*
  lymphocytic (Hashimoto's) 85–6, *87*, *88*
  Riedel's 86–7, *88*
  subacute 85
thyrotoxicosis, hyperactive goitre 84
toxic goitre 84–5, *84*
toxoplasmosis 122, 126–7, *128*
  granulomatous lymphadenitis *125*
training in FNAC interpretation 12
trisomies, lymphocytic lymphoma 144
tuberculosis
  granulomatous lymphadenitis 122, *122*, *123*, 124
  granulomatous sialadenitis 23
  HIV infection/AIDS 131
  lipoma *177*
tularaemia 122, 125

ultrasound guidance, thyroid lesions 72–4, **73**
undifferentiated carcinoma, salivary gland 59

vimentin 41, 60, 103

Waldenström's macroglobulinaemia 144
Warthin's tumour *see* adenolymphoma, salivary gland

zellballen 189